E–Health, Assistive Technologies and Applications for Assisted Living:
Challenges and Solutions

Carsten Röcker
RWTH Aachen University, Germany

Martina Ziefle
RWTH Aachen University, Germany

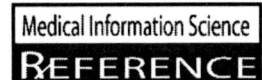

MEDICAL INFORMATION SCIENCE REFERENCE

Hershey · New York

Director of Editorial Content:	Kristin Klinger
Director of Book Publications:	Julia Mosemann
Acquisitions Editor:	Lindsay Johnston
Development Editor:	Myla Harty
Typesetters:	Michael Brehm, Milan Vracarich Jr.
Production Editor:	Jamie Snavely
Cover Design:	Nick Newcomer

Published in the United States of America by
Medical Information Science Reference (an imprint of IGI Global)
701 E. Chocolate Avenue
Hershey PA 17033
Tel: 717-533-8845
Fax: 717-533-8661
E-mail: cust@igi-global.com
Web site: http://www.igi-global.com/reference

Library of Congress Cataloging-in-Publication Data

E-health, assistive technologies and applications for assisted living: challenges and solutions / Carsten Röcker and Martina Ziefle, editors.
    p. cm.
  Includes bibliographical references and index.
  Summary: "This book reviews existing literature in assistive technologies and provides suggestions and solutions for improving the quality of assisted living facilities and residences through the use of e-health systems and services"--Provided by publisher.
   ISBN 978-1-60960-469-1 (hardcover) -- ISBN 978-1-60960-471-4 (ebook) 1. Medical informatics. 2. Assistive computer technology. 3. Congregate housing. I. Röcker, Carsten, 1975- II. Ziefle, Martina, 1962-
  R858.E225 2011
  610.285--dc22
                                    2010048865

British Cataloguing in Publication Data
A Cataloguing in Publication record for this book is available from the British Library.

Table of Contents

Section 1
Challenges of Future E-Health Systems

Brett Harnett, University of Cincinnati, USA

Milan Petković, Philips Research Europe & Eindhoven University of Technology, The Netherlands
Luan Ibraimi, University of Twente, The Netherlands

Cynthia L. Corritore, Creighton University, USA
Beverly Kracher, Creighton University, USA
Susan Wiedenbeck, Drexel University, USA
Robert Marble, Creighton University, USA

Martina Ziefle, RWTH Aachen University, Germany
Carsten Röcker, RWTH Aachen University, Germany
Wiktoria Wilkowska, RWTH Aachen University, Germany
Kai Kasugai, RWTH Aachen University, Germany
Lars Klack, RWTH Aachen University, Germany
Christian Möllering, RWTH Aachen University, Germany
Shirley Beul, RWTH Aachen University, Germany

Detailed Table of Contents

Section 1
Challenges of Future E-Health Systems

The first section of this book hosts five chapters addressing different challenges of future e-health systems. In the first chapter, the concept of "patient centeredness" in healthcare is discussed. The second chapter analyzes privacy and security requirements in healthcare and reviews both classical and novel security technologies that could fulfill these requirements. In chapter 3, the nature of trust in e-health systems is explored. Chapter 4 illustrates the different disciplinary design challenges of smart healthcare systems and presents an interdisciplinary approach toward the development of an integrative Ambient Assisted Living environment. The last chapter of this section presents an analysis of various Wireless Sensor Networks (WSN) security techniques in the context of healthcare applications.

Healthcare across the globe varies in capability and complexity. In some parts of the world healthcare is seen as an inalienable right, in other areas it is a privilege. Despite how medical expertise is allocated, there are logical processes that dictate an intervention. To accurately diagnose and treat a condition, many factors are considered. These include information about the patient's history, allergies, current medications and surroundings, in other words, data. The more that is known about a patient, the more quickly and efficiently an accurate diagnosis can be rendered as well as an appropriate treatment plan. In many locations throughout the world, the optimal process is non-existent or has broken down. The situation has become inefficient because of poorly coordinated, acute-focused, episodic care. The solution lies in the most basic role of the healthcare continuum, primary care. However, to achieve maximum effectiveness and efficiency, adoption of various technologies need to be embraced. While it is referenced by different terms, the concept is often termed "patient centered medicine".

Milan Petković, Philips Research Europe & Eindhoven University of Technology, The Netherlands
Luan Ibraimi, University of Twente, The Netherlands

The introduction of e-health and extramural applications in the personal healthcare domain has raised serious concerns about security and privacy of health data. Novel digital technologies require other security approaches in addition to the traditional "purely physical" approach. Furthermore, privacy is becoming an increasing concern in domains that deal with sensitive information such as healthcare, which cannot absorb the costs of security abuses in the system. Once sensitive information about an individual's health is uncovered and social damage is done, there is no way to revoke the information or to restitute the individual. Therefore, in addition to legal means, it is very important to provide and enforce privacy and security in healthcare by technological means. In this chapter, the authors analyze privacy and security requirements in healthcare, explain their importance and review both classical and novel security technologies that could fulfill these requirements.

Cynthia L. Corritore, Creighton University, USA
Beverly Kracher, Creighton University, USA
Susan Wiedenbeck, Drexel University, USA
Robert Marble, Creighton University, USA

Trust has always been an important element of healthcare. As healthcare evolves into e-health, a question arises: What will the nature of trust be in e-health? In this chapter the authors provide the reader with a foundation for considering this question from a research perspective. They focus on one e-health domain: online websites. The chapter begins with a high-level overview of the body of offline trust research. Next, findings related to online trust are presented, along with a working definition. Trust research in the context of online healthcare is then examined, although this body of work is in its infancy. A detailed discussion of our research in the area of online trust is then presented. Finally, with this background, the authors take the reader through some possible research questions that are interesting candidates for future research on the nature of trust in e-health.

Martina Ziefle, RWTH Aachen University, Germany
Carsten Röcker, RWTH Aachen University, Germany
Wiktoria Wilkowska, RWTH Aachen University, Germany
Kai Kasugai, RWTH Aachen University, Germany
Lars Klack, RWTH Aachen University, Germany
Christian Möllering, RWTH Aachen University, Germany
Shirley Beul, RWTH Aachen University, Germany

This chapter illustrates the different disciplinary design challenges of smart healthcare systems and presents an interdisciplinary approach toward the development of an integrative Ambient Assisted Living environment. Within the last years a variety of new healthcare concepts for supporting and assisting users in technology-enhanced environments emerged. While such smart healthcare systems can help to minimize hospital stays and in so doing enable patients an independent life in a domestic environment, the complexity such systems raises fundamental questions of behavior, communication and technology acceptance. The first part of the chapter describes the research challenges encountered in the fields of medical engineering, computer science, psychology, communication science, and architecture as well as their consequences for the design, use and acceptance of smart healthcare systems. The second part of the paper shows how these disciplinary challenges where addressed within the eHealth project, an interdisciplinary research project at RWTH Aachen University.

Wireless sensor networks (WSNs) in e-health applications are acquiring an increasing importance due to the widespread diffusion of wearable vital sign sensors and location tags, which can track both healthcare personnel and patient status location continuously in real-time mode. Despite the increased range of potential application frameworks the security breach between existing sensor network characteristics and the requirements of medical applications remains unresolved. Devising a sensor network architecture, which complies with the security mechanisms is not a trivial task since the WSN devices are extremely limited in terms of power, computation and communication. This chapter presents an analysis of various WSN security techniques from the perspective of healthcare applications, and takes into consideration the significance of security to the efficient distribution of ubiquitous computing solutions.

Section 2
User-Centered Design of Assistive Technologies

The second section comprises four chapters illustrating user studies, conceptual frameworks and novel design approaches in the field of assistive technologies. In chapter 6, a new approach for supporting the adoption of personal health record systems is presented. Chapter 7 illustrates a novel technique for studying the relationship of movement to health changes. Chapter 8 reports on the development of a multi-level model for understanding assimilation of e-health systems. The last chapter of this section presents a user study exploring the acceptance of mobile home automation devices by elderly people.

Healthcare delivery is undergoing radical change in an attempt to meet increasing demands in the face of rising costs. Among the most intriguing concepts in this effort is shifting the focus of care management to patients by means of Personal Health Record (PHR) systems, which can integrate care delivery across the continuum of services and also coordinate care across all settings. However, a number of organizational and behavioral issues can delay PHR adoption. This chapter presents a general approach to breaking down barriers that exist at the level of individual healthcare professionals and consumers. According to this approach, user participation in PHR system development is considered essential for achieving successful system implementations. Realizing a participative PHR system development, where users are full members of the development team, requires not only choosing an appropriate methodology, but also organizing the participation process in a way that is tailored to the particular situation in order to achieve the desired results.

Everything that happens to a person during their lifetime happens in the context of place, and the movements made by the person through and within that place. Persons begin life with a birthplace, they remember exactly where they were when they first laid eyes on their true love, the street address of their first home, etc. New research suggests that changes in movement patterns, which occur in home and public spaces, may be significant indicators of declining mental and physical health. In this chapter, the authors discuss efforts to measure natural human movement and present a novel technique that uses a referential grid system to study the relationship of movement to health changes. The authors then present several syndromes, whose understanding may be increased by a more thorough analysis of movement. They conclude with a discussion of how location-aware technologies can play a role in identifying problems and solutions in the design of living spaces for the elderly.

With increased use of tele-health to provide healthcare services, bringing tele-health technology out of experimental settings into real-life settings, it is imperative to gain a deeper understanding of the mechanisms underlying the assimilation of tele-heath systems. Yet, there is little understanding of how information systems are assimilated by organizations, more work is then warranted to understand how tele-health can be integrated into administrative and clinical practices and to identify factors that may impinge onto tele-health integration. Borrowing from institutional, structuration and organizational learning theories, the authors develop a multi-level model for understanding assimilation of tele-health systems. Their study addresses limitations of past work and will be helpful for guiding research and managerial actions while integrating tele-health in the workplace.

The aim of "Ambient Assisted Living" devices is to increase comfort and safety and to provide support for elderly people in their homes. In a housing estate in Kaiserslautern, Germany, a touch-screen tablet PC called PAUL (Personal Assistive Unit for Living), sensors and an EIB/KNX-Bus were installed in 20 apartments. Within the framework of the project Assisted Living, urban sociologists from the Technical University of Kaiserslautern analyzed the elderly peoples' experiences and acceptance of the implemented home automation devices, especially of the tablet PC over a period of two years of usage. Besides technical aspects social issues like community building are focused in the project. The main results of the project are presented in the paper.

Section 3
Applications for Assisted Living

In the third section, several examples of prototype systems and applications for assisted living are presented. Chapter 10 illustrates the research project SOPRANO, which aims at developing supportive environments for elderly people. Chapter 11 discusses the applicability of wearable motion-sensing technologies for mobility assessment and monitoring in clinical contexts. In chapter 12, a new emergency tele-medical service system is presented, which increases the quality of care for emergency patients by operationalizing rescue processes. The section closes with chapter 13, which presents the Smart Condo project, an environment for supporting seniors and rehabilitating patients.

This chapter is based on results from the European research project SOPRANO, which is developing supportive environments for older people based on the concept of Ambient Assisted Living (AAL). The project adapts and applies Experience and Application Research methods involving active participation of older users throughout an iterative development and design process. Innovative participatory methods enable developers to thoroughly focus on the users when defining the system requirements, generating design solutions and evaluating these design solutions in both lab and real-life settings. The example chosen to best demonstrate how the character and detail of user ideas changed in the different stages of the research and development process is the design of an exercise support system, which uses an avatar showing exercises on TV in the home of an older person.

Wiebren Zijlstra, University Medical Center Groningen, The Netherlands
Clemens Becker, Robert Bosch Gesellschaft für medizinische Forschung, Germany
Klaus Pfeiffer, Robert Bosch Gesellschaft für medizinische Forschung, Germany

Monitoring the performance of daily life mobility-related activities, such as rising from a chair, standing and walking may be used to support healthcare services. This chapter identifies available wearable motion-sensing technologies, discusses their potential clinical application for mobility assessment and monitoring, and addresses the need to assess user perspectives on wearable monitoring systems. Given the basic requirements for application under real-life conditions, this chapter emphasizes methods based on single sensor locations. A number of relevant clinical applications in specific older populations are discussed, including risk assessment, evaluation of changes in functioning, and monitoring as an essential part of exercise-based interventions. Since the application of mobility monitoring as part of existing healthcare services for older populations is rather limited, this chapter ends with issues that need to be addressed to effectively implement techniques for mobility monitoring in healthcare.

In-Sik Na, University Hospital Aachen, Germany
Max Skorning, University Hospital Aachen, Germany
Arnd T. May, University Hospital Aachen, Germany
Marie-Thérèse Schneiders, RWTH Aachen University, Germany
Michael Protogerakis, RWTH Aachen University, Germany
Stefan Beckers, University Hospital Aachen, Germany
Harold Fischermann, University Hospital Aachen, Germany
Nadja Frenzel, University Hospital Aachen, Germany
Tadeusz Brodziak, P3 Communications GmbH, Germany
Rolf Rossaint, University Hospital Aachen, Germany

The aim of the project Med-on-@ix is to increase the quality of care for emergency patients by operationalizing rescue processes. Currently available technologies will be integrated into a new emergency tele-medical service system. The aim is to capture all necessary information including electrocardiograms, vital signs, clinical findings, images and necessary personal data of patients at an emergency scene and transmit these data in real time to a centre of competence. This would enable a "virtual presence" at the site of an Emergency Medical Services (EMS) physician. Thus, it would be possible to raise the quality of EMS in total and counteract the growing problem of EMS physician shortage by exploiting the existing medical resources. In addition, this system offers EMS physicians and paramedics the possibility of consulting a centre of competence.

Chapter 13

Nicholas M. Boers, University of Alberta, Canada
David Chodos, University of Alberta, Canada
Pawel Gburzynski, University of Alberta, Canada
Lisa Guirguis, University of Alberta, Canada
Jianzhao Huang, University of Alberta, Canada
Robert Lederer, University of Alberta, Canada
Lili Liu, University of Alberta, Canada
Ioanis Nikolaidis, University of Alberta, Canada
Cheryl Sadowski, University of Alberta, Canada
Eleni Stroulia, University of Alberta, Canada

Providing affordable, high-quality healthcare to older adults, while enabling them to live independently longer, is critical. To this end, Ambient Assisted Living environments have been developed that are able to non-intrusively monitor the health of people at home and to provide them with improved care. The authors have designed an environment, the Smart Condo, to support seniors and rehabilitating patients. They embedded a wireless sensor network into a model living space, which was developed according to Universal Design principles. Information from the sensor network is archived in a server, which supports a range of views via APIs. One such view is a virtual world, which is realistic and intuitive, while remaining non-intrusive. The authors begin this chapter by examining computing technologies for smart healthcare-related environments as well as the needs of elderly patients. They then discuss the Smart Condo architecture and review key research challenges. Finally, they present lessons learned through the project.

Preface

Due to increased life expectancy and improved general health states of citizens, more and more old and frail people will need medical care in the near future. At the same time, considerable bottlenecks arise from the fact that increasingly fewer people are present, who may take over the nursing. In order to master the requirements of an aging society, innovations in information and communication as well as medical engineering technologies come to the forefront, which offer novel or improved medical diagnosis, therapy, treatments and rehabilitation possibilities. Nevertheless, recent research shows that acceptance barriers are prevalent, which might be due to the fact that current development praxis predominately focuses on technical feasibility, while the "human factor" in these systems is fairly underdeveloped. In order to fully exploit the potential of future healthcare applications, acceptance and usability issues of assistive technologies need to be considered, especially for older users, who have specific needs and requirements regarding usability and acceptance issues. As the knowledge about the antecedents of acceptance and utilization behavior is restricted, it is necessary to explore acceptance and the fit of emerging healthcare technology within homes and private spheres. In order to meet the needs future patients and care givers, an integrative and multidisciplinary approach is required, which combines engineering and medical knowledge with theoretical and methodological contributions from the social sciences and humanities. This book will address these challenges by providing an in-depth introduction into medical, social, psychological, and technical aspects of assistive e-health technologies as well as their consequences for the design, use and acceptance of future systems.

The knowledge and insights provided in this book will help students as well as systems designers to understand the fundamental social and technical requirements future healthcare technologies have to meet. By providing a well-rounded introduction within one single volume, this book is equally suited as a library reference and upper-level course supplement, but also represents a first-class resource for independent study.

The book **"E-Health, Assistive Technologies and Applications for Assisted Living: Challenges and Solutions"** consists of 13 chapters, which are clustered in three sections: (1) Challenges of Future E-Health Systems, (2) User-Centered Design of Assistive Technologies, and (3) Applications for Assisted Living.

The first section on **Challenges of Future E-Health Systems** provides an introduction in the field of e-health and assistive technologies and illustrates the design challenges of future healthcare systems. In **Chapter 1**, *"Patient Centered Medicine and Technology Adaptation"*, by Brett Harnett from the University of Cincinnati, USA, the concept of "patient centeredness" in healthcare is discussed. Healthcare across the globe varies in capability and complexity. In some parts of the world healthcare is seen as an inalienable right, in other areas it is a privilege. Despite how medical expertise is allocated, there are logical processes that dictate an intervention. To accurately diagnose and treat a condition, many factors are considered. These include information about the patient's history, allergies, current medications and surroundings, in other words, data. The more that is known about a patient, the more quickly and efficiently an accurate diagnosis can be rendered as well as an appropriate treatment plan. In many locations throughout the world, the optimal process is non-existent or has broken down. The situation has become inefficient because of poorly coordinated, acute-focused, episodic care. The solution lies in the most basic role of the healthcare continuum, primary care. However, to achieve maximum effectiveness and efficiency, adoption of various technologies need to be embraced. While it is referenced by different terms, the concept is often termed "patient centered medicine".

Chapter 2 on *"Privacy and Security in E-Health Applications"*, authored by Milan Petković and Luan Ibraimi from Philips Research Europe, The Netherlands, analyzes privacy and security requirements in healthcare and reviews both classical and novel security technologies that could fulfill these requirements. The introduction of e-health and extramural applications in the personal healthcare domain has raised serious concerns about security and privacy of health data. Novel digital technologies require other security approaches in addition to the traditional "purely physical" approach. Furthermore, privacy is becoming an increasing concern in domains that deal with sensitive information such as healthcare, which cannot absorb the costs of security abuses in the system. Once sensitive information about an individual's health is uncovered and social damage is done, there is no way to revoke the information or to restitute the individual. Therefore, in addition to legal means, it is very important to provide and enforce privacy and security in healthcare by technological means. In this chapter, the authors analyze privacy and security requirements in healthcare, explain their importance and review both classical and novel security technologies that could fulfill these requirements.

In **Chapter 3** entitled *"Foundations of Trust for E-Health"*, Cynthia L. Corritore and colleagues from Creighton University, USA, explore the nature of trust in e-health systems. Trust has always been an important element of healthcare. As healthcare evolves into e-health, a question arises: What will the nature of trust be in e-health? In this chapter the authors provide the reader with a foundation for considering this question from a research perspective. They focus on one e-health domain: online websites. The chapter begins with a high-level overview of the body of offline trust research. Next, findings related to online trust are presented, along with a working definition. Trust research in the context of online healthcare is then examined, although this body of work is in its infancy. A detailed discussion of our research in the area of online trust is then presented. Finally, with this background, the authors take the reader through some possible research questions that are interesting candidates for future research on the nature of trust in e-health.

Chapter 4, *"A Multi-Disciplinary Approach to Ambient Assisted Living"*, authored by Martina Ziefle et al. from RWTH Aachen University, Germany, illustrates the different disciplinary design challenges of smart healthcare systems and presents an interdisciplinary approach toward the development of an integrative Ambient Assisted Living environment. Within the last years a variety of new healthcare concepts for supporting and assisting users in technology-enhanced environments emerged. While such smart healthcare systems can help to minimize hospital stays and in so doing enable patients an independent life in a domestic environment, the complexity such systems raises fundamental questions of behavior, communication and technology acceptance. The first part of the chapter describes the research challenges encountered in the fields of medical engineering, computer science, psychology, communication science, and architecture as well as their consequences for the design, use and acceptance of smart healthcare systems. The second part of the paper shows how these disciplinary challenges where addressed within the *eHealth* project, an interdisciplinary research project at RWTH Aachen University.

In **Chapter 5**, *"Security in E-Health Applications"*, Victor Pomponiu from the University of Torino in Italy presents an analysis of wireless sensor networks (WSN) security techniques in the context of healthcare applications. Wireless sensor networks in e-health applications are acquiring an increasing importance due to the widespread diffusion of wearable vital sign sensors and location tags, which can track both healthcare personnel and patient status location continuously in real-time mode. Despite the increased range of potential application frameworks the security breach between existing sensor network characteristics and the requirements of medical applications remains unresolved. Devising a sensor network architecture, which complies with the security mechanisms is not a trivial task since the WSN devices are extremely limited in terms of power, computation and communication. This chapter presents an analysis of various WSN security techniques from the perspective of healthcare applications, and takes into consideration the significance of security to the efficient distribution of ubiquitous computing solutions.

The second section on **User-Centered Design of Assistive Technologies** comprises four chapters illustrating user studies, conceptual frameworks and novel design approaches in the field of assistive technologies. In **Chapter 6**, *"An Approach to Participative Personal Health Record System Development,"* Vasso Koufi and colleagues form the University of Piraeus in Greece present a new concept for supporting the adoption of personal health record systems. Healthcare delivery is undergoing radical change in an attempt to meet increasing demands in the face of rising costs. Among the most intriguing concepts in this effort is shifting the focus of care management to patients by means of Personal Health Record (PHR) systems, which can integrate care delivery across the continuum of services and also coordinate care across all settings. However, a number of organizational and behavioral issues can delay PHR adoption. This chapter presents a general approach to breaking down barriers that exist at the level of individual healthcare professionals and consumers. According to this approach, user participation in PHR system development is considered essential for achieving successful system implementations. Realizing a participative PHR system development, where users are full members of the development team, requires not only choosing an appropriate methodology, but also organizing the participation process in a way that is tailored to the particular situation in order to achieve the desired results.

Chapter 7 entitled *"How Knowing Who, Where and When Can Change Health Care Delivery"* by William D. Kearns et al. from the University of South Florida, USA, illustrates a novel technique for studying the relationship of movement to health changes. Everything that happens to a person during their lifetime happens in the context of place, and the movements made by the person through and within that place. Persons begin life with a birthplace, they remember exactly where they were when they first laid eyes on their true love, the street address of their first home, etc. New research suggests that changes in movement patterns, which occur in home and public spaces, may be significant indicators of declining mental and physical health. In this chapter, the authors discuss efforts to measure natural human movement and present a novel technique that uses a referential grid system to study the relationship of movement to health changes. The authors then present several syndromes, whose understanding may be increased by a more thorough analysis of movement. They conclude with a discussion of how location-aware technologies can play a role in identifying problems and solutions in the design of living spaces for the elderly.

In **Chapter 8**, *"Integrating Tele-Health into the Organization's Work System"*, Joachim Jean-Jules and Alain O. Villeneuve from the Université de Sherbrooke, Canada, report on the development of a multi-level model for understanding assimilation of e-health systems. With increased use of tele-health to provide healthcare services, bringing tele-health technology out of experimental settings into real-life settings, it is imperative to gain a deeper understanding of the mechanisms underlying the assimilation of tele-heath systems. Yet, there is little understanding of how information systems are assimilated by organizations, more work is then warranted to understand how tele-health can be integrated into administrative and clinical practices and to identify factors that may impinge onto tele-health integration. Borrowing from institutional, structuration and organizational learning theories, the authors develop a multi-level model for understanding assimilation of tele-health systems. Their study addresses limitations of past work and will be helpful for guiding research and managerial actions while integrating tele-health in the workplace.

Chapter 9 on the *"Acceptance of Ambient Assisted Living Solutions in Everyday Life,"* authored by Annette Spellerberg and Lynn Schelisch from the Technical University of Kaiserslautern in Germany, presents a user study exploring the acceptance of mobile home automation devices by elderly people. The aim of so-called Ambient Assisted Living devices is to increase comfort and safety and to provide support for elderly people in their homes. In a housing estate in Kaiserslautern, Germany, a touch-screen tablet PC called *PAUL* (Personal Assistive Unit for Living), sensors and an EIB/KNX-Bus were installed in 20 apartments. Within the framework of the project Assisted Living, urban sociologists from the Technical University of Kaiserslautern analyzed the elderly peoples' experiences and acceptance of the implemented home automation devices, especially of the tablet PC over a period of two years of usage. Besides technical aspects social issues like community building are focused in the project. The main results of the project are presented in the paper.

In the third section on **Applications for Assisted Living**, several examples of prototypes and applications of Ambient Assisted Living systems are presented. **Chapter 10** entitled *"Iterative User Involvement in Ambient Assisted Living Research and Development Processes: Does It Really Make a Difference?"* authored by Sonja Müller and colleagues from empirica - Gesellschaft für Kommunikations- und Technologieforschung in Germany, reports on the research project *SOPRANO*, which aims at developing supportive environments for elderly people. The chapter is based on results from the European research project *SOPRANO*, which is developing supportive environments for older people based on the concept of Ambient Assisted Living (AAL). The project adapts and applies Experience and Application Research methods involving active participation of older users throughout an iterative development and design process. Innovative participatory methods enable developers to thoroughly focus on the users when defining the system requirements, generating design solutions and evaluating these design solutions in both lab and real-life settings. The example chosen to best demonstrate how the character and detail of user ideas changed in the different stages of the research and development process is the design of an exercise support system, which uses an avatar showing exercises on TV in the home of an older person.

In **Chapter 11**, *"Wearable Systems for Monitoring Mobility Related Activities: From Technology to Application for Healthcare Services,"* Wiebren Zijlstra et al. from the University Medical Center Groningen, The Netherlands, discuss the applicability of wearable motion-sensing technologies for mobility assessment and monitoring in clinical contexts. Monitoring the performance of daily life mobility-related activities, such as rising from a chair, standing and walking may be used to support healthcare services. This chapter identifies available wearable motion-sensing technologies, discusses their potential clinical application for mobility assessment and monitoring, and addresses the need to assess user perspectives on wearable monitoring systems. Given the basic requirements for application under real-life conditions, this chapter emphasizes methods based on single sensor locations. A number of relevant clinical applications in specific older populations are discussed, including risk assessment, evaluation of changes in functioning, and monitoring as an essential part of exercise-based interventions. Since the application of mobility monitoring as part of existing healthcare services for older populations is rather limited, this chapter ends with issues that need to be addressed to effectively implement techniques for mobility monitoring in healthcare.

In **Chapter 12**, *"Med-on-@ix: Real-time Tele-Consultation in Emergency Medical Services – Promising or Unnecessary?"* a new emergency tele-medical service system is presented by In-Sik Na and colleagues from the University Hospital in Aachen, Germany. The aim of the illustrated project *Med-on-@ix* is to increase the quality of care for emergency patients by operationalizing rescue processes. Currently available technologies will be integrated into a new emergency tele-medical service system. The aim is to capture all necessary information including electrocardiograms, vital signs, clinical findings, images and necessary personal data of patients at an emergency scene and transmit these data in real time to a centre of competence. This would enable a "virtual presence" at the site of an Emergency Medical Services (EMS) physician. Thus, it would be possible to raise the quality of EMS in total and counteract the growing problem of EMS physician shortage by exploiting the existing medical resources. In addition, this system offers EMS physicians and paramedics the possibility of consulting a centre of competence.

The section closes with **Chapter 13**, *"The Smart Condo Project: Services for Independent Living,"* in which Nicholas M. Boers et al. from the University of Alberta, Canada, present the *Smart Condo* project, an environment for supporting seniors and rehabilitating patients. Providing affordable, high-quality healthcare to older adults, while enabling them to live independently longer, is critical. To this end, Ambient Assisted Living environments have been developed that are able to non-intrusively monitor the health of people at home and to provide them with improved care. The authors have designed an environment, the *Smart Condo*, to support seniors and rehabilitating patients. They embedded a wireless sensor network into a model living space, which was developed according to Universal Design principles. Information from the sensor network is archived in a server, which supports a range of views via APIs. One such view is a virtual world, which is realistic and intuitive, while remaining non-intrusive. The authors begin this chapter by examining computing technologies for smart healthcare-related environments as well as the needs of elderly patients. They then discuss the *Smart Condo* architecture and review key research challenges. Finally, they present lessons learned through the project.

Carsten Röcker
RWTH Aachen University, Germany

Martina Ziefle
RWTH Aachen University, Germany

Acknowledgment

A number of people have contributed to the successful completion of this book project. We would like to use this opportunity to express our sincere appreciation to all persons, who provided us with their useful and helpful assistance throughout the last 12 months, in which this book endeavor lasted. Without their consideration and support, this book would most likely not have matured.

First of all, we would like to express our gratitude to all chapter authors for their interest in this book, and the time and effort they invested to go through several revision cycles in order to share their research outcomes with us. We are especially thankful for their patience during the editing and peer-reviewing process, which surely was a quite difficult and time-consuming task. We are extremely thankful for this fruitful collaboration and the confidence they had in us.

We would also like to thank our editorial board members, all renowned experts from academia and industry coming from nine different countries all over the world, for their competent assistance during the editing of this book. Furthermore, we thank our research assistants Luisa Bremen, Simon Himmel, Stefan Ladwig, Johanna Kluge, Oliver Sack, Lena Taube, and Christina Vedar from RWTH Aachen University for their editorial support as well as Christine Bufton, Erica Carter, Myla Harty, Dave de Ricco and Jan Travers from IGI Global for their fast, professional and sensible assistance throughout the entire publication process.

And last but not least, we would like to thank the board of directors of the Human Technology Center at RWTH Aachen University for financial and organizational support as well as the freedom to work on this project.

Carsten Röcker
RWTH Aachen University, Germany

Martina Ziefle
RWTH Aachen University, Germany

Section 1
Challenges of Future E-Health Systems

Chapter 1
Patient Centered Medicine and Technology Adaptation

Brett Harnett
University of Cincinnati, USA

ABSTRACT

Healthcare across the globe varies in capability and complexity. In some parts of the world healthcare is seen as an inalienable right; in other areas it is a privilege. Despite how medical expertise is allocated, there are logical processes that dictate an intervention. To accurately diagnose and treat a condition, many factors are considered. These include information about the patient history, allergies, current medications and surroundings, in other words, data. The more that is known about a patient, the more quickly and efficiently an accurate diagnosis can be rendered as well as an appropriate treatment plan.

In many locations throughout the world, the optimal process is non-existent or has broken down; the United States is no exception as explained from a national, (Sarfaty, 2010) as well as an international perspective by Zwar (2010). The situation has become inefficient because of poorly coordinated, acute-focused, episodic care. The solution lies in the most basic role of the healthcare continuum; primary care. However, to achieve maximum effectiveness and efficiency, adoption of various technologies need to be embraced. While it is referenced by different terms, the concept is often termed patient centered medicine.

INTRODUCTION

The concept of the "patient centeredness" and the patient centered medical home is not new. It is a model of care originating 40 years ago and refers

DOI: 10.4018/978-1-60960-469-1.ch001

to a migration from episodic care to a longitudinal plan, a continuum of care that involves the patient and a team to not just deal with illness, but to promote wellness.

The objective of this chapter is to illuminate the issues that plague a specific sector of the healthcare system and how technology can begin to cultivate opportunity for significant improvement. While the discussions largely revolve around the issues within the United States, the principles echo across the globe (Sisko, Truffer, Smith, Keehan & Cylus, 2008). Some nations have been using the patient centered model for years and have found success. In an interview with Dr. Paul Grundy, the Global Director of Healthcare Transformation for IBM, (personal communication, December 28, 2009) he discussed how Denmark has made great strides in the new care model as well as Spain, New Zealand and others. The reader should take away from this a broad perspective on the issues that currently face the foundering primary care industry and in particular the proposed technological adoption to support patient centered medicine.

BACKGROUND

In a message to Congress, the President of the United States said "Millions of our citizens do not now have a full measure of opportunity to achieve and to enjoy good health. Millions do not now have protection or security against the economic effects of sickness. And the time has now arrived for action to help them attain that opportunity and to help them get that protection." The President was Harry S. Truman - in 1945.

Indeed, how times have not changed.

The current financial model for healthcare stems from business rules of the 1800s. People get sick. Clinicians fix them. They get paid for the service. It's a business. Healthcare is like any other business, it requires cash. A constant revenue flow means a constant flow of customers (the industry calls them patients). We have what is better-termed a "sickcare" system. Beyond pure altruism, physicians have little incentive to keep patients healthy. Healthier patients, on the other hand, need less episodic care and more longitudinal care such as annual physicals, care treatment or monitoring plans.

Patient centered medicine is often correlated with the application called the Patient Centered Medical Home (PCMH), the terms are nearly interchangeable. This is a model based on enhanced primary care meaning comprehensive, timely and patient-centered care that embraces preventative tactics and suitable reimbursement where healthcare professionals can practice at the "top of their licenses," a term used to outline a professional's activities to perform services at the fullest extent possible stipulated by the license. This is accomplished using a team that includes not only the physician staff but also family members and social entities. Patient centered medicine is more than a model; it is a healthcare setting that promotes partnerships between those participants to create a team-oriented and supportive environment. In other words, the care spectrum spans various settings. To facilitate this requires more than a change in culture, it requires technology.

ISSUES, CONTROVERSIES, PROBLEMS

While the medical interventions have moved forward, how we document them has not. Saying electronic medical records (EMRs) are sorely needed is an obvious understatement, so are the frustrations. It has been well documented that migration to an EMR, even in small practices, is met with resistance because it presently slows down the process (Robeznieks, 2005). Cataloging a visit with sidebar activities such as prescriptions is traditionally done with a few notes in a manila folder and a prescription pad. On the other hand, using a tablet PC to populate an EMR that boots slowly, is prone to lockups and stalls between applications exacerbates the problems. Now add the front-end costs of hardware, software, training and risks of data security and we have a woeful candidate for replacement of paper and pen.

But what we have to remember are lessons from the past. In the early 1900s, a novel mechanical device to travel from point A to point B was introduced. The automobile, compared to the horse, had constant machinery problems, was noisy, required fuel that was not widely available, and there were no roads smooth enough for them to work! Yet the benefits were realized by the masses and eventually the automobile took its place in the transportation infrastructure; the rest is history.

The migration from the hand-written medical record to a digital one faces a rough road as well. But like the automobile compared to the equine, the benefits will outweigh the struggles and a new order will prevail. And it will not just be EMRs that energize this industry; it will be a wide array of technology, interfaces and revised practice regiments that will move healthcare out of the Stone Age and into the digital domain.

BACKGROUND

Primary Care Physicians (PCPs) in the United States feel they are becoming the "repairers of American indiscretion." Patients are poorly educated and pay little attention to details, even critical issues like what type of medications they use. A recent study by Commins (2009) showed that almost half of hospital patients thought they were receiving a medication they were not, and 96% could not remember the name of at least one medication that they had been prescribed during their hospitalization. This is indeed disturbing and a good example of the apathetic attitude people have towards their healthcare. This creates expensive problems. In the U.S., healthcare costs are approaching 20% of the gross domestic product. In 2010, the government endorsed controversial, overhauled healthcare legislation that embraces a budget of over $800 billion (U.S.) over ten years (Hitt & Adamy, 2009).

Part of the future lies in the past; the American Academy of Pediatrics (AAP) introduced the medical home concept in the late 1960s to assist parents with a child's care at home including a copy of the medical record. The model received more attention in the 1980s and then, in a 2002 policy statement, the AAP revisited the medical home concept and outlined the following characteristics: accessible, continuous, comprehensive, family-centered, coordinated, compassionate, and culturally effective care (American Academy of Pediatrics, 2007). Since then, other medical professional organizations have begun to embrace patient centered medicine.

Within the U.S. healthcare plan, billions of dollars are earmarked for healthcare information technology (HIT). It is not enough that processes and reimbursement mechanism are changed. Technology will play a vital role as it has in countless other industries. From monolithic electronic medical records to tiny sensors worn on the skin, technology will be integrated into the infrastructure of comprehensive medical programs.

Through a combination of operational changes, reimbursement enhancements and technical adoption, the system can evolve into an elegant and efficient platform that not only provides better care, but promotes better health. Consumers, armed with tools discussed later, will fuel market forces in exchange for more responsible clinical management. The bi-directional flow of data will be one of the key ingredients to a leaner and more successful healthcare environment.

The Patient, Not the Process

To characterize the patient flow at an abstract layer we can use a simple circular analogy. In properly administered primary or family care practice models, the PCP is the target location, a focused and narrow point of entry for healthcare. See Figure 1. This is where a person's history is known, uses of current medications are identified, relationships are built, communication is open and self-management is cultivated. If the patient needs specialty care they would be referred to a qualified clinical care echelon, armed with the data to best facilitate care. That is the next outer care layer. The PCP is consulted as needed and a streamlined care plan continues. Then there is the emergent care scenario. Emergencies happen even to the best patients; this is the third and currently most accessible level of the care spectrum. It is broad and comprehensive. This could be a local hospital's emergency room or a walk-in care center. Here, the patient is cared for with minimal background information. Due to the lack of information, everything is often thrown at them from a barrage of tests to needless, expensive imaging.

The current system, however, does little to promote coordinated and efficient care, and has no mechanism in place to assist in this process. People who do not follow even the most basic rules of maintaining themselves tend to end up using the emergency room as their primary care provider. The model is largely and inappropriately inside-out.

The patient centered model will help to guide people back to the center. In the PCMH, access is enhanced such as same day scheduling, after hours access coverage, better prevention, screening processes, and a scope to include local populations (not just current customers.) This involves the community, local organizations and employers - a shared mission of promoting wellness, and addressing illness.

To migrate from episodic to continual care will require improved communications an order of magnitude over what is currently used. Similar to software engineering, a process-driven architecture is required where the state of a patient is indexed, variables are injected and response mechanisms are applied. This process requires a very different operational framework than is now in place.

Traditionally the healthcare session in primary care is based on the practitioner's outdated methodology. An appointment is made, the patient

Figure 1. Because care is currently episodic, the patient is distanced from the center. To minimize access to the outer layer, the patient must be kept close to the clinical core

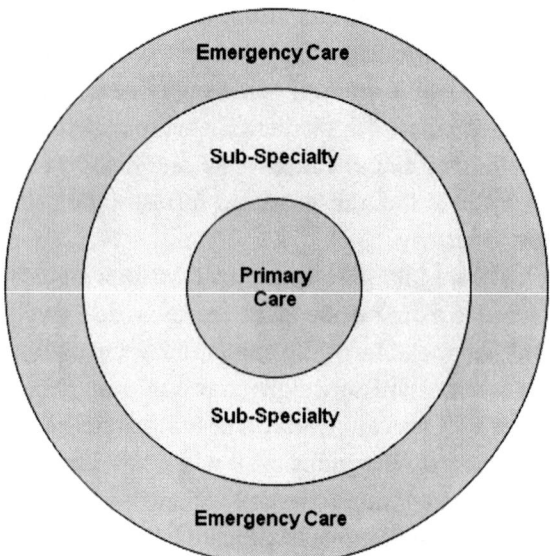

arrives, insurance information is updated and the wait begins. So appropriate was waiting that the term "waiting room" was coined decades ago and is synonymous with the traditional family medicine healthcare episode. When your name is called you are weighed and escorted to another room where your blood pressure is taken and a few questions are asked by the nurse as to why you are there. And then you wait – again. As a process, it is well-tolerated but not efficient. But it is not the fault of the physician or the clinical staff; it is the fault of this outdated process.

Like most specialties, the classic family practice subscribes to fixing the problem and then goes on to the next problem. Even the language of the clinical intervention is procedural. When a patient goes to the doctor they state what the problem is. In the medical world we call that the chief complaint. The chief complaint may be a very simple response such as "blurred vision" or it may be a series of related issues. That is the process that leads to procedures.

The PCMH still has a process, it has to. But what it also has is a culture change embedded within its fabric that preventative care is equally important. The Institute of Medicine uses the phrase "Continuous Healing Relationships" that embody patient centered medicine. There are many terms that can be used to support that broad phraseology. While the exact words used to graphically represent the overall concept are debatable, the concept is well-embraced. See Figure 2.

Notice in the center is the primary issue – the patient. Closely aligned to the patient is the physician who fosters interactive communications, striving for quality and a positive experience. Next to this is special relationship are coordinated and integrated services that promote wellness and positive trajectories through efficient and coordinated teams.

The environment includes internal and external locations facilitated by technology including interoperable data, telemedicine, if appropriate, and patient portals for improved communications where the security of a patient's information is ensured. The community portion dictates how the PCP interacts with outside business and reporting agencies, sharing de-identified data to populate registries and public health reporting.

These interactions are facilitated by both processes and people. While the physician is the key clinical player in a patient's medical home, the support staff - such as nurses, physician assistants and mid level associates - plays critical roles in the longitudinal process. The team-oriented ingredient is extraordinarily important because it facilitates a patient's experience and subsequent actions. Dr. Grundy (personal communication, December 28, 2009) referred to the term "partialists." While a general practitioner oversees the patient's entire health spectrum, a partialist does just what the term implies: focuses on a part of the body such as the backbone. This could be contrived as a sub-specialty within a person's medical home. As teams become a more crucial role in the health plan of a

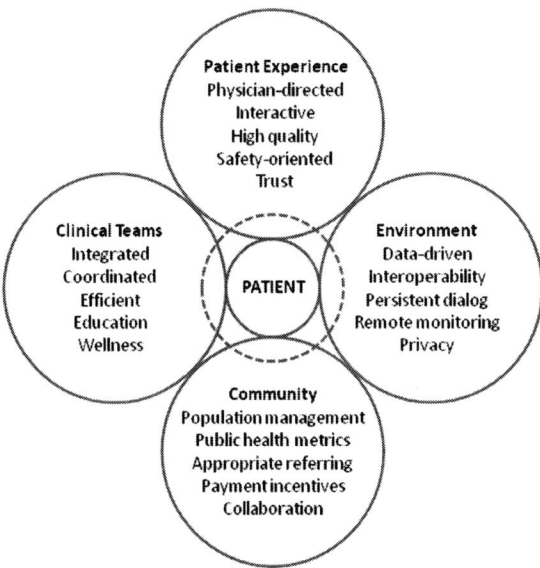

Figure 2. The focus is the patient, in the center, surrounded by conceptual procedures and activities

patient, it is important to note that effectiveness will be measured much more comprehensively.

Dr. Robert Graham at the University of Cincinnati, College of Medicine knows a few things about quality and effectiveness. Dr. Graham (personal communication, December 16, 2009) categorized the PCMH as not only clinical practice that embodies patient-centeredness, but also the community. This population-based medicine approach embraces the healthcare of a region by creating a community of caregivers. "The PCMH is focused not just on curing but also caring." The episodic care translates to longitudinal care and cuts across the social fabric of communities. Dr. Graham also points out that the PCMH – with its digital dimension – will elevate the traditional patient registry to a new level. Registries provide single-threaded summaries of disease states, but with new data-driven algorithms; physicians will have a new armamentarium of capabilities. See Figure 3. Click once, and a list of all patients with Type 2 diabetes is presented, click again and a consolidated analysis of the aggregate treatment plans is compiled. A third click and the real time

Figure 3. Data from disparate EMRs can feed a new generation of registries that can be used for local, regional, national and global purposes

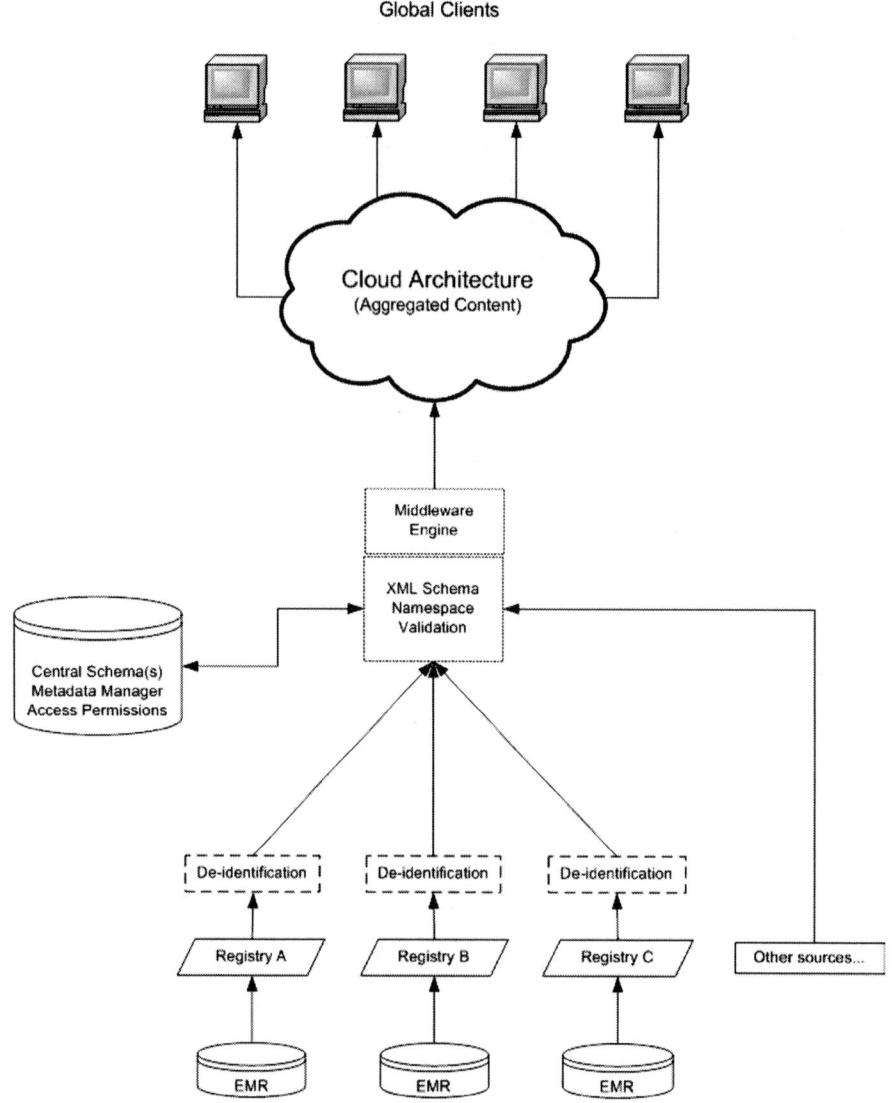

results of blood sugar management based on the established plans appear. These digital dashboards based on the field of informatics will provide a composite graphical view of the data that was never before available.

The classic primary care episode often includes periods of isolation and inefficiencies. The PCMH concept neutralizes this unproductive time and integrates the patient as an active participant in the process. For example, due to the added effi-

ciencies of the visit, the wait time is minimized. When the patient does wait, processes are in action. Educational components are contextualized and delivered either by a clinician or device, likely a kiosk. Access to one's EMR may be a part of that so that a patient can not only review the data but add to it. This could be presented in many forms such as a survey or free-form retrospective on an issue. This may be where the chief complaint could be posted with detail. The kiosks will take the form of stand-alone workstations, portable PC-tablets or interactive tables with highly intuitive and icon-driven touch screens that can even read an insurance identification card. In the event the patient has a condition such as diabetes, a certified Diabetes Educator may intervene after a brief kiosk module and have a conversation before the patient even steps on a scale. But to fully realize the benefits, the clinician must be armed with data. This data should come from a history of glucose readings and other parameters that affect the blood sugar levels of the patient. The type of interaction this lends itself to is highly coordinated care.

All of the components in the grid above will not always be evident. The goal is to elegantly weave as many as possible into an orchestrated, continuous process that follows the patient – even as they leave the medical domain.

Technology: The Great Enabler

Technology spans our world. As a very generic term, technology enables us to do more with less effort, hopefully resulting in better outcomes. It is now time for us to embrace the energy of technology to process and to promulgate better healthcare.

The technology to be used for patient centered medicine and the PCMH is initially very specific but ultimately will be comprehensive. The most important piece of technology that will enable the PCMH to be as effective as it can, will be the EMR and the networks it is connected to. To achieve and maintain a close and personal relationship with a patient, the clinical team needs to stay in contact long after the patient leaves the medical office. Data sent to and from a patient in the form of written words, automated instructions or physiological data from a patient's sensor will be facilitated by the EMR; it is the digital diary of a patient's health.

For years, patients with heart problems who required surgery often wore monitors that measured cardiac rhythm. Atrial fibrillation, for example, is a condition where the heart beats erratically for a period of time. The patient wears a monitor for weeks that hopefully picks up the arrhythmia and stores the event. At the next medical appointment, the data is downloaded and evaluated. This data would help to pinpoint the problem and extent assisting the surgeon in planning the procedure. This is a form of asynchronous monitoring. Data is collected while the patient is outside the clinical environment and evaluated for the optimal treatment plan. But this type of monitoring is not real time. A new generation of sensors is emerging that can be worn continuously – and not just by those identified as needing a surgical intervention - rather, can be worn by those identified as "high risk." These inexpensive, non-invasive, unobtrusive sensors can send data over existing digital wireless networks. Smarter sensors will have the ability to store normal patterns and when an event occurs outside expected parameters, such as an atrial fibrillation event, the sensors send the data and an alert.

And people support the use of technology. According to a survey by Siemens Medical Solutions and the Center for Health Transformation (2004), 97% of consumers polled said new healthcare information technology will be important in contributing to overall better healthcare and 60% of healthcare opinion leaders believe new medical technologies and equipment can actually reduce the costs of healthcare.

Continua (www.continuaalliance.org) is an industry alliance that promotes interoperability of devices, medical sensors in particular. This allows for a myriad of devices to interoperate. This type of business logic promotes not only economies of scale but also provides consumers with "best of breed" options for different conditions. Soon the individual's mobile phone will be the communications platform for transmitting one's vital signs. The EMR is the destination for these clinical signatures that are incorporated into the clinical support algorithm.

But significant questions remain such as who will hold and maintain the public's electronic health records. While the concept of a person's complete medical record on their person would be convenient, it is not plausible. People are not responsible enough to keep their medical records on a portable drive or optical disk that they constantly carry and carefully protect. A centralized concept is not ideal either. The U.S. Veteran's Administration (VA) is an exception to this rule. The VA's system is connected, and a patient's data in that system can be accessed at any VA facility across the country. Such a government-based organization holding the public's medical records would meet with significant resistance because of the fears of many believing the government knowing too much about us. In other nations, this is a non-issue.

More recently, however, as we move forward with actual implementation of EMRs – much like any capitalistic society – the market comes to bear. There are now well over two hundred EMRs available and the healthcare community is wrestling with which is the best choice. Other options are available from the consumer perspective. Large employers are offering forms of electronic health records to their workers. Software giants, such as Microsoft and Google now offer Personal Health Records (PHRs) that is a simplified version of an EMR and often managed by the individual.

Another issue is unique identification. In the U.S., every person is assigned a social security number. This is a unique identifier. But in the wake of new threats such as identity theft, the social security number along with date of birth, mother's maiden name and place of birth fall under the category of sensitive data that if compromised, can lead to identity theft. The HIPAA legislation in the U.S. and similar laws in other nations are designed to protect this information to minimize this risk. What is needed is another unique identifier that indexes a person's medical data. How this identifier is created is still in debate. It is likely it will be a constellation of personal attributes in some type of alpha-numeric structure. Another option is purely biometric such as finger prints, retina scan or voice signature. The trouble with biometrics is that hardware is needed to authenticate the mode and this is expensive.

To date, a solution for nationwide unique patient identifiers has been elusive. Global uniqueness is a larger challenge. Most numbers today are location or enterprise specific referred to as Enterprise-wide Master Patient Indexing (EMPI). New efforts called Registry Master Patient Indexes (RMPI) are being investigated by standards bodies such as HL7. RMPI forms a framework for searching and matching identifiers across disparate domains. It may be necessary to call for a Central Trusted Authority to aggregate a Universal Health Identifier (UHID). Or is it possible to serialize one's DNA profile? The solution required to facilitate interoperability of EMRs is from both and organizational and technical perspective.

Once a unique identifier is agreed upon there needs to be a centralized registry. Again, who maintains this critical inventory of data? There exists in the computing world a specification that defines a uniform resource namespace for Universally Unique Identifiers (UUIDs). Also known as Globally Unique Identifier, a UUID is a 128-bit long character set that guarantees uniqueness in the global community of web locations. The number of possibilities is 2^{128} or more than 340,000,000,000,000,000,000,000,000,000,000,000,000! With only seven billion people on the planet, this "googolian" number far exceeds absolute unique identification. But what is most intriguing is that the UUID system requires no centralized authority to administer or maintain them. As a result, generation of an identifier can be automated and on-demand. An identifier such as this can also be used to create unique transaction numbers essential to data interoperability. Since UUIDS are unique and persistent, they could be considered a candidate for medical identification numbers. The challenge is some kind of recipe is needed to feed the system to generate the number, this goes back to the constellation of personal parameters mentioned above.

There will be a significant array of both EMRs and PHRs that will incorporate our medical data. One of the larger challenges will be how they interoperate, exchange messages and even synchronize. This topic is discussed shortly. Suffice to say, having islands of medical data that do not interchange with other systems will prove little more valuable than existing paper-based systems.

Even without EMRs, selected data has been collected in list format for years. Patient registries have been used with success to categorize disease states and disease cohorts from a single provider to a large geographic area. For example, a physician may want to know what percentage of his patients are Type 2 diabetics. This number not only assists in operational guidelines and staff requirements within the office but, also when shared with regional or national repositories, provides aggregated public health data. To drill down further, ontologies and taxonomy refer to the relationships of data elements, often in heterogeneous environments. This is more appropriately used in the computer science of medical analysis and health informatics. Other industries have been using complex data relationships to visualize large data sets to look for trends and opportunities through business intelligence tools. By adding the element of time, two-dimensional data evolves into three-dimensional panoramas called cubes that are presented with elegant, user-friendly interfaces we now call dashboards. This data warehousing and data mining will begin to integrate seamlessly into the measurement and reporting mechanisms so closely tied to medicine.

A prominent organization in this area is the National Committee for Quality Assurance (NCQA) which is a U.S.-based non-profit organization widely accepted as an authoritative force in the area of healthcare quality. The NCQA has worked tirelessly for nearly 20 years to ascertain what is important, how to measure it and how to improve. NCQA's Patient-Centered Medical Home program

emphasizes the systematic, multi-disciplinary approach of patient-centered, coordinated care management processes with appropriate recurring revenues (Thompson, Bost, Ahmed, Ingalls & Sennett, 1998).

The measurement of outcomes will be carefully monitored - not only to justify payment for quality healthcare but also for public health reporting and the continued development and best practices. Cabral (2009) indicates one of the advantages of embracing best practices from a clinical standpoint is that a doctor is basing a treatment plan on established protocols and methodologies. According to the data; this is the best course of action to follow. But another advantage of having a directory of best practice guidelines is automation. Clinical Support Systems (CSS) and Decision Support Systems (DSS) are becoming increasingly more sophisticated and will accelerate as more electronic data about our health emerges. These programs guide a caregiver on the steps required to address a particular ailment. CSS are based on established clinical protocols, use rules and associations to provide detailed instructions and suggest medication options if appropriate. Sometimes these steps are extremely simple but other times, such as cancer treatment, they are exceedingly complicated and timing is a critical issue. An EMR with DSS can provide timely and automated prompts to clinicians and patients.

While the implementation of EMRs is clearly an important issue, the ability to monitor and interface with patients from locations outside the practice will also be an asset. As an extremely rudimentary and practical instantiation, the use of email (or a digital equivalent) seems prudent. It is unlikely doctors will ever open their email box to their patients simply because email is too convenient. People may feel they have a 24x7 access account to their "doc's box." The patient centered approach promotes communication but with logical restraints. There are those who will not be able restrain themselves from forwarding a humorous cartoon about healthcare. What about security? Email is natively unsecure and not advised for medical data. A secure web form is a simple solution. Much like many organizations already do, these forms have controls built in to limit choices, ensure interchangeable formats and limited options for free text. All the content of the message is encrypted using Transport Layer Security (TLS) or equivalent. In addition, algorithms and DSS can allow for automated responses and routing to the appropriate caregivers.

As EMRs are installed, they will have the ability to communicate with electronic scheduling applications and many other operational interfaces. E-prescribing is increasingly well-embraced (Friedman, Schueth & Bell, 2009). But one particular application will be what really attracts the consumer: the patient portal. Portals have been in use for years by many industries as a conduit to customers. These personalized sites not only allow for people to interact in a one-to-one relationship with a business entity, but also lower operational costs by permitting users to perform tasks that normally would be done by an employee. An example would be online banking where customers can move money from one account to another with a few clicks of a mouse. Healthcare deserves and requires the same degree of functionality.

The Ina-bilities

When it comes to building enterprise software applications, four "bilities" [sic] are often referenced. They are interoperability, scalability, portability and extensibility. This is underscored when sharing medical data between providers.

The term enterprise is not actually appropriate in this context. Enterprise traditionally means within an organization; that organization could be one location or a dispersed entity with regional offices. The data and the interfaces have to be modeled consistently. But how will hundreds of commercial systems and select government systems work together?

Although Regional Health Information Exchange (RHIOs) and Health Information Networks (HINs) have been filling some of the large gaps that have emerged over the years, the real breakthrough will be the comprehensive adoption of digital record keeping. So a large challenge remains in that most vendors of EMRs have little reason to be "open." By that we mean they have open system architecture and seamlessly interoperate with competing vendor products. Developers of software (and hardware) often respond to market pressures by attempting to carve out a competitive edge using proprietary technology, using components that are unique to their product. This is an easy thing to do because they are unfettered by the rules of interoperability. This appears to give the application an advantage such as better and less bandwidth-intensive video streams, but at a cost of not being able to communicate with other systems. In the world of requisite data interexchange, proprietary formats should be avoided at all costs. One can use an automated teller machine card to get cash from locations all over the world. This is possible because the banking industry and vendors agreed long ago to established data exchange protocols and formats often referred to as non-proprietary or open source.

The medical paradigm differs greatly around the world. Like the U.S., many countries offer quality medical care but, unlike the U.S, being a physician does not guarantee a large paycheck and enhanced lifestyle. In many areas of the world, compensation is merely adequate. People do not go into medicine for the money; they do it because of passion. They want to help other people and feel fulfilled. But because of this, many people who go into healthcare stay in urban settings where a second job is more likely - doctor by day and computer programmer by night as an example. Because of this geography restriction, fewer clinicians venture to the rural areas. This by definition creates underserved communities. Even if technology is unavailable, components of the patient centered approach can be utilized, such as better education, teamwork and a focus on wellness. Simple tasks such as teaching people to better wash their hands before handing food has been proven to be successful (Bilterys, 2008). Areas that are better equipped to integrate technology allow for more clinical care. Wireless phone services around the globe are adding data capabilities to the network so remote areas without wires can still talk and even send data. This again echoes the need for standards-based formats.

Earlier the issue of PHRs was discussed. The future of PHRs are highly debated since they rely heavily on the patient themselves to populate the data. But a pragmatic question arises. How will these PHRs communicate with a PCMH's EMR? If, for example you are working in the yard on Saturday afternoon and step on a rusty nail, you may need medical assistance for not only the wound but you may also need a tetanus shot if you cannot remember when you received your last shot. If you go to a local walk-in emergency center, they may or may not have an EMR to post your clinical intervention. You may also have a PHR with your employer. Your provider's EMR needs to be updated to reflect the new tetanus shot. Other issues remain such as free-form text that is considered unstructured data - digital information that is not modeled or is not easily processed by software applications. Unstructured data is easy to exchange but difficult to quantify. Rules are needed to govern use of these data snippets. What about your medical home – how will your primary care physician know you have been injured and had an inoculation? Medical treatment can take place anywhere you are. Records are kept but today, they do not "talk to each other."

Therefore, having a PHR and a clinical EMR complicates the system. But it is not the technology itself that poses the problem. Other factors are in play, such as funding, politics or poor management. There are established, mature technologies such as eXtensible Markup Language (XML), Health Level 7 (HL7), service oriented architectures, web services, schemas and namespaces, etc. that are designed to process data across disparate entities. Whether the need is exchanging lab results or creating metadata for warehousing applications, metadata harvesting or data mining, the technologies are available.

Take for example XML. The extensible markup language is an extremely powerful and flexible format that was designed to be self-describing. Unlike the hypertext markup language (HTML), XML is not constrained by predefined and limiting tags; rather, XML can be created with tags that appropriately structure the data. So long as the document is properly structured, or well-formed, the data can be exchanged in associations with associated published schemas. The latest version of HL7 is a relevant example. HL7 is a legacy system for the exchange of clinical data. Instead of programmers writing individual connectors to facilitate data exchanges, the new HL7 will permit exchange through XML schemas.

HIEs are models for how data is becoming interoperable. Classically stored in disparate silos, data is being cleansed, normalized, distilled to standardized formats and delivered in near real time. This data, and metadata, facilitates better decision making at the point of care. Even unstructured data is beginning to be distilled through semantic interpretation.

Equally important is the extensibility of information. This refers to systems having the ability to do more things. In some cases, the extensible factor is pre-designed, such as an option to add modules. Other times it refers to something more ad hoc, or unplanned. Contemporary principles in software design such as Object Oriented applications tend to be more extensible because of software classes and inheritance. As the systems evolve they must not only accommodate the clinical needs specific to the patient, but must also subscribe to a high level abstraction such as public health monitoring and bio surveillance.

The Neighborhood: Extending the Home

The use of the word "home" already confuses some people into thinking that this relates to a nursing home. The semantics of the word home really means the physician practice that is evolved to an environment where the patient is the center of the visit. But the existence of the PCMH is designed to migrate outwardly to the patient's actual home.

So why do we need a more patient centered approach and medical homes? What is fundamentally wrong with the current primary care system? There are many issues:

- Costs continue to rise, outstripping inflation
- There is an increase in chronic illnesses
- Access to care is not unified and considered poor, especially for the uninsured
- The payment system rewards volume and repeat customers, not health
- Purchasers of care are demanding accountability and better processes
- Pandemics such as the H1N1 virus underscore global public health reporting needs
- In the U.S., fewer and fewer medical graduates are entering primary care
- This model can be used not only in the U.S., but anywhere
- The world is connected, our healthcare is not

To ensure our population has access to the center of the circular target diagram, the models of the 19th century must be abolished and fresh, contemporary models such as the PCMH need to be adopted. As primary care practices evolve and join hands across the country and the globe, a new paradigm in coordinated care becomes evident: the patient centered medical neighborhood (PCMN). The PCMN is simply a term to describe the interconnection with other aspects of one's social world such as community programs or even social media.

The concept of the neighborhood, like the home, is not new. In fact a raw version of it has been in use for years in disparate locations. The RHIOs and HINs are network-based information exchange mechanisms where data, such as from a lab, can be sent digitally to a physician's office but in bits and pieces. These existing architectures will allow the system to scale up and scale out as integration becomes more important.

In the U.S., as the mandate for EMRs becomes reality in 2014, the tem "meaningful use" is being used as a metric for actually using the EMRs to receive financial incentives from government sources (Medicare and Medicaid). At the time of this writing, only the preliminary definition has been released. It references the use of computerized physician order entry (CPOE), implementing drug interaction and formulary checks, maintaining updated problem lists, recording demographic data, incorporating lab results as structured data and implementing at least five clinical decision support rules. This sets the stage for more enhanced functions.

A patient's personal health portal will be the digital extension of the relationship to his or her doctor and according to Terry (2009), consumers will demand them. This personalized and secure site permits bidirectional communications and is, in essence, a subset of the patient's EMR. The secure patient portal is a conduit and not yet widely deployed. There are so many opportunities to maintain connections between patient and the healthcare team. When a patient leaves the confines of the PCP's office, they will not be out of touch. Messages (both automated and personal), nutritional issues, exercise, medication management can all delivered that reflect a patient's personal plan. Here too, will be options to communicate back to the doctor. These communications will also be autonomous through asynchronous devices such as smart scales and home blood pressure cuffs for transmission of vital signs. And the portal platform does not stop at the computer screen; the CSS energized by patient needs, will have the ability to send digested content that can be pushed to a mobile phone and even the new generation of web-enabled digital photo frames. Some have termed this "ubiquitous healthcare." It is unlikely the self-service continuum such as pumping fuel, online banking and grocery store self-checkout will ever migrate to self-service medicine, what we expect is a much higher level of personal attention to one's heath – coached by a clinical team. The experience of dealing with your doctor evolves from a periodic encounter to part of your daily life. And this is one of the mainstays of the concept: the patient is the center of care and becomes more personally proactive.

Even though the PCMH does not explicitly define the patient's "home", by definition it implies care is extended outside the primary care clinic. The transfer of clinical data from the patient to a remote location is called telemetry. This is common in critical care environments such most hospital rooms. When it extends outside the facility it is broadly termed telemedicine - evaluating and affecting clinical care from a distance. Telemedicine, or the more recent term telehealth, has been around since NASA's Gemini program in the late 1950s (Nicogossian, Pober & Roy, 2001). While not a new concept, telemedicine has only succeeded in pockets of activity. The most successful is arguably tele-radiology and the implementation of the Digital Imaging and Communications in Medicine protocol (DICOM). For the past decade and more, radiographic images have been read at distant locations. A great example is expertise from the opposite of the globe in India where their day is another's night and the cost may be a fraction of what it is in the referring location. The Institute of Medicine, however, is examining how tele- or e-health can be applied after consideration of health literacy (Institute of Medicine workshop proceedings, 2009).

Other specialties, for example, include tele-dermatology, tele-mental health/psychiatry, tele-ultrasound and tele-cardiology. Many prison systems have implemented telehealth for all kinds of ailments because transport costs are prohibitive, the concern for security is high, and it lowers the incidents of "complaints" by inmates. Instead of traveling to a hospital to look at new faces, the telemedicine consult occurs in the prison infirmary and is far less adventurous (Brady, 2004).

Dr. Grundy is enthusiastic about asynchronous telehealth technologies. The covenant of changes, as he refers to it, includes the breakdown of geographic barriers where people are no longer trapped and data will be exchanged. Despite the physical distance, smart devices in concert with DSS and robust networks will permit better self management of chronic diseases, with the physician performing the functions of a navigator. Self management is a critical role for sustainability (Routasalo, Airaksinen, Mäntyranta & Pitkälä, 2009).

Telehealth will have a profound effect on how patients and clinicians communicate. Telehealth will not only be used to connect rural or frontier communities, but as telemetry devices become less expensive and show up at department stores in shrink-wrapped packages, the benefits of monitoring the chronically ill, even in urban settings, will prove worthy. It will take some time for the reimbursement mechanisms to catch up with the technologies however. This unfortunately will slow development of such inexpensive solutions.

But there is another powerful participant that will leverage the new patient-centered paradigm – the pharmaceutical industry. Armed with deep pockets and phenomenal expertise in patient behavior, the "pharmas" will take keen interest in the asynchronous care delivered to patients since they already have a foothold in the evolving medical home. One of the primary goals will be adherence. If patients would better adhere to drug regimens prescribed by their doctors, the outcomes would improve. Forthcoming smart pill bottles are just one tool to assist consumers with better adherence practices. Using standards-based data formats and communication protocols, data from the programmable bottles update the patient's

EMR. Expect significant interest and action from the pharmaceutical industry across the board.

The implementation of technology will be challenging and evolutionary. As the patient centered medicine gains momentum the nascent market in wearable and portable technology will expand. PCPs will utilize the technology that provides not only better health but more revenue. For those who embrace technology the rewards will be significant. For those who ignore it, the outlook may be bleak.

Social Media and the Home

As social media sites such as Facebook, MySpace, Twitter and others, grow in popularity and complexity, it seems natural to snap in healthcare components. Terry (2009) implies that what is appearing is not socialized medicine, but rather social medicine. These locations in cyberspace are becoming a double-edged sword. On the one hand, the details of one's health are confidential, between a caregiver and the patient. But the far-reaching benefits of online interactions offer value that may trump privacy. For example, discussion threads about pancreatic cancer help patients cope by connecting with others with the same diagnosis. While these forums do not require disclosure of your name or use of an online alias, the data sent across the wire is likely not encrypted and could be intercepted and traced. Users may or may not understand this, but one thing is obvious: people want information about their health and will take some chances to get it.

So the question remains: what can you believe in the online world beyond a message from your clinical confidants? This is debatable, but people still do it. Accessing information about health or specific ailments is now commonplace. The knowledge, although not necessarily completely accurate, is part of what makes a patient empowered.

Location-based technology will play an obvious role in the selection of a PCP. For those that have an existing relationship with a doctor this will rarely come into play, but for families that change locations, have children or seek more specialty care, geography will dictate what is available within a reasonable distance. Simple web searches with starting addresses will deliver maps with pins just as we see in almost every other industry. As data pours in the information is "mashed up" and compiled. This is called mashing. Links within the directories will point to online videos of testimonials and complaints. On the business side, other industries have been posting Facebook and Twitter accounts to not only provide a platform for people to blog but also to promote themselves. Unlike the medical establishment, prone to communication blackout, these industries continually strive to outperform and out-market competitors. Healthcare has rarely done this in the new media world, but it will.

Pay for Performance (P4P) has been debated for years and it will take hold (Pearson, Schneider, Kleinman, Coltin & Singer, 2008). Just like the restaurants, you will judge the customer service, quality of care and capabilities. Unlike a restaurant, your expectations are much higher. Are you still sick? The PCMH entails a little secret in its architecture: we rate our outcomes. If, for example, you go in to have a plantar wart removed and six weeks later the wart is back, what kind of job did your doctor do? And for that matter, did the doctor follow up with you to even ask? This will change. If the wart comes back, the doctor does not get paid. Business rules will change because it will be required to report patient outcomes for the online community to see (Duberstein, Meldrum, Fiscella, Shields & Epstein, 2007). Related to P4P, doctor report cards are now beginning to appear (Matthews, 2009). Online feedback about the quality of a provider will be a powerful mechanism and marketing metric by which people choose a care provider.

Unfortunately for the doctor, there is little recourse. While patients have every right to disclose their medical issues, medical professionals can not due to (in most places) privacy laws. This means dissatisfied patients can post negative comments (short of libel) online and the clinical professionals cannot respond other than broad statements. Under no circumstances can a doctor respond directly to a disgruntled patient in the social media. This is yet another example of the patient becoming more empowered that will drive change in the industry.

There is another dilemma in this dimension. Many institutions specialize in high risk cases; the outcomes for those types of organizations are typically lower. It is likely that some type of sliding scale will be employed to level the playing field. But primary care is largely level already since family medicine is geographic. It serves a community and all communities have a wide array of patients. How this population is serviced will dictate how well the physician practice is compensated. According to Dr. Grundy, population dynamics will be a critical measure by which outcomes are based. Patient centered medicine will force improved communications about outcomes.

Patient Privacy and Security

The issue of privacy and security of one's protected health information is due to receive much more attention as the PCMH becomes more widespread. With the 2014 requirement in the U.S. for practices to have and use EMRs, the amount of electronic patient data is poised to explode. With an increase in the volume of data come increased security risks. The source of data does not stop at clinical locations. RHIOs, healthcare clearinghouses, insurance carriers, even employers and the PHRs all house and transmit electronic protected health information (ePHI). As already mentioned, data from the PCMH must be transportable. If you are traveling far away from your home and become injured, the emergency department will need as much information about you as possible. Perhaps you have lost consciousness. How is the clinical staff to learn even the most basic information such as allergies and current medications? Few people

carry an accurate list of current medications. Accessing an online record is the only way. This is clinical mobility and involves security.

Therefore, in a vastly connected medical environment, appropriate access to ePHI is decisive. From one perspective, a clinician may need to have rapid access such in an emergency. This may not require a complete medical history but rather those that affect critical care issues. If the patient is moved to a specialty unit such as a catheter lab, additional information will be required. The same applies to other actions such as surgery. Along the way, clinician access is expanded on a "need-to-know" basis. At each clinical layer, access can be granted based on the diagnosis codes indexed to a physician ID number (Unique Physician Identification Number (UPIN)) which is indexed to permissions. This cascading access protocol ensures timely data availability with rules-based granular security.

In the U.S., privacy and security laws (Health Insurance Portability and Accountability Act of 1996 (HIPAA) have been in place for years. Other nations have similar laws. Furthermore, these laws are continuously being tightened in an effort to protect information for both clinical privacy and identity theft. As EMRs become required for all clinical practices, the regulations are sure to become more stringent. This poses another challenge: most small practices do not have, and will not have, the financial capability to have experienced network/server security personnel on staff. Many primary care practices likely have no idea as to the cost and effort required to protect data. Unlike larger organizations that have information technology departments, the clinics will struggle with the moral and federal requirements to protect data that is not only stored but also in transit. It is likely many will use hosted solutions obviating the need for digital security staff, but many will opt for in-house systems.

To address the governmental requirements, third-party entities will emerge to assist with implementation of HIPAA security polices and procedures. Any organization that houses ePHI must have polices in place that say what they are going to do and procedures that dictate how they will do it. The documentation is complicated and must evolve to address changes in the environment. As new risks appear, data volume changes and portability will constantly be pressed by the marketplace.

Having the ability to outsource will allow smaller clinics to remain compliant and strive towards best practices for data security. Examples would be to perform risk assessments on assets/servers, periodic network checks on servers to look for open ports that can pose risks, detect breaches, periodic user training and audit trails for document changes. These types of activities are far outside the scope of a primary care practice but, nonetheless will have to be addressed.

Revenue Requirements

People tend to look at healthcare as altruism. Doctors take an oath to care for patients. The truth is it is a business. Budgets, revenue projections, compensation and general discussions about money are issues in most settings.

As the data from primary physicians become more public, the pressures to perform well will become more important. Through wellness programs and better outcomes, we should theoretically expect better health across all spectrums. The classic "fee for service" will begin to show its age. A healthier population should result in fewer clinical interventions from the primary care entry point to the emergency room visit. A population-based approach includes not only improving quality and but reducing inequities.

One of the challenges of the PCMH is an appropriate compensation model. In the U.S., doctors are generally well compensated; this will be very hard to change. The classic fee-for-service model is far from going away, but new reimbursement mechanisms will be interwoven. Recurring supplements will likely be offered such as quar-

terly payments based on quality, efficiency, and satisfaction improvements through a contractual arrangement with payers. These contracts will be difficult to draft since outcome metrics are still nebulous. The goal of the PCMH is to provide more comprehensive, coordinated care to reduce the delivery of services in suboptimal settings such as the emergency room.

Primary care providers will have to address a very different business paradigm and will have to build new service lines to address patient-centered care to replace revenues lost from traditional procedures (as the population becomes healthier). As consumers become more knowledgeable about their personal health, PCPs should expect to face low-cost competition from non-healthcare companies selling tools and services that are skilled in consumer marketing. Home telemonitoring will be a significant example and would be considered a medical "vertical" that expands the traditional healthcare service mix. If properly administered, revenues will increase through efficiencies and better throughput.

Currently, the healthcare domain uses International Statistical Classification of Diseases and Related Health Problems (ICD-9) codes for diagnosis and Current Procedural Terminology (CPT) codes for billing. While GT and GQ code modifiers are permitted in some cases for telehealth reimbursement, the processes in the U.S. are so mired in legalities and state differentials it is difficult for anyone to clearly understand what can and cannot be reimbursed. The ICD codes are scheduled to migrate to ICD-10 by 2013. This change alone will morass the system as the code sets increase from 17,000 to over 155,000. This simply represents yet another change to processes.

Many changes will occur, issues will unfold and controversy will continue. Dr. Graham (personal communication, December 16, 2009) believes the largest obstacle faced by the industry is the change in culture. "Practices are faced with dataset issues and mindset issues." Those that embrace the changes from purely hands-on or synchronous care to including persistent asynchronous care will persevere. This asynchronous care powered by a new generation of home healthcare devices, affordable computing, available networks and interoperable EMRs will give doctors a much more accurate portrayal of a patient's health, and how to manage it.

Doctors will begin to advertise their PCMH much like the cosmetic surgery industry has done for years. Price lists will show up on their websites, emphasizing healthcare services as a commodity. Initially, many will frown on this practice but, in an age of consumerism, it will happen. As mentioned earlier, social media will drive traffic to sites that offer certain services that are perhaps better at Doctor A versus Doctor B. What about my medical home - the place where I have built a personal and trusting relationship with my doctor and her team? The 21st century medical home will have to be adaptable to market pressures like any other competitive industry.

The healthcare marketplace has considerable room to evolve and expand. Because technology is beginning to be implemented on a much broader scale, traditional one to many relationships between doctor and patients will move to a 1:1 relationship much like other industries. PCPs will be incentivized to improve individual health. The cost of chronic disease perpetuated by poor individual health management is a core issue. For example, an obese patient who smokes is a prime candidate for heart disease and diabetes. By working closely with that patient, on a continual basis, the physician can have more influence over the patient's day-to-day activities; not necessarily from the doctor but from the team that includes virtual renditions that can convey information over various medium such as a website or mobile phone, referred to as avatars. These computer generated entities distill data from the asynchronous data points, information posted by the patient in their portals and best practices to apply gentle pressure to the patient to keep them on course. The avatars appear not only though the portal but in the form of email, text messaging and voice prompts.

The healthcare industry can learn from another existing medical community for guidance: the clinicians that care for our pets in veterinary offices. The ones that care for your canine companion are more likely to have digital documentation, to send reminders, and to follow-up about a procedure than the average PCP's office. True, animals do not have the complexity, interoperability and legal issues associated with humans, but it was recognized years ago that efficient processes were needed to compete effectively and to maximize profits.

What was once a political construct will become a thriving industry based on health, but dealing with illness. Things will continue to improve. Best practices will be shared, and the market will lean on the practices to be efficient and effective. It will take much more than hardware and software to culturally shift the industry, it will require thoughtware – an iconoclastic change in of how we think and operate. The sickcare system of old will finally evolve to a pure healthcare system.

SOLUTIONS AND RECOMMENDATIONS

Change is difficult for the healthcare industry. To make the transformation, PCPs face many obstacles. A century ago doctors made house calls as a regular course of business. Those days are virtually gone. Small pockets of door-to-door doctors still exist, but usually to the wealthy that pay large sums of money to be cared for at home. But the PCMH is a type of resurrection of the "housecall" and the nomenclature "medical home" even echoes this. While the physician does not actually go to the home, they are there in concept. Telehealth technologies that have failed to gain traction the past over 20 years will now play a critical role in supporting data capture, virtual visits and enhanced communications.

The information about our individual health-care is largely stored in metal filing cabinets on paper. We are 10% through the 21st century and a tiny percentage of medical records are electronic. Some countries are further ahead than others, but overall our data is far from interoperable. Clinical intervention tools continue to march forward but our records do not. We can, however, finally say this is changing.

The amount of data that will be collected about our bodies will not only be voluminous, it will also be combined with others. Subsets of data will be extracted for research and reported in aggregate for outcomes called research informatics. These outcomes will drive best practice guidelines and track trends for public health. Superbugs that develop resistance to many or all known antibiotics will continue to plague our global society, and identifying outbreaks of disease as early as possible is our best defense. But we need extremely sophisticated and robust information exchange mechanisms to do so. The interoperable EMR is not only the data foundation of patient centered medicine; it also will feed the global conduit for messaging and reporting.

Consumerism is one ingredient that will force change – patients want better care at lower prices with more convenience. It will no longer be a fee for a service no matter how well the service is performed. Pressure will mount on all fronts to transform the practice into an elegantly managed curing and caring dimension.

FUTURE RESEARCH DIRECTIONS

Patient-centered medicine is sure to persist. In the digital world we have already seen how the Internet has changed how business is conducted – as mentioned earlier, medicine is a business. How this concept will propagate throughout the international community is much more difficult to predict. The excessive cost of EMRs will begin to align with free PHRs. These, as in other indus-tries, will morph into software as a service (SaaS). Hosted versions of medical data will arise for our burgeoning global village as clinicians recognize they are in healthcare, not information technology.

On the clinical side, fascinating new technology will enter the arena of asynchronous health monitoring. Personal area networks (PANs) will surround our bodies, sending vital signs across the network. In the coming years we will see incredible capabilities such as micro-machines. You may drink orange juice that has microscopic sensors floating within. These miniature robots will circulate through your system and seek out dangers or markers far sooner than we can today. As you step on the scale, a burst of energy may contact these roving machines. Any suspicious activity, such as excessive cell reproduction indicating a birth of cancer, could be reported to the scale. This information, along with traditional vital signs such as weight and temperature, could be sent to your individual health profile and processed using a DSS. Patient centered medicine would surround this process and the appropriate actions would be taken by the team. This type of process is broadly termed "individualized healthcare" and specifically termed "nanomedicine." It is likely that eventually we will have full-body image sets at the molecular or DNA level. An annual checkup would include a new scan. Using algorithms such as subtractive modeling, image sets could be compared and differences analyzed. Predictive analytics based on genomically-determined patient profiles will take the core concept of the PCMH to the next level. Predictive analytics and taking preventive action will save vast amounts of money and improve overall health. But without a robust patient centered approach, the economies of scale needed to manufacture devices at huge volume and low cost will never exist.

A scenario: In the near future, the PCP will change significantly how they interact with patients. Each day he logs into his service portal using a biometric ID on a lightweight and durable tablet PC. Here, all appointments are listed, clearly marked are those that are virtual. For each patient, a click of the mouse displays a summary about the patient. Every patient is required to answer a short questionnaire prior to the visit that can be from home or in the waiting room. If the patient has specific questions, the CSS automatically pulls relevant data from trusted sources. For those that utilized home health monitoring equipment, the data is automatically sent to the EMR and summarized by the CSS. Prior to being posted on the physician portal, members of the clinical team review the appointment file and append the data. Based on the reason for the visit, the CSS presents questions and options for a care plan. Historical data can be immediately accessed on the tablet PC and shown to the patient. If-then scenarios can be run with projected outcomes. If routine tests are due, a flag is displayed. A click of the mouse sends a message to the patient; email, phone or both depending on user preferences. If appropriate, the patient encounter posts de-identified data to central registries and public health agencies. The CSS suggests a certain medication based on research outcomes, and matched against current medications and allergies, prescriptions are sent as well with a reminder with possible side effect to watch for. Using Natural Language Processing (NLP), the physician adds notes that are transcribed to the EMR. At the end of the visit, the patient checks out and reviews an encounter summary. Diagnostic and billing codes are generated and are forwarded to the billing application. Even after the patient leaves, continual communications occur between the clinical team and the patient occurs. If parameters exceed a predetermined range, alerts are sent. Over time, the condition of the patient is mapped. Positive outcomes result in higher reimbursement rates, poor outcomes demand more attention. For the virtual visits, the encounter is performed using software video applications similar to online meeting tools used by corporations regularly. Select data and images can be pushed to the patient. This is an example of how technology can assist in centering the patient.

CONCLUSION

Healthcare is the responsibility of the person. Medical intervention is the responsibility of the physician. How the two come together at the family medicine level is poised to change dramatically. No longer will healthcare rely on poorly coordinated, isolated episodic care sans technology. It will be a continual relationship in multiple directions. The proliferation of patient centered medicine and market forces will do what the managed care approach has failed to do; successfully integrate the primary care physician as the gatekeeper for managing healthcare for not only individuals, but for local populations as well (Bodenheimer, 2006). The approach is primed and in need of reengineering with technology at its core. The issues are not just in the U.S.; they are prevalent all over the world. We must care locally and think globally.

REFERENCES

American Academy of Pediatrics, American Academy of Family Physicians, American College of Physicians, American Osteopathic Association. (2007). *Joint principles of the patient-centered medical home.* Retrieved January 6, 2010, from http://www.medicalhomeinfo.org/joint 20Statement.pdf.

Bilterys, R., & Milord, F. (2008). Preventing nosocomial infections: a topic of concern in developing countries as well. *Perspective Infirmiere, 5*(7), 21–26.

Bodenheimer, T. (2006). Primary care – will it survive? *The New England Journal of Medicine, 355*(9), 861–864. doi:10.1056/NEJMp068155

Brady, J. L. (2005). Telemedicine behind bars: a cost-effective and secure trend. *Biomedical Instrumentation & Technology, 39*(1), 7–8.

Cabral, K. P. (2009). How to meet national quality initiatives: best practices. [Epub ahead of print]. *Journal of Thrombosis and Thrombolysis*, (Nov): 12.

Commins, J. (2009). *Patient knowledge of their meds woeful, says stud: Health leaders media*, December 10, 2009. Retrieved January 5, 2010, from http://www.healthleadersmedia.com/content/243355/topic/WS_HLM2_QUA/Patient-Knowledge-of-Their-Meds-Woeful-Says-Study.html.

Duberstein, P., Meldrum, S., Fiscella, K., Shields, C. G., & Epstein, R. M. (2007). Influences on patients' ratings of physicians: Physicians demographics and personality. *Patient Education and Counseling*, 65(2), 270–274. doi:10.1016/j.pec.2006.09.007

Friedman, M. A., Schueth, A., & Bell, D. S. (2009). Interoperable electronic prescribing in the United States: a progress report. *Health Affairs*, 28(2), 393–403. doi:10.1377/hlthaff.28.2.393

Hitt, G., & Adam, J. (2009, December 25). Senate passes sweeping health-care bill. *Wall Street Journal*. Retrieved January 5, 2010, from http://online.wsj.com/article/SB126165317923104141.html.

Institute of Medicine. Workshop Proceedings. *Health literacy, eHealth, and communication: Putting the consumer first.* (March 24, 2009). Retrieved January 6, 2010, from http://www.iom.edu/Reports/2009/Health-Literacy-eHealth-and-Communication-utting-the-Consumer-First-Workshop-Summary.aspx.

Mathews, A. W. (2009, October 27). Compare and contrast. *Wall Street Journal*, R4.

National Archives and Records Administration. *President Truman's proposed health program.* November 19, 1945. Retrieved January 5, 2010, from http://www.trumanlibrary.org/publicpapers/index.php?pid=483&st=&st1.

Nicogossian, A. E., Pober, D. F., & Roy, S. A. (2001). Evolution of telemedicine in the space program and earth applications. *Telemedicine Journal and e-Health*, 7(1), 1–15. doi:10.1089/153056201300093813

Pearson, S. D., Schneider, E. C., Kleinman, K. P., Coltin, K. L. & Singer, J. A. (2008). The impact of pay-for-performance on health care quality in Massachusetts, 2001-2003. *Health Affairs*.

Robeznieks, A. (2005). In no big hurry. Physicians still slow to adopt EMR systems: survey. *Modern Healthcare*, 35(38), 17.

Routasalo, P., Airaksinen, M., Mäntyranta, T., & Pitkälä, K. (2009). Supporting a patient's self-management. *Duodecim*, 125(21), 2351–2359.

Sarfaty, M. (n.d.). American Public Health Association. *The Rise of the patient centered medical home: What is it? What does it mean?* Retrieved January 6, 2010, from http://www.apha.org/membergroups/newsletters/sectionnewsletters/medical/winter09/pcmh.htm.

Sisko, A., Truffer, C., Smith, S., Keehan, S., Cylus, J., et al. (2009). OECD health data 2008: statistics and indicators for 30 countries. Organisation for economic co-operation and development; Health spending projections through 2018: Recession effects add uncertainty to the outlook. *Health Affairs*.

Terry, M. (2009). Twittering healthcare: social media and medicine. *Telemedicine Journal and e-Health*, 15(6), 507–510. doi:10.1089/tmj.2009.9955

Thompson, J. W., Bost, J., Ahmed, F., Ingalls, C. E., & Sennett, C. (1998). The NCQA's quality compass: Evaluating managed care in the United States. A brief look at the NCQA's comparison of health plan performance. *Health Affairs*, 17(1).

Zwar, N. A. (2010). Health care reform in the United States: An opportunity for primary care? *The Medical Journal of Australia*, 192(1), 8.

ADDITIONAL READING

American Academy of Family Physicians. (2009). The Robert Graham Center. *Policy Studies in Family Medicine and Primary Care*. Retrieved January 5, 2010, from http://www.graham-center. org/online/graham/home.html.

American Academy of Family Physicians. (2009). *Ten Steps to a Patient-Centered Medical Home*. Retrieved January 5, 2010, from http://www. aafp.org/online/en/home/membership/initiatives/ pcmh.html.

Bazarko, D. (2008). *Framing the medical home model of care: Blueprint from early adopters*. Bath, UK: M2 Communications Ltd.

Christensen, C. M., & Grossman, J. H. (2009). *The innovator's prescription: A disruptive solution for health care*. Columbus, OH: The McGraw-Hill Companies.

Davis, K., Schoenbaum, S. C., & Audet, A. M. (2005). A 2020 vision of patient-centered primary care. *Journal of General Internal Medicine, 20*(10). doi:10.1111/j.1525-1497.2005.0178.x

Donovan, P. P., Greene, L. M., & Salmon, J. (2009). *Model medical homes: Benchmarks and case studies in patient-centered care*. Manasquan, NJ: The Healthcare Intelligence Network.

Earp, J. A., French, E. A., & Gilkey, M. B. (2009). *Patient advocacy for healthcare quality: Strategies for achieving patient centered care*. Sudbury, MA: Jones and Bartlett Publishers.

Frampton, S. B., & Charmel, P. A. (2009). *Putting patients first: Best practices in patient-centered care*. San Francisco, CA: Planetree.

Hayes, T. L., Cobbinah, K., Dishingh, T., Kaye, J. A., Kimmel, J., Labhard, M., & Leen, T. (2009). A study of medicine-taking and unobtrusive, intelligent reminding. *Telemedicine and e-Health, 15*(8), 770-776. Retrieved January 5, 2010, from http:// www.liebertonline.com/doi/pdfplus/10.1089/ tmj.2009.0033.

Hicks, L. L. (2009). The application of remote monitoring to improve health outcomes to rural area. *Telemedicine and e-Health, 15*(7), 664-671. Retrieved January 5, 2010, from http:// www.liebertonline.com/doi/pdfplus/10.1089/ tmj.2009.0009.

Naditz, A. (2009). Coming to your senses: Future methods of patient monitoring and home healthcare. *Telemedicine and e-Health, 15*(6), 511-516. Retrieved January 5, 2010, from http:// www.liebertonline.com/doi/pdfplus/10.1089/ tmj.2009.9953.

National Committee for Quality Assurance. (2009). *Physician practice connections-patient-centered medical home*. Retrieved January 5, 2010, from http://www.ncqa.org/tabid/631/default.aspx.

Ponte, P. R., Conlin, G., Conway, J. B., Grant, S., Medeiros, C., & Nies, J. (2003). Making patient-centered care come alive: Achieving full integration of the patient's perspective. *The Journal of Nursing Administration, 33*(2), 82–90. doi:10.1097/00005110-200302000-00004

Rosenthal, T. C. (2008). The medical home: Growing evidence to support a new approach to primary care. *Journal of the American Board of Family Medicine, 21*(5), 427–440. doi:10.3122/ jabfm.2008.05.070287

Siemens Medical Solutions and the Center for Health Transformation. (2004). *Survey Findings Contradict Conventional Wisdom About Healthcare Costs*. Retrieved March 15, 2010, from http:// www.medical.siemens.com/webapp/wcs/stores/ servlet/PSGenericDisplay~q_catalogId~e_-1~a_ catTree~e_100005,18301,18902~a_langId~e_- 1~a_pageId~e_53129~a_storeId~e_10001.htm

Stewart, M., Brown, J. B., Weston, W. W., Mcwhinney, I. R., & McWilliam, C. L. (2003). *Patient-centered medicine: Transforming the clinical method*. Salem, MA: Radcliffe Medical Press Ltd.

Terry, M. (2009). The Personal Health Dashboard: Consumer Electronics Is Growing in the Health and Wellness Market. *Telemedicine and e-Health, 15*(7), 642-645. doi:10.1089/tmj.2009.9947.

KEY TERMS AND DEFINITIONS

Asynchronous Communications: Data transmission without timing criteria, meaning in this case non-real-time sessions such as physiologic data parameter transfer (see synchronous).

Data Warehousing: A repository of stored data within an organization for aggregate reporting, often with the element of time.

EMR: Usually institutional, an electronic medical record.

ePHI: Electronic Patient Health Information that resides in numerous formats and states.

Health Level 7 (HL7) Interface: A software interface based on established standards for the exchange of information within healthcare settings.

Metadata: Information about the data and its structure itself.

Namespaces: A method for qualifying element and attribute names used in XML documents by associating them with other locations on a network.

Open Source: A practice that promotes access to a product's source materials, often the source code, to facilitate collaborative, interoperable development.

Patient Registries: Lists within a clinical domain to track key measures within a specific realm.

Proprietary Technology: Technology that is typically owned exclusively by a single company based on non-standard, non-shared and carefully guarded processes.

Schemas: A description of the structure of a document type, often XML.

Synchronous Communications: data transmission with timing criteria, meaning in this case real-time sessions such as videoconferencing (see asynchronous).

Web Services: A software approach to support interoperable machine-to-machine interactions over a network.

XML: Extensible Markup Language, a set of specifications for encoding documents to facilitate data exchange across heterogeneous environments.

Chapter 2
Privacy and Security in e–Health Applications

Milan Petković
Philips Research Europe & Eindhoven University of Technology, The Netherlands

Luan Ibraimi
University of Twente, The Netherlands

ABSTRACT

The introduction of e-Health and extramural applications in the personal healthcare domain has raised serious concerns about security and privacy of health data. Novel digital technologies require other security approaches in addition to the traditional "purely physical" approach. Furthermore, privacy is becoming an increasing concern in domains that deal with sensitive information such as healthcare, which cannot absorb the costs of security abuses in the system. Once sensitive information about an individual's health is uncovered and social damage is done, there is no way to revoke the information or to restitute the individual. Therefore, in addition to legal means, it is very important to provide and enforce privacy and security in healthcare by technological means. In this chapter, the authors analyze privacy and security requirements in healthcare, explain their importance and review both classical and novel security technologies that could fulfill these requirements.

INTRODUCTION

Recently, many e-Health applications are proposed worldwide. They include initiatives on creation of national/regional electronic health record (EHR) infrastructures such as RHIO's in the US, the NHS Spine project in the United Kingdom and NICTIZ in the Netherlands, as well as efforts on creating commercial Web-based personal health record (PHR) systems such as Microsoft HealthVault and Google Health. These applications process, store and exchange patient's medical information. Next to that, there is an increasing number of extramural telemedicine applications in the personal healthcare domain such as remote patient monitoring. On the one hand these technologies

DOI: 10.4018/978-1-60960-469-1.ch002

improve the quality of health care by providing faster and cheaper health care services, on the other hand they are exposed to different security threats as it becomes simpler to collect, store, and search electronic health data, thereby endangering people's privacy. Therefore, they pose new security and privacy challenges towards the protection of medical data.

In contrast to other domains, such as financial, which can absorb the cost of the abuse of the system (e.g. credit card fraud), healthcare cannot. Once sensitive information about an individual's health problems is uncovered and social damage is done, there is no way to revoke the information or to restitute the individual. Therefore e-Health applications must implement safeguards in place to protect the privacy of patients' health data.

This is recognized by legislation. There are a number of laws around the world designed to protect the electronic health data that the healthcare institutions maintain about their patients, such as the Health Insurance Portability and Accountability Act (HIPAA) in the US, which specifies rules and standards to achieve security and privacy of health data, or directive 95/46/EC in the EU for protecting personal data processed by information systems. Furthermore, there are a number of sophisticated security mechanisms, such as access control mechanisms, encryption techniques and auditing tools which are applicable for e-Health applications.

In this chapter, we address the issues of security and privacy in e-Health applications. Firstly, we survey different types of digital health records and describe examples of human-centered e-Health applications which use them. Next we overview their privacy and security requirements such as data availability, data confidentiality, data integrity, accountability, anonymity and user awareness and discuss the state-of-the-art technologies which address these requirements. The focus is put on the technologies centered around the patient.

DIGITAL HEALTH RECORDS: CURRENT SITUATION AND TRENDS

To reduce cost and improve accuracy there is a pressure on healthcare providers to start managing and sharing patient information in digital form. This implies a revolution in the way health information is managed. Paper-based records are becoming obsolete as with the increasing complexity of the healthcare system the paper systems cannot fulfill the complicated requirements and ensure that the right information is available at the point of care when needed. Therefore, digital records are increasingly used within hospitals in departmental information systems (DIS) as well as at the hospital level in hospital information systems (HIS). However, the use of digital records will go beyond the walls of the hospital. General practitioners (GP), pharmacies, remote patient monitoring systems and other home e-Health services are increasingly using them.

In this section, we give an overview of digital health records and describe two main purposes they have: (i) to serve healthcare providers and (ii) to empower the patient/consumer. To make the differences clear, we describe the architecture of a national/regional EHR system, as well as an example of a PHR system. However, there are a number of dedicated services such as remote patient monitoring systems that collect and use some types of health data, such as blood pressure, pulse, weight, etc. These systems share a number of security and privacy concerns with EHR and PHR systems, but we do not describe them in this chapter as their architectures are in most cases related to the EHR and PHR architectures. For a good example, the interested reader can check the architecture of the Philips Motiva system (Simons, 2006).

Electronic Health Records (EHR)

Digital health records are used at different levels in healthcare. First, they are used in hospitals at the departmental level (e.g., at a radiology department) where medical data related to examinations or treatments are stored in the so-called electronic medical records (EMR). To improve sharing of information within institutions, different departmental systems are increasingly integrated into hospital information systems (HIS) such that digital health or patient records can span over different departments. Such records, which also include administrative data, are often called electronic health records (EHR).

The Healthcare Information and Management Systems Society[1] (HIMSS, 2003) defines EHRs as follows:

"The Electronic Health Record (EHR) is a secure, real-time, point-of-care, patient centric information resource *for clinicians*.

- The EHR aids clinicians decision making by providing access to patient health record information *where and when they need* it and by incorporating evidence-based decision support.
- The EHR *automates and streamlines the clinician's workflow*, closing loops in communication and response that result in delays or gaps in care.
- The EHR also *supports the collection of data for uses other than direct clinical care*, such as billing, quality management, outcomes reporting, resource planning, and public health disease surveillance and reporting."

The next step after implementation of hospital centric EHR systems is integration of information systems of larger institutions that have multiple sites, or systems of co-operating care-providers in a region. This is an important first step towards the creation of a real EHR, as it is about increased availability of healthcare data and sharing among different healthcare providers and organizations. Sometimes this intermediate step is referred to as Continuity of Care Records (CCR), because it supports care chains (also known as care pathways) within a region.

Finally, the EHR term[2] is often used in relation to national electronic health record infrastructures. Spine (Spine, 2009), InfoWay (InfoWay, 2007) and NICTIZ (NICTIZ, 2007) are examples of such infrastructures that are currently under development in the UK, Canada and the Netherlands. A national EHR infrastructure connects various entries that a patient has in the various hospital EHR systems deployed by different healthcare providers. The EHR is meant to provide an integrated, holistic, *patient-centric* and life-long (across multiple disease episodes) view on the healthcare contents of all these systems.

Figure 1 shows the generic structure of a service-based architecture of the EHR implementations. These systems are based on a communications bus that provides access between all EHR system components.

Health information about patients and their demographics is distributed over several (medical) databases (DB). These databases are run by either independent organizations or by the different participating healthcare providers (like a GP's office or hospital). As most patients return to the same medical professional, the latter option has the benefit that most relevant (detailed) data can be found locally, reducing the need to access information over the communication bus.

As the information is distributed over several databases, a number of problems must be solved. The first problem is locating where EHR entries of a patient are stored. For this purpose, EHR systems typically contain a location register. This registry stores an index and perhaps a summary of the entries and can be queried by applications. The second problem relates to a patient who may have several identifiers across the different EHR components. Within a regional or national EHR infrastructure, sometimes a national patient security number is used, but each component may use its own (legacy) set of identifiers. The patient registry provides the means to translate identifi-

Figure 1. Generic EHR system structure

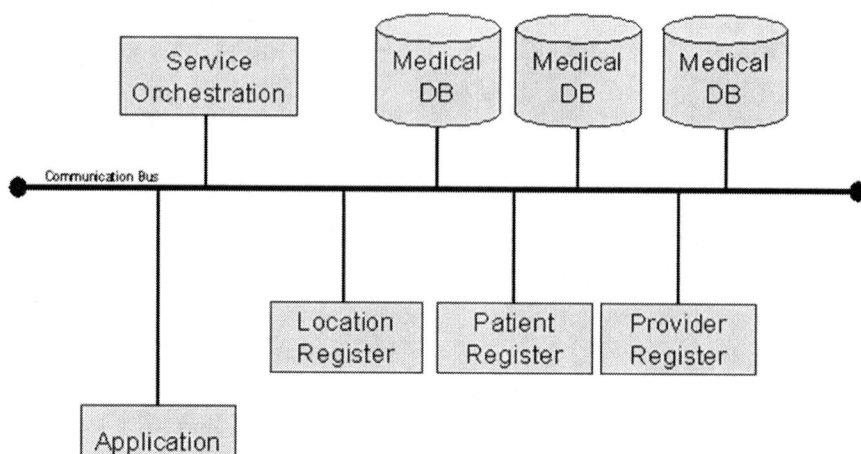

ers. This means that an application has to map its identifier to the different identifiers of the patient at the corresponding medical databases before being able to query those databases.

Then, there is the problem of access control. Not all care-providers may access all data. For this reason, the EHR has its own provider registry that contains the access privileges of the different users from different institutions. This means that applications (or the different databases) have to check with the provider registry if a certain request of the care provider that uses the application is allowed. The provider registry is typically based on existing registries that list all qualified professionals (individuals) and amongst others their roles (e.g. doctor, nurse, etc.). Finally, there is a problem of interoperability between different databases – the application should be able to understand the data coming from the databases. For that reason communication is usually done using HL7 standard (HL-7, 2007). HL7 provides the vocabulary/data formats (such as Clinical Document Architecture) to communicate about relevant medical 'acts'. This implies that the medical databases produce HL7 formatted output. Furthermore, HL7 has standardized the protocols to query and invoke the different functions of the EHR system. This includes querying and filling the various registries.

The efforts that an application has to go through to obtain EHR information are quite extensive. This process becomes worse when several EHR systems are coupled, as it is in the Canadian Info-Way system (InfoWay, 2007). In such a case, an application has to query several patient registries, search for medical information, and do cross-system user authentication and authorization. To simplify this process, orchestration services are added to the system. These orchestration services take over a number of responsibilities from the applications.

Personal Health Records (PHR)

Nowadays, patients are taking a more active role in their own healthcare management. They track symptoms, perhaps take themselves their vital body signs, discus them with doctors, and manage their illnesses. They are becoming much more responsible and aware of their own health. However, currently patients can hardly access their electronic health records (they have rights to access it, but in practice the processes are difficult). Furthermore, they are not able to add their own data to EHRs. Therefore, patients have very limited possibilities to manage their health data in general. To overcome this problem, a number of

Figure 2. Typical architecture of personal health systems

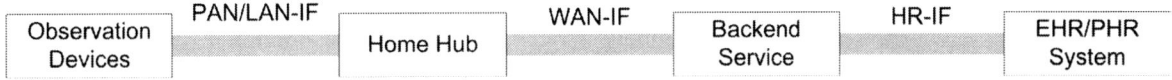

solutions are introduced in the market that allows patients to collect their own information and to store them on portable devices, PCs, and more importantly on online services. These solutions are often referred to as personal health record (PHR). While EHRs are mainly meant for clinicians, PHRs empower the patient and allow him to gather, maintain and share his health records and consequently have complete control over them.

The Markle foundation (Markle, 2003) defines PHRs as follows:

"An electronic application through which individuals can access, manage and share their health information, and that of others for whom they are authorized, in a private, secure, and confidential environment.

- An *Internet-based set of tools* that allows people to access and coordinate their life-long health information and make appropriate parts of it available to those who need it
- Provides an *integrated view* encompassing health status, medical and treatment history, communications with healthcare providers
- Includes data from clinical systems, data received from monitoring devices, and information entered by providers and the individual himself/herself
- A *communications hub*: to send email to doctors, transfer information to specialists, receive test results and access online self-help tools."

As mentioned, already a number of products in the market allows patients to take their vital body signs and enter them together with other medical data into their PHR database. Depending on the solution, this database is stored on the patient's PC, a special storage device (typically USB-based), or preferably in an online service such as Microsoft HealthVault, Google Health or WebMD. The large benefit is that the data is electronically available (through the online connections with the service, or the fact that the patient carries all data with him on the portable device).

To ease the data collection process, some of the measurements that the patient undertakes can be automated. For example, a weight-scale can send the measurement wirelessly to the application or service that collects the data (e.g. Philips Telemonitoring Services). Another example is a system that allows the collection of ECG data using a wireless connection to a mobile phone (MyHeart, 2003). Similar applications and architecture are used in ambient assisted living domain (i.e. aging independently) where sensors and services help elderly to live longer in their own homes. As an increasing number of the monitoring devices and healthcare and wellness services are appearing, a big industry alliance called Continua (Continua, 2007) was formed to provide interoperability in these domains.

The components and interfaces of typical architectures shown in Figure 2, which are used in the domains of personal healthcare, wellness, and ambient assisted living include:

1. Observation devices: these devices measure patient's vital signs, such as blood pressure, heart rate, weight, ECG, or environment,

e.g. presence in a room. They are stationary, portable, or worn by patients.

2. Home hub: this is a stationary or portable device such as PC, dedicated medical device, set top box or a mobile phone. It collects the measurements (e.g. vital-signs observations) from observation devices, possibly stores them and forwards them to a service.

3. Personal/local area network interface (PAN/LAN-IF): this interface connects observation devices with a home hub. This could be wired or wireless (low-power) interface. For example, Continua health alliance provides interoperability guidelines for using medical profiles of USB and Bluetooth standards on top of which IEEE 11073-20601 base framework protocol and ten device specializations (e.g. IEEE 11073-10407 for blood pressure) are used. Low power radios such as ZigBee can also be used.

4. Backend service: this system collects the data from subscribed patients/consumers and makes it available to healthcare/wellness providers. It typically offers data processing, representation and decision support (e.g. identification of trends) to increase efficiency of healthcare/wellness providers.

5. Wide area network interface (WAN-IF): this interface provides connectivity between the home hub (or patient's mobile phone) and the backend service. In the telemedicine domain this is typically a medical data format (such as one provided by HL-7) over TCP/IP.

6. PHR/EHR system: this is the electronic or personal health record system (e.g. at a hospital) that eventually can receive the measured data.

7. Health records interface (HR-IF): this is the interface between the backend service and the electronic/personal health record system. Typically this connection also uses the Internet. Different health record standards can be used. For example, Continua health alliance provides interoperability guidelines for this interface by using IHE XDR - Integrated Healthcare Enterprise cross-enterprise document reliable exchange (IHE, 2005) on top of which HL-7 Personal Health Monitoring profile (PHM) is used.

SECURITY AND PRIVACY REQUIREMENTS OF E-HEALTH APPLICATIONS

Although there is a whole range of security issues related to e-Health application, given the significance of digital health data for e-Health applications we focus in this chapter on digital health data related requirements. As already mentioned, health data is usually stored by different entities at different places of healthcare IT systems. For instance, researchers need health data for clinical research, doctors exchange health data for a second opinion, and patients send their medical histories to doctors to get right treatments. The most important security requirements for e-Health applications are described as follows:

- **Availability.** The health data and applications should be available to the authorized users upon request. While for wellness applications not so critical, time delays in accessing patient data is unacceptable in professional healthcare as it can be fatal for the life of the patient. The most dangerous threat to data availability is the so called Denial-of-Service (DoS) attack which prevents the normal function of the system by overloading the system with automated bogus information requests. In addition to DoS attacks, data availability can be impaired by natural disasters, technical problems or human error.

- **Confidentiality.** The Individually Identifiable Health Information (IIHI) should be protected when it moves from one place to another, when it is stored in centralized or decentralized servers, and when someone operates it. In the EU, this is the case in any domain (wellness or e-Health), while in the US this is one of the HIPAA requirements relevant to HIPAA covered entities.

The access policy specifies who is authorized to access the data. The access policy can be specified by the patient to whom the data refers, by means of patient consent or his PHR privacy preferences, by national legislation, and/or by a healthcare provider with whom the patient has a predefined contract. In healthcare, the access to patient data should be provided on a "need-to-know" basis (e.g. only healthcare providers that are involved in the treatment of a patient have access to his information). Another specific confidentiality related requirement in healthcare is a "break-the-glass" functionality that allows care providers to exceed their rights and get access to data which they normally would not be able to access. This functionality has to be implemented together with non-repudiation mechanisms for its usage. Healthcare professionals, following their professional obligations, are usually trusted by patients to keep their health information confident. Wellness providers or web-based e-Health services are typically less trusted by consumers.

- **Integrity.** The health data should be correct and should not be modified in an unauthorized manner. Moreover, the party operating with health data has to ensure that the data is not lost or altered in an improper way. This implies that only authorized users should be able to create new records, add them, and later update. Different health data have different integrity requirements. For instance, in healthcare, it is not acceptable to compress an original chest x-ray photo using lossy data compression algorithms and later use the compressed photo to give opinions. The compressed photo can impact the patient care; therefore it is necessary to have the absolute integrity of the original chest x-ray photo. On the other hand, there are some others type of health data used by wellness services which do not require absolute integrity.

  ○ Data integrity, as well as data confidentiality, is an important HIPAA requirement as part of the HIPAA Security Rules. HIPAA asks from covered entities to implement procedures to protect health data from improper alteration and destruction.

- **Accountability and non-repudiation.** e-Health services and other entities operating with health data should be legally responsible for their actions. Therefore, these information systems should log user actions. Accountability also implies the property of non-repudiation. Non-repudiation means that a user cannot deny a particular action performed. Accountability and non-repudiation are very important requirements in any healthcare information system that improve patient safety (all actions of healthcare providers are traceable) but also enhance patient's privacy (healthcare providers who may intentionally access patients data which they are not authorized to access, cannot deny their action). HIPAA implicitly asks from cover entities to have information systems to support accountability. According to HIPAA patients have the right to receive an accounting of their data disclosures.

- **Anonymity.** The electronic health records must be anonymized before they are released to the public. For instance, the health data used for a medical research should not reveal the identity of the patient who is a subject of the health data. Data anonymization is the process of removing all personal identification information (PII) of an individual from the data. To truly anonymize data, not only removing identifiable references to the individual is necessary, but also the context and content information should be altered in such a way that it would be impossible for an attacker to indentify an individual.

- **User awareness and control on data use.** Patients have the right to define the access control policies to their personal health records. They also have the right to provide their consent on the use of their records by healthcare providers. Recent trends in the healthcare sector towards personal and user-focused healthcare demand more patient involvement at all levels of healthcare. This is also observed in practice where patients are taking a more active role in managing their health (e.g. obtaining educational information about diseases from the Internet, taking measurements and monitoring symptoms of their illnesses). This also has some backing in legislation such as HIPAA which gives patients more rights with respect to EHRs. Consequently, a patient could request additional restrictions on the disclosure of their records to certain individuals involved in his care that otherwise would be permitted (based on role-based access control governed by the care institution). If the care institution agrees with his request, it is required to comply and enforce the agreement. Furthermore, the privacy policies (e.g. patient consent or organizational policies) can define next to access control also usage and disclosure control, purpose, obligations and other advanced features which call for mechanisms that go beyond traditional access control.

Next sections discuss the state-of-the-art solutions which address the privacy and security requirements discussed above.

DATA AVAILABILITY

There are no healthcare specific mechanisms to ensure availability that differ from traditional solutions such as **redundancy**. Redundancy means to have multiple copies of the same data in multiple independent locations which can be accessed via multiple independent paths. Redundancy is used to prevent DoS attacks against the full system. If one location is unavailable due to a DoS attack, then the access to the information is possible via other independent sub-systems.

Redundancy is important not only for data availability, but also for availability of a system as whole. Traditionally, system availability has been ensured through the use of a technique called fault-tolerance. Fault-tolerant systems use a hardware system configuration to prevent the system to fail. If one component of the system fails, then redundant components are used to ensure the system availability. The main goals of redundant components are to prevent single point of failure in a system and to provide: a) continuous service in case of system maintenance, and b) system recovery in case of unexpected events. Next to that, remote maintenance of medical devices is often used to decrease the out of operation time.

"Clustering" is a technology which allows redundancy at the application level where different servers in the same cluster are configured to provide backups during system failures. RAID (Redundant Array of Independent Disks) is a technology which provides redundancy when hardware fails. RAID is a way of storing the same data into multiple hard disks. If one hard disk fails, then the data is accessed through the other available disk.

DATA CONFIDENTIALITY

Access Control

Access-control mechanisms are very important for protecting the confidentiality of electronic health records. They comprise a very large set of technologies, which include mechanisms to authenticate and authorize individuals or systems to access resources. Currently, there are many authentication and authorization mechanisms, ranging from simple username-password combinations to federated role-based access schemes (the next section discusses in more details authentication methods). After a user is authenticated in a system, the access control system enforces access policies or authorization rules associated with the authenticated users. Access policies are defined as relationships between subjects, objects and actions. Subjects are the authenticated users, objects are the documents/files (data) that the users want to access, and actions are the action that the user can perform on the data, e.g. read, write, etc. Note that, based on the access control mechanism (which are explained below), the subject can be the identity of a user, the role of a user, the attributes that a user posseses, etc.

Access control mechanisms can be grouped into three main classes: *discretionary*, *mandatory*, and *role/attribute-based*. In a discretionary access control (DAC) model (Graham, 1972), access is controlled based on user identities and a number of rules, called *authorizations. The authorization rules* explicitly state which subjects can execute which actions on which resources. After a user makes an access request, the access control is enforced based on the identity of the requester and on the authorization rules involving the requester and the requested object and action. In a mandatory access control (MAC) model (Jajodia, 1991), access is controlled based on mandated policies determined by a central authority. These policies are based on *classifications* associated with subjects and objects (*security levels* and a set of *categories*). Finally, in a role-based access control (RBAC) model (Ferraiolo, 1992), access is controlled based on the roles that users are assigned to within the system and on rules defining which roles can execute which actions on which resources. Role-based access control (or its gen-

eralization called attribute-based access control) has become the predominant model for advanced access control in healthcare. It is often the best choice for healthcare systems as it has a number of particular advantages compared to the previously described classes of access control. First of all, access permissions are naturally assigned to roles in healthcare (e.g. the doctor who treats the patient has access to his information whoever it is, John Smith or Arjen de Vries). Furthermore, the RBAC model reduces the complexity and cost of security administration in large networked applications. The process of defining roles should be based on a thorough analysis of how an organization operates and should include input from a wide spectrum of users in the organization. For example, within a hospital system, the role of GP can include operations to perform diagnosis, prescribe medication, and order laboratory tests. In contrast, the role of researcher can be limited to gathering anonymous clinical information for studies. ISO TS 21298 (ISO 21298, 2007) defines a model that distinguishes between structural and functional roles and populates it with a basic set of roles for international use in healthcare applications. This standard builds upon ISO/IS 22600 - Privilege Management and Access Control (ISO 22600, 2007) which defines privilege management and access control services required for communication and use of distributed health information over different security domains (typically across hospitals/care organizations). Most healthcare information systems implement the role-based access control model, sometimes together with discretionary and group-based access control such as in the Canadian InfoWay (Ratajczak, 2005).

Attribute-Based Access Control (ABAC) is another technique, similar to RBAC, to manage access to system resources. Compared to Role-Based Access Control (RBAC) where the permissions are defined directly between user roles and objects, in ABAC, permissions are defined between user or environmental attributes (e.g. department, role, location, etc.) and objects. The access decisions are

Figure 3. Access control mechanism

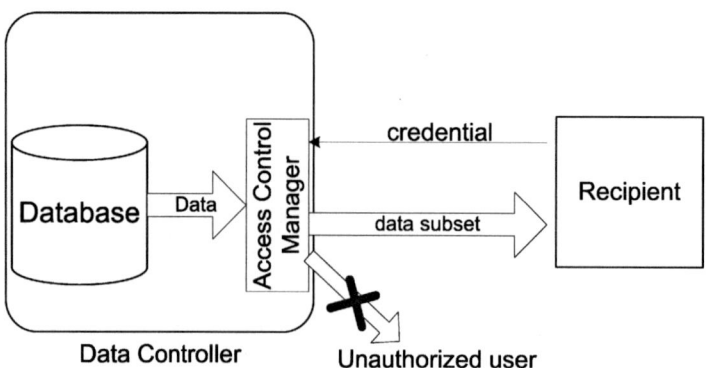

based on the attributes that individual users have. The attempts to provide a uniform framework for attribute-based access control and enforcement include the works of Bonati and Samarati (Bonati, 2002) and Yu et al. (Yu, 2000). The most notable authorization framework which supports ABAC is OASIS eXtensible Access Control Markup Language (XACML) (XACML, 2007). Recently OASIS has developed Cross Enterprise Security and Privacy Authorization (XSPA) profile of XACML that standardizes the way healthcare providers, pharmacies, and insurance companies exchange privacy policies, consent directives and authorizations. These models and standards have high potential to be used in the personal health domain too.

In dynamic environments such as healthcare, the access right may depend not only on the role's entity, but also on the contextual attributes such as the place from where the request comes and the time when the request is made. Such access control models are known as context-dependent RBAC.

Another variation of access control is the so-called "purpose-based access control" (Byun, 2005). In this model, the data is associated with the "intended purpose" which specifies the purpose (e.g. medical treatment, billing, etc.) for which the data can be used. When a user requests to access the data, the user specifies the "access purpose" for which the data in needed. The access is granted if the "access purpose" is same as the

"intended purpose". The purpose attribute is also added to XACML in the XACML privacy profile (XACML, 2007).

In any access-control mechanism the receiving end of the information must authenticate (e.g. by providing a set of credentials). The access-control manager (ACM), responsible to enforce access control policies, checks whether user credentials satisfy the access control policy assigned to protect the resource. If the user credentials satisfy the access policy then the user can access the data, otherwise not. This is shown in Figure 3. On the basis of this credential, a selection of the data may become accessible.

Note that no control is applied on how the data is used by the recipient. The recipient can use the data in any way as soon as he has access to it. Limitations on the use of the data can still be specified in the contract, but access control mechanisms cannot monitor or control its use. For this, some additional measures are necessary such as auditing or digital/information management.

Break-the-Glass

Advanced hospital information systems support emergency access to the data through a "break-the-glass" functionality. They allow healthcare providers to exceed their rights and get access to data which they normally would not be able to access. The "break-the-glass" functionality is implemented together with non-repudiation mechanisms. A care provider that accesses data through this mechanism is warned that he is accessing data beyond his normal rights and that this access will be subject to auditing. An audit-log is created and a notification that the user exceeded his rights is sent to a responsible officer or his superior. Examples of such systems are described in (Lovis, 2006) and (Ferreira, 2006). A mechanism that provides this functionality for more advanced systems which encrypt the data is presented in (Künzi, 2009).

Authentication

The access-control mechanism must authenticate or verify the identity of the user who wants to access the data. In most current PHR systems (including Microsoft Health Vault and Google Health) a user is authenticated using a username (i.e. an email address) and a password. Even though the username-password approach is widely used, for more sensitive applications it is recommended to use multiple-factor authentication where two or three different types of information are used to verify the identity. This provides stronger security than one-factor authentication methods. For example, using a username/password in combination with a token device, is more secure than just using a username/password because it will be harder for an attacker to simultaneously crack the password and steal the token. The username-password is one type of information that can be used for authentication. This type is known as *something the user knows*. The security token is another type of information that can be used for authentication which is known as *something the user has*. A typical example is a smart card which is often used in healthcare to authenticate doctors and/or patients. A good examle is a German healthcard (Marschollek, 2006). The third type of information which can be used for authentication is known as *something the user is*. Such kind of

information are the biometric identifications such as fingerprint, retinal pattern, voice recognition, etc. This authentication method is becoming more popular in healthcare (Marohn, 2006) as it allows seamless and fast authentication (no lost badges, or forgotten passwords). See (SharpHealthcare, 2009) for an example of a healthcare delivery system in San Diego that utilizes biometrcis.

An important issue related to authentication is a single sign-on property which allows a user to log in once and then gain access to different systems without being required to log in at each of them. The main concern that raises here is that the identity of a user being authenticated should be the same in each healthcare system. Identity federation allows the same identity to be portable on different autonomous institutions (e.g. hospitals). This is important for the following reasons: different healthcare providers can easily identify and exchange their opinions about a patient treatment, and a patient/doctor can use the same type of information to be authenticated by different hospitals. The identity federation is not applicable only to users.

Authentication protocols are used to authenticate users across a network. The well-known client-server authentication protocol is Kerberos (Kohl, 1993), invented at the Massachusetts Institute of Technology (MIT). Kerberos protocol allows both the client and the server to authenticate each other. To make a protocol run, each entity on the network (both the client and the server) has to be registered with a username and password in a database maintained by the Key Distribution Server (KDC). The KDC is maintained by a trusted security administrator and consists of two components the Ticket Granting Server (TGS) and the Authentication Server (AS).

Similar functionality can be achieved using the Security Assertion Markup Language (SAML) standard (SAML, 2005). SAML defines a common XML framework for exchanging security assertions between entities. An assertion is a declaration of facts about subjects according to the assertion issuer. SAML assertions include authentication, attribute and authorization decision statements. For example, a user is authenticated by an authentication authority that generates a SAML assertion token (containing the user information). The token is passed to a desired service that looks for the SAML token, reads assertion data and makes a decision as to whether access is allowed or not. Recently OASIS (XSPA, 2008) has developed Cross Enterprise Security and Privacy Authorization (XSPA) profile of SAML 2.0 which is healthcare specific. It allows cross-enterprise authorization of entities operating within a healthcare workflow by providing common semantics and vocabulary for interoperable access control.

The Enterprise User Authentication (EUA) profile (EUA, 2005) of Integrated Healthcare Enterprise (IHE) defines a means for single sign-on authentication in the healthcare environment. This profile assumes a single enterprise which is governed by a single security policy. This profile builds upon Kerberos and HL7 CCOW (Clinical Context Object Workgroup). The same authentication issue but across different healthcare institutions is addressed by the IHE Cross-Enterprise User Authentication (XUA) profile (XUA, 2005), which is based on SAML 2.0.

Encryption Mechanisms

When medical data is sent from one to another entity the communication channel has to be protected. It should be impossible for an attacker to sniff the communication channel and learn the health data. Encrypting the data is a straightforward method to securely transfer information in the presence of an adversary. Encryption is a process of converting information (known as plaintext) into an unreadable text (known as ciphertext). To convert the information the encryptor needs an encryption key. Decryption is a reverse process of encryption. It converts the ciphertext into plaintext. Only users who have a decryption key can convert the ciphertext into plaintext.

Symmetric key cryptography is a method which uses the same key for encryption and decryption. The sender of the information runs the encryption algorithm, and the recipient runs the decryption algorithm. The encryption algorithm takes as input a secret key and a message to be encrypted, and outputs a ciphertext. The decryption algorithm takes as input the ciphertext to be decrypted and the secret key, and outputs the plaintext. The drawback of the symmetric key cryptography is that the sender and the receiver have to meet and agree on a secret keys before the secure communication takes place. Nowadays, the most common used symmetric key algorithm is AES (Daemen, 2002).

Asymmetric key cryptography (known as public key cryptography) is a method which uses a key pair (the private key and the public key) for encryption and decryption. Everyone can encrypt a message using a public key but only users who have the associated secret (private) key, can decrypt the encrypted message. This method does not require the sender and receiver to meet and exhange a secret key. However, it requires the use of digital certificates to certify that the public key used in a public key encryption belongs to an user. Public Key Infrastructure (PKI) is a system for distribution and revocation of digital certificates. The digital certificate is created by the trusted third party known as Certificate Authority (CA). ISO 17909 defines the essential elements of a healthcare public key infrastructure that supports the secure transmission of healthcare information. Nowadays, the most commonly used public key algorithm is RSA (Rivest, 1978).

In practice, symmetric key cryptography is faster than public key cryptography. Therefore, the public key cryptography is used to exhchange a symmetric key, which is then used to encrypt and decrypt messages. Transport Layer Security (TLS) is a cryptographic protocol which uses both symmetric key cryptography and public key cryptography. The main application of TLS is to secure communications over insecure channels (such as the Internet). In practice, websites which use TLS protocol have a URL which begins with "https://". TLS consists of two layers: the TLS Record Protocol and the TLS Handshake Protocol. The TLS Record Protocol, to secure the client-server connection, uses symmetric encryption algorithms such AES, IDEA, DES, etc., and uses hash-based message authentication code to preserve the integrity of a message, e.g., HMAC-MD5 or HMAC-SHA. The TLS Handshake Protocol, to allow the server and client to authenticate each other and to negotiate protocol parameters, use public key cryptography such RSA, DSA, etc.

New Approaches to Data Confidentiality in e-Health Applications

In Figure 3, the ACM is responsible to verify whether the data requester has the appropriate credentials to access the data. Therefore, patients who store their health data on the PHR servers of Microsoft HealthVault or Google Health have to trust Microsoft or Google not to misuse their data, to keep their data confidential and to properly enforce their privacy preferences (access control policies). Even if the PHR service is trustworthy with respect to the use and sharing of patients health data the servers that store the PHR data can be compromised and therefore the patient health data can be revealed.

To address this problem, recent proposals on enforcing access control policies suggest removing the need for an ACM and exploiting the use of cryptography to enforce access control policies. In such systems, the data is stored in encrypted form at the server and the server does not hold the decryption key. Only authorized users who have decryption keys can access the data. Therefore, if an attacker succeeds to compromise the server, he cannot reveal patients' private data. If cryptography is used to enforce the policy, then the encrypted data can be made publicly available and there is no need for the ACM to check whether the user who gets the data has enough credentials to satisfy the policy.

Ciphertext-Policy Attribute-Based Encryption (CP-ABE)

The most notable cryptographic technique that is used to enforce access control is called ciphertext-policy attribute-based encryption (CP-ABE). CP-ABE allows encrypting the data using a policy which can be defined as a logical expression of attributes. Instead of encrypting the data with someone's public key the data is encrypted based on an access control policy, which establishes a strong link between the encryption and the policy. The encryption algorithm of CP-ABE takes as an input i) the master public key, ii) an access control policy defined over the set of attributes and iii) the data to be encrypted, and based on this the algorithm encrypts the data. Only the users, who have a secret key with enough attributes to satisfy the access control policy, can decrypt the encrypted data. The attributes of the secret key are mathematically incorporated into the key itself. In CP-ABE users do not have individual public keys, but there is a master public key generated by a trusted authority which is used for each encryption.

In general, a CP-ABE scheme is based on bi-linear mappings and secret sharing and it consists of the following four algorithms (Bethencourt, 2007; Ibraimi, 2009):

- Setup algorithm (**MK, PK**) ← **Setup (1^k):** is run by the trusted authority (TA) or the security administrator. The algorithm outputs a master secret key MK and a master public key PK. MK is used by the TA to generate user secret keys and PK is used by all users to encrypt the data.
- Encryption algorithm (**CT**) ← **Encrypt (m, PK, P):** is run by the encryptor. The input of the algorithm consist of a message *m*, the PK and an access control policy P defined over the set of attributes, and out-

puts a ciphertext CT encrypted under the access control policy P.

- Key Generation algorithm **(SK) ← Key Gen (MK, ω)**: is run by the TA. The algorithm takes as input a set of attributes ω for which a user wants to have a secret key and the MK. The algorithm outputs a user secret key SK associated with the attribute set ω.

- Decryption algorithm **(m) ← Decrypt (CT, SK)**: is run by the decryptor. The input of the algorithm is a ciphertext CT to be decrypted and a user secret key SK. The output of the algorithm is a message *m* if the attributes of the secret key satisfy the access policy P under which the message was encrypted, or an error symbol $\perp$ otherwise.

In the context of healthcare, each healthcare provider can employ its own TA to generate the master public key PK and assign attributes to their staff and patients. For example, in Figure 4, the TA from Healthcare Provider 1 runs the Setup algorithm and distributes the PK to the patient. It is assumed that there is a secure channel between the TA and patient. Next (2), the patient encrypts the data according to the policy "A AND B". Everyone, including the doctor (3) can download the encrypted data. However, only users who have a secret key associated with attributes which satisfy the policy "A AND B" can decrypt the encrypted data. For this reason, the doctor makes a secret key request (4) associated with attributes [A,B]. The TA of Healthcare Provider 1 authenticates the doctor and verifies whether the doctor has credentials which show that the doctor indeed has attributes [A,B]. After the verification is finished, the TA sends the secret key (5) associated with attributes [A,B] to the doctor. Using the secret key, the doctor can decrypt the encrypted data locally.

The major drawback of CP-ABE is its slow speed of operation. For this reason, it is recommended to encrypt the data using symmetric key cryptography (e.g. AES) and then use the CP-ABE to encrypt and distribute the symmetric keys.

Multi-authority CP-ABE. It is important to allow users from one healthcare provider to share electronic health data with the users from a different healthcare provider, based on attributes generated by multiple authorities. For example, a patient can encrypt her data such that it can be accessed by some individuals from a professional domain 1, as well as some other individuals from the professional domain 2. In the literature, schemes which allow attributes to be generated by different TAs are known as multi-authority attribute-based encryption (Ibraimi, 2009).

Attribute and User Revocation. Attribute and user revocation is an important requirement in the domain of electronic health data. An attribute may be valid until a specific date and after the expired date the attribute becomes invalid and has to be revoked. This means that all users who hold an expired attribute cannot use it in the future to decrypt the encrypted data. Users can be revoked as well. A user might be revoked if the user is misusing her secret key by giving a copy to illegitimate users. When one user is revoked then the other non-revoked users are not affected. We illustrate the attribute and user revocation with the following example. Suppose there is a system with two users: Alice who has a secret key SK_{Alice} associated with attributes [A,B,C], and Bob who has a secret key SK_{Bob} associated with attributes [A,B,F]. In case of attribute revocation, if the attribute A is revoked then both Alice and Bob are affected. After the revocation, Alice will have a secret key SK_{Alice} associated with attributes [B,C], and Bob will have a secret key SK_{Bob} associated with attributes [B,F]. In case of user revocation, if Bob is revoked then Bob cannot use any attribute from the set [A,B,F], while Alice is not effected and can use all attributes [A,B,C] of her secret key SK_{Alice}.

In CP-ABE, attribute and user revocation can be achieved by using an online semi-trusted mediator (Ibraimi, 2009). In this model, the secret

Figure 4. Ciphertext-Policy Attribute-Based Encryption

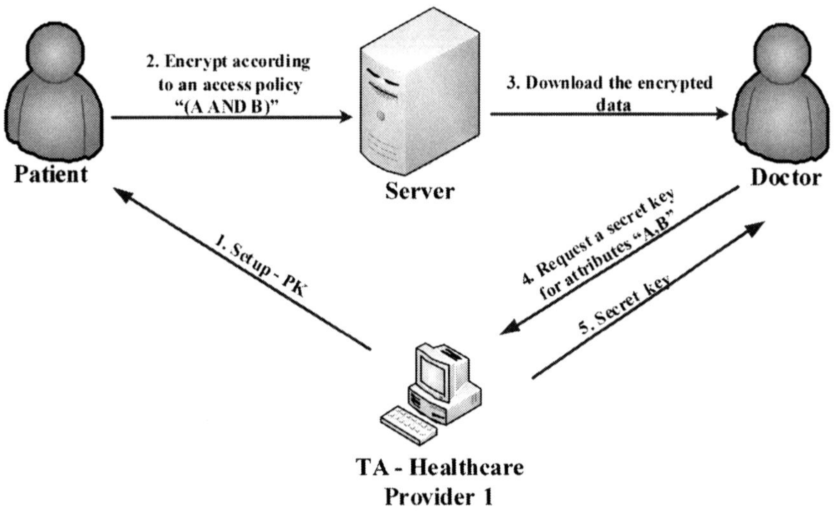

key is divided into two shares, one share for the mediator and the other for the user. The trusted authority or the security administrator generate an attribute-user revocation list and send it to the mediator. To decrypt the data, the user must contact the mediator to receive a decryption token. On each request, the mediator checks whether the requester is in the attribute-user revocation list and refuses to issue the decryption token for revoked users or attributes. Without the token, the user cannot decrypt the ciphertext, therefore the attribute is implicitly revoked.

DATA INTEGRITY

Digital Signature is a powerful cryptographic primitive which can be used to preserve the data integrity. Digital signatures use a key pair - the private key and the public key. The signature algorithm takes as input the signer's private key and a message to be signed. The verification algorithm takes as input the signature, the message, and the public key. To check if the signature is valid, the verifier encrypts the signature with the public key and check if the result is equal to the message.

When the signer uses his private key to sign a message, usually the signer applies a hash function to the message, and then uses his private key to encrypt the hashed value. Actually, the signer signs the hash of the message instead the message itself. The property of the hash functions is that it is one-way function for which it is infeasible to find two messages which have the same output. This implies that if the message is altered, then the verifier during the signature check will get a different hash result than the signed hash value. Therefore, the verfier can detect if the message has been altered. A good example of a healhcare implementation is the digital signature service of the Canadian InfoWay system (Ratajczak, 2005).

The XML Signature (Simon, 2001) specification provides a very flexible digital signature mechanism for XML documents or everything that can be referenced from a URL. XML signatures apply either to a part or to a complete XML document. This is very relevant in the healthcare domain when a single XML document may have a long history, in which different components are authored at different times by different parties. XML signatures provide the basis for the IHE Document Digital Signature (IHE, 2005) profile that applies signatures to medical documents exchanged between healthcare organizations.

In addition to digital signatures, a keyed hash function, known as *Message Authentication Code* (MAC) is used to protect both data integrity and data authenticity. MAC, unlike digital signatures, requires a single secret key to generate and verify a MAC value. To generate the MAC value, a MAC generation algorithm takes as input a message to be authenticated and the secret key. The MAC value and the message are then sent to the MAC verifier. The MAC verifier runs the MAC verification algorithm which takes as input the message to be authenticated and the secret key and outputs the MAC value. Next, the MAC verification algorithm checks if the outputted MAC value is the same as the MAC value created by the MAC generation algorithm. If MAC values are the same, then both message authenticity and integrity are not compromised.

ACCOUNTABILITY AND NON-REPUDIATION

It is very hard to control how the data is used by the recipient. The recipient can use the data in any way as soon as he has access to it. For example, the owner may want that the recipient should not store the data, but should request the data from the owner before each use. While this is a good way to limit the risks, the access control mechanisms have no means to allow the data owner to prevent or monitor the storage of the data at the recipient side. For this, some additional measures are necessary: *auditing* that allows for monitoring the use of data or *usage control* that enforces certain use of data (see for usage control the section on user awareness and control on data use).

Accountability is often addressed by contracts that allow the owner of the data to inspect or audit the recipient. In other cases, the recipient can be audited by the government or other third parties (for example when required by law). In any case, the party to be trusted (trustee) needs to be accountable for its actions. If the trustee is never inspected, the 'trust-giver' can never know if the trustee is really trustworthy.

In practice, information systems are equipped with monitoring techniques that create logs describing who used which data when and where. This monitoring allows for audits to take place. By inspecting the logs, misuse may be detected after or even during the event. Furthermore, the logs allow the owner of the data to trace who had access to information, which might be valuable when data has been compromised. Figure 5 shows a simplified model of an audit mechanism, where the owner verifies the audit logs of the data recipient. In practice, much more complex audit systems can be applied, where the audit can be performed by a (trusted) third party. In any case the recipient of the data must install monitoring mechanisms that securely collect information to allow for audits to take place. These monitoring systems typically require (amongst others):

- user identification,
- extensive management of user authorizations to control access to data or functions,
- integration with information databases and other resources to monitor data access patterns,
- security measures to prevent tampering with the audit trails.

The recipient also has to install organizational structures to reduce the risk of tampering with the audit mechanisms. For example, ordinary users should not have access to the audit databases, including physical access to the servers where those databases are hosted.

The main application of audit logs is to support non-repudiation. Using non-repudiation one can prove or disprove that a specific user has performed a specific action. For instance, if there is a system which supports non-repudiation, then a doctor who intentionally has emailed patients

Figure 5. Audit mechanisms

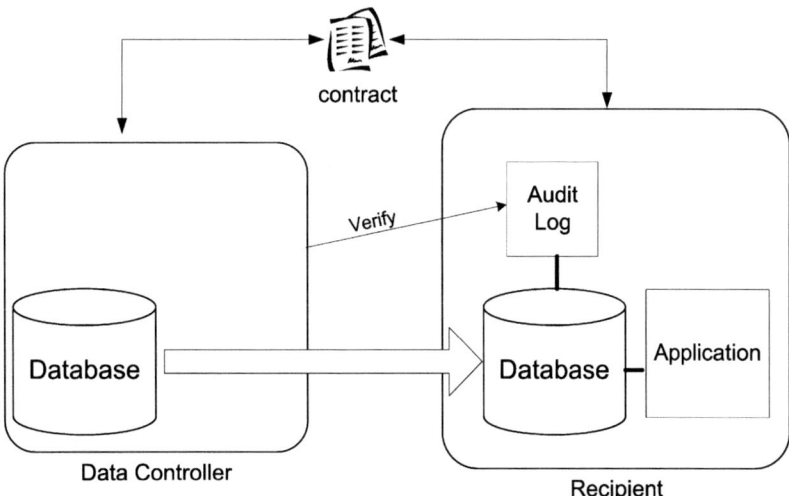

data to unauthorized users cannot deny his actions since all actions taken by the doctor are recorded by the audit log mechanism. Digital signatures can also be used to support non-repudiation. Only the holder of the secret (private) key can sign a message, therefore the signer cannot successfully prove that he did not sign a message (the secret key is known only to the signer).

Auditing is very important for healthcare, where different legislations, such as HIPAA in the US require that organizations implement mechanisms that record and examine activity in information systems that contain or use protected health information, as well as mechanisms to regularly review records of information system activity, such as audit logs, access reports, and security incident tracking reports. To address these requirements several standards have been developed including IHE Audit Trial and Node Authentication (IHE, 2005) and ASTM E2147 Specification for Audit and Disclosure Logs for Use in Health Information Systems (ASTM, 2009).

Anonymity

Health data is very valuable for medical research. In practice there are a lot of situations when medical researchers need patients' health data to perform investigations that lead to the invention of new medicines and/or healthcare procedures. However, as mentioned above, the health data is very sensitive and should not reveal the identity of the subject. Removing from the database only patient's name, social security number (SSID) and the telephone number will not completely anonymize the data. Other attributes known as quasi-identifiers, such as date of birth (DOB), gender and zip code can be used to de-anonymize the data (identify the subject of the health data). For example, a database with attributes [DOB, gender, zip code] containing medical records of the governor of Massachusetts was completely de-anonymized by joining attributes [DOB, gender, zip code] with attributes [name, gender, zip code, DOB] of the database containing Massachusetts voters (Sweeney, 2002). To address this problem, several concepts and techniques are proposed such as k-anonymity, *l*-diversity, indistinguishability, etc. In the sequel, we explain k-anonymity and l-diversity as the most general techniques which are the easiest to understand.

k-anonymity is a technique proposed by Samarati and Sweeney (Samarati, 1998) to prevent attacks using quasi-identifiers. To obtain k-anonymity for a private table, firstly, the data controller (in the context of healthcare in most cases the data controller is the healthcare provider) has to categorize all attributes into three categories: key attributes, quasi identifiers attributes and sensitive attributes. Key attributes are removed before the table is published. Such attributes might be explicit identifier such as [name, SSID]. If the attribute is in the private database and the same attribute is in other public databases, then the attribute is qualified as a quasi identifier. Quasi identifiers might be [gender, zip code, DOB]. Sensitive attributes are the values that the researchers need, and actually these are the values that might harm an individual if someone discovers the subject of the health data.

A table satisfies k-anonimity if each sequence of values in quasi identifiers of the table appears at least k times. This implies that there are at least k records which share the same values of the quasi identifier.

k-anonymity can be achieved using two techniques: generalization and suppression. To generalize a value means to replace part of the value with a less specific value. For example the last digit of the ZIP code is replaced with *. The ZIP code 213* is more general and covers all geographic area that at the last digit start with 0 and end with 9. See for an example of generalization the anonymization service of the InfoWay system (Ratajczak, 2005). Suppression means not to release the value at all. Generalization and suppression are applied as long as each row is identical with at least k-1 other rows.

A similar concept to k-anonymity is *l*-diversity. Machanavajjhala et al. (Machanavajjhala, 2007) pointed out that k-anonymity also suffers from the homogeneity attack. Homogeneity attack happens when k-tuples share same values of their quasi identifiers as well as same value of their sensitive attributes (e.g. if all male patients with ZIP code 213* and age between 30 and 35 have as sensitivity attribute that they are positive on

AIDS – the attacker gains important information about the specific male patient who lives in 2136 and is 32 years old). To prevent this attack, the data owner in addition to k-anonymity, should use diverse values for their sensitive attributes. k-tuples sharing the same values of their quasi identifiers are *l*-diverse if they contain at least *l* values for their sensitive attributes.

Privacy Preserving Data Mining

The k-anonymity and *l*-diversity models are techniques which can provide privacy when the database owner publishes the database in such a way that no one should be able to learn who the subject of the information is. In practice, there are situations where one can run (preselected) data mining algorithms (statistical queries) to extract patterns from data sets and deduce knowledge from those patterns. In the healthcare domain, the mined data sets may contain sensitive health information, the confidentiality of which, as explained above is required by legislations. Privacy-preserving data mining (Agrawal, 2000) is a technique which addresses the problem of protecting the confidentiality of sensitive information in this situation. The main objective of these algorithms is to modify the original data in such a way that the sensitive data remain private while the results of the mining algorithm are correct. The first technique to protect the confidentiality of sensitive information is to randomize the original data before it is minded. Data randomization is achieved by aggregation, swapping or adding enough noise (Evfimievski, 2002). Another technique used with distributed databases is secure multiparty computation (Goldreich, 1987). It allows each party in the protocol holding a private data to compute a function. The protocol ensures that parties do not learn anything else except the output of the function and their private data.

Private Information Retrieval

Let's consider a situation when a patient, who suffers from a specific disease, searches a disease database of a service to obtain information or help. In such situations the patient does not want to reveal his query to the database administrator, since from the query the administrator can deduce some information about patient's health condition. This problem was first introduced by Chor et al. (Chor, 1998) where a database is modeled as n-bit string $x = x_1 x_2 x_3 \ldots x_i \ldots x_n$, and the user wants to retrieve x_i without the database administrator learning x_i. A naive solution is to send the whole database to the patient. However, the drawback of this approach is that the communication cost is n. Chor et al. showed how to design a better protocol and achieve less communication than n in the settings with multiple copies of the database. They showed that if there are two copies of the same database which are modeled as n-bit string $x = x_1 x_2 x_3 \ldots x_i \ldots x_n$, then the user can retrieve x_i with communication cost of $n^{1/3}$.

USER AWARENESS AND CONTROL ON DATA USE

As already mentioned a patient should have control over the disclosure of his data. The system operating electronic health records should have mechanisms to support patient consent. Similarly, personal health record systems should support patients' privacy preferences. There are some data which are considered to be very sensitive by the patient (e.g. mental health record or records related to sexually transmitted diseases) and require explicit patient involvement in order to be disclosed to a third party. The patient has the right to request additional restrictions on the disclosure of their records to certain individuals involved in his care (for example, it may occur that the patient wishes to deny access to a specific physician who would have default rights to access

his data). Patient consent can be expressed in a privacy/consent policy signed by the patient and given to the EHR/PHR system (i.e. ACM) that controls the patient data. Every time healthcare providers request access to the data, next to organizational policies of the healthcare institution and national regulations, the ACM takes into account the patient consent policy when deciding upon the request. As already mentioned, an interoperable way to express privacy and access control policies is by using XACML. A very basic mechanism to capture scanned versions of paper-based consent is provided by the IHE Basic Patient Privacy Consents (BPPC) profile (BPPC, 2006). HL-7 in Composite Privacy Consent Directive provides specifications for system interactions during consent management as well as information model for management of consent directives. The same SDO introduces several use cases that describe the requirements for the creation and use of privacy consent directives to express client preferences in Composite Privacy Consent Directive Domain Analysis Model (CPC-DAM, 2009).

Next to access control, the policies (e.g. patient consent or organizational policies) can also define usage and disclosure control, as well as purpose of the data use and obligations. Therefore, it is an important requirement to enforce that the data is used at the client (data receiver) according to the defined policies. Traditional access control mechanisms cannot fulfill this requirement. The domain of digital content distribution has a similar requirement which is addressed by the Digital Rights Management (DRM) technology. This technology provides digital content protection by enforcing the use of digital content according to granted rights expressed by one of the rights description languages such as eXtensible rights Markup Language (XrML, 2009) or Open Digital Rights Language (ODRL, 2009). DRM controls what consumers can do with digital content once they have it (play, copy, edit, etc.). A very important building block that is used by DRM to provide this functionality is a compliant infrastructure, i.e. compliant clients and trusted modules that make piracy too difficult for most consumers. Commercial DRM systems include Apple FairPlay, Microsoft Media DRM (in each Windows Media Player), Open Mobile Alliance DRM for mobile phones, and Marlin DRM for consumer electronics. Digital Rights Management technology extends to information management in enterprises where it is called Information/Enterprise Rights Management. There, conceptually the same technology solves the regulatory requirements defined by HIPAA or Sarbannes-Oxley laws. For example, the author can specify a set of rules on how a document (or parts of it) may be used by whom and bind this to the document (e.g. a policy can be that a specific user can view the document with a password but not print it). Commercial IRM/ERM systems, which include Microsoft Rights Management System (MS RMS), Adobe LiveCycle Rights Management and Oracle Rights Management Solution, allow protection of PDF, MS Word and other documents.

A general architecture of IRM/ERM system, which also resembles the architecture of Microsoft RMS, is shown in Figure 6. To protect a document using Microsoft RMS, the author (data publisher) has to register and receive a client licensor certificate from the RMS server. Then, as shown on the Figure 6, the author creates a publishing license that contains the rights – access and usage policies. The DRM packager sends that license to the License Server. The DRM packager application then encrypts the file with a symmetric key which is then encrypted using the public key of the author's Windows RMS server. The publishing license is bound to the file which is distributed to the users. To be able to use the protected document the user (denoted as client/recipient on Figure 6) has to request a usage license (this request is sent to the License server). The license server checks the publishing license and creates a personalized usage license which is returned to the user (client). After receiving the usage license the user can exercise the rights which have been granted. The

compliant client enforces these rights. In a similar way, healthcare documents can be protected by applying the digital rights management technology which has been recently proposed in (Petkovic, 2007; Sheppard 2009).

CONCLUSION

Throughout this chapter we were focused on security and privacy issues of e-Health applications. We gave an overview of digital health records such as Electronic Health Records (EHR) and Personal Health Records (PHR) and described their purposes: to serve healthcare providers and to empower the patient. Next we made an overview of the privacy and security requirements of digital health records such as data availability, data confidentiality, data integrity, accountability, anonymity, and user awareness. Finally, we discussed the state-of-the-art technologies and security standards which address these requirements. Given this discussion we can conclude that a number of healthcare requirements are met by traditional security technologies. However, the healthcare domain has certain specific requirements such as the trade-off between data availability and confidentiality (e.g. a specific data access rules in emergency situations), multiple complex policies including patient consent that govern access to health data, and enforcement of these policies. These requirements call for adjustment and extensions of traditional security technologies as well as for novel security mechanism (such as CP-ABE) that ensure compliance with legislation and increase usability and seamless integration of security mechanisms in standard healthcare workflows. Still there are interesting security topics related to e-Health which need to be considered such as: (i) advanced policy management which includes specification and translation of high-level patient's privacy policies into machine readable security policies, (ii) policy enforcement where technologies such as informa-

Figure 6. Architecture of information rights management system

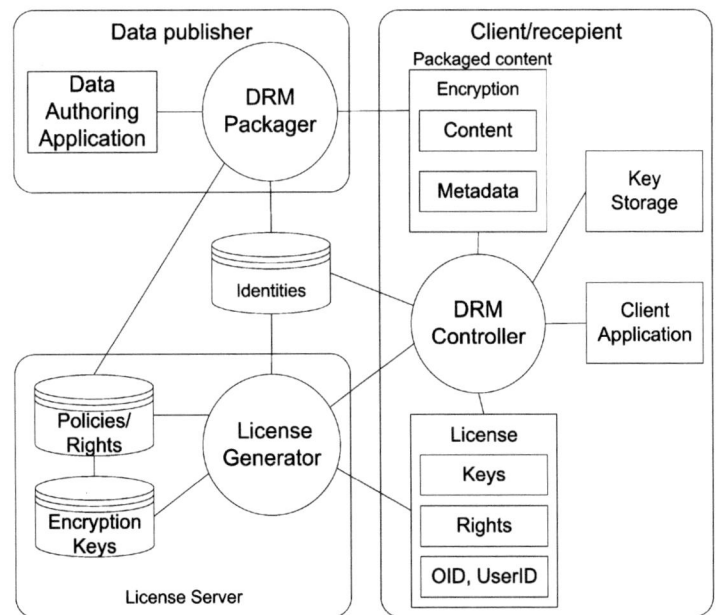

tion rights management might help organizations to enforce privacy and security policies in an end-to-end manner, (iii) practical implementations of advance privacy enhancing technologies such as one presented in (Katzenbeisser, 2008), which can protect consumer privacy when interacting with organizations that are not professional healthcare providers but for example wellness applications, and iv) usable privacy and security mechanisms that allow seamless workflows and are not seen as additional burden by healthcare providers and patients.

REFERENCES

Agrawal, R., & Srikant, R. (2000). Privacy-preserving data mining. [New York: ACM.]. *SIGMOD Record*, 29(2), 439–450. doi:10.1145/335191.335438

ASTM E2147 - 01(2009). *Standard Specification for Audit and Disclosure Logs for Use in Health Information Systems.* Retrieved from http://www.astm.org/Standards/E2147.htm

Benaloh, J., Chase, M., Horvitz, E., & Lauter, K. (2009). *Patient Controlled Encryption: Ensuring Privacy of Electronic Medical Records.* Retrieved December 20, 2009, from: http://research.microsoft.com/en-us/um/people/horvitz/ccsw_2009_benaloh_chase_horvitz_lauter.pdf.

Bethencourt, J., Sahai, A., & Waters, B. (2007). Ciphertext-policy attribute-based encryption. In *Proceedings of the 28th IEEE Symposium on Security and Privacy (Oakland)* (pp. 321-334).

Bonatti, P., & Samarati, P. (2002). A unified framework for regulating access and information release on the web. [Amsterdam: IOS Press.]. *Journal of Computer Security*, 10(3), 241–271.

Boneh, D., & Franklin, M. K. (2001) Identity-based encryption from the weil pairing. In *J. Kilian, editor, Advances in Cryptology - CRYPTO 2001, 21st Annual International Cryptology Conference* (pp 213–229), vol. 2139 of LNCS.New York: Springer.

BPPC (2006). *IHE, Patient Care Coordination Technical Framework, Supplement 2005-2006, Basic Patient Privacy Consents (BPPC)*, Trial Implementation Version, Draft

Byun, J. W., Bertino, E., & Li, N. (2005). Purpose based access control of complex data for privacy protection. *In Proceedings of the tenth ACM symposium on Access control models and technologies* (pp. 102-110). New York: ACM.

Chor, B. Z., & Goldreich, O. Kushilevitz, E. (1998). Private Information Retrieval. *Journal of the ACM, 45* (6), 965-982. Retrieved December 20, 2009, from: http://citeseerx.ist.psu.edu/viewdoc/download?doi=10.1.1.126.9441&rep=rep1&type=pdf.

Continua. (2007). Retrieved from http://www.continuaalliance.org/home.

CPC-DAM. (2009). *HL-7 Composite Privacy Consent Directive Topic.* Retrieved from http://www.hl7.org/v3ballot/html/domains/uvmr/uvmr_CompositePrivacyConsentDirective.htm#RCMR_DO000010UV-Privacyconsent-ic.

Daemen, J., & Rijmen, V. (2002). *The design of Rijndael: AES-the Advanced Encryption Standard.* New York: Springer Verlang.

EUA (2005). *IHE, "IT Infrastructure Technical Framework Volume 1 (ITI TF-1) Integration Profiles; Revision 2.0 - Final Text.* August 15, 2005

Evfimievski, A., Srikant, R., Agrawal, R., & Gehrke, J. (2002). *Privacy preserving mining of association rules,* In Proceedings of the 8th ACM SIGKDDD International Conference on Knowledge Discovery and Data Mining.

Ferraiolo, D. F., & Kuhn, D. R. (1992). Role Based Access Control. In *Proceedings of the NIST–NSA National (USA) Computer Security Conference* (pp. 554–563).

Ferreira, A., et al. (2006). How to break access control in a controlled manner. *19th IEEE International Symposium on Computer-Based Medical Systems (CBMS 2006)*, IEEE Press, 2006, pp. 847–854.

Gentry, C., & Silverberg, A. (2002). Hierarchical ID-based cryptography. In *Asiacrypt 2002* (LNCS, vol. 2501, pp. 149-155). Berlin: Springer Berlin / Heidelberg.

Goldreich, O., Micali, S., & Wigderson, A. (1987). How to play ANY mental game. In *Proceedings of the nineteenth annual ACM conference on Theory of computing* (pp. 218-229), New York: ACM Press.

Graham, G. S., & Denning, P. J. (1972). *Protection: principles and practice.* In Proceedings of AFIPS (pp. 417-429). Montvale, NJ, USA.

HIMSS. (2003). *EHR Definition, Attributes and Essential Requirements.* Retrieved from: http://www.himss.org/content/files/EHRAttributes.pdf.

HL-7. (2007). Retrieved from http://www.hl7.org.

Ibraimi, L., Asim, M., & Petkovic, M. (2009). *Secure Management of Personal Health Records by Applying Attribute-Based Encryption.* Centre for Telematics and Information Technology, University of Twente.

Ibraimi, L., Petkovic, M., Nikova, S., Hartel, P., & Jonker, W. (2009). Mediated Ciphertext-Policy Attribute-Based Encryption and Its Application. In *Information Security Applications: 10th International Workshop-WISA* (pp. 309-323), Springer-Verlag.

Ibraimi, L., Tang, Q., & Hartel, P. Jonker. W. (2009). Efficient and provable secure ciphertext-policy attribute-based encryption schemes. In *Proceedings of Information Security Practice and Experience* (pp. 1-12), vol. 5451 of *LNCS,* Springer.

IHE. (2005). *IHE IT Infrastructure, Technical Framework, Volume 3 – Document Content Profiles.* Retrieved December 20, 2009, from: http://www.ihe.net/Technical_Framework/upload/IHE_ITI_TF-Supplement_Digital_Signature-TI_2005-08-15.pdf.

InfoWay. (2007). Retrieved from http://www.infoway-inforoute.ca.

ISO 21298 (2007). *ISO/TC 215/WG 4, ISO TS 21298 Health Informatics - Functional and structural roles.*

ISO 22600 (2007). *ISO/TC 215/WG 4, ISO/IS 22600 Privilege management and access control.*

Jajodia, S., & Sandhu, R. (1991). Toward a multilevel secure relational data model. *In Proceedings of the ACM SIGMOD Conference on Management of Data* (pp. 50-59). Denver, CO, USA.

Katzenbeisser, S., & Petkovic, M. (2008). *Privacy-preserving recommendation systems for consumer healthcare services ARES 2008* (pp. 889–895). Washington, DC: IEEE Computer Society Press.

Kohl, J., & Neuman, C. (1993). *RFC 1510: The Kerberos network authentication service (v5).* Citeseer.

Künzi, J., Koster, P., & Petkovic, M. (2009). Emergency Access to Protected Health Records. In Adlassnig, K.-P. (Eds.), *Medical Informatics in a United and Healthy Europe, MIE 2009* (pp. 705–709). IOS Press.

Lovis, C. (2006). Comprehensive management of the access to the electronic patient record: Towards trans-institutional networks. *International Journal of Medical Informatics, 176*(5-6), 466–470.

Machanavajjhala, A., Kifer, D., Gehrke, J., & Venkitasubramaniam, M. (2007). l-diversity: Privacy beyond k-anonymity. In *ACM Transactions on Knowledge Discovery from Data (TKDD), 1,* (3), New York: ACM.

Markle. (2003). *The personal health working group. Markle foundation. Connecting for health: a public-private collaborative, final report.* Retrieved December 20, 2009, from: http://www.connectingforhealth.org/resources/wg_eis_final_report_0704.pdf.

Marohn, D. (2006) Biometrics in Healthcare. *Biometric Technology Today, 14*(9), 9-11. New York: Elsevier.

Marschollek, M., & Demirbilek, E. (2006). Providing longitudinal health care information with the new German Health Card—a pilot system to track patient pathways. [New York: Elsevier]. *Journal of Computer Methods and Programs in Biomedicine, 81,* 266–271. doi:10.1016/j.cmpb.2006.01.001

Marshall. P. (2007). *Personal Health Records - An Overview.* Retrieved December 20, 2009, from: http://www.ncvhs.hhs.gov/050106p1.pdf.

MyHeart. (2003). Retrieved from http://www.hitech-projects.com/euprojects/myheart/.

NICTIZ. (2007). Retrieved from http://www.nictiz.nl.

ODRL. (2009), *Open Digital Rights Language.* Retrieved from http://odrl.net/

Petković, M., Katzenbeisser, S., & Kursawe, K. (2007). *Rights Management Technologies: A Good Choice for Securing Electronic Health Records?* International Conference on Information Security Solutions Europe (ISSE), Warsaw, Poland

Ratajczak, S. (2005). *Electronic Health Record Infostructure (EHRi) Privacy and Security Conceptual Architecture, v1.1* (p. 171). Canada Health Infoway Inc.

Rivest, R. L., Shamir, A., & Adleman, L. (1978). A method for obtaining digital signatures and public-key cryptosystems. [ACM]. *Communications of the ACM, 21*(2), 120–126. doi:10.1145/359340.359342

Samarati, P., & Sweeney, L. (1998). Protecting privacy when disclosing information: k-anonymity and its enforcement through generalization and suppression. *In Proceedings of the IEEE Symposium on Research in Security and Privacy* (pp. 384-393), Citeseer.

SAML. (2005). *Security Assertion Markup Language. Version 2.0.* OASIS Security Service TC. Retrieved from http://www.oasis-open.org/specs/index.php#saml2.0.

SharpHealthcare. (2009). *Enabling strong authentication with biometrics.* Retrieved from http://www.sourcesecurity.com/markets/healthcare/application/co-854-ga.64.html

Sheppard, N. P., Safavi-Naini, R., & Jafari, M. (2009). A Digital Rights Management Model for Healthcare. *Policies for Distributed Systems and Networks, IEEE International Workshop on*, pp. 106-109, 2009 IEEE International Symposium on Policies for Distributed Systems and Networks

Simon, E., & Madsen, P. Adams, C., (2001). *An Introduction to XML Digital Signatures.* Retrieved from http://www.xml.com/pub/a/2001/08/08/xmldsig.html.

Simons, D., Egami, T., & Perry, J. (2006). Remote Patient Monitoring Solutions. In Spekowius, G., & Wendler, T. (Eds.), *Advances in Health care Technology* (pp. 505–516). The Netherlands: Springer. doi:10.1007/1-4020-4384-8_30

Spine (2009). *NHS Connecting for Health.* Retrieved from http://www.connectingforhealth.nhs.uk/systemsandservices/spine

Sweeney, L. (2002). k-anonymity: A model for protecting privacy. *International Journal of Uncertainty Fuzziness and Knowledge Based Systems*, *10*(5), 557–570. doi:10.1142/S0218488502001648

Van Deursen, T., Koster, P., & Petkovic, M. (2008). Hedaquin: A reputation-based health data quality indicator. In *Electronic Notes in Theoretical Computer Science* (pp. 159-167). Elsevier.

WeightWatchers. (2007). Retrieved from http://www.weightwatchers.com.

XACML. (2007). *OASIS eXtensible Access Control Markup Language (XACML) TC.* http://www.oasis-open.org/committees/download.php/2406/oasis-xacml-1.0.pdf.

XrML. (2009). *Extensible Rights Markup Language.* Retrieved from http://www.xrml.org/

XSPA. (2008). *OASIS Cross-Enterprise Security and Privacy Authorization (XSPA) TC.* http://www.oasis-open.org/committees/tc_home.php?wg_abbrev=xspa.

XUA. (2005). *IHE, Cross-Enterprise User Authentication (XUA) Integration Profile; Rev 1.1.* Public Comment II Version.

Yu, T., Winslett, M., & Seamons, K. E. (2000). Prunes: An Efficient and complete strategy for automated trust negotiation over internet. *In Proceedings of the 7th ACM Conference on Computer and Communications Security* (pp. 210-219). New York: ACM.

ADDITIONAL READING

Agrawal, R., Grandison, T., Johnson, C., & Kiernan, J. (2007). Enabling the 21st century health care information technology revolution. [New York: ACM Press]. *Communications of the ACM*, *50*(2), 34–42. doi:10.1145/1216016.1216018

Agrawal, R., Kiernan, J., Srikant, R., & Xu, Y. (2002). Hippocratic Databases. In *Proceedings of Very Large Databases*, pp. 143-154.

Agrawal, R., & Srikant, R. (2000). Privacy-preserving data mining. [New York: ACM.]. *SIGMOD Record, 29*(2), 439–450. doi:10.1145/335191.335438

Anderson, G. J. (2007). Social, ethical and legal barriers to E-health. [New York: Elsevier.]. *International Journal of Medical Informatics, 76*(5), 480–483. doi:10.1016/j.ijmedinf.2006.09.016

Anderson, R. J. (1996). A security policy model for clinical information systems. In *Proceedings of the 1996 IEEE Symposium on Security and Privacy*, pp. 30. Washington, DC: IEEE Computer Society Press.

Becker, M. (2005). *Cassandra: flexible trust management and its application to electronic health records.* Technical Report UCAM-CL-TR-648. Cambridge, UK: University of Cambridge.

Daskala, B. (Ed.). (2009). *Being diabetic in 2011 – Identifying Emerging and Future Risks in Remote Health Monitoring and Treatment.* European Network and Information Security Agency.

Deursen van. T., Koster, P., Petković, M. (2008). Reliable Personal Health Records. In *eHEalth Beyond the Horizon – Get IT There Proceedings of Medical Informatics Europe,* pp.484-489. Amsterdam: IOS Press.

Ibraimi, L., Asim, M., & Petković, M. (2009). *Secure Management of Personal Health Records by Applying Attribute-Based Encryption.* Centre for Telematics and Information Technology, University of Twente.

Katzenbeisser, S., & Petković, M. (2008). Privacy-preserving recommendation systems for consumer healthcare services. In *ARES.* Washington, DC: IEEE Computer Society Press, pp. 889-895.

Künzi, J., Koster, P., & Petković, M. (2009). Emergency Access to Protected Health Records. In Adlassnig, K.-P. (Eds.), *Medical Informatics in a United and Healthy Europe* (pp. 705–709). Amsterdam: IOS Press.

Künzi, J., Petković, M., & Koster, P. (2009). Data-centric Protection in DICOM. In *Medical Imaging, Advanced PACS-based Imaging Informatics and Therapeutic Applications, Progress in Biomedical Optics and Imaging.* SPIE Vol. 10, No. 40, pp.726419-1 – 726419-11

Petković, M. (2009). *Remote Patient Monitoring: Information Reliability Challenges. 9th International Conference on Telecommunications in Modern Satellite, Cable and Broadcasting Services,* pp. 295-301. Washington, DC: IEEE Press.

Petković, M., & Jonker, W. (2007). Privacy and Security Issues in a Digital World. In Petković, M., & Jonker, W. (Eds.), *Security, Privacy and Trust in Modern Data Management* (pp. 3–10). New York: Springer. doi:10.1007/978-3-540-69861-6_1

Petković, M., Katzenbeisser, S., & Kursawe, K. (2007). Rights Management Technologies: A Good Choice for Securing Electronic Health Records? In *International Conference on Information Security Solutions Europe,* Warsaw, Poland

Sandhu, R., Coyne, E., Feinstein, H., & Youman, C. (1996) Role-based access control models. In *IEEE Computer, 29*(2),38–47.

Sheppard, N. P., Safavi-Naini, R., & Jafari, M. (2009). A Digital Rights Management Model for Healthcare. IN *Policies for Distributed Systems and Networks, IEEE International Workshop on,* pp. 106-109.

Win, K., & Fulcher, J. (2007). *Consent Mechanisms for Electronic Health Record Systems: A Simple yet unresolved issue. Journal of Medical Systems, 31(2).* New York: Springer.

KEY TERMS AND DEFINITIONS

Electronic Health Record (EHR): A longitudinal electronic record of patient health information generated by one or more encounters in any care delivery setting. It includes patient demographics, progress notes, problems, medications, vital signs, past medical history, immunizations, laboratory data and radiology reports.

Personal Health Record (PHR): An electronic record of health-related information on an individual that can be drawn from multiple sources while being managed, shared, and controlled by the individual.

Individually Identifiable Health Information (IIHI): Health data that is transmitted by or maintained in electronic media or any other form or medium that can be uniquely associated with an individual.

Consent Directive: A record of a patient's consent or dissent to collection, access, use or disclosure of individually identifiable health information.

Data Availability: The prevention of the unauthorized withholding of information, so that the information is available for the authorized purposes.

Data Confidentiality: The prevention of the unauthorized disclosure of the information, for example individual identifiable health information (IIHI) to the unauthorized individuals.

Data Integrity: The detection of the unauthorized or improper modification of the information assets.

Authentication: The act of establishing or confirming that someone or something is authentic, that claims made by or about the subject are true.

Access Control: The process of controlling every request to a system and determining, based on specified rules, whether the request should be granted or denied.

Audit Trail: A record of access attempts and resource usage to verify enforcement of business, data integrity, security, and access-control rules.

ENDNOTES

[1] HIMSS is not-for-profit healthcare industry's organization dedicated to promoting a better understanding and the optimal use of healthcare information and management systems.

[2] Sometimes the term "virtual EHR' is used instead.

Chapter 3
Foundations of Trust for e-Health

Cynthia L. Corritore
Creighton University, USA

Beverly Kracher
Creighton University, USA

Susan Wiedenbeck
Drexel University, USA

Robert Marble
Creighton University, USA

ABSTRACT

Trust has always been an important element of healthcare. As healthcare evolves into ehealth, a question arises: What will the nature of trust be in ehealth? In this chapter the authors provide the reader with a foundation for considering this question from a research perspective. The authors focus on one ehealth domain: online websites. The chapter begins with a high-level overview of the body of offline trust research. Next, findings related to online trust are presented, along with a working definition. Trust research in the context of online health care is then examined, although this body of work is in its infancy. A detailed discussion of our research in the area of online trust is then presented. Finally, with this background, we take the reader through some possible research questions that are interesting candidates for future research on the nature of trust in ehealth.

INTRODUCTION

Sixty-one percent of American adults in 2008 used the Internet to obtain health information, up 21 percent from 2001 (Fox & Jones, 2009). The information they sought ranged from identifying ways to stay healthy to descriptions of specific disease symptoms and treatments. In addition to this fast growing, widespread use, ehealth consumers report that they consider the Internet to be a better, more accurate, and more reliable source of information than television or print. Forty-one percent also consider the Internet to be a 'frequently accessed, useful source of [medicine-related] information', second only to health care providers (Werbler & Harris, 2009).

DOI: 10.4018/978-1-60960-469-1.ch003

These figures indicate an underlying trust in online health information by consumers. But what is the nature of this trust? Our focus in this chapter will be on this key factor of trust, which we believe must be considered when dealing with information dissemination of any type online. Online trust is important in the business transactions occurring online every day, but in the context of health, we believe it will take on even more significance.

Building trust is particularly important in ehealth since a lack of trust can be so harmful. We all know that trust is an important factor in traditional health care systems. One need only to look at the relationship between patients and their healthcare providers to illustrate this point. Trust has repeatedly been shown to be critical to such things as patient engagement and compliance. However, what happens to trust when millions of people go online for their healthcare information? A simplistic example illustrates this question.

Bob is 49 years old – 50 is looming in his near future, a fact on which he regularly reflects. His age is even more poignant to him as his father died of a heart attack at the age of 55. So Bob decides that he needs to start taking better care of himself. He begins by going online for health information about how to improve his heart health. He visits a website that recommends reducing cardiac risk by reducing his salt intake. Though this information is accurate, he is very skeptical of the website. He notices that the 'last updated' date on the website is three years ago and assumes the information on the site is outdated. The website also seems very amateurish to him. So he does not trust the site or the information on it, and does not follow up on the recommendation to reduce his sodium intake. He picks up a bag of potato chips, downs a couple of handfuls, and promises himself that he'll search online again another time.

In Bob's case, he did not follow a correct recommendation because of a lack of online trust. How often does this occur? No one knows. But

these kinds of scenarios made us wonder about trust and ehealth. How will *offline* health care trust translate into *online* health care trust? How could online trust be developed? While it is obvious to us that trust is very important in the context of ehealth, we found that it is equally unclear what the nature of trust will be as health information and care move online.

The intention of this chapter is to examine the concept of online trust and to consider its place in ehealth research. In order to do so, we begin by examining the nature of trust in the real world, that is, the offline world. We will then move to an overview of research that has studied trust in the online world, and finally we will take a look at the state of trust research in ehealth. Along the way, we will examine the concept of trust itself, touch on some of the confusions that exist with other similar concepts, and provide a working definition of online trust. Then we discuss some of the research we have conducted related to online trust. Finally, we examine the implications for ehealth researchers, and speculate about some of the research questions that could help us understand and maximize the effectiveness of ehealth trust.

Before moving on to a discussion of trust, we pause to clarify our terminology. In this chapter, we will use the term 'online' to indicate websites that are hosted on the Internet and are accessed across a network using a browser. Online trust refers to trust assigned to a website online. While the term ehealth generally is a broader term that includes all possible ways to digitally deliver health care-related activities, we will use it more narrowly to simply refer to health information being delivered via online websites.

A DEFINITION OF TRUST

Before talking about the state of online trust research, we need to take a look at the concept of trust itself. Trust is complex, and as a complex concept it has been possible to study it from several different (and often divergent) angles. For example, Barber (1983) focused on the generality of trust. She noted that there are different generalities of trust, moving from a specific trust for an individual person or thing to a general trust that applies to all things in a group or even all of humankind. There are also kinds of trust. For example, a slow trust that develops over time or a swift trust that occurs almost instantaneously and often disappears just as quickly (Meyerson, Weick & Kramer, 1996). In addition, there are degrees of trust that describe how much trust is given in a situation. In this case, trust can range from a blanket trust (basic), to a trust that is restrained and cautious (guarded), to a trust that is whole, unmitigated and true (extended) (Brenkert, 1998). Stages of trust have also been proposed (Lewicki & Bunker, 1996) that correspond to varying levels of trust. These start with initial trust given because there is protection by laws and agreements (deterrence-based), moving to an intermediate trust based on some knowledge acquired over time for the object of trust (knowledge-based), then finally to a deeper, mature trust that is based on overall perceived shared values and beliefs (shared-identification-based trust).

In the face of all of these ways of thinking about trust, we have defined what we mean by trust. Our definition has been developed by analyzing and synthesizing existing trust literature. We start by distinguishing what trust is from what it is not. Trust is not the same thing as trustworthy or trustworthiness (Blois, 1999). Though they are essentially related, as two sides to the same coin, they are different concepts. Trust is an *attitude* of a trustor, that is, a person who is giving the trust. In contrast, trustworthiness is an attribute of the trustee, that is, that which is trusted. Though it is hopeful that a person gives trust only to that which is trustworthy, it is not always the case. Sometimes, that which is trusted is not trustworthy. For example, a person might trust that a "doctor" who advertises online is authentic but the "doctor" could be fake and not trustworthy. However, it would not be surprising to postulate that what is trusted is *perceived* to be trustworthy (think again of a "doctor" advertising online). To put this last point another way, when we trust, we *expect* that the object of our trust is trustworthy.

We also maintain that trust is not the same thing as faith, though they both necessarily involve an element of *risk* since without risk there is no occasion to have either (Mayer, Davis, & Schoorman. 1995). Trusting one's health with a doctor who advertises online is risky. However, saying "I trust you" is not synonymous with "I have faith in you." Faith requires taking a leap as in "leap of faith." Faith is *believing* in something that we cannot understand. Faith is akin to hope: it goes beyond reason. But trust does not. Generally speaking, trust is grounded in reason. It is achieved when we have *confidence* in a thing based on its reliability, credibility, competence, etc (Lewicki & Bunker, 1995). Trust is an expectation that what we perceive to be trustworthy, really is.

Thus, by looking at what trust is not, we have begun to craft a definition of what trust is. Fundamentally, trust is an attitude of confident expectation in a situation of risk. However, this definition is not yet sufficient. In order to complete this definition we must include the concepts of vulnerability and exploitation (Deutsch, 1962; Mayer et. al. 1995; Zand, 1972). These two concepts elucidate the risks that distinguish trust from other forms of confident attitudes. For example, I may be confident that I will win a hand of poker because, risky as is any game of chance, I am playing at a reputable casino, I have been practicing, and I have been playing well all night long. But I do not trust that I have a chance of winning a hand of poker unless I believe that I am vulnerable. My confident attitude relates to the chance that my hand beats all the others at the table, whereas my trust relates to the chance that my better hand will be recognized and paid. Trust is relevant to poker only when there is a possibility that I may be exploited in some way as when cheating may be involved.

Herein we arrive at a definition of trust based on the literature that can be applied in the online world. Note that this definition assumes the object of trust (ie. that which is being trusted) to be a website. We will expand upon the idea of 'website trust' in a later section. For now, online trust is

an attitude of confident expectation towards a website in an online situation of risk that one's vulnerabilities will not be exploited.

In other words, people have online trust when they expect that accessing a website will not harm them even though they know that there is a risk that they could be harmed. The implications of this online trust are enormous for ehealth.

TRUST IN THE REAL (OFFLINE) WORLD

Researchers in a wide variety of fields, including psychology, sociology, philosophy, business (marketing, management, etc.), and human-computer interaction have studied trust. They all agree that trust is essential and fundamental to human interactions (Barber, 1983; Good, 1988; Dasgupta, 1988; Giddens, 1990; Buskens, 1998) and that trust provides a means for people to decrease the complexity of their world by reducing the number of options they must consider in a given situation (Barber, 1983; Lewis & Weigert, 1985). Trust is also seen as a key mechanism that enables people to function in risky and uncertain situations (Deutsch, 1962; Mayer et al., 1995). Early researchers showed that trust has a strong relationship with risk (Deutsch, 1962; Luhmann, 1988). That is, there is no need for trust if risk is not present (Mayer et al., 1995). Therefore, if trust is present, so is risk. While the exact relationship between the two concepts is unclear, trust researchers agree that people are able to accept risky and uncertain situations by employing trust (Deutsch, 1962; Mayer et al., 1995). Sociologists

also view trust as a form of social capital that makes coordination and cooperation between people even possible (Misztal, 1996; Putnam, 1995). So it should come as no surprise that trust in the real (offline) world has been extensively studied for decades. Yet to date, in spite of such widespread study of trust, it is still not clearly or deeply understood.

Researchers agree that trust is important, and they believe that it is complex. However, this is where the agreement ends. Most trust researchers have developed their own definitions of trust, contexts of study, and research methodologies. This eclectic approach has delivered correspondingly eclectic findings, making understanding and generalizing the concept of trust very difficult. Of course, the complexity of the concept of trust itself is likely partially to blame. A multifaceted concept such as trust gives researchers many different aspects to study, perhaps minimizing overlap in their work. In spite of this, we will take a look at some of the key offline trust research that we believe have implications for online trust.

Many early trust researchers focused on interpersonal trust. Their work either 1) attempted to identify factors that led to a trusting personality (for example, see Erickson, 1963), or 2) focused on examining trust in interpersonal relationships, interactions, and collaborative efforts (for example see Deutsch, 1962; Lewicki & Bunker, 1995). While no definitive results regarding the first were clearly demonstrated, the second has yielded some interesting findings. This body of work is built upon the premise that trust is a basic feature of all social situations that demand cooperation and interdependence, and is vital to social life and personality development (Kee & Knox, 1970; Rotter, 1971). Very early on, foundational trust researcher Morton Deutsch (Deutsch, 1958; Deutsch, 1962) identified two types of trust: interpersonal and mutual. Interpersonal is trust that a person has for another person, while mutual trust is the complementary trust that two people share for each other with respect to their behavior (ie. each trusts the other to behave in a certain way, and is willing to do what the other trusts her to do).

Early researchers went on to study these types of trust in the context of mixed-motive games such as Prisoner's Dilemma (Deutsch, 1962; Kee & Knox, 1970; Rotter, 1971). The Prisoner's Dilemma (and its variants) is a type of non-zero sum game in which pursuing a strategy of self-interest loses the game, while cooperation and mutual trust win. Using this methodology, Deutsch (1958; 1962) found that communication appeared to promote trust. He stated that effective communication contained: 1) intention and expectations, 2) an outline of the basic features of the trusting relationship, 3) an indication of how violations will be treated, and 4) an outline of a method of absolution from violations of trust. This line of research also elucidated several aspects of trust and factors that can influence the development of trust. For example, Deutsch (1962) found that shared goals and mutual benefits with an expectation of reciprocation were important to trust. Control over another's behavior, as well as the ability to predict behavior and perceive intentions and motivations of another, were also important to the formation of trust (Barney & Hansen, 1994; Deutsch, 1958; Lewicki & Bunker, 1995; Rotter, 1967). Experience, expectations, and confidence in another's abilities have also been found to be central in making decisions based on trust (Deutsch, 1958; Lewicki & Bunker, 1995; Rotter, 1967). Another interesting finding in this body of work is the effect of psychological simultancity, the degree to which both parties know what the other is doing. Psychological simultaneity has been found to be important to trust (Kee & Knox, 1970; Deutsch 1958; Deutsch, 1962). Kee and Knox (1970) grouped many of these factors that had been shown to be important to trust into three categories: structural (i.e., incentives, power, communication), situational (i.e., degree of control in a given situation), and dispositional (i.e., motivational orientation, personality, attitudes).

Other researchers examined the interplay between cognition and affect in the context of trust. During the 1950s through the 1970s, most researchers viewed affect and cognition as intertwined, or alternatively affect was viewed as subservient to cognition. Out of this body of work arose several different ways of understanding trust. For example, Shapiro, Sheppard, and Cheraskin (1992) proposed that people make decisions to trust based on a cognitive calculation of trustworthiness that entailed a rational calculation of costs and benefits. They termed this type of trust calculative. Other researchers focused on the affective component of trust. Zajonc (1980) paved the way for such research, with his proposition that cognition and emotion are separable and partly independent. He argued that affective responses could even precede cognitive ones. Consequently, some trust researchers began to study affective elements of trust. Two of these, McKnight and Chervany (2000), found that affective elements such as a *feeling* of security and safety were important elements of trust. These same researchers defined a type of trust they called Perceptual Trust, also referred to as Beliefs. Perceptual Trust is based on the extent to which a trustor *perceives* [not solely calculates] a trustee to be competent or benevolent. This type of trust has been found to be an important element in determining trustworthiness of others.

Again, while all of these studies have merit, it is hard to see how they combine into one overarching view of trust. Instead, a significant outcome of this body of work is the many frameworks, models, and measurement tools produced. Two widely recognized tools are the Rotter Scale (Rotter, 1967) and the Dydactic Trust Scale (Larzelere & Huston, 1980). While these scales provided a way for researchers to measure the same concept, they were not without criticism as some felt that they conflated trust with other concepts such as benevolence or honesty (i.e., see Johnson-George & Swap, 1982; Schumm, Bugaighis, Buckler, Green & Scanton, 1985). In addition, their exclusive focus on interpersonal trust made them of little use in studying other types of trust.

Trust has also been studied extensively by researchers who examined it in the larger context of society. These researchers tended to be sociologists and philosophers. They identified trust as essential social capital, which is used to improve the efficiency of society by facilitating coordination and decreasing social complexity (Barber, 1983; Buskens, 1998; Dasgupta, 1988; Giddens, 1990; Good, 1988). Generally they made a distinction between personal, or face-to-face, trust and trust in some type of societal structure (Barber, 1983; Giddens, 1990; Good, 1988). Many of these researchers studied face-to-face trust in the context of games. These researchers viewed trust as a rational process, and, like their psychology counterparts, believed that cooperation in a two-person gaming situation defined trust (Barber, 1983; Buskens, 1998). They found that social perception, which is the ability to read others' intentions and inclinations, the stakes involved, and the importance of the stakes all play a role in trust (Barber, 1983; Macy & Skvoretz, 1998; Snijders & Keren, 1999). Their ideas were later extended to include the factors of situational context and trust variability based on context, which were recognized as important to trust (Barber, 1983; Buskens, 1998; Good, 1988; Lewis & Weigert, 1985; Macy & Skvoretz, 1998). Other social researchers examined face-to-face trust between individuals during social interactions. Underlying some of this work was the idea that interpretation bias underlies all human interactions. In this vein, Giddons (1990) identified a cognitive inertia in individuals that acts to preserve trust. Social expectations underlie the classic experiments conducted by Garfinkel (1963). He found that the removal of seemingly inconsequential features of everyday conversation led to significant disruption of the social interaction that people 'trusted' to be in place.

Business researchers have conducted a great deal of research around trust. Most active in this area are marketing researchers. They have an obvious interest in trust, as building trusting relationships between organizations, their representatives, and customers can be crucial. In the last two decades, this research has narrowed its focus to one of trust in Relationship Marketing. Relationship Marketing is centered on the establishment and maintenance of long-term relations with customers. These researchers have identified many trust antecedents. Among these are credibility (defined in terms of expertise) and benevolence (positive intentions toward the customer) (Ganesan, 1994). Marketing researchers have also examined practices that appear to engender trust. In this light, fair treatment of customer information was found to create trust (Milne & Boza, 1999). Trust was also evoked by employing practices that increase information to customers, make multi-organization interactions seamless for customers, and increase the use of known brands (Davis, Buchanan-Oliver, & Brodie, 1999; Lau & Sook, 1999; Urban, Sultan, & Qualls, 1998). Finally, the size of an organization, the level of communication, and the presence and degree of shared values between a vendor and customer have all been found to affect trust (Doney & Cannon, 1997; Morgan & Hunt, 1994).

Summary of Trust Research in the 'Real' World

At this point, it should be clear that while trust has been extensively studied in the offline world, no unifying theory of trust has emerged. The most descriptive thing that can be said for this body of work is that the findings are eclectic, in part due to the complexity and depth of the concept of trust. Trust has been studied in interpersonal relationships, in mixed-motive (zero-sum) games, in social contexts. In an attempt to summarize the findings, we would point out that trust 1) can be applied to inanimate objects such as organizations as well as other people, 2) it is a perceptual process (in the eyes of the trustor), 3) is likely affected by emotions or affect, 4) is likely assigned based on application of specific criteria used to evaluate the trustworthiness of an object, and that these criteria differ depending on the context and the trustor. Antecedents such as credibility, experience, shared goals, expectations of reciprocation, and benevolence are some of these.

TRUST IN THE ONLINE WORLD

A significant factor in the nature of *online* trust research is its timeframe. The World Wide Web began in 1991, and researchers began to study trust in this new online environment shortly after that. Thus, one can see that *online* trust is a relatively new research topic. As with the offline trust researchers, a confounding aspect for online trust researchers has been the plurality of different ways in which trust is defined, conceptualized, and operationalized. This makes comparison and amalgamation of findings difficult. For example, Gefen, Karahanna, and Straub (2003b) expanded the concept of online trust to include the measurement of four hypothesized types of trust: calculative-based, institution-based, structural assurances, and institution-based situational normality. In contrast, McKnight, Choudhury and Kacmar (2000), in their widely cited study, defined trust as a composite of benevolence, integrity, and competence. But in spite of this difficulty, we will examine some of the main studies of online trust that have been done.

Much of the online trust research has been conducted in the context of ecommerce. This body of work has focused on the trust of a customer for a specific online vendor, and how trust affected transaction-related behaviors. These researchers consistently found that trust positively impacted the intention to make a purchase from a vendor (Gefen, 2000; Einwiller, 2003; Gefen, Karahanna, & Straub, 2003a; Gefen, Karahanna, & Straub, 2003b; McKnight, Choudhury, & Kacmar, 2002b), customer satisfaction with a vendor (Kim & Stoel, 2004), and customer loyalty for a vendor (Harris

& Goode, 2004). The nature of the entire shopping experience has also been shown to impact a consumers' trust of a vendor website (Cheskin Research and Studio Archetype/Sapient, 1999; Fogg, Marshall, Laraki, Osipovich, Varma, Fang, Paul, Rangnekar, Shon, Swani & Treihen, 2001; Ribbink, vanRiel, Lijander & Streukens, 2004). In their study, "shopping" included availability of company information, range of merchandise, branding, promotions, security, fulfillment, quality and quantity of customer service. In the course of this research, most of these researchers developed valid trust measures and models that were supported by their data.

The effect of different technologies on online trust has also been studied. This is important because, today, consumers often have the opportunity to interact with vendor representatives or others online. A good example of this body of work is that done by Bos, Olson, Gergle, Olson & Wright (2002), who found that members of virtual teams who do not know each other have higher trust when collaborators use rich media. Video, audio, and text chat were compared to face-to-face communication, and the results showed that the richer video and audio technologies were almost as good as the face-to-face, whereas text chat lagged behind. Similarly, Riegersberger, Sasse, and McCarthy's study (2005) involved expert advice and non-expert advice on financial issues presented in several media: video, audio, avatar, and photo+text. Their results showed that participants preferred the expert advice, and that participants believed that video or audio presentation would provide most detailed advice about financial issues than the avatar or photo+text options. Even within a single technology, trust can be affected by its fidelity. For example, in widely used group video conferencing technologies trust issues arose because of distortions of nonverbal cues, such as poor eye contact and gaze awareness (Nguyen & Canny, 2007). In their empirical study of group conferencing, trust formation was found to be affected negatively by the lack of "spatial faithfulness" of the system -- it failed to preserve spatial relationships.

Not only is online trust affected by various technologies, but aspects of a technology can distinguish possible *objects* of trust in the online environment. First, a user can trust (or distrust) the underlying technology infrastructure and control mechanisms that allow communication and transactions between customers and vendors. These include the Internet technology itself as well as technological security safeguards and protection mechanisms such as digital signatures and encryption. This kind of online trust is called technology trust and is an important focus of some trust research (Lee & Turban, 2001; Ratnasingam & Pavlov, 2003). It is possible that baseline trust in technological infrastructure may be required for customers to accept online information. Second, customers can trust the organizations with which they interact via the Internet. In this case, technology is a means or conduit for the trust between them. This kind of online trust is called computer-mediated trust and has been the object of a significant amount of study (Jarvenpaa, Tractinsky, & Saarinen, 1999; Olson & Olson, 2000a; Olson & Olson, 2000b; Koehn, 2003). Third, customers can trust an organizations website, regardless of whether or not they trust the organization. This kind of online trust is called website trust because trust is placed in the website which represents or stands for an organization. Indeed, because of this representative relationship between the website and the organization some researchers take website trust to be a dimension of computer-mediated trust. They posit that a website is akin to a salesperson or an organization's facility, and interaction with it can enhance formation of a consumer's trust in an organization (Jarvenpaa, Tractinsky & Saarinen, 1999; McKnight et al., 2002a). However, the trust a consumer can have in a website is conceptually distinct from the trust a consumer can have in an organization, and online providers must manage both. We will return to the concept of website trust when discussing our own online trust research.

Some researchers have focused on how characteristics of the website itself affects trust. This body of work typically takes one of two approaches: 1) focusing on the effect of superficial, or visual, characteristics of a website, e.g., color and clipart, or 2) focusing on deeper, substantive aspects of a website such as perceived expertise and reputation. While we recognize that important findings do exist in the first body of work and will provide a brief overview of this body of work, we see it as more a stylistic issue and one that is subject to frequent change. So our main focus will be on the second, as we believe the implications are more significant and more stable over time. Two of these are of particular interest as they are supported by findings from offline trust research and early online trust research indicates that they appear to translate to the online world. These are 1) credibility, and 2) risk (Lewis & Wiegert, 1985; Giddons, 1990; McKnight et.al., 2002a). We also posited that moving trust online might also create a new factor to impact trust: ease of use of the website.

Design has been shown to affect online trust, although this appears to be more extreme in non-experts (Stanford, Tauber, Fogg & Marable, 2003). Some studies have focused specific design elements, and have found an effect on trust. These elements include good use of visual design elements (Kim & Moon, 1998), professional images of products (Nielsen, Molich, Snyder & Farell, 2000), freedom from small grammatical and typographical errors (Fogg, Marshall, Laraki, Osipovich, Varma, Fang, Paul, Rangnekar, Shon, Swani, & Treinen, 2001), an overall professional look of the website (Belanger, Hiller & Smith, 2002; Kim & Stoel, 2004; McKnight et al., 2002b), and ease of carrying out transactions (Nielsen et al., 2000). The effect of graphics on online trust is mixed. Some researchers have found images to increase assignment of trust (Fogg, Marshall, Kameda, Solomon, Rangnekar, Body & Brown, 2001; Steinbrück, Schaumburg, Duda & Krüger, 2002). In contrast, others have found either no effect or a slight negative effect on trust (Riegels-gerger & Sasse, 2001). Not surprisingly, Nielsen et al. (2000) found that poor website maintenance, i.e., broken links and outdated information, tends to decrease trust.

Now we will consider the more substantive aspects of websites. We start with credibility. As we have discussed, credibility has been identified as an antecedent to trust in the offline world. However, like trust, credibility is not a simple, unary factor. It appears to be a complex, multi-faceted construct. Therefore, credibility must be studied in terms of its component parts. Credibility appears to be comprised of three subfactors: expertise (Giffen, 1967; Fogg & Tseng, 1999; Wathen & J. Burkell, 2002), honesty (Fogg et.al, 2001; Lee, Kim, & Moon, 2000), and reputation (DasGupta, 1988; Good, 1988; Ganesen, 1994; Kim, Xu, & Koh, 2004). Specifically, Giffen (1967) identified expertise and reputation as sub-factors of credibility. In fact, simply conveying expertise, providing comprehensive information, and projecting honesty and shared values between a website and a user have been found to be positive cues for promoting the perceived trustworthiness of a website (Fogg et al., 2001; Kim & Moon, 1998; Lee et. al, 2000). Interestingly, researchers have found that an authors' photograph can suggest credibility based on the interpretation of the customer (Fogg et al., 2001; Johnson & Wiedenbeck, 2009; Riegerlsberger, Sasse & McCarthy, 2003). With respect to reputation, Ganesan (1994) found that vendor reputation and the perception that a vendor has made investments on the buyers' behalf, e.g., product customization, are important precursors for customer trust. Similarly, Kim et.al. (2004) found that reputation significantly impacted early and ongoing trust for online vendors, explaining 52% of the variance of the online trust measured. The research of many others has supported these findings (see Ganesen, 1994; Grazioli & Jarvenpaa, 2000; McKnight et al., 2002a; Einwiller, 2003).

Next we consider risk, another important antecedent of trust. Most theoretical definitions of trust include a discussion of risk and the fact that trust ameliorates risk. But the object of risk has varied between research studies. In the context of business, the focus has been almost exclusively on the perception of risk in transactions, online vendors, or the Internet itself rather than of a given website. Given this focus, researchers have found that a relationship does exist between online trust and perceived risk (Jarvenpaa, Tractinsky, & Vitale, 2000; Salam, Rao, & Pegels, 2003). However, the nature of this relationship was not clear. McKnight et. al. (2002a), in their study of 'perceived web risk' found that risk indirectly impacted trust, although their definition of risk centered on the risk of transacting over the web in general (the Internet environment) rather than the risk of trusting a given website. They also found that a perception of high risk (of the Internet environment) was associated with a reduction in trust of a particular online vendor. Einwiller (2003) found that assessment of vendor risk strongly impacted the development of a trusting intention to act. Although they did not study trust specifically, Grazaioli and Jarvenpaa (2000) found that perceived risk of an online store negatively affected customers' willingness to purchase from the store. Likewise, Briggs, Burford, DeAngeli and Lunch (2002) found that willingness to trust a site was higher if perceived risk (related to the domain) was low. A surprising finding related to online risk is that the effect of privacy and security assurances such as third party seals have not been shown to be important in establishing trust by reducing the perception of risk (Belanger, Hiller and Smith, 2002).

Finally, many researchers have studied the effect of ease of use on online trust of websites. Ease of use typically refers to something that is free of effort. Researchers operationalize this as ease of navigation, transaction, and searching as well as an indication of the efficiency, effectiveness, learnability, and fun of an application.

Today, most researchers would agree that ease of use of software or a website has been shown to increase trust (for example, see Davis, Bagozzi, & Warshaw, 1989; Snijders & Keren, 1999; Pavlou, 2001; McKnight, V. Choudhury, and C. Kacmar, 2002a; Gefen, et al., 2003a). In fact, the positive effect of ease of use on user interaction with technology and software is the basis for the field of Human-Computer Interaction (HCI).

Summary of Trust Research in the Online World

In summarizing the state of online trust research, we see the same issues as noted in the body of work studying offline trust. That is, the research is eclectic. With this noted, we can identify some key points. First, online trust research has primarily examined trust related to the Internet infrastructure (including security), trust between people mediated by technology, and trust in websites themselves. Online trust has been shown to positively impact a decision to purchase (from a vendor), customer satisfaction, and customer loyalty. Similarly, risk has been shown to decrease such behaviors. The fidelity of the technology used to portray an object of trust also has been shown to affect the assignment of trust (rich media being the best). Both superficial characteristics of the object of trust as well as deeper traits such as credibility and risk, have been shown to impact online trust. Finally, research indicates that like trust, credibility is a complex concept, and may be composed of expertise, honesty, and reputation.

THE OBJECT OF TRUST

Earlier we referred to the fact that in the online world, what a person is trusting, ie. their object of trust, could be one of several different things. One of these, the website itself, has recently become an item of interest in some online trust research (Corbitt, Thanasankit & Yi, 2003; Kim, Song,

Braynov & Rao, 2001). While a consideration of the object of trust is tangential to our discussion, we will take a moment to examine it briefly as it is an important issue that must be addressed when studying online trust.

Much of the offline trust research deals with either some variant of person-to-person trust (ie. interpersonal trust) or trust in an organization [made up of people]. However, when trust research moves to the online environment, the object of trust becomes less clear. While some online trust researchers have continued to study trust using interpersonal or organizational frameworks, a few others are considering trust in the website itself, ie. website trust. However, to be clear, this distinction had not been clearly addressed in the online trust literature to date. There are researchers on both sides of the issue. Researchers in the field of philosophy have long examined the issue of whether people can trust something that is inanimate, such as a website. Based on their work, they would object to an assertion that people can trust websites. Their objection would be that people cannot trust websites in the same way they can trust humans or human institutions. While some might think that websites are reliable, predictable, or have some other human-like characteristic, they admonish that trust can only exist between agents, that is, things that can act with intention. In essence, according to philosophers Friedman, Kahn, and Howe (2000), people can only trust other people, not machines. Perhaps Solomon and Flores put it most succinctly when they wrote, "Trust, properly understood, is a function of human interaction" (2001, p. 70).

However, others disagree with the notion that trust can only occur between *human* agents. They see trust as a strongly perceptual experience (Deutsch, 1958; Kee & Knox, 1970; Rotter, 1980; Giddens, 1990; Muir & Moray, 1996). So what would impact trust is how a potential object of trust is perceived. When taking into account perception, researchers have found that people actually do trust even non-human objects that are perceived to have a social presence (Muir & Moray, 1996; Nass, Fogg & Moon, 1996; Kim & Moon, 1998). Of particular relevance is work done by Reeves and Nass (1996). In a series of experiments in which they studied peoples' responses to computers, they found that people do enter into relationships with computers, websites, and other non-human media. Their findings indicate that people appear to respond to computers, for example, based on rules that apply to social relationships in general. In their studies, people were polite or rude to their computers, identified them as assertive, timid, or helpful, and had physical responses to them. Reeves and Nash take a strong position, based on their findings, that computers are social actors or agents. They found that people tend not to look beyond the technology to consider the creators or operators of the technology in responding socially to the technology.

Trust in E-Health

Up to this point, we have focused exclusively on trust in non-health settings. We have two reasons for doing this. First, to provide the reader with a broad foundation of the complex concept of trust. Second, because that trust research in ehealth is still very new. While we suspect that all health care professionals would agree that patient trust is a key factor in successful patient outcomes, satisfaction, engagement, and empowerment (for example, see Kao, Gree, Zaslavsky, Koplan & Cleary, 1998; Thorne & Robinson, 1998; Mechanic, 2004), its role in ehealth is little studied to date. Not surprisingly, given the newness of ehealth, much of the research that does exist is descriptive. It has either focused on depicting the characteristics of ehealth consumers and noting what their online activities involve (see Baker, Wagner, Singer & Bundorf, 2003; Mohan, 2004), examining the quality and accuracy of online health information and websites (see Impicciatore, Pandolfini, Casella & Bonzti, 1997; Kisely, 2002), or investigating the effectiveness of specific

online health programs and treatment strategies (see Walther, Pingree, Hawkins & Buller, 2005). We will take a look at both the current state of this body of research, as well as the nascent empirical work that is developing.

In a study investigating the consequences of trust in online healthcare services, Gummerus and Liljander (2004) found that trust is significant in driving consumer satisfaction and loyalty. Other researchers have been interested in how specific characteristics of health information websites themselves could promote trust. For example, Rippen (1999) posited that the trustworthiness of a health information website could be increased by disclosure on the site of 1) the mission and purpose of the site, 2) potential conflicts of interest, 3) collection processes, 4) absence of plagiarism, and 5) disclaimers that the site facilitates but does not replace traditional medical care. However, no empirical investigation of his posits was conducted. Likewise, Luo and Najdawi (2004) examined 12 health information portals, looking for inclusion of their defined "trust-building features" such as seals of approval from accrediting bodies. They found that most portals contained some of their identified features. Similarly, an interesting and disturbing finding of Werbler and Harris' (2009) research is that four in 10 health care consumers do not pay attention to provided risk information. While their study was done using print and television, the finding is important as the same lack of attention has been noted in online trust research in general. Therefore, it might be expected to translate online in the context of ehealth. Another aspect of the online environment and its effect on trust was studied by Becker (2004). While not examining trust specifically, Becker examined a possible antecedent of trust – ease of use – as related to older Americans. Using the Web Guidelines of the National Institute on Aging, he evaluated the ease of use of 125 ehealth websites. He identified poor ease of use, manifested as small font size, no help feature, and information that spanned multiple pages.

ehealth researchers are beginning to investigate factors that may be involved in the assignment of trust by online consumers. Credibility in ehealth is particularly germane given that most people search for health information using search engines, thus arriving at websites that may not be reliable sources (Pew Internet Research, 2002). As a result, they must determine credibility of the site and its information on their own. Some of this research has looked at credibility as a unary concept, while others have addressed some of the sub-factors of credibility, i.e., honesty, expertise and reputation. Findings are mixed. Some researchers have found that credibility of health websites is based more on the nature and quality of the website information than on surface and design aspects (Stanford, Tauber, Fogg, & Marable, 2003; Hong, 2006). This is reassuring, and what health professionals would hope. However, other researchers have found that the first impression made by a website, based on the superficial aspects of the website such as design, visual appeal, and presence of errors, was the most important factor in a patient deciding whether or not to explore the site further (Sillence, Briggs, Fishwick, & Harris, 2004; Sillence, Briggs, Fishwick, & Harris, 2007). While these researchers did not directly measure credibility, they did show that the superficial aspects of a website can render its true credibility irrelevant. This is certainly not good news. However, these same researchers did find that once a given website was chosen for further investigation, i.e., had passed a 'first impression' step, patients changed their evaluation criteria to a focus on expertise and non-commercial intent. They also found that expertise and honesty had a positive effect on the assignment of trust. The positive effect of expertise on trust was even more evident in participants with more at stake, i.e., more serious health problems. Such expertise and honesty in information has also been shown to be key in trust of traditional health care information providers, i.e., physicians (Semmes, 1991; Thom & Campbell, 1997).

Some have also studied the relationship between trust and reputation, a sub-factor of credibility. In one study, reputation was found to be a key factor in the determination of the quality of ehealth information websites by health professionals (Jenkins, Corritore & Wiedenbeck, 2003). However, this study used health care providers, not health consumers. These findings were supported by Stanford et al. (2003), who saw an effect for reputation, along with information source and company motive, in establishing credibility.

Summary of Trust Research in ehealth

The study of online trust in the context of ehealth is a new research topic. As such, there is not yet development of a clear picture of the role of trust in ehealth. Many existing studies are descriptive, focusing on characteristics of health websites, online health consumers, and the quality of online health information. Some researchers simply posit what could be important, ie. nature of the content, superficial characteristics of a health website, risk, and ease of use. But some commonalities with general trust research seem to be emerging. Like trust in ecommerce, health consumer trust appears to drive satisfaction and loyalty. Of particular interest is research demonstrating that the most important factors in patients exploring a website further are superficial, ie. design, visual appeal, error rate. But once a website passed this first impression step, patients change their criteria for trust to focus on expertise, non-commercial intent, and honesty. Finally, reputation has been shown to be a key factor in assignation of trust online by health professionals.

OUR RESEARCH

Our online trust research on ehealth is based on our proposals of how we believe credibility, risk, and ease of use impact trust of a website that a given person is visiting. These beliefs have been built upon the foundation of previous trust research. We see credibility as very important in online informational websites, and expect that honesty, expertise, and reputation offer a good representation of the higher order characteristic of website credibility. Setting aside strict research thinking for a moment, we would like to give a feel for some of the thinking we did about online trust, credibility, risk, and ease of use. Consider that when people visit an informational website, such as an ehealth website, they investigate topics of interest and evaluate information as best they can. If the information is plausible, they are likely to accept the information and subsequently may act on it. The more a person finds credible information, the more they are likely to revisit the website.

These repeated episodes can then lead to a more generalized trust in the website. On the other hand, if a person does not perceive the information as credible, the person is unlikely to delve into other topics in the website. They will not trust the website, and they will likely perceive risk at some level. At some point their perception of risk will negatively affect their trust in the website. Consequently, the person will likely go to a different website. Ease of use, too, is important. In this case, the issue is not the content of the website per se, but the presentation of it. If people visit an ehealth informational website and find that it is easy to search, navigate, browse, read content, and print or share information, we posit that they will perceive credibility and consequently be more likely to trust the website. The opposite scenario is that people notice website problems – search does not find the desired topics, navigation is non-standard, and browsing leads the person into deep levels of the website without finding the desired information. Further, when the person does find an article of interest, they may notice that the article is poorly written, badly edited, cannot be printed, and cannot be shared with others online. These lacks reduce the person's trust of the website and the perceived credibility of the content.

In our research, we consider trust to be a social phenomenon that can occur between an agent and any medium that is *perceived* to have a social presence, so long as it occurs within a social context. Therefore, we considered the object of trust to be a website, although we did not rule out the notion that people may also think about the person or organization behind the website. The initial goal of our online trust research was to develop and validate a model of online trust, and in the process develop a valid tool that could be used to measure trust in websites. This was motivated by the lack of an online trust model that we felt was adequate as well as a related measurement tool. Our proposed model focuses on three antecedents of trust: *credibility*, *risk*, and *ease of use*. Credibility is represented by the three sub-factors honesty, expertise, and reputation. The risk factor was characterized by notions of negative consequences and caution. We included ease of use [of the website] as a third factor because it is an important concept that affects user experiences interacting with software. Also, researchers have consistently found that website ease of use affects trust (Pavlou, 2001; Gefen, Karahanna, & Straub, 2003a).

In our first step we developed a 34-item Likert-type questionnaire, with several questions for each of the predictors as well as the outcome variable, trust. The three credibility sub-factors were each measured separately along with ease of use and risk, for a total of five measured factors. Where possible, questions were adapted from previous validated research on their corresponding factors. We chose to focus on online well health information (health promotion), as trust in ehealth is highly personal as well as important, and a well population was readily available. The participants were 176 undergraduate and graduate students enrolled in a variety of programs at a medium-sized university in the United States. The participants were regular computer users who were comfortable using the

Web. Demographic statistics indicated that the average age of participants was 22.1 years and males comprised 44.1 percent of the participants. The participants were healthy individuals with no medical conditions, consistent with our focus on health wellness. Participation in the study was voluntary.

In several large rooms, the participants visited a health information website, WebMD (http://www.webmd.com). Our choice of WebMD for the study was based on its extensive and detailed information, the health tools available on the website, and recognitions of WebMD over the years. Participants carried out three tasks on WebMD in order to become familiar with the website. For example, one of the assigned tasks was navigating to the location in WebMD in which family medical histories could be created. When a participant finished the tasks, the research questionnaire was presented online. Participants filled out the questionnaire, submitted it, and left the classroom. The entire session took 30 to 40 minutes.

We conducted a statistical validation of the research questionnaire using a two-phase process: 1) principle component factor analysis (PCA), followed by 2) confirmatory factor analysis (CFA). In the PCA the questions generally grouped as they were intended, although the questions about honesty and expertise merged, indicating that participants essentially considered honesty and expertise the same. Next, the CFA was carried out. This allowed us to identify questions that had cross-correlations that could perturb multiple factors as well as identify redundancies in the questions. As a result of the CFA, one of the predictive factors was removed (reputation), leaving credibility to be represented solely by expertise and honesty. Therefore, credibility, ease of use, and risk were identified as the predictors with trust the outcome variable. The final 15-question instrument resulted from this process and is shown in Figure 1. The CFA resulted in a more concise instrument, which we then used to refine our predictive model.

Next we moved on to analysis of our model. We used structural equation modeling (SEM) to test our predictive model (see Figure 2). In the figure, the ovals represent the factors we studied, and the arrows represent the predicted relationships between the factors. The solid arrows show relationships that were validated as statistically significant by our data. Following the arrows, one sees that ease of use affects both trust and credibility, and risk affects trust. Furthermore, credibility affects both risk and trust. Our hypothesized predictive relationship of ease of use on risk (shown by the dotted arrow) was non-significant. The R^2 statistic of trust, the outcome variable, is 0.73, indicating that credibility, ease of use, and risk explained 73% of the variance of trust – a very strong result.

The outcome of this study was a model for trust in online websites that has strong reliability, discriminant validity and unidimensionality (Corritore et al., 2007). In addition, a concise measurement tool with strong validity was also an outcome of this work.

The research described above is a first effort in predicting trust in e-Health. Therefore, there are limitations of this research. First, we utilized a single health care website in the experiment. In order to generalize from our study, the experiment should be replicated using other health care websites. In addition, there are issues of access. We used personal computers in our study, but there are other ways to access the website, e.g., mobile phones or smart phones. Results may differ if the participants consider the website to be awkward for navigating and reading using a mobile phone. Results may also differ if there are concerns of privacy on the part of the user who accesses e-Health information using a mobile phone in contexts such as public spaces. Alternative devices to access the website must be taken into account because some cultures rarely use personal computers as their preferred device. A further study should include mobile devices for e-Health information. More

Figure 1. Measurement tool for Online Trust

Credibility
1. The website provides truthful information.
2. The information provided by the website is believable.
3. The website content reflects mastery of knowledge.
4. The website is qualified in this field.
5. The website content reflects expertise.
Ease of Use
6. Learning to operate this website was easy for me.
7. I found it easy to get this website to do what I wanted it to do.
8. I found it easy for me to become skillful at using the site.
9. I found the website easy to use.
Risk
10. I believe that there could be negative consequences from using this website.
11. I feel that the risks outweigh the benefits of using this website.
12. I feel I must be cautious when using this website.
13. It is risky to interact with this website.
Trust
14. I believe this website is trustworthy.
15. I trust this website.

Figure 2. Path Analysis of the Online Trust Model of Health Information Websites

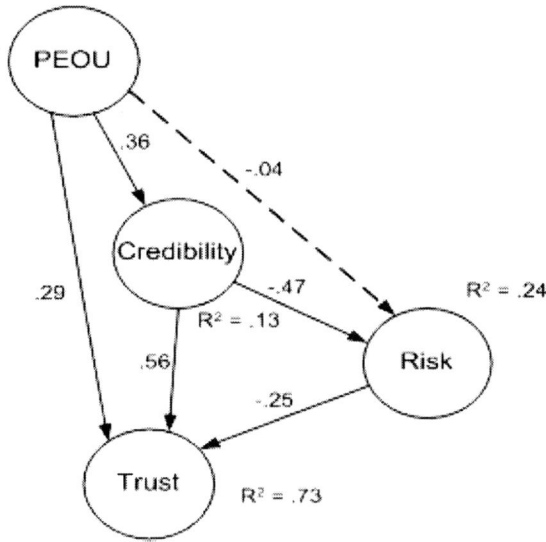

generally, we acknowledge that e-Health can be delivered by ways other than accessing a website.

Further limitations of the study are related to our model, the participants, and the tasks. The model included credibility, risk, ease of use, and trust. Emotion is likely to be related to some of these constructs; for example, an individual who perceives risk in the website may also have an emotional reaction to it. For conciseness we did not include emotion as a factor in the model, but there is a possibility that emotion mediates the relationship between risk and trust. This question can be determined empirically in a future study. With respect to the subject population, we used students to represent the general adult population who seek well health information. Our student population is likely to have interests similar to other adults, for example, diet, weight, exercise, etc. Nevertheless, a broader population is needed. A future study should include a range of healthy adults, and the analysis should compare the differences of age, gender, education, and socioeconomic status. Finally, future work should consider the scope of tasks on an e-Health website. Tasks on e-health websites are normally information tasks, searching for desired information and evaluating the resulting information. Since our tasks were well health information tasks, we did not include users who search for information about ill health information. A study of ill health information is also needed. In particular, we want to find out whether ill patients perceive credibility, risk, and trust differently than healthy individuals.

IMPLICATIONS

The survey of trust research along with an overview of our research that has been presented in this chapter provides an indispensable foundation upon which future trust research in ehealth can be built. An essential insight is the recognition that the field of ehealth trust must move beyond descriptive research and into more experimental studies. This will allow for deeper and richer insights into the complex nature that ehealth trust likely has. Within this context, we see many directions online trust research in ehealth could take.

The general study of online trust of websites is, of course, of great importance as an umbrella theory. Its discovered principles are highly relevant to each of its different areas of application, ehealth included. However, most of the online trust research to date has been conducted in application areas that are *not* ehealth-specific. Thus, one avenue of future research would be replica-

tion of previous online trust work in the context of ehealth. As an example, our model of online trust and our measurement tool could be used to conduct a study that examines the role of trust in breast cancer survivors pursuing online health care information. The benefit of replication is two-fold. On the one hand, it allows applied research to move forward quickly since a tested methodology is already available, along with a tested model to confirm and a valid tool to employ. Replication studies can also help refine and fine-tune the model of online trust and the measurement tool in the context of ehealth. For example, perhaps the model will only explain 30% of the variance in website trust for patients who have breast cancer. Such a finding would open other variables for inspection regarding the nature of their trust, with a possible end result of refining the online trust model and tailoring it to different contexts. Ultimately, the unique characteristics of the ehealth application area deserve a rigorous look for the role they might play as a lens, through which to view the general principles of online trust of websites.

Another avenue of study is to develop new research questions that are relevant for trust in the context of ehealth. While this area could still make use of our trust model and measurement tool, like Gummerus and Liljander (2004), it can also begin to look at relationships between online trust and important ehealth outcomes. After all, in the end, ehealth trust is important because of the effect on outcomes it can produce. We can think of several interesting questions. Does online trust increase patient compliance with ehealth information? Does it increase engagement in treatment plans? Does it improve actual health or reduce health risk factors? These are interesting new questions that deserve exploration. In addition, the relationship between online trust and various outcomes may differ based on an assortment of aspects that pertain to the population under study. For example, gender, age, educational level, attitudes towards health care, finances, or insurance coverage may impact compliance with a treatment regime that is either online or that has online components. The type of infirmary, as well as severity and timeframe, i.e., newly diagnosed or chronic, may also impact the relationship between online trust and compliance with ehealth information. Poor access to health care, e.g., people with no health insurance or limited mobility to access health, may have to use online health resources as their sole contact with health information. How does their status affect the relationship between online trust and their use of the healthcare information, and perhaps differ from those in other groups? This is a potentially rich area of research. Indeed, the context in which the online ehealth resources are being used can go beyond a consumer orientation, evincing further questions. For example, the issue of trust is also important for health care providers and caregivers, as their interventions increasingly involve online methods.

A third, and significant, area for using and extending our trust model and measurement tool in the context of ehealth is the impact of social networking. This line of research wasn't even conceivable when we began to conduct online trust research in the late 1990s. Today there is a growing pervasiveness of social networking online. The underlying technologies, coined Web 2.0, may even lead to a new ehealth model, referred to as Health 2.0. Health 2.0 is the confluence of health care, online health information, and Web 2.0 technologies that encourage everyday people to actively interact with each other, build content, participate in online communities, and share information (Schreeve, 2007). As ehealth transitions from primarily passive access to increasingly active engagement, what are the implications for online trust? When people can interact online, share their health information, disease concerns and treatment experiences with each other around the world, what will be the role of online trust? Will the role of online trust reflect its role in non-social websites, or will it change? How can it be affected in a way that improves health and desired outcomes? Will other variables such as

nature of the disease, primacy, or well health vs. disease treatment nature affect the online trust of a person? These are all fascinating questions that researchers are just beginning to frame and explore.

Then there is the question of delivery. The term ehealth is an open term that does not specify delivery modality. So one area of interest might be mobility – will our model of online trust and measurement tool be applicable when ehealth is delivered via portable devices, anytime, anywhere? This question can get complicated when considering specific populations, environments, or contexts within ehealth. In developing nations, such mobility-facilitated health information and treatment may be the dominant delivery method for ehealth. Although current approaches to information delivery via hand-held devices and smart phones have sought to emulate the methods provided by Internet interfaces, this will not always be the case. Interesting investigations might pursue the degree to which factors of online trust enjoy a device-independent significance. How will the mobility and size characteristics of alternative delivery methods affect the requirements of users for trusted use. The simulation and visualization capabilities that some technologies now provide may drastically change some aspects of ehealth delivery. Will this render game consoles and tablet PCs a preferred medium for trusted health explanations, for instance? Another fertile area for new online trust research.

On the other side of the coin is the question of losing trust. If building trust is important in ehealth, what about breaking established trust? Most agree that while trust is hard to establish, it is easy to break (McKnight & Chervany, 2001). It has also been asserted that broken trust is extremely difficult to rebuild (Lewicki and Bunker, 1995). A classic illustration of this concept in relation to humans and technology was conducted by Lee and Moray (1992) in a study of human operators of automated equipment. They found that trust declined immediately and sharply after a fault.

Subsequently, in the absence of more faults, operators' trust in the automation recovered slowly to prior levels. Would this finding apply to trust in the context of ehealth? This is an open question; certainly knowing how to avoid breaking established trust in the context of ehealth is important.

Methodological questions also emerge from our investigations. Increased reliance on ehealth in the future will very likely impact an increasingly broader segment of the general population. This is something that online trust researchers must pursue. As ehealth continues to expand beyond websites that are purely informational, researchers can sample more widely. Perhaps new research methodologies will arise that are also online – i.e., eDataCollection. An example of this already in progress is research conducted by Gummerus and Liljander (2004). Their ehealth website offered their research survey to all users of the site (as part of the log-out process) during a specific period of four days. While research methodological issues exist surrounding the self-selection characteristics of their sample and loss of control of extraneous variables, e.g., length of time, we find this to be nevertheless an interesting, innovative means of gathering otherwise difficult to find data. Indeed, approaches like this would also foster another circumstance that we would view as an advance in the field, namely, enhanced relationships between researchers of ehealth issues and purveyors thereof.

Finally, in addition to health information websites, our research could be extended to studies that examine the role of online trust in ehealth systems such as health consultation websites (paid and free), health maintenance sites, insurance carriers' websites, electronic medical records system (EMR) interfaces, disease support group sites, and active health intervention systems such as those that monitor blood sugar or pacemakers. The degree to which our model of online trust might be applicable in any of the many facets of ehealth would definitely be of interest. It is our expectation that increased dependence on the World Wide Web for healthcare will witness an increase in the risk that users perceive is associated with that dependence. The demands it places on healthcare websites, in order to engender trust, remains to be seen.

CONCLUSION

ehealth can be effective only if patients can trust the health websites they access. As early research is showing, people will quickly leave a website if they are not able to easily find what they want or are not confident in its information. Healthcare information is too risky to get wrong or do shoddily. It can be a matter of life and death. For this reason, perhaps no other online trust research is as important as that rooted in ehealth.

The overall intention of this chapter was to examine the nature of online trust. We hope that you have achieved the three goals we had for you. First, after reading this chapter, that you possess a knowledge base about the state of trust research in general, as well as the current state of online trust and its state within ehealth. Second, that you have an understanding of our validated online trust model and measurement tool that provides a framework and understanding of three factors (perceived ease of use, credibility and risk) that appear to explain a high percentage of trust in websites. Third, that your curiosity and imagination have been stimulated to consider the rich variety of research questions that revolve around understanding trust in the context of ehealth.

REFERENCES

Baker, L., Wagner, T., Singer, S., & Bundorf, K. (2003). Use of the Internet and e-mail for health care information: Results from a national survey. *Journal of the American Medical Association*, *289*, 2400–2406. doi:10.1001/jama.289.18.2400

Barber, B. (1983). *The Logic and Limits of Trust*. New Brunswick, NJ: Rutgers University Press.

Barney, J., & Hansen, M. (1994). Trustworthiness as a source of competitive advantage. *Strategic Management Journal*, *15*, 175–190. doi:10.1002/smj.4250150912

Becker, S. (2004). A study of web usability for older adults seeking online health resources. *ACM Transactions on Computer-Human Interaction*, (April): 11, 387–406.

Belanger, F., Hiller, J., & Smith, W. (2002). Trustworthiness in electronic commerce: the role of privacy, security, and site attributes. *The Journal of Strategic Information Systems*, *11*(3&4), 245–270. doi:10.1016/S0963-8687(02)00018-5

Bhattacherjee, A. (2002). Individual trust in online firms: Scale development and initial test. *Journal of Management Information Systems*, *19*(1), 211–241.

Blois, K. J. (1999). Trust in business to business relationships: an evaluation of its status. *Journal of Management Studies*, *36*(2), 197–215. doi:10.1111/1467-6486.00133

Bos, N., Olson, J., Gergle, D., Olson, G., & Wright, Z. (2002). *Effects of four computer-mediated communications channels on trust development. Proceedings of Human Factors in Computing Systems. CHI2002* (pp. 135–140). ACM.

Brenkert, G. G. (1998). Trust, morality and international business. *Business Ethics Quarterly*, *8*(2), 293–317. doi:10.2307/3857330

Briggs, P., Burford, B., DeAngeli, A., & Lunch, P. (2002). Trust in online advice. [March.]. *Social Science Computer Review*, *20*, 321–334.

Buskens, V. (1998). The social structure of trust. *Social Networks*, *20*(3), 265–289. doi:10.1016/S0378-8733(98)00005-7

Cheskin Research & Studio Archetype/Sapient. (1999). *Ecommerce trust study*. Retrieved May 5, 2007 from http://www.sapient.com/cheskin.

Corbitt, B. J., Thanasankit, T., & Yi, H. (2003). Trust and ecommerce: a study of consumer perceptions. *Electronic Commerce Research and Applications*, *2*, 203–215. doi:10.1016/S1567-4223(03)00024-3

Corritore, C., Kracher, B., & Wiedenbeck, S. (2003). On-line trust: concepts, evolving themes, a model. *International Journal of Human-Computer Studies*, *58*, 737–758. doi:10.1016/S1071-5819(03)00041-7

Dasgupta, P. (1988). Trust as a commodity. In Gambetta, D. (Ed.), *Trust: Making and Breaking Cooperative Relations* (pp. 49–72). New York: Basil Blackwell.

Davis, F. (1989). Perceived usefulness, perceived ease of use and user acceptance of information technology. *Management Information Systems Quarterly*, *13*(3), 319–340. doi:10.2307/249008

Davis, F., Bagozzi, R., & Warshaw, P. (1989). User acceptance of computer technology: A comparison of two theoretical models. *Management Science*, *35*(8), 982–1003. doi:10.1287/mnsc.35.8.982

Davis, R., Buchanan-Oliver, M., & Brodie, R. (1999). Relationship marketing in electronic commerce environments. *Journal of Information Technology*, *14*, 319–331. doi:10.1080/026839699344449

Denning, P., Horning, J., Parnas, D., & Weinstein, L. (2005). Wikipedia risks. *CACM*, *48*, 152.

Deutsch, M. (1958). Trust and suspicion. *Conflict Resolution*, *2*(4), 265–279. doi:10.1177/002200275800200401

Deutsch, M. (1962). Cooperation and trust: Some theoretical notes. *Nebraska Symposium on Motivation. Nebraska Symposium on Motivation*, *10*, 275–318.

Doney, P. & Canon, J. (1997). An examination of the nature of trust in buyer-seller relationships. *Journal of Marketing*, February, 61, 35-51.

Einwiller, S. (2003). When reputation engenders trust: An empirical investigation in business-to-consumer electronic commerce. *Electronic Markets*, (March): 13, 196–209.

Erickson, E. G. (1963). *Childhood and Society*. New York: W.W. Norton.

Fishbein, M., & Ajzen, I. (1975). *Belief, Attitude, Intention and Behavior: An Introduction to Theory and Research*. Reading, MA: Addison-Wesley Publishing Company.

Fogg, B., Marshall, J., Kameda, T., Solomon, J., Rangnekar, A., Body, J., & Brown, B. (2001). Web credibility research: A method for online experiments and early study results. *Proceedings of Human Factors in Computing Systems*, CHI2001, ACM, 295-296.

Fogg, B., Marshall, J., Laraki, O., Osipovich, A., Varma, C., Fang, N., et al. (2001). What makes web sites credible? A report on a large quantitative study. *Proceedings of the Conference on Human Factors in Computing Systems* CHI 2001, ACM, 3(1), 61-8.

Fogg, B., Marshall, J., Laraki, O., Osipovich, A., Varma, C., Fang, N., et al. (2001) What makes web sites credible? A report on a large quantitative study, in *Proceedings of the Conference on Human Factors in Computing Systems CHI 2001*, 61-68. New York: ACM Press.

Fogg, B., Osipovich, A., Varma, C., Laraki, O., Fang, N., Paul, J., et al. (2000). Elements that affect web credibility: Early results form a self-reported study. *Proceedings of the 2000 Conference on Designing for User Experiences*, CHI 2000, ACM, 287-288.

Fogg, B., Soohoo, C., Danielson, D. R., Marable, L., Stanford, J., & Tauber, E. R. (2003). How do users evaluate the credibility of web sites? A study with over 2500 participants. *Proceedings of the 2003 Conference on Designing for User Experiences*, ACM, 1-15.

Fogg, B. & Tseng, H. (1999). The elements of computer credibility. *Proceedings of Human Factors in Computing Systems*, CHI1999, ACM, 80-87.

Fox, S., & Jones, S. (2009). *The social life of health information: Americans' pursuit of health takes place within a widening network of both online and offline sources*. PEW Report. Retrieved December 15, 2009 from http://www.pewInternet.org/Reports/2009/8-The-Social-Life-of-Health-Information.aspx.

Friedman, B., Kahn, P. H., & Howe, D. C. (2000). Trust online. *Communications of the ACM*, *43*(12), 34–40. doi:10.1145/355112.355120

Fromkin, H. L., & Streufert, S. (1976). Laboratory experimentation. In Dunnette, B. (Ed.), *Handbook of Industrial and Organizational Psychology* (pp. 415–465). Chicago: Rand McNally College Publishing Company.

Ganesen, S. (1994). Determinants of long-term orientation in buyer-seller relationship. *Journal of Marketing*, *58*, 1–19. doi:10.2307/1252265

Garfinkel, H. (1963). A conception of, and experiments with, 'Trust' as a condition of stable concerted actions. In Harvey, O. J. (Ed.), *Motivation and Social Interaction: Cognitive Determinants* (pp. 187–238). New York: Ronald Press.

Gefen, D. (2000). Ecommerce: The role of familiarity and trust. *Omega*, *28*(6), 725–737. doi:10.1016/S0305-0483(00)00021-9

Gefen, D., Karahanna, E., & Straub, D. (2003a). Inexperience and experience with online stores: The importance of TAM and trust. *IEEE Transactions on Engineering Management*, *50*(3), 307–321. doi:10.1109/TEM.2003.817277

Gefen, D., Karahanna, E., & Straub, D. (2003b). Trust and TAM in online shopping: an integrated model. *Management Information Systems Quarterly, 27*(1), 51–90.

Gefen, D. & Straub, D. (2003). Managing user trust in B2C e-services. *e-Service Journal,* 7-24.

Giddens, A. (1990). *The Consequences of Modernity.* Cambridge, U.K.: Polity Press.

Giffen, K. (1967). The contribution of studies of source credibility to a theory of inter-personal trust in the communications process. [February.]. *Psychological Bulletin, 68,* 104–120. doi:10.1037/h0024833

Good, D. (1988). Individuals, interpersonal relations, and trust. In Gambetta, D. (Ed.), *Trust: Making and Breaking Cooperative Relations* (pp. 32–47). New York: Basil Blackwell.

Grazioli, S., & Jarvenpaa, S. L. (2000). Perils of Internet fraud: An empirical investigation of deception and trust with experienced Internet consumers. *IEEE Transactions on Systems, Man, and Cybernetics, 30*(4), 395–410. doi:10.1109/3468.852434

Gummerus, J., & Liljander, V. (2004). Customer loyalty to content-based Web sites: The case of an online health-care service. *Journal of Services Marketing, 18*(2/3), 175–186. doi:10.1108/08876040410536486

Harris, L. C., & Goode, M. M. H. (2004). The four levels of loyalty and the pivotal role of trust: A study of online service dynamics. *Journal of Retailing, 80,* 139–158. doi:10.1016/j.jretai.2004.04.002

Hong, T. (2006). The influence of structural ad message features on web site credibility. [January.]. *Journal of the American Society for Information Science and Technology, 57,* 114–127. doi:10.1002/asi.20258

Impicciatore, P., Pandolfini, C., Casella, N., & Bonzti, M. (1997). Reliability of health information for the public on the World Wide Web: Systematic survey of advice on managing fever in children at home. *British Medical Journal, 314,* 1875–1881.

Jarvenpaa, S., Tractinsky, N., & Vitale, M. (2000). Consumer trust in Internet store. *Information Technology Management, 1*(1-2), 45–71. doi:10.1023/A:1019104520776

Jarvenpaa, S. L., Tractinsky, N., & Saarinen, L. (1999). Consumer trust in an Internet store: A cross-cultural validation. *Journal of Computer-Mediated Communication 5*(2). Retrieved on March 3, 2010 at http://www.ascusc.org/jcmc/vol5/issue2.

Jenkins, C., Corritore, C., & Wiedenbeck, S. (2003). Patterns of information seeking on the web: A qualitative study of domain expertise and web expertise. *Information Technology & Society, 1*(3), 64–89.

Johnson, K., & Wiedenbeck, S. (2009). Enhancing perceived credibility of citizen journalism web sites. *Journalism & Mass Communication Quarterly, 86*(2), 332–348.

Johnson-George, C., & Swap, W. (1982). Measurement of specific interpersonal trust: Construction and validation of a scale to assess trust in a specific other. *Journal of Personality and Social Psychology, 43*(6), 1306–1317. doi:10.1037/0022-3514.43.6.1306

Kao, A., Gree, D., Zaslavsky, A., Koplan, J., & Cleary, P. (1998). The relationship between method of physician payment and patient trust. *Journal of the American Medical Association, 280,* 1708–1715. doi:10.1001/jama.280.19.1708

Kee, H., & Knox, R. (1970). Conceptual and methodological considerations in the study of trust and suspicion. *Conflict Resolution, 14*(3), 357–366. doi:10.1177/002200277001400307

Kim, D. J., & Ferrin, D. L. (2009). Trust and satisfaction, two stepping stones for successful ecommerce relationships: A longitudinal exploration. *Information Systems Research, 20*(2), 237–257. doi:10.1287/isre.1080.0188

Kim, D. J., Song, Y., Braynov, S. B., & Rao, H. R. (2001). A B-to-C trust model for on-line exchange. *Proceedings for the Seventh Americas Conference on Information Systems*, 784-787.

Kim, H., Xu, Y., & Koh, J. (2004). A comparison of online trust building factors between potential customers and repeat customers. *Journal of the Association for Information Systems*, (October): 5, 392–420.

Kim, J., & Moon, J. Y. (1998). Designing towards emotional usability in customer interfaces-trustworthiness of cyber-banking system interfaces. *Interacting with Computers, 10*(1), 1–29. doi:10.1016/S0953-5438(97)00037-4

Kim, S., & Stoel, L. (2004). Apparel retailers: Website quality dimensions and satisfaction. *Journal of Retailing and Consumer Services, 11*(2), 109–117. doi:10.1016/S0969-6989(03)00010-9

Kisely, S. (2002). Treatments for chronic fatigue syndrome and the Internet: a systematic survey of what your patients are reading. *The Australian and New Zealand Journal of Psychiatry, 36*, 240–245. doi:10.1046/j.1440-1614.2002.01017.x

Klein, H. K., & Myers, M. D. (1999). A set of principles for conducting and evaluating interpretive field studies in information systems. *Management Information Systems Quarterly, 23*(1), 67–93. doi:10.2307/249410

Koehn, D. (2003). The nature of and conditions for online trust. *Journal of Business Ethics, 43*, 3–19. doi:10.1023/A:1022950813386

Larzelere, R. E., & Huston, T. L. (1980). The dyadic trust scale: Toward understanding interpersonal trust in close relationships. *Journal of Marriage and the Family*, (Aug): 595–604. doi:10.2307/351903

Lau, G. T., & Sook, H. L. (1999). Consumers' trust in a brand and the link to brand loyalty. *Journal of Market Focused Management, 4*, 341–370. doi:10.1023/A:1009886520142

Lee, J., Kim, J. & Moon, J. (2000). What makes Internet users visit cyber stores again? Key design factors for customer loyalty. *Proceedings of Human Factors in Computing Systems,* CHI2000, ACM, 305-312.

Lee, J., & Moray, N. (1992). Trust, control strategies and allocation of function in human-machine systems. *Ergonomics, 35*(10), 1243–1270. doi:10.1080/00140139208967392

Lee, M. K. O., & Turban, E. (2001). A trust model for consumer Internet shopping. *International Journal of Electronic Commerce, 6*(1), 75–91.

Lewicki, R. J., & Bunker, B. (1996). Developing and maintaining trust in work relationships. In Kramer, R., & Tyler, T. (Eds.), *Trust in Organizations: Frontiers of Theory and Research* (pp. 114–139). Newbury Park, CA: Sage.

Lewicki, R. J., & Bunker, B. B. (1995). Trust in relationships: A model of development and decline. In B.B. Bunker & J.Z. Rubin (Eds.), *Conflict, Cooperation, and Justice: Essays Inspired by the Work of Morton Deutsch* (pp. 133-173). San Fransicso: Jossey-Bass.

Lewis, D., & Weigert, A. (1985). Trust as a social reality. *Social Forces, 63*(4), 967–985. doi:10.2307/2578601

Luhmann, N. (1979). *Trust and Power*. Chichester, UK: Wiley.

Luo, W., & Najdawi, M. (2004). Trust-building measures: A review of consumer health portals. *Communications of the ACM, 47,* 108–113. doi:10.1145/962081.962089

Macy, M. W., & Skvoretz, J. (1998). The evolution of trust and cooperation between strangers: A computational model. *American Sociological Review, 63*(10), 638–660. doi:10.2307/2657332

Marcus, M. L. (1983). Power, politics, and MIS implementation. *Communications of the ACM, 26,* 430–444. doi:10.1145/358141.358148

Mayer, R. C., Davis, J. H., & Schoorman, F. D. (1995). An integrative model of organizational trust. *Academy of Management Review, 20*(3), 709–734. doi:10.2307/258792

McKnight, D., & Chervaney, N. (2001). Trust and distrust definitions: One bit at a time. In Falcone, R., Singh, M., & Tan, Y. (Eds.), *Trust in Cybersocieties* (pp. 27–54). Berlin: Springer-Verlag. doi:10.1007/3-540-45547-7_3

McKnight, D., Choudhury, V., & Kacmar, C. (2000). Trust in ecommerce vendors: A two-stage model. *Proceedings of the Twenty First International Conference on Information Systems,* 532-536.

McKnight, D., Choudhury, V., & Kacmar, C. (2002a). The impact of initial consumer trust on intentions to transact with a web site: A trust building model. *The Journal of Strategic Information Systems, 11,* 297–323. doi:10.1016/S0963-8687(02)00020 3

McKnight, D., Choudhury, V., & Kacmar, C. (2002b). Developing and validating trust measures for ecommerce: An integrative typology. *Information Systems Research,* (March): 13, 334–359.

McKnight, D. H., & Chervany, N. L. (2000). What is trust? A conceptual analysis and an interdisciplinary model. In Chung, M. H. (Ed.), *Proceedings of the Americas Conference on Information Systems,* August, 2000, (pp. 827-833). Long Beach, California.

McKnight, D. H., & Kacmar, C. J. (2007). Factors and effect of information credibility. *Proceedings of the ninth international conference on Electronic commerce,* ICEC2007, ACM, 423-432.

Mechanic, D. (2004). In my chosen doctor I trust. *British Medical Journal, 329*(7480), 1418–1419. doi:10.1136/bmj.329.7480.1418

Meyerson, D., Weick, K. E., & Kramer, R. M. (1996). Swift trust and temporary groups. In Kramer, R. M., & Tyler, T. R. (Eds.), *Trust in Organizations: Frontiers of Theory and Research* (pp. 166–195). Thousand Oaks, CA: Sage Publications.

Milne, G. R., & Boza, M.-E. (1999). Trust and concern in consumers' perceptions of marketing information management practices. *Journal of Interactive Marketing, 13*(1), 5–24. doi:10.1002/(SICI)1520-6653(199924)13:1<5::AID-DIR2>3.0.CO;2-9

Misztal, B. A. (1996). *Trust in Modern Societies: The Search for the Bases of Social Order.* New York: Polity Press.

Mohan, J. (2004). Health attitudes, health cognitions, and health behaviors among Internet health information seekers: Population-based survey, *Journal of Medical Internet Research,* vol. 6. Retrieved January 14, 2009 from http://www.jmir.org/.

Morgan, R. M., & Hunt, S. D. (1994). The commitment-trust theory of relationship marketing. *Journal of Marketing, 58,* 20–38. doi:10.2307/1252308

Muir, B. M., & Moray, N. (1996). Trust in automation: Part II, Experimental studies of trust and human intervention in a process control simulation. *Ergonomics*, *39*(3), 429–460. doi:10.1080/00140139608964474

Nass, C., Fogg, B. J., & Moon, Y. (1996). Can computers be teammates? *International Journal of Human-Computer Studies*, *45*, 669–678. doi:10.1006/ijhc.1996.0073

Nguyen, D. & Canny, J. (2007). MultiView: Improving trust in group video conferencing through spatial faithfulness. *Proceedings of Human Factors in Computing Systems*, CHI 2007, ACM, 1465-1474.

Nielsen, J., Molich, R., Snyder, C., & Farrell, S. (2000) E-commerce user experience: trust. Fremont, CA, USA, Nielsen NormanGroup, http://www.nngroup.com/reports/ecommerce, accessed 3/2001.

Olson, G., & Olson, J. (2000a). Distance matters. *Human-Computer Interaction*, *15*(2&3), 139–178. doi:10.1207/S15327051HCI1523_4

Olson, J., & Olson, G. (2000b). i2i trust in ecommerce. *Communications of the ACM*, *43*(12), 41–44. doi:10.1145/355112.355121

Orlikowski, W., & Baroudi, J. (1991). Studying information technology in organizations: Research approaches and assumptions. *Information Systems Research*, *2*(1), 1–28. doi:10.1287/isre.2.1.1

Pavlou, P. (2001). Integrating trust in electronic commerce with the technology acceptance model: Model development and validations. *Proceedings of the Seventh Americas Conference on Information Systems, Association of Information Systems*, 816-822.

Pew Internet Research. (2002).Vital decisions: How Internet users decide what information to trust when they or their loved ones are sick. Retrieved November 22, 2008 from http://www.pewInternet.org.

Putnam, R. D. (1995). Bowling alone: America's declining social capital. *Journal of Democracy*, *6*(1), 3–10. doi:10.1353/jod.1995.0002

Ratnasingam, P., & Pavlov, P. (2003). Technology trust in Internet-based interorganizational electronic commerce. *Journal of Electronic Commerce in Organizations*, *1*(1), 17–41.

Reeves, B., & Nass, C. (1996). *The Media Equation: How People Treat Computers, Television, and New Media Like Real People and Places*. California: CSLI Publications and Cambridge: Cambridge University Press.

Ribbink, D., van Riel, A., Liljander, V., & Streukens, S. (2004). Comfort your online customer: Quality, trust and loyalty on the Internet. *Managing Service Quality*, *16*(6), 446–456. doi:10.1108/09604520410569784

Riegelsberger, J., & Sasse, M. (2001) Trust builders and trustbusters: the role of trust cues in interfaces to e-commerce applications, in *Towards the E-Society: Proceedings of the First IFIP Conference on E-Commerce, E-Society, and E-Government*,17-30.London: Kluwer.

Riegersberger, J., Sasse, M., & McCarthy, J. (2003). Shiny happy people building trust? Photos on e-commrece websites and consumer trust. *Proceedings of Human Factors in Computing Systems*, CHI2003, ACM, 1465-1474.

Riegersberger, J., Sasse, M., & McCarthy, J. (2005). Rich media: Poor judgments? A study of media effects on users' trust in expertise. *Proceedings of the British HCI Conference*, British Computer Society, 267-284.

Rippen, H. (1999). Criteria for assessing the quality of health information on the Internet. *Health Summit Working Group*, Retrieved November 24, 2009 from http://hitiweb.mitretek.org/docs/policy.html.

Rotter, J. (1967). A new scale for the measurement of interpersonal trust. *Journal of Personality, 35*, 651–665. doi:10.1111/j.1467-6494.1967.tb01454.x

Rotter, J. (1971). Generalized expectancies for interpersonal trust. *The American Psychologist, 26*, 443–452. doi:10.1037/h0031464

Rotter, J. (1980). Interpersonal trust, trustworthiness, and gullibility. *The American Psychologist, 35*(1), 1–7. doi:10.1037/0003-066X.35.1.1

Salam, A., Rao, H., & Pegels, C. (2001). Consumer-perceived risk in ecommerce transactions. *Communications of the ACM*, (December): 46, 325–331.

Schumm, W., Bugaighis, M., Buckler, D., Green, D., & Scanton, E. (1985). Construct validity of the dyadic trust scale. *Psychological Reports, 56*, 1001–1002.

Semmes, C. (1991). Developing trust: Patient-practitioner encounters in natural health care. *Journal of Contemporary Ethnography, 19*, 450–470. doi:10.1177/089124191019004004

Shapiro, D. L., Sheppard, B. H., & Cheraskin, L. (1992). Business on a handshake. *Negotiation Journal, 8*(4), 365–377. doi:10.1111/j.1571-9979.1992.tb00679.x

Shreeve, S. (2007). http://scottshreeve.blogspot.com. Retrieved on December 31, 2009.

Sillence, E., Briggs, P., Fishwick, L., & Harris, P. (2004). Trust and mistrust of online health sites. *Proceedings of the Conference on Human Factors in Computing Systems* CHI 2004. New York: ACM Press.

Sillence, E., Briggs, P., Harris, P., & Fishwick, L. (2007). Health websites that people can trust – the case of hypertension. *Interacting with Computers, 19*(1), 32–42. doi:10.1016/j.intcom.2006.07.009

Snijders, C., & Keren, G. (1999). Determinants of trust. In Budescu, D.V., Erev, I., Zwick, R. (Eds.) *Games and Human Behavior: Essays in Honor of Amnon Rapoport*(355-383). Mahwah, NJ: Lawrence Erlbaum.

Solomon, R., & Flores, F. (2001). *Building Trust in Business, Politics, Relationships, and Life*. New York: Oxford University Press.

Stanford, J., Tauber, E., Fogg, H., & Marable, L. (2003). Experts vs. online consumers: A comparative credibility study of health and finance Web sites. *Consumer WebWatch Research Report*, Retrieved May 20, 2007 from http://www.consumerwebwatch.org/dynamic/web-credibility-reports-experts-vs-online-abstract.cfm.

Steinbrück, U., Schaumburg, H., Duda, S., & Krüger, T. (2002) A picture says more than a thousand words – photographs as trust builders in e-commerce websites, in *Proceedings of Conference on Human Factors in Computing Systems CHI 2002, Extended Abstracts*, 748-749. New York: ACM Press

Thom, D., & Campbell, B. (1997). Patient-physician trust: an exploratory study. *The Journal of Family Practice, 44*, 169–177.

Thorne, S., & Robinson, C. (1998). Reciprocal trust in health care relationships. *Journal of Advanced Nursing, 13*, 782–789. doi:10.1111/j.1365-2648.1988.tb00570.x

Urban, G., Sultan, F., & Qualls, W. (1998). Trust-based marketing on the Internet. *MIT Sloan School of Management Working Paper* #4035-98.

Walsham, G., & Waema, T. (1994). Information systems strategy and implementation: A case study of a building society. *ACM Transactions on Information Systems, 12*(2), 150–173. doi:10.1145/196734.196744

Walther, J., Pingree, S., Hawkins, R., & Buller, D. (2005). Attributes of interactive online health information systems. *Journal of Medical Internet Research,* March, *7,* Retrieved December 4, 2008 from http://www.jmir.org.

Wathen, C., & Burkell, J. (2002). Believe it or not: Factors influencing credibility on the web. *Journal of the American Society for Information Science and Technology, 53,* 134–144. doi:10.1002/asi.10016

Werbler, C., & Harris, C. (2009). *Consumers pay little or no attention to drug company's advertised risk disclosures.* Retrieved on December 21, 2009 from http://www.orcguideline.com/about_us_news.aspx.

Yoon, C., & Kim, S. (2009). Developing the causal model of online store success. *Journal of Organizational Computing and Electronic Commerce, 19*(4), 265. doi:10.1080/10919390903262644

Zajonc, R. B. (1980). Feeling and thinking: Preferences need no inferences. *The American Psychologist, 35*(2), 151–175. doi:10.1037/0003-066X.35.2.151

Zand, D. E. (1972). *Trust and managerial problem solving.* Administrative Science.

ADDITIONAL READING

Becker, S. (2004). A study of web usability for older adults seeking online health resources. *ACM Transactions on Computer-Human Interaction,* (April): 11, 387–406.

Corritore, C. L., Kracher, B., & Wiedenbeck, S. (2003). Online trust: concepts, evolving themes. *International Journal of Human-Computer Studies, 58*(6), 737–758. doi:10.1016/S1071-5819(03)00041-7

Corritore, C. L., Marble, R. P., Wiedenbeck, S., Kracher, B., & Chandran, A. (2005). Measuring online trust of websites: credibility, perceived ease of use, and risk. *Proceedings of the Eleventh Americas Conference on Information Systems, Omaha, NE, USA August 11th-14th 2005, 2419-2427.*

Fogg, B. J. (2003). *Prominence-interpretation theory: Explaining how people assess credibility online. Proceedings of CHI'03,* Extended Abstracts on Human Factors in Computing Systems, 722-723.

Gefen, D. (2000). Ecommerce: The role of familiarity and trust. *Omega, 28*(6), 725–737. doi:10.1016/S0305-0483(00)00021-9

Grazioli, S., & Jarvenpaa, S. L. (2000). Perils of Internet fraud: an empirical investigation of deception and trust with experienced Internet consumers. *IEEE Transactions on Systems, Man, and Cybernetics, 30*(4), 395–410. doi:10.1109/3468.852434

Hoffman, D. L., Novak, T. P., & Peralta, M. (1999). Building consumer trust online. *Communications of the ACM, 42*(4), 80–86. doi:10.1145/299157.299175

Jenkins, C., Corritore, C. L., & Wiedenbeck, S. (2003). Patterns of information seeking on the web: A qualitative study of domain expertise and web expertise. *IT and Society, 1*(3), 64–80.

Kracher, B., Corritore, C. L., & Wiedenbeck, S. (2005). A foundation for understanding online trust in electronic commerce. *Journal of Information. Communication and Ethics in Society, 3,* 131–141. doi:10.1108/14779960580000267

McKnight, D. H., & Kacmar, C. J. (2007). Factors and effect of information credibility. Proceedings of the ninth international conference on Electronic commerce. *ICEC2007,* pp. 423-432. New York: ACM

Pew Internet Research. (2002).*Vital decisions: How Internet users decide what information to trust when they or their loved ones are sick.* Retrieved November 22, 2008 from http://www.pewInternet.org.

Ridings, C. M., Gefen, D., & Arinze, B. (2002). Some antecedents and effects of trust in virtual communities. *The Journal of Strategic Information Systems, 11*(3-4), 271–295. doi:10.1016/S0963-8687(02)00021-5

Riegelsberger, J., Sasse, M., & McCarthy, J. D. (2005). The mechanics of trust: A framework for research and design. *International Journal of Human-Computer Studies, 62*(3), 381–422. doi:10.1016/j.ijhcs.2005.01.001

Sillence, E., Briggs, P., Fishwick, L., & Harris, P. (2006). A framework for understanding trust factors in web-based health advice. *International Journal of Human-Computer Studies, 64,* 697–713. doi:10.1016/j.ijhcs.2006.02.007

Sillence, E., Briggs, P., Harris, P., & Fishwick, L. (2006). Going online for health advice: Changes in usage and trust practices over the last five years. *Interacting with Computers, 19*(3), 32–42.

Thorne, S., & Robinson, C. (1998). Reciprocal trust in health care relationships. *Journal of Advanced Nursing, 13,* 782–789. doi:10.1111/j.1365-2648.1988.tb00570.x

KEY TERMS AND DEFINITIONS

Online Trust: Trust in the context of websites and users on the Internet.

Trust: Attitude of confident expectation toward an object of trust in a context of risk.

Health Care: Prevention, Management, Treatment of illness.

ehealth: Health care processes supported by digital technologies.

Websites: Set of inter-connected webpages accessed over the Internet via a browser.

Credibility: Capable of being believed; antecedent of online trust.

Ease-of-Use: Capable of being learned and used easily.

Risk: Exposure to the chance of loss or injury; antecedent of online trust.

Chapter 4
A Multi–Disciplinary Approach to Ambient Assisted Living

Martina Ziefle
RWTH Aachen University, Germany

Carsten Röcker
RWTH Aachen University, Germany

Wiktoria Wilkowska
RWTH Aachen University, Germany

Kai Kasugai
RWTH Aachen University, Germany

Lars Klack
RWTH Aachen University, Germany

Christian Möllering
RWTH Aachen University, Germany

Shirley Beul
RWTH Aachen University, Germany

ABSTRACT

This chapter illustrates the different disciplinary design challenges of smart healthcare systems and presents an interdisciplinary approach toward the development of an integrative Ambient Assisted Living environment. Within the last years a variety of new healthcare concepts for supporting and assisting users in technology-enhanced environments emerged. While such smart healthcare systems can help to minimize hospital stays and in so doing enable patients an independent life in a domestic environment, the complexity of such systems raises fundamental questions of behavior, communication and technology acceptance. The first part of the chapter describes the research challenges encountered in the fields of medical engineering, computer science, psychology, communication science, and architecture as well as their consequences for the design, use and acceptance of smart healthcare systems. The second part of the chapter shows how these disciplinary challenges were addressed within the eHealth project, an interdisciplinary research project at RWTH Aachen University.

DOI: 10.4018/978-1-60960-469-1.ch004

INTRODUCTION

The increased life expectancy and improved general health states of citizens in most western countries will inevitably result in more and more elderly people requiring medical care in the near future (Wittenberg et al., 2006). At the same time, considerable bottlenecks arise from the fact that increasingly fewer people are present, who may take over the nursing (Leonhardt, 2005). In order to master the requirements of an aging society, innovations in information and communication as well as medical engineering technologies come to the fore, which offer novel or improved medical diagnosis, therapy, treatments and rehabilitation possibilities (Weiner et al., 2003; Warren & Craft, 1999). Though, recent research shows that acceptance barriers are prevalent, which might be due to the fact that development praxis predominately focuses on technical feasibility, while the "human factor" in these systems is fairly underdeveloped. In order to fully exploit the potential of e-health applications, acceptance and usability issues of e-health applications need to be considered, especially for older users, who have specific needs and requirements regarding usability and acceptance issues (Melenhorst et al., 2006; Arning & Ziefle, 2009; Zimmer & Chappell, 1999). As the knowledge about the antecedents of e-health acceptance and utilization behavior is restricted, it is necessary to explore the acceptance and fit of e-health technologies within homes and private spheres (Wilkowska & Ziefle, 2009; Gaul & Ziefle, 2009; Röcker & Feith, 2009).

DISCIPLINARY CHALLENGES

The following sections outline the research challenges encountered in the fields of medical engineering, computer science, psychology, communication science, and architecture as well as their consequences for the design, use and acceptance of smart healthcare systems.

Medical Engineering

Major changes in the demographic and social structure of most western countries bring up new challenges, not only for the health care systems in general, but also for the development of new medical technologies. In such an aging society, where medical progress leads to a considerably increased life expectancy, age-related chronic diseases require constant medical assistance by a new generation of medical care equipment (Röcker et al., 2010). In situations, where patients cannot be treated in institutional setting alone anymore, individual and personalized care in the patients' home environment plays a more and more important role (Ziefle et al., 2009).

Those technologies and devices have to provide the essential, established attributes of today's medical devices, to be *functional, safe and reliable*, but furthermore in the future they also have to be *mobile* (can be used in professional and home environments), *adaptive* (can be run by patients and professionals) and *ergonomic* (easy to use and accepted by users). To implement those new aspects in medicine technology is a great challenge because most medical devices influence the patients´ health in a direct way and are highly critical in terms of patient safety. The decentralized application of such devices puts users in the centre of attention and it will give them a high degree of independency and self-control of the therapy, but also a high degree of responsibility.

The most important modification in the development approaches in the field of medical engineering is to include the user actively in the design process. A coherent user-centered design of medical devices will result in a medical technology, which is not only functional in an engineering way of thinking, but also addresses fundamental user needs in terms of appearance, ease of use and privacy.

Especially medical assistance devices for the elderly are often perceived to be stigmatizing and therefore not used efficiently. One example is the

Figure 1. Unobtrusive measurement of vital parameter through embedded sensor technologies

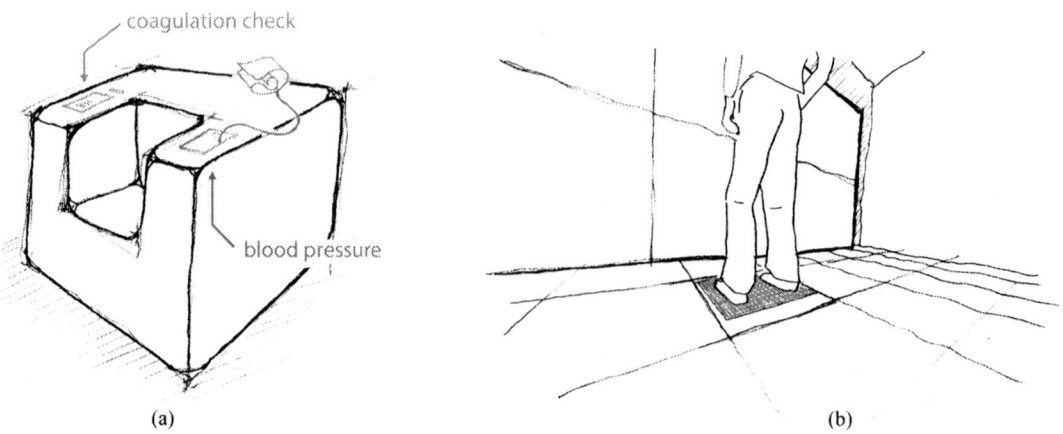

(a)

(b)

emergency button, which is supposed to be used by fragile patients in case of an emergency event (e.g., fall) where external help is required (Beul et al., under revision; Klack et al., under revision). Most of the users don't carry that device with them because it marks them as *diseased* or *dependent*. Another example is rehabilitation therapy, where the therapy success is often decelerated because patients do not want to wear medical equipment in public or even at home because they feel stigmatized. But even in life critical situations patients sometimes decide against the implantation of a medical device because their fear of a loss of control or independency is to high. In the light of these problems, a user-centered design approach bears a high potential for the optimization of therapy compliance and overall therapy success.

With a focus on an aging society, one of the most striking challenges for medical engineers is to develop medical support devices for the needs of the elderly, and especially for chronically diseased people in their home environments. The development of sensor devices, which can monitor the patients vital data, identify emergency situations, as well as discover slow changes or trends in the patients health state and give preventive advise is promising. In order to achieve a broad user acceptance and even a desire for those systems

within the population, it is necessary to take hedonic aspects into account when it comes to the integration of sensor devices into existing home environments. The sensors should be primarily invisible and passive, while the results of the processed data can be provided in a way that was previously customized by the user. In many cases, a passive and even invisible measurement is possible (e.g., temperature, weight, movement behavior, see Figure 1 left), while it is inevitable that other cases the medical sensor devices remain visible (e.g., blood pressure measurement, pulse, coagulation measurement, see Figure 1, right). In those cases, higher acceptance can be achieved by a device design, which includes usability aspects and hedonic components from the very beginning. In that way a medical device can turn into something that patients are proud to wear or to possess, just like a watch or a mobile phone, which are also assistive devices in a persons` daily life.

Computer Science

Middleware

Many devices of our everyday life are equipped with processors. In special technical environments or in the field of mobile phones you can find

Figure 2. Conceptual design of the middleware framework

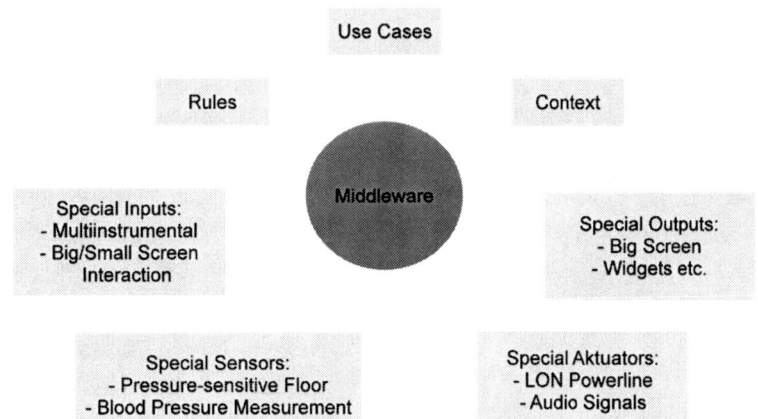

some specific communication, but in broad areas inter-device communication is not taking place (Bottaro & Gérodolle, 2008). In order actively support people in their homes integrated sensors and actuators have to communicate intensively, giving the system context information on what is going on. This task is a huge challenge in technical sense. Within the context of our project, we do not only look at the technical integration of different devices, spatial sensors, multimedia, personal and medical devices, but also on the usability and acceptance of smart homecare applications based on these new systems (Röcker et al., 2010).

One of the main goals of our investigations is the generation of reliable context. While a considerable amount of work has been done on context awareness, usability aspects are largely unexplored due to their tremendous complexity (Ye et al., 2008). Furthermore, capturing and aggregating personal data could lead to serious privacy infringements, especially in home environments, which are traditionally perceived as very private places (Armac et al., 2009; Röcker & Feith, 2009). Thus, the integration of privacy aspects in context-adapted frameworks is another focus of our work.

As a precondition of further steps, the contextual data of all input devices has to be integrated

on a middleware platform. Besides the OSGi-based *OpenAAL* platform, which has been developed in the *SOPRANO* project (Wolf et al., 2008), a follow-up of the *AMIGO* project (Vallée et al., 2006), there are also other interesting approaches. The *Distributed Wearable Augmented Reality Framework* (DWARF) developed at the Technical University Munich (Bruegge & Klinker, 2005), has its focus on mobile nodes. Another framework focusing on mobile, autonomous nodes is the *OpenWings* framework, which is hosted by General Dynamics and mainly used for military purposes. The Java Context Awareness Framework (JCAF) by Badram (2005) is still not very broadly implemented. Similar commercial frameworks are *COBA* of LONIX Ltd., Finland, or the *dSS* of digitalSTROM.org, Switzerland, where the latter mainly aims on energy management at home.

While many projects are working on different approaches toward the integration of context data within smart home environments, the JAVA originated OSGi-platform has evolved into a de-facto standard over the last years. After an intensive evaluation period, we have decided on using the community based OpenAAL framework working on top of OSGi (Wolf et al., 2010) as a basis for our own developments. Besides the definition of use cases, formulating rules and methods on aggregating and analyzing the vast amount on input data towards reasonable context will lead to higher acceptance of the suggested technologies. In addition to usual sensors and actuators, our lab covers work on big screens and their usability as well as the seamless integration of medical devices, starting with chronic heart diseases and evolving into ambient assistance in a wider sense (Klack et al., 2010).

User Interfaces

In contrast to traditional information and communication technologies, assistive medical devices are mostly used by older and diseased persons, who have very specific needs (Ziefle, 2010). Compared to the average computer user, older people differ considerably regarding their cognitive as well as motor skills. As known from a vast body of literature (see, e.g., Craik & Salthouse, 1992 or Fisk & Rogers, 1997) the ageing process impedes the interaction of older users with technical devices to a considerable extent. Age-related changes in the cognitive system usually lead to a decline in working-memory capacities and cause a general slow down in processing speed as well as a reduction of spatial abilities (Pak, 2001). As a result, persons with reduced spatial abilities frequently experience disorientation when navigating through menu structures of computer systems. A reduced working memory capacity hampers the untroubled menu navigation additionally, especially when using small screen devices, where the provision of optimized or additional information is often not possible due to the limited screen estate (Ziefle & Bay, 2006). In the context of medical technology usage such declines become especially critical when task demands are high, as for instance when using novel or complex devices, or when it is the matter of sensitive data like in health-related context. As a result, older people face greater difficulties in extracting relevant information from technical systems or they are simply overwhelmed by the high information density in applications and technical devices.

When discussing aging and technology usage, the willingness of older people to use computer technology or to interact with medical systems is a crucial aspect that needs to be carefully considered. A number of earlier studies (e.g., Wilkowska & Ziefle, 2009) examining the interaction with technology have shown that the success of technological innovations is largely influenced by the extent to which users accept the technology. Empirical evidence suggests that different age groups have different reasons to accept or reject medical technologies. In this context, it is very likely that the actual impulse to use a specific device is largely influenced by motivational factors. On the one hand, usage motives are related to perceived advantages and gains, which at the same time support the positive attitude toward the technology. However, disadvantages and barriers can overshadow the intended interaction, and – as a consequence – provoke an averseness to accept and use the system. On the other hand, user motives to employ medical technologies might also interact with the their individual characteristics such as gender, educational level, previous technical learning history or the resulting technical self-confidence. Thus, emotional factors need to be carefully considered in the analyses of usability and acceptability aspects of medical systems.

Psychology

In the history of information technology (IT) there was long enough a perfunctory development of technical devices, systems and applications that disregarded or simply did not include users and their opinions about the products' usability, acceptance or design. From an economical perspective, this resulted frequently in higher expenditure and additional costs in comparison to the yielded benefits. Nowadays, it seems indeed to be increasingly realized that technical products are accepted and utilized by the people only if usability issues are appropriately considered within device designs (e.g., cognitive complexity, key design, navigation structure, icon usage, language usage - naming and categorizing of function names -, and communication dialogues), because technical end products without such framework conditions are foredoomed to fail in an age of global economical crisis with keen competition in IT sector.

Thus, integrating potential customers into development of technical systems from the beginning on is indispensable. Especially in case of Ambient Assisted Living and Smart Healthcare systems this is of great importance for at least two reasons. Firstly, for most people there is no other place, which is more intimate and confiding than "the own four walls". Yet, according to Maslow's Hierarchy of Needs (Maslow, 1954) accommodation is extremely important in human's life for reasons of perceived safety, and it belongs to the basic human needs to feel protected, stable and secure. Secondly, health is the greatest wealth and therefore a very sensitive and delicate topic – there is no higher good than this and everyone tries to protect it as long as somehow possible. Thus, putting these two relevant aspects of human life together, it is all the more understandable that the involvement of end users, their perspectives, wishes and needs, into every step of the development process plays a great role for a successful rollout. The integration, though, is connected with some considerable challenges.

First of all, Ambient Assisted Living enhanced by modern health supporting technologies is connected with plenty of emotions: barriers and restraints on the one hand, as well as motivational aspects and positive stimuli to perceive the advantages of such a tool on the other hand. Also, in contrast to traditional information technologies, medical assistance devices address mostly older, frail and diseased people, whose health condition, i.e. some of their vital parameters (e.g., blood pressure, body temperature, weight), have to be regularly controlled. However, elderly as well as chronically ill or handicapped persons have very

specific and wide-ranged needs requiring from modern medical systems individually adapted input and output devices. For instance, there is another need regarding the communication with the system for a mobility-impaired person in comparison to a user with hearing deficiencies but otherwise unlimited mobility. The same problem applies to the cognitive skills, or more specifically to their degree of decline, to technical self-confidence and not at least to the willingness to use such modern technologies in the own home. Hence, there is a great necessity for a comprehensive and sensible identification of factors that influence the usage behavior of such medical systems. In addition, it should be kept in mind that all the processes, trends and meanings about technology as well as health states and abilities may change over the years. This fact alone demands an enormous flexibility and adaptability from the assistive devices. Reflecting this dynamic character of human progress it follows that different input and output modalities are necessary for covering the broadest possible range of existing requirements in order to assure the users' straightforward interaction with a system. While sophisticated technological solutions are on the threshold to merge, the analysis of actual user needs and the identification of appropriate interaction modalities still remains a challenge from a psychological perspective.

In order to meet the complexity of users' demands and to understand the resulting acceptance patterns, complex methodology is necessary. Thereby, not only for satisfaction reasons of scientific ethos, but especially because of preferably highest effectiveness of psychological analysis, both qualitative and quantitative methods are essential.

For the examination of different aspects influencing acceptance and usage behavior of medical assistance technology (e.g., users' diversity, requirements, motivational factors, barriers) a user-centered approach is needed that considers characteristics of highly heterogeneous user

Figure 3. Psychological research model

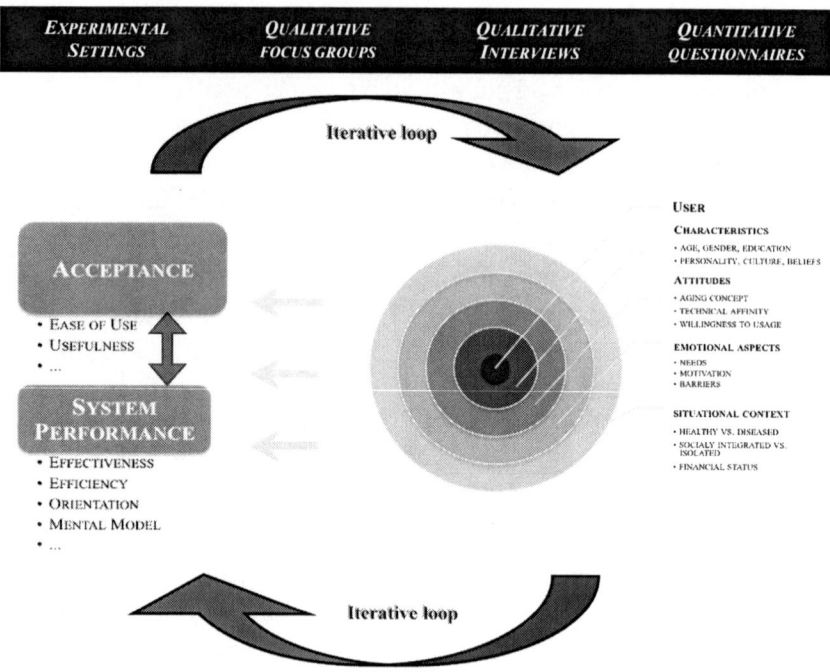

groups. Thereby, to ensure user-oriented development and continuous implementation of newly acquired knowledge an iterative process (see Figure 3) characterized by a consequent dialogue between developers and users is necessary. Such cooperation enables to continuously integrate user feedback into the design process and helps to tailor the system to the specific needs of the target population.

In the explorative phase of the psychological research, a combination of proven methods like focus groups, interviews and questionnaires is applied in order to collect user data, which provide first insights into the acceptance and perceived usefulness of the tested technology. The intention is to identify the special needs and wants of older and/or diseased people as well as the barriers and perceived obstacles regarding the interaction with the system. Moderated focus groups with a small number of participants as well as interviews with individuals are highly suitable for discussions about functionality, navigation

issues, and communication options with the assistive technology. In quantitative surveys, large-scale influences of different user characteristics on the persons' reported acceptability and the effects of various other aspects (e.g., ageing concepts, coping strategies, attitude towards technology, context of usage, role of trust, privacy, security, etc.) on usage behavior are examined. Finally, in experimental studies in a living lab environment, the users' direct interaction with the system (e.g., navigational effectiveness and efficiency) and evaluation of systems' usability can be observed in realistic usage situations in order to analyze the influences of the described factors.

As illustrated above, the usage of assistive medical technologies is defeated by multi-faceted factors. An optimal interaction with the system does not only depend on the users' physical abilities or personal preferences, instead it is also likely to be impacted by other factors, like the social situation, societal norms, and individual wishes with respect to privacy and intimacy. Moreover,

Figure 4. Possible perspectives of patients on the doctor

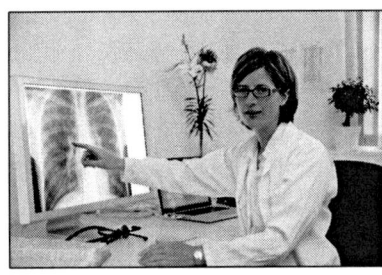 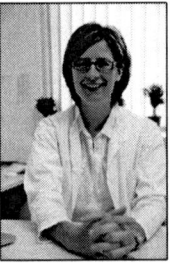 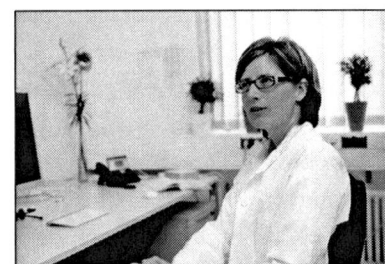

different users face various difficulties in this interaction. Thus, the understanding of users' capabilities and limitations as well as the detection of possible influences, which determine a smooth and ergonomically favorable interaction with the assistive technology, is the task and the goal of psychology in this multidisciplinary approach.

Communication Science

Monitoring older and/or chronically ill people requires the implementation of tele-medical services in an AAL system. Physicians and patients have to communicate regularly with each other for exchanging and discussing medical data concerning the patients' conditions, adjusting their treatment (e.g., medication) and negotiating their conditions. Due to the demographic change, the number of medical professionals declines while the number of (older) patients increases (Beul et al., 2010). Moreover, older patients' mobility diminishes because of the appearance of senescence or disease phenomena (Mollenkopf et al., 2004). Therefore, the human resources of doctors have to be allocated as efficient as possible, while at the same time the treatment of patients has to be organized as comfortable as possible. For this reason, tele-medical services between doctors and patients in their homes are a promising solution. To put this vision into practice, three major challenges have to be met: grasping and operationalizing the communicative scenario, realizing face-to-face interactions on novel types of information and

communication technologies (ICT) like, e.g., wall-sized interactive displays, and enhancing the participants trust in the tele-medical service.

Doctor-patient communication is traditionally taking place in a face-to-face interaction (Roter & Hall, 1989): Patients either consult doctors in their surgery or doctors visit patients in their home environment. With the implementation of an ICT-based communication channel, both parties can stay in their original location. Because neither party moves physically, their perspectives on the communicative scenario diverge. Thus, it cannot be classified clearly as a surgery visit by the patient or a home visit by the physician, which leads to the challenge of characterizing the communicative scenario in this tele-medical service.

Furthermore, the formerly physically realized interaction has to be transferred into a media-supported interaction with an interactive wall. For this, it is necessary to identify patients' and doctors' requirements on the design of the communication channel. The appropriate communicative modes dependent on user types have to be detected (e.g., verbal only interaction, combination of images and verbal interaction, or video interaction). In addition, the usage of an interactive wall for the realization of doctor-patient communication opens up new opportunities with respect to the presentation of the interlocutor: Owing to the size of the screen, it is possible to interact while walking, standing or sitting in the room. Additional media (e.g., X-ray images) can be integrated into the interaction to facilitate the participants understanding.

On account of these new possibilities of presentation, personal preferences of the interlocutors have to be identified. The support of individual communicative skills, styles and strategies of the participants should be considered, too.

Lastly, the patients' and doctors' requirements on the design and the features of the tele-medical service, realized as an application, should be investigated. One key feature of the tele-medical service is the exchange of medical data (e.g., blood pressure and blood coagulation data) between doctor and patient as a precondition for the medical consultation. The data can be seen as the subject of their talk. Therefore, privacy and trust issues must be regarded. Feedback reports have to be implemented to inform patients about the transfer of their medical data and to give them a feeling of control over their data. Besides feedback, the graphical user interface must be designed user-friendly to increase the participants' trust in the system (Fruhling & Sang, 2006). Cognitive-ergonomic issues as well as linguistic and semiotic means have to be considered to contribute to a pleasurable usage of the application (Wirtz et al., 2010).

Architecture

In the course of advancements in sustainable building design, buildings are changing from being static to dynamic. Building automation and intelligence are allowing for automated maintenance making buildings adaptable and reactive to environmental changes. Temperature, humidity, and position of the sun are typical parameters that an intelligent building reacts to, in order to optimize climate and ergonomics of the working or living environment it houses. Apart from adaptability to environmental changes, technological advances provide more potential in integrating modern technology into buildings and homes. Especially, elderly and ill inhabitants can benefit considerably from medical technology that is seamlessly integrated into their apartments. The concept of Ambient Assisted Living integrates information

and communication technology, and sensors into the everyday living environment. Buildings will no longer "only" react to environmental changes, but also to the context and the situation of the user.

As described earlier, medical technology can be stigmatizing if visually prominent with explicit focus on the disease of the patient. This stigma can be potentially minimized especially with information and communication technology that has long overcome exclusiveness in purpose. Hence, hedonic aspects have to be taken into account along with ergonomics and usability when designing health technology, as they will greatly affect the acceptance and actual use of the device or the system. The less medical technology is visible, the more it becomes part of the room and eventually the architecture. But how do users interact with rooms and architecture in general? Human-Computer Interaction (HCI) covers the broad field of research and development between technology and technical products on the one hand and human factors on the other hand (Dix et al., 2003). With the technological advances, research in HCI today includes addressing challenges in creating intuitive, easy to use and elegant interfaces for mobile, wearable and ubiquitous technology. As information and communication technologies are not longer restricted to technical products but increasingly enter living spaces, HCI research will also need to cover architectural issues.

Rapid advances in display technology in the recent years, large displays are entering our everyday urban experience. Important information is displayed in train stations and airports, advertisements are shown on facades and LED billboards, and events are broadcasted on large screens for public viewing. It is only a matter of time before large displays will also find their way into our homes. As walls become displays, they become part of an architectural space. Kasugai et al. (2010) introduce the concept of spatially, functionally and socially extending a space through large screen technology in an Ambient Assistive Living environment.

Wenger et al. (1996) state that lack of social support and networks as well as changing health can lead to the feeling of loneliness and secludedness, which is correlated with old age, often resulting in the emergence of depression. Socially extending a space can potentially help overcome these feelings. Creating social network ties may help people to protect their health and to develop coping strategies (Penninx et al., 1999).

By spatially extending a room and seamlessly merging virtual and physical spaces, new standards of communication between doctors and patients can be established (Kasugai et al., 2010). This provides an opportunity to immerse users into a life-like videoconference, who were previously not exposed to any video chat technology.

In this context, the main architectural challenge we seek to address in our research is to combine, integrate and answer medical demands, as well as usability and technology acceptance aspects in an architecturally satisfying space.

TOWARDS A MULTI-DISCIPLINARY SOLUTION

eHealth – Enhancing Mobility with Aging

The project "eHealth – Enhancing Mobility with Aging" aims at approaching the disciplinary challenges outlined above in an integrative and multidisciplinary fashion. The project started in January 2009 as part of the Human Technology Centre, a newly established project house, funded by the Excellence Initiative of the German federal and state governments. Its main focus is on the design of adaptive immersive interfaces for personal healthcare systems and the development of novel, integrative prototypes of user-centered healthcare systems. This includes new concepts of electronic monitoring systems within ambient living environments, suited to support persons individually (according to user profiles), adaptively

(according to the course of disease) and sensitively (according to living conditions).

Threefold Strategy

Due to the complexity of the topic, the interdisciplinary research concept includes three complimentary strategies: (1) *Methodological Strategy*: The project bridges competencies of different disciplines in order to develop a truly interdisciplinary approach for a human-centered development of future healthcare technologies. (2) *Spatial Strategy*: As a continuous exchange of ideas is needed, and the disciplinary perspectives have to be transformed into an interdisciplinary methodology, a new research house, the Human Technology Centre, was created that allows the teams to research under one roof. At the same time, researchers maintain close relationships to their "home" institutes, enabling continuous exchange of disciplinary and interdisciplinary knowledge. (3) *Educational Strategy*: Through its integration into the academic context, the e-health program offers young academics the opportunity to participate in interdisciplinary research quite early in the educational process. In addition, new teaching concepts, as, e.g., the interdisciplinary school of methods, foster holistic education concepts and form the next generation of researchers.

Overall Research Goals

The three-year research plan focuses on homecare solutions for patients with chronic heart disease as a key application with high clinical demand, recurrent hospital stays, high morbidity, and mortality. Due to ageing, incidence and prevalence is considerably increasing (Murray et al., 1994). The project follows a multidisciplinary approach regarding the development of user-centered smart healthcare technologies, which integrate perspectives of different disciplines, including computer science, medicine, engineering, psychology, communication science and architecture.

The research duties aim at age-sensitive concepts for technical devices within living environments enabling old and ill patients suffering from chronic heart disease to live independently at home. Devices should be perceived as personally helpful, supportive, safe and secure, and should evoke feelings of trust and reliability, while at the same time respect patients' desire for intimacy, independence, and dignity. In addition, the way devices are communicating with their owners must be easily understandable at any time. Devices are conceptualized as context-adaptive, smart and immersive. Thus, they are not only communicating with patients, but also with the environment (furniture, walls, floor), family members, doctors or emergency personnel. The main issues addressed within the project are the systematic evaluation and consecutive optimization of the interrelation of medical, environmental, technical, communicative, psychological and social factors, and their consequences for the design, use and acceptance of personal healthcare systems.

Integrative Approach

To examine how patients communicate with smart homecare environments, how they deal with invisible technology, and how the information is to be delivered such that it meets the requirements of timeliness, data protection, dignity as well as medical demands, an experimental space is necessary, which enables to study patients "life at home". It is planned to develop a full-scale prototype room as part of a smart apartment in order to test various smart healthcare systems. The room will consist of a simulated home environment, which enables researchers to use experimental interfaces with test persons of different ages and health states. Out of validity reasons, the experimental space is of central importance, as patients and care givers need to experience and "feel" the technology to be used, in order to fairly evaluate it (Woolham & Frisby, 2002). Further, persons might overemphasize their sensitiveness towards privacy violations

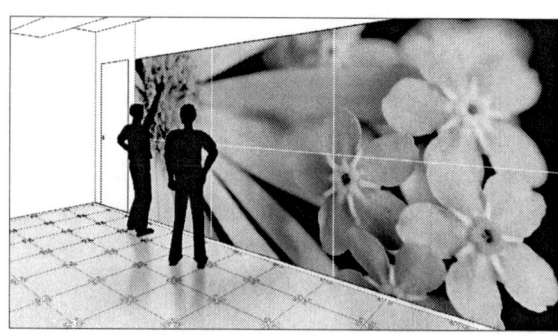

Figure 5. Iterative design cycle illustrating the interdisciplinary research approach

if their judgments only rely on the imagination of using it (Cvrcek et al., 2006).

Therefore, different evaluation methods and scenarios will be used, ranging from empirical and experimental procedures, psychometric testing, questionnaire methods and behavioral observations. In order to realize this ambient living concepts, which represent the daily situation of patients at home, communication and interaction mechanisms as well as bio signals have to be integrated into architectural concepts and components (furniture, walls, floor).

The design will follow several cycles, in which the technological design is carefully harmonized and weighted with acceptance and/or usability demands. Patients differing in gender, age, health status, emotional and cognitive factors, and severity of disease will be involved in the design cycles. In a first step, we will concentrate on the two opposite ends of the design space, a small personal device ("a medical helper") and an interactive wall, with which patients can directly interact. In a second step, a smart floor will be included to complement the smart environment.

The complexity of the topic and the concurrent research of many different disciplines need a specific working rationale, in which each discipline has its own research focus (following disciplinary research habits), but at the same time an inter- and transdisciplinary working mode, in which the different parts are combined and harmonized.

Figure 6. Vision scribble of the interactive environment

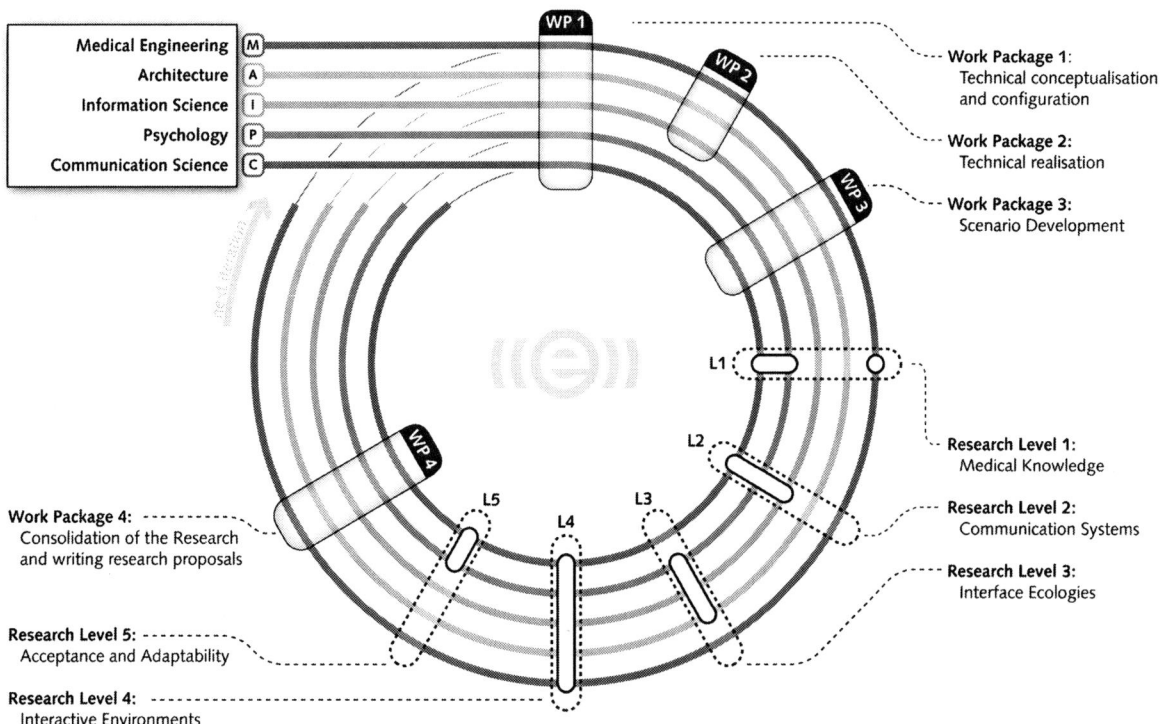

Visualizing this novel approach, in Figure 5, the working mode of the different disciplines, their interlocking within the iterative cycle of user-centered designs is pictured.

First Steps towards a Living Lab Environment

Currently, first technical components of the intelligent home environment are built. As such, interacting mechanisms, cognitive ergonomic issues of the interface, but also spatial, architectonical and communication demands are discussed, conceptualized, realized and iteratively tested. Figure 6 shows a vision scribble of the interactive environment with a large-scale interactive wall and a smart floor.

From a medical-engineering perspective, a flexible, home-based therapy assistance system for people with different health and life conditions has to be created. The medical focus considers a

broad range of disease states, ranging from persons with beginning coronary, ischemic or hypertensive heart diseases, heart failures or congenital heart diseases up to high-urgency transplant patients. Though the medical focus is on chronic heart patients, the system is open for a much larger range of users. The sensoric part of the system consists of biosensors that acquire patients' vital data. A special middleware merges different data streams and analyses the data on a central processor unit. The actoric part provides therapeutic advises to the patient and, in case of blood pump patients, optimizes the performance of the mechanical assistive device based on patients' actual vital conditions. Our field studies (Alagöz et al., 2010) in leading heart centers (Bad Oeynhausen, Germany and Leuven University, Belgium) showed that four prominent vital parameters are essential: blood pressure, blood coagulation, body temperature, and weight. To achieve this, various state-of-the-art sensor technologies for noncontact or minimal invasive vital data monitoring will be evaluated in our living lab. In parallel, first studies regarding users' acceptance of medical home technology are currently running, which take users of different age, upbringing and health states into account.

OUTLOOK & FUTURE WORK

The insights gained during the formative studies will be used to design the "Future Care Lab", an experimental space for studying users' "life" at home and examining how they interact and communicate with invisible technology (Ziefle et al., 2009). The lab will enable to explore how future homecare environments have to be designed such that they meet technical and medical requirements and at the same time satisfy fundamental user needs regarding data protection, dignity, and intimacy.

Within the Future Care Lab, the development of user-centered smart healthcare technologies will be realized by a truly multidisciplinary team of individuals coming from the fields of psychology, communication science, computer science, medicine, engineering, and architecture. The Future Care Lab will provide a full-scale technical infrastructure to test various immersive systems. It will consist of a simulated home environment, which allows researchers to use various prototype interfaces with test persons of different ages and health states.

The lab will provide an intelligent care infrastructure, consisting of different mobile and integrated devices, for supporting elderly people in technology-enhanced home environments. The setup of the lab will enable in-situ evaluations of new care concepts and medical technologies by observing different target user populations in realistic usage situations. As the lab will rely on a modular technical concept, it will be possible to expand it with other technical products, systems and functionalities, in order to address different user groups as well as individuals with differ-

ences in their cognitive, health-related or cultural needs. By this the lab will have the potential to be sensibly adapted to new technical developments as well as societal changes and needs.

ACKNOWLEDGMENT

This research was funded by the Excellence Initiative of the German federal and state governments.

REFERENCES

Alagöz, F., Wilkowska, W., Roefe, D., & Klack, L. Ziefle, M. & Schmitz-Rode (2010). Technik ohne Herz? Nutzungsmotive und Akzeptanzbarrieren medizintechnischer Systeme aus der Sicht von Kunstherzpatienten. *In Proceedings of the Third Ambient Assisted Living Conference (AAL'10)*, Berlin, Germany: VDE. CD-ROM.

Armac, I., Panchenko, P., Pettau, M., & Retkowitz, R. (2009). Privacy-Friendly Smart Environments. In K. Al-Begain (Ed.). *Proceedings of the Third International Conference and Exhibition on Next Generation Mobile Applications, Services and Technologies (NGMAST 2009)*, Cardiff, U (pp. 425-431). London: IEEE Computer Society, 2009.

Arning, K., & Ziefle, M. (2009). Effects of cognitive and personal factors on PDA menu navigation performance. *Behaviour & Information Technology*, *28*(3), 251–268. doi:10.1080/01449290701679395

Arning, K., & Ziefle, M. (2009). Different Perspectives on Technology Acceptance: The Role of Technology Type and Age. In Holzinger, A., & Miesenberger, K. (Eds.), *Human – Computer Interaction for eInclusion. LNCS 5889* (pp. 20–41). Berlin, Heidelberg: Springer.

Bardram, J. E. (2005). (JCAF) – A Service Infrastructure and Programming Framework for Context-Aware Applications. In *Pervasive Computing* (pp. 98–115). The Java Context Awareness Framework. doi:10.1007/11428572_7

Beul, S., Klack, L., Kasugai, K., Möllering, C., Röcker, C., Wilkowska, W., & Ziefle, M. (2010). Between Innovation and Daily Practice in the Development of AAL Systems: Learning from the experience with today's systems. *3rd International ICST Conference on Electronic Healthcare for the 21st century* (ehealth 2010).

Beul, S., Mennicken, S., Ziefle, M., & Jakobs, E.-M. (2010). What Happens After Calling the Ambulance: Information, Communication, and Acceptance Issues in a Telemedical Workflow. In C.A Shoniregun & G.A. Akmayeva (Eds.). In *Proceedings of the International Conference on Information Society* (pp. 111-116). London: Infonomics Society.

Bruegge, B., & Klinker, G. (2005). *DWARF - Distributed Wearable Augmented Reality Framework* (White Paper). Technische Universität München, Chair for Applied Software Engineering.

Craik, F. I. M., & Salthouse, T. A. (1992). *Handbook of Ageing and Cognition*. Hillsdale, NJ: Lawrence Erlbaum Associates.

Cvrcek, D. Kumpost, M., Matyas, V., & Danezis, G. (2006). A Study on the Value of Location Privacy. In: *Proceedings of the ACM Workshop on Privacy in the Electronic Society* (pp. 109-118). New York: ACM.

Dix, A., Finlay, J., Abowd, G., & Beale, R. (2003). *Human-Computer Interaction* (3rd ed.). Upper Saddle River, NJ: Prentice Hall.

Fisk, A. D., & Rogers, W. A. (1997). *Handbook of Human Factors and the Older Adult*. San Diego, CA: Academic Press.

Fruhling, A., & Lee, S. M. (2006). The Influence of User Interface Usability on Rural Consumers' Trust of e-Health Services. *International Journal of Electronic Healthcare, 2*(4), 305–321.

Gaul, S., & Ziefle, M. (2009). Smart Home Technologies: Insights into Generation-Specific Acceptance Motives. In Holzinger, A. (Eds.), *Human–Computer Interaction for eInclusion. LNCS 5889* (pp. 312–332). Berlin, Heidelberg: Springer.

Hauber, J., Regenbrecht, H., Billinghurst, M., & Cockburn, A. (2006). Spatiality in videoconferencing: trade-offs between efficiency and social presence. In CSCW '06: *Proceedings of the 20th anniversary conference on computer supported cooperative work* (pp. 413–422). New York: ACM.

Kasugai, K., Ziefle, M., Röcker, C., & Russell, P. (2010). Creating spatio-temporal contiguities between real and virtual rooms in an assistive living environment. In Bonner, J., Smyth, M., O'Neill, S., & Mival, O. (Eds.), *Proceedings of create 10* (pp. 62–67). Loughborough, UK: Institute of Ergonomics & Human Factors.

Klack, L., Kasugai, K., Schmitz-Rode, T., Röcker, C., Ziefle, M., Möllering, C., et al. (2010). A Personal Assistance System for Older Users with Chronic Heart Diseases. In: *Proceedings of the Third Ambient Assisted Living Conference (AAL'10)*. Berlin, Germany: VDE (CD-ROM).

Klack, L., Möllering, C., Ziefle, M., & Schmitz-Rode, T. (2010). Future Care Floor: A sensitive floor for movement monitoring and fall detection in home environments, *1st International ICST Conference on Wireless Mobile Communication and Healthcare* - MobiHealth 2010.

Leonhardt, S. (2005). Personal Healthcare Devices. In S. Mekherjee et al. (Eds.), *Malware: Hardware Technology Drivers of AI* (pp. 349-370). Dordrecht, NL: Springer.

Maslow, A. (1954). *Motivation and Personality*. New York: Harper.

Melenhorst, A.-S., Rogers, W., & Bouwhuis, D. (2006). Older Adults' Motivated Choice for Technological Innovation. *Psychology and Aging, 21*(1), 190–195. doi:10.1037/0882-7974.21.1.190

Mollenkopf, H., Marcellini, F., Ruoppila, I., & Tacken, M. (2004). *Ageing and Outdoor Mobility. A European Study*. Amsterdam: IOS Press.

Murray, D., Hannan, P. J., Jacobs, D. R., McGoven, P. J., Schmid, L., Baker, W. L., & Gray, C. (1994). Assessing Intervention Effects in the Minnesota Heart Health Program. *American Journal of Epidemiology, 139*, 91–103.

Pak, R. (2001). A Further Examination of the Influence of Spatial Abilities on Computer Task Performance in Younger and Older Adults. In *Proceedings of the Human Factors and Ergonomics Society 48th Annual Meeting* (pp. 1551 – 1555). Santa Monica, CA: The Human Factors and Ergonomic Society.

Penninx, B., van Tilburg, T., Kriegsman, D., Boeke, A., Deeg, D., & van Eijk, J. (1999). Social network, social support, and loneliness in older persons with different chronic diseases. *Journal of Aging and Health, 11*(2), 151–168. doi:10.1177/089826439901100202

Riva, G. (2003). Ambient intelligence in health care. *Cyberpsychology & Behavior, 6*(3), 295–300. doi:10.1089/109493103322011597

Röcker, C., & Feith, A. Revisiting Privacy in Smart Spaces: Social and Architectural Aspects of Privacy in Technology-Enhanced Environments. *Proceedings of the International Symposium on Computing, Communication and Control* (2009) 201-205.

Röcker, C., Wilkowska, W., Ziefle, M., Kasugai, K., Klack, L., Möllering, C., & Beul, S. (2010). Towards Adaptive Interfaces for Supporting Elderly Users in Technology-Enhanced Home Environments. In *Proceedings of the 18th Biennial Conference of the International Communications Society: Culture, Communication and the Cutting Edge of Technology*. Tokyo, Japan. CD-ROM.

Roter, D. L., & Hall, J. A. (1989). Studies of Doctor-Patient Interaction. *Annual Review of Public Health, 10*, 163–180. doi:10.1146/annurev.pu.10.050189.001115

Singh, V. K., Pirsiavash, H., Rishabh, I., & Jain, R. (2008). Towards environment-to-environment (e2e) multimedia communication systems. *In Same '08: Proceeding of the 1st ACM international workshop on semantic ambient media experiences* (pp. 31–40). New York: ACM.

Vallée, M., Ramparany, F., & Vercouter, L. (2005). A Multi-Agent System for Dynamic Service Composition in Ambient Intelligence Environments. In: *Advances in Pervasive Computing, Adjunct Proceedings of the Third International Conference on Pervasive Computing* (Pervasive'05), May 8-11, 2005, Munich, Germany.

Warren, S., & Craft, R. L. (1999). Designing Smart Health Care Technology into the Home of the Future. *Engineering in Medicine and Biology, 2*, 677–681.

Weiner, M., Callahan, C., Tierney, W., Overhage, M., Mamlin, B., Dexter, P., & McDonald, C. (2003). Using Information Technology To Improve the Health Care of Older Adults. *Annals of Internal Medicine, 139*, 430–436.

Wenger, G. C., Davies, R., Shahtahmasebi, S., & Scott, A. (1996). Social isolation and loneliness in old age: Review and model refinement. *Ageing and Society, 16*(03), 333–358. doi:10.1017/S0144686X00003457

Wilkowska, W., & Ziefle, M. (2009). Which Factors Form Older Adults' Acceptance of Mobile Information and Communication Technologies? In Holzinger, A., & Miesenberger, K. (Eds.), *Human–Computer Interaction for eInclusion. LNCS 5889* (pp. 81–101). Berlin: Springer.

Wirtz, S., Jakobs, E.-M., & Beul, S. (2010) Passenger Information Systems in Media Networks – Patterns, Preferences, Prototypes. *In Proceedings of the International Professional Communication Conference 2010 – Communication in a self-service society (IPCC 2010)*, Twente, Netherlands.

Wittenberg, R., Comas-Herrera, A., King, D., Malley, J., Pickard, L., & Darton, R. (2006). Future Demand for Long-Term Care, 2002 to 2041: Projections of Demand for Long-Term Care for Older People in England (PDF). *PSSRU Discussion Paper 2330*. London: London School of Economics.

Wolf, P., Schmidt, A., & Klein, M. (2008). SO-PRANO - An Extensible, Open AAL Platform for Elderly People Based on Semantic Contracts. Paper presented at the *3rd Workshop on Artificial Intelligence Techniques for Ambient Intelligence (AITAmI'08)*, 18th European Conference on Artificial Intelligence (ECAI 08), Patras, Greece.

Woolham, J., & Frisby, B. (2002). Building a Local Infrastructure that Supports the Use of Assistive Technology in the Care of People with Dementia. *Research Policy and Planning, 20*(1), 11–24.

Wright, P., McCarthy, J., & Meekison, L. (2005). Making sense of experience. In Blythe, M., Overbeeke, K., Monk, A., & Wright, P. (Eds.), *Funology: from usability to enjoyment* (pp. 43–53). Norwell, MA: Kluwer Academic Publishers.

Ziefle, M. (2010). Modeling Mobile Devices for the Elderly. *Proceedings of the 3rd International Conference on Applied Human Factors and Ergonomics* (AHFE'10): Miami, Florida.

Ziefle, M., & Bay, S. (2006). How to Overcome Disorientation in Mobile Phone Menu. A Comparison of Two Different Navigation Aids. *Human-Computer Interaction, 21*(4), 393–432. doi:10.1207/s15327051hci2104_2

Ziefle, M., Röcker, C., Kasugai, K., Klack, L., Jakobs, E.-M., Schmitz-Rode, T., et al. (2009). eHealth – Enhancing Mobility with Aging. In M. Tscheligi, B. de Ruyter, J. Soldatos, A. Meschtscherjakov, C. Buiza, W. Reitberger, N. Streitz, T. Mirlacher (Eds.), *Roots for the Future of Ambient Intelligence, Adjunct Proceedings of the Third European Conference on Ambient Intelligence* (AmI'09 (pp.25-28). Salzburg, Austria.

Zimmer, Z., & Chappell, N. (1999). Receptivity to New Technology among Older Adults. *Disability and Rehabilitation, 21*(5/6), 222–230.

ADDITIONAL READING

Aarts, E., Harwig, R., & Schuurmans, M. (2002). Ambient Intelligence. In Denning, P. J. (Ed.), *The Invisible Future - The Seamless Integration of Technology in Everyday Life* (pp. 235–250). New York: McGraw-Hill.

Aarts, E., & Marzano, S. (2003). *The New Everyday - View of Ambient Intelligence*. 010 Publishers.

Adam, S., Mukasa, K. S., Breiner, K., & Trapp, M. (2008). An apartment-based metaphor for intuitive interaction with ambient assisted living applications. *Proceedings of the 22nd British HCI Group Annual Conference on HCI 2008: People and Computers XXII: Culture, Creativity* [Liverpool: United Kingdom.]. *Interaction, 1*, 67–75.

de Ruyter, B., & Aarts, E. (2004). Ambient intelligence: visualizing the future. *Proceedings of the working conference on advanced visual interfaces* (pp. 203 – 208). New York: ACM.

Ellis, D., & Allaire, J. (1999). Modelling Computer Interest in Older Adults: The Role of Age, Education, Computer Knowledge and Computer Anxiety. *Human Factors, 41*, 345–364. doi:10.1518/001872099779610996

Fuchsberger, V. (2008). Ambient assisted living: elderly people's needs and how to face them. *Proceeding of the 1st ACM international workshop on Semantic ambient media experiences* (pp.21-24). Vancouver, British Columbia, Canada.

Gaul, S., Ziefle, M., Arning, K., Wilkowska, W., Kasugai, K., Röcker, C., & Jakobs, E.-M. (2010). Technology Acceptance as an Integrative Component of Product Developments in the Medical Technology Sector. In: *Proceedings of the Third Ambient Assisted Living Conference (AAL'10)*. Germany: VDE. CD-ROM.

Jähn, J., & Nagel, K. (2003). *e-Health*. Heidelberg: Springer.

Kasugai, K., Ziefle, M., Röcker, C., & Russell, P. (2010). Creating Spatio-Temporal Contiguities Between Real and Virtual Rooms in an Assistive Living Environment. In J. Bonner, M. Smyth, S. O' Neill, & O. Mival (Eds.). *Proceedings of Create 10 innovative interactions* (pp. 62-67). Loughborough: Elms Court.

Röcker, C. (2010). Living and Working in Automated Environments - Evaluating the Concerns of End-Users in Technology-Enhanced Spaces. In V. Mahadevan, & Z. Jianhong (Eds.), *Proceedings of the Second International IEEE Conference on Computer and Automation Engineering* (pp.513-551), Singapore: IEEE.

Röcker, C., & Feith, A. (2009). Revisiting Privacy in Smart Spaces: Social and Architectural Aspects of Privacy in Technology-Enhanced Environments. In *Proceedings of the International Symposium on Computing, Communication and Control* (ISCCC'09) (pp. 201 – 205), Singapore: IACSIT.

Röcker, C., Hinske, S., & Magerkurth, C. (2008). Information Security at Large Public Displays. In Gupta, M., & Sharman, R. (Eds.), *Social and Human Elements of Information Security: Emerging Trends and Countermeasures*. Hershey, PA: IGI Publishing.

Salthouse, T. A. (1991). *Theoretical Perspectives on Cognitive Aging*. Hillsdale, NJ: LEA.

Tan, J. (2005). *E-Health Care Information Systems*. San Francisco: Jossey-Bass.

Weiser, M. (1991). The Computer for the Twenty-First Century. *Scientific American*, *265*(3), 94–104. doi:10.1038/scientificamerican0991-94

Ziefle, M. (2008). Age Perspectives on the Usefulness on eHealth Applications. In *Proceedings of the International Conference on Health Care Systems, Ergonomics, and Patient Safety* (HEPS'08). CD-ROM.

Ziefle, M., & Röcker, C. (2010). Acceptance of Pervasive Healthcare Systems: A comparison of different implementation concepts. Full paper on the Workshop User-Centred-Design of Pervasive Health Applications (UCD-PH'10). In Proceedings of the *4th ICST Conference on Pervasive Computing Technologies for Healthcare 2010*. CD-ROM.

KEY TERMS AND DEFINITIONS

Ambient Intelligence: The concept of Ambient Intelligence (AmI) describes the integration of a variety of tiny microelectronic processors and sensors into almost all everyday objects, which enables an environment to recognize and respond to the needs of users in an almost invisible way. The term Ambient Intelligence was coined within the European research community as a reaction to the term 'Ubiquitous Computing' (see above), which was introduced and frequently used by American researchers. In contrast to the more technical notion of Ubiquitous Computing, Ambient Intelligence includes also aspects of Human-Computer Interaction and Artificial Intelligence. Hence, the emphasis of AmI developments is usually on greater user-friendliness, more efficient services support, user-empowerment and support for human interactions. Ambient Intelligence applications are generally characterized by a high degree of embeddedness, using computers integrated into the physical environments in order to provide a variety of context-adapted user services.

Ambient Assisted Living: Ambient Assisted Living (AAL) is one domain of Ambient Intelligence and integrates information and communication technology, and sensors into the living space to enable context awareness and to assist inhabitants in everyday situations.

Intracorproral Technology: Medical, technical devices that are implanted in the human body or any structure anatomically called the corpus. Such devices can range from functional support structures like stents placed in blood vessels to guarantee a good blood flow or prothesis that functionally replace bone structures up to implanted mechanical machines like for example an artificial heart.

Smart Materials: Smart Materials or Textiles can be defined as the materials and structures, which have sense or can sense the environmental conditions or stimuli and can react or respond on those stimuli. These stimuli as well as response, could be thermal, chemical, mechanical, electric, magnetic or from other source.

User Diversity: The term user diversity describes in this context users' characteristics like age, gender, physical condition as well as the moderating influence of users' level of education and financial status.

Ease of Use: The ease of use describes the extent to which users believe a technical system to be free from effort and easy to handle.

Usability: The term describes users' effectiveness, efficiency, and satisfaction with which users achieve specified goals in a technical system.

Aging Concept: Aging concept described here refers to the comprehensive view of aging process and its consequences to the person concerned. It includes 1) the perceived quality of life regarding autonomy, social life and healthcare, 2) misgivings about aging concerning dependency of others, social loneliness and health issues, as well as 3) the active vs. passive attitude towards aging itself.

Technology Acceptance: Technology acceptance deals with the approval, favorable reception and ongoing usage of newly introduced devices and systems, and explores the relation of end-users using motives, cognitive and affective attitudes toward the respective technology and the technological impact assessment.

Middleware: Part of a information system which integrates software components in an inter-process way, in our field especially between sensors and actuators on one hand and abstract tasks, context information, human machine interaction on the other.

Chapter 5
Security in E–Health Applications

Victor Pomponiu
University of Torino, Italy

ABSTRACT

Wireless sensor networks (WSNs) in e-health applications are acquiring an increasing importance due to the widespread diffusion of wearable vital sign sensors and location tags which can track both healthcare personnel and patient status location continuously in real-time mode. Despite the increased range of potential application frameworks the security breach between existing sensor network characteristics and the requirements of medical applications remains unresolved. Devising a sensor network architecture which complies with the security mechanisms is not a trivial task since the WSN devices are extremely limited in terms of power, computation and communication. This chapter presents an analysis of various WSN security techniques from the perspective of healthcare applications, and takes into consideration the significance of security to the efficient distribution of ubiquitous computing solutions.

INTRODUCTION

Nowadays in modern communication age, health and its related issues are very important since they involve all people. Actual health care system recompenses the medical doctors and hospitals for treating sick people, but does not prevent people from being sick. Due to the raising costs of health

DOI: 10.4018/978-1-60960-469-1.ch005

care services together with the growth of elderly population, the current medical system is subject to reform that requires several major changes in insurance companies, hospitals and patients.

The idea that emerges is that healthcare needs to move toward a more *proactive* behavior, which implies prevention and early detection of severe events, combined with the availability of scalable and accessible medical solutions. These requirements create a great need for pervasive electronic health (e-Health) environments, accessible from everywhere and that commit reduced financial and human resources (Aziz et al., 2008; Savastano, Hovsto, Pharow, & Blobel, 2008). As a consequence, e-Health has become an important research topic with developments in multiple domains like, health care, public health, data management, image processing, wireless networking and telecommunications.

Recently, networking and computing technologies started to penetrate the health care and medical treatment, bring important benefits, e.g., deployment of quality healthcare services at lower costs (BioHealth, 2008). The modern networks and communications technologies such as Wireless Sensor Networks (WSNs), Global System for Mobile communications (GSM), Universal Mobile Telecommunications System (UMTS), WiMAX, and Wireless, offer high data rates, and allow time-efficient transmission and processing of medical data.

Owing to these benefits Wireless Sensor Networks, that consist of several connected device called smart senor nodes, began to be widely used in medical environments (Fragopoulos, Gialelis, & Serpanos, 2009; Lorincz et al., & 2004; Malasari et al., 2007; Waterman et al., 2005; Wood et al., 2006). The sensors within a WSN are able to communicate with each other through wireless technologies, like IEEE 802.15.4/ZigBee and IEEE 802.15.1/Bluetooth, which are intended for cable replacement, ad hoc connectivity and low-rate medical applications (e.g., those provided near the patient's bed). Instead, 2.5G (e.g., GPRS) and 3G (e.g., UMTS) technologies are used to transmit information to devices residing on another network.

A particular case of WSNs are Body Area Networks (BANs), which are also called Wireless Body Area Networks (WBANs). Briefly, a BAN consists of several mobile and dense connected sensors, either wearable or implanted into the human body, which permanent monitors and logs patient vital body parameters, e.g., the

blood-pressure, the blood-oxygen, and the ECG. The sensors are attached to the patient's body and connected, through Bluetooth and ZigBee technologies, to a central data-collecting unit. e-Health applications based on BANs (Konstantas, Jones, & Herzog, 2002; Lupu et al., 2007; Marti, Delagado, & Perramon, 2004; Ng et al., 2004; Stingl & Slamanig, 2008; Stoa, Balasingham, & Ramstad, 2007; Vouyioukas et al, 2008; S. Warren et al., 2005) are extremely valuable since they allow doctors and hospitals to monitor remotely, in real-time the patient health condition.

However, shifting from wires to wireless networks impose a deep analysis of the available technologies in order to find the most suitable ones for e-Health environment. Moreover, in order to increase the users' acceptance of these new technologies, protection and security mechanisms of sensitive data should be of the highest standard (Chevrollier & Golmie, 2005; Chhanabhai & Holt, 2007).

The characteristics of the modern e-Health applications impose security requirements such as protection, integrity and confidentiality of sensitive medical data, i.e., of the electronic health records (EHRs) and electronic personal records (EPRs) (Agrawal & Johnson, 2007; Katsikas, Lopez, & Pernul, 2008; Savastano et al., 2008). Considering the limited resources of such applications, is challenging to devise and distribute efficient solutions that are able to satisfy the security requirements.

In this chapter we discuss the security challenges and techniques for e-Health applications delivered over WSNs. To provide useful insights, we structure the rest of this chapter as follows: first, we give a brief overview of the wireless sensor networks along with a description of their main characteristics. Second, an overview of the latest healthcare applications based on WSNs is provided. A particular attention is devoted to the intrinsic vulnerabilities of wireless networks which can affect the effectiveness of medical applications. Then, we present the potential malevolent users in the pervasive healthcare environments together with an overview of the most significant threats. Furthermore, the most important security techniques are analyzed, highlighting both advantages and disadvantages. We conclude the chapter by presenting future research directions towards secure e-Health applications.

BACKGROUND

This section offers a brief introduction to wireless networking by presenting its fundamental components and architectures. A special attention will be given to the wireless sensor networks. However, this section only provides a high-level overview of wireless networking, as background information for the security mechanisms in e-Health applications.

Wireless Networking

The wireless communication is bringing crucial changes to data networking and telecommunication services, making integrated networks a reality. By removing the wires, personal communications networks, local area networks, mobile radio networks and cellular systems, give the promise of entirely distributed mobile computing and communications, anywhere, anytime.

Wireless networking facilitates devices with wireless capabilities to communicate without being connected physically to a network. The involved devices need only to be within the range of the wireless network infrastructure. A collection of wireless nodes within a limited range, which are capable to transmit data through radio communications, forms a *wireless local area network* (WLAN). Typically, WLANs are devised to extend the existing wired local area networks (LANs), increasing the user mobility.

Generally, WLAN architecture comprises two important components: *stations*, which are mobile devices that act as endpoints (e.g., personal digital assistants (PDA), portable computers and other electronic devices with wireless capabilities) and the *access points* that connect the wireless *stations* with a wired network infrastructure or an external network like the Internet. The networks which use access points to coordinate the communication among them are called infrastructure (centralized) wireless networks, and offer the advantages of scalability and reliability of transmission.

Unlike to the infrastructure architecture, wireless ad hoc networks consist of a group of mobile nodes (peers) which are able to communicate with each other without the intervention of an access point. Depending on their application, wireless ad hoc networks can be further classified into: *mobile ad hoc networks* (MANETs) which are autonomous systems of mobile nodes; *wireless mesh networks* (WMNs) that are multihop systems in which devices, organized in a mesh topology, assist each other in transmitting packets through the network, and *wireless sensor networks* (WSNs).

The dynamic changing topology and lack of centralized management and monitoring, together with the reduced capacity of the communication medium are the main characteristics of the wireless ad hoc networks (Raghavendra, Sivalingam, & Znati, 2004). Applications that exploit these features range from military operations to civil exploitation, such as rescue missions in case of disasters, data acquisition and healthcare (Chevrollier & Golmie, 2005; Hadim & Mohamed, 2006; Neves, Stachyra, & Rodrigues, 2008).

Wireless Sensor Networks

A Wireless sensor network consists of many spatially distributed autonomous devices, called smart sensor nodes, which cooperatively analyze the environmental or physical conditions at different locations (Karl & Willing, 2005). Each of these smart nodes comprises several components (Raghavendra, Sivalingam, & Znati, 2004):

Figure 1. The block diagram of a sensor node within a WSN

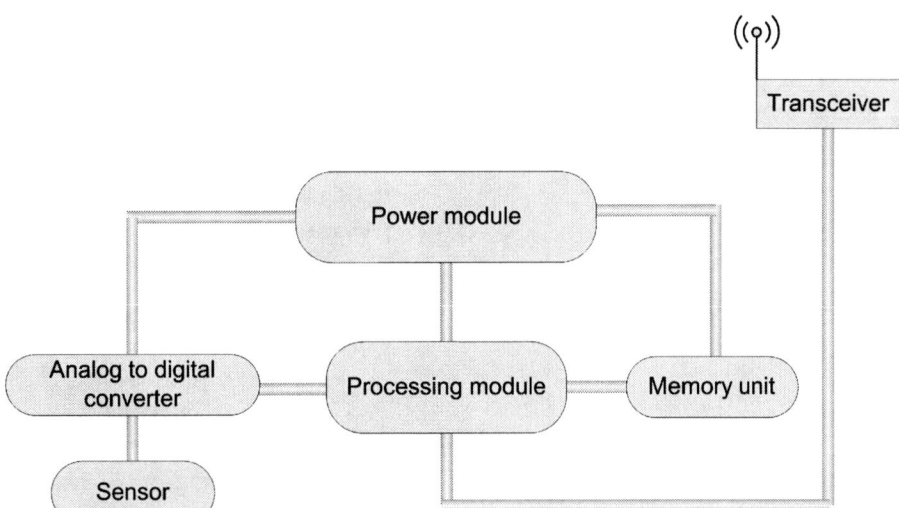

- Transceiver which is used by the sensor to send and receive information over a wireless channel.
- A processing unit which analyze all important data.
- A memory unit for storing data and programs.
- The sensing unit which represents the interface to the physical world, being composed of one or more sensors and an analog-to-digital converter (ADC).
- The power unit that consents autonomous operation.

To better understand the interconnection between these components, a block diagram of the wireless sensor node is given in Fig. 1.

Depending on their intended applications, the size of a sensor node can vary from the size of a box to the size of a microscopically small particle while the cost of a sensor node ranges from hundreds of dollars to a few cents. The size and cost greatly depend on its resources and the sensor itself. This leads to different architectures and functionality for the sensor node (Karl & Willing, 2005).

A sensor network may have one or more gateway nodes (also referred as base station or sink) that collect data from the sensors and forward it to an end-user application. In some rare circumstances, the sensor network can be without any sink node. The purpose of the sink node is to receive information from the network and to allow data aggregation and consumption. Figure 2 presents the typical working principle of a wireless sensor network.

WSNs are largely deployed in physical environments for fine-grain monitoring since they require just the placement of tiny smart sensor nodes in order to gather, process and send the information to the desired location through accessible wireless communication links, e.g., Bluetooth and ZigBee (Zhao & Guibas, 2004).

MANETs and WSNs share many characteristics. Nevertheless, there are some major differences between these networks, which can be summarized as follows (Karl & Willing, 2005; Stojmenovic & Olariu, 2005):

- *Role.* Unlike to sensor networks, MANETs are associated with different applications. For instance, the MANET is applied for voice communication between nodes

Figure 2. A wireless senor network equipped with a sink node

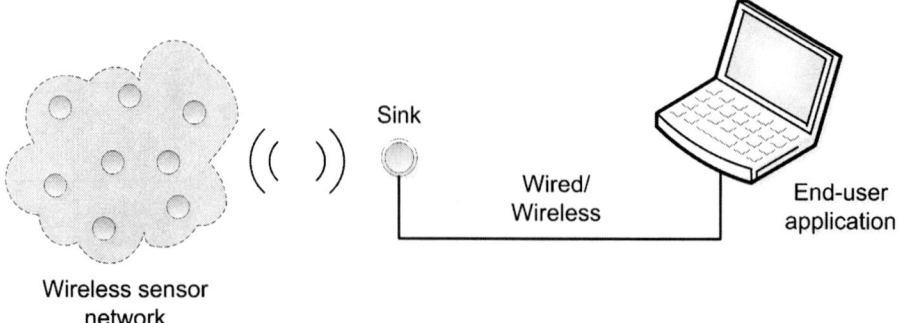

(peers) or to access remote infrastructures (e.g., file or web servers).

- *Equipment.* Due to their use in high energy consumption applications, the terminals of the MANETs are fairly powerful, e.g., laptops or PDAs, with a quite large power supply.
- *Traffic features.* Since WSNs need to interact with environment, they traffic properties are very different from human-driven networks such as MANETs. Thus, the traffic of WSNs is characterized by long periods of inactivity followed by short periods of high network activity.
- *Scalability.* Sensor networks should be more scalable than other types of ad hoc networks since it is expected that thousands of WSNs will be deployed in the current decade.
- *Energy.* Both WSNs and MANETs have constrained power supply. However, WSNs have tighter energy requirements, while recharging or replacing the power unit is a rarely option. Thus, the impact of the energy aspects on the entire network imposes unique challenges and limitations for WSNs.
- *Self-configurability.* Similar to MANETs, sensor networks are capable to arrange themselves into connected networks. Nevertheless, traffic, energy and scale

characteristics determine new solutions for the network self-configuration.

- *Dependability and quality of service (QoS).* Considering their intended applications, for MANETs the node reliability and the QoS aspects are extremely important. Instead, for WSNs the reliability is irrelevant while the QoS solutions should take into considerations the energy limitations.
- *Data centric.* Redundant deployment will make data centric protocols (i.e., sink node sends queries to certain regions and waits data from the sensors located in that regions) suitable for WSNs. Instead, in case of majority of MANETs data centric approaches are inappropriate.
- *Mobility.* The mobility issue in MANET is due to the moving nodes, which determines permanent changes of the multihop routes in order to manage the network. This behavior can also occur in WSNs if the sensor nodes are considered mobile for a given context. Furthermore, two specific situations should be considered in WSNs:
  - In the first scenario, the sensor which is used to detect and monitor a physical environment possesses mobility features.
  - The second case considers the mobility of the nodes that collect and aggregate the network information,

i.e., the sink nodes. By assuming this kind of mobility within a WSN, several difficulties can occur by adopting static routing protocols for data transmission.

The idea that emerges is that even if there are some common properties, MANETs are different form WSNs. By taking into account their specific features, and in particular the energy constraints, WSNs need to support critical applications, such as military and healthcare applications.

E-HEALTH APPLICATIONS BASED ON WSNS

Healthcare is always a big concern, since it encompasses the quality of life a given individual can have. It is always better to prevent an illness than to treat it, therefore individual monitoring is required as a periodic activity. An appropriate incorporation of medical sensor networks would improve the healthcare services from emergency response and in-hospital communications to out-hospital monitoring. An illustration of the generic architecture for WSNs in various healthcare environments is given in Fig. 1.

However, the distribution of WSNs in the context of pervasive healthcare applications should meet strict privacy and security requirements (De Moor & Claerhout, 2004; Halperin, Heydt-Benjamin, Fu, Kohno & Maisel, 2008). These requirements differ depending of the usage scenarios, and include (COM, 2004): *authorization* which encompasses the access control mechanisms; *data integrity* and *authentication* that assure the protection of medical data and of the communication links between the sensors nodes, and *availability* which represents the ability to maintain the network accessible for its intended use.

Actual healthcare applications of WSNs regard heart problems, asthma, emergency response,

stress and post-operator period monitoring, among others. To compare and quantify the existing security solutions, in the following some of these developments are described.

MobiHealth (Konstantas, Jones & Herzog, 2002), an fremawork developed within the European Commission co-founded project MobiHealth, provides mobile value-added services in the healthcare context through 2.5G (e.g., GPRS) and 3G (e.g., UMTS) wireless technologies. This is achieved by integrating the sensors and actuators into a wireless body area network. These sensors nodes and actuators permanently measure and communicate vital signs data to health service providers. The value-added services offered include disease prevention and diagnostics, remote assistance and physical state monitoring. Additionally, by enabling transmission of the vital signs data between the paramedics and the accident site the MobiHealth system supports the fast and reliable deployment of remote assistance in case of accidents.

CodeBlue (Lorincz et al., 2004) is a WSN for medical purpose developed by Harvard University. It is devised for deployment in emergency care and incorporates low-power, wireless vital sign sensors, PDAs, and PC systems. It facilitates efficient allocation of hospital resources and augments the first responders' ability to assess patients where they are found, ensuring a seamless transfer of data between healthcare personnel.

Ubiquitous Monitoring Environment for Wearable and Implantable Sensors (UbiMon) (Ng et al., 2004) is a framework which uses wearable/implantable devices for distributed health services. The architecture comprises the following modules: body sensor network node (BSN), the local processing module, the main server, the patient database and the workstation. BSN nodes are autonomous sensors on a patient that form network connectivity by using the processing module (e.g., a PDA or a laptop). The processing module acts as a router by forwarding the sensor readings to the server through Bluetooth or GPRS wireless

Figure 3. The generic architecture of WSNs in various healthcare scenarios

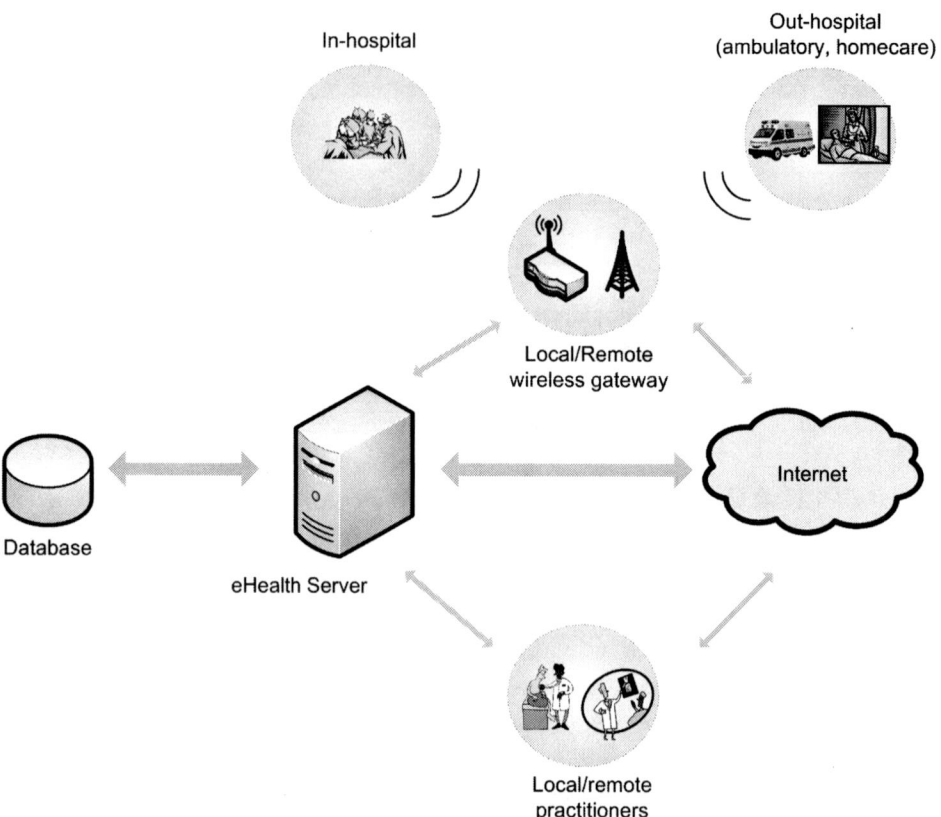

technologies. The purpose of medical database is to store and analyze the sensitive data received while the workstation is used by medical personnel for real-time monitoring.

Waterman et al. (2005), proposed a scalable medical alert response technology (SMART) for patient tracking and monitoring which initiates at the emergency site and follows through transport, triage, stabilization, and transfer between external sites and healthcare facilities. The system is based on a scalable location-aware monitoring architecture with: remote transmission from medical sensors and display of information on PDAs, detection based on logic for recognizing events requiring action, and logistic support for optimal response. Patients and providers, as well as critical medical equipment, will be localized by SMART on demand, while the remote alerts from

the medical sensors could trigger the responses from the available providers.

Wood et al. (2006) introduced ALARM-NET that is a WSN which integrates physiological and environmental sensors in a heterogeneous architecture for pervasive, adaptive healthcare services. A query protocol allows real-time collection and processing of sensor data for authorized health care providers and analysis programs.

SNAP (Malasri & Wang, 2007) is an architecture for medical WSNs where several wireless sensors are attached to each patient. The received data are forwarded by a number of wireless relay nodes throughout the hospital area. These nodes are categorized into limited and unlimited-powered nodes. Leaving apart the routing, mobility or congestion problems, the main concern of this approach is that related to security

Warren et al. (2005) developed wearable health monitoring systems using off-the-shelf ZigBee wireless sensor platforms (i.e., Telos platforms from Moteiv), custom signal processing boards, and the open-source operating system for WSNs TinyOS (TinyOS, 2004). Sensor nodes that are strategically placed on the users' body sample, process, and store the physiological signals information.

Sensium (Wong, McDonagh, Omeni, Nunn, Hernandez-Silveira, & Burdett, 2009) is a system-on-chip for wireless body sensor networks, which integrates a transceiver, a hardware MAC protocol, a microprocessor, IO peripherals, memories, ADC and custom sensor interfaces. Addressing the challenges in the design, one application is described: LifePebble that provides real-time measurement of vital signs optimized for ambulatory conditions.

To determine cardiovascular risk factors earlier, Vogel et al. (2009) devised a permanently in-ear monitoring system (IN-MONIT) of vital signs. The micro-optic reflective sensor positioned inside the auditory canal measures the photoplethysmographic curves through which the heart activity and rate can be computed.

Apart from these developments there are other ongoing projects such as that devised by the Norwegian National Hospital which uses the sensors integrated hardware platform Tmote Sky. Another example is the BAN technology platform presented in (Penders, van de Molengraft, Brown, Grundlehner, Gyselinckx, & van Hoof, 2009), which integrates technology from the Human++ research program on autonomous wireless sensors. The target of this technology is the development of miniaturized body sensor nodes powered by the body-energy that foresees the need of emerging personal health applications. However, these projects aim to optimize the wireless communication and the data throughput, while ignoring the security issues that can arise in the healthcare context.

The Main Security Attacks on WSNs

Due to their inherent properties, such as resource constrains, uncontrollable environment, and dynamic network topology, an adversary can mount many attacks on WSNs which could cripple them. Following the approach introduced in (Halperin et al., 2008), the potential malevolent users in the healthcare environments can be classified into:

- *Active adversaries*, which have direct access to a sensor node such as wearable or implanted sensors.
- *Passive adversaries* that have implicit interferences with a sensor node by eavesdropping its communication links.
- *Insiders*, which encompass healthcare personnel, nurses, doctors, IT experts or even the patients.

As a direct consequence, the attacks can be as well subdivided into active and passive ones (see Fig. 4). Passive attacks, such as eavesdropping and traffic analysis, consist of illegitimate stealing and disclosure of medical information such as the patient's EHR. Regarding the traffic analysis attack, it is usually performed on the captured packets. It is worth to point out that these attacks involve an adversary which has gained access to the wireless links between the sensor nodes.

Contrasts to passive attacks, the active attacks are more harmful since the adversary modifies or spoof packets, or interferes with the wireless signals in order to perturb the network. Even if the information is protected by encryption, the attacker may blindly modify the encrypted information (i.e., message corruption attack) transforming it into gibberish. Instead, by exploiting the weaknesses of the authentication process, an attacker may counterfeit false data, misleading the recipient by making him to believe that data come from a different originator.

Exchanges of the location information might lead attackers to identify the node positions. Fur-

Figure 4.Classification of security threats which affect WSNs

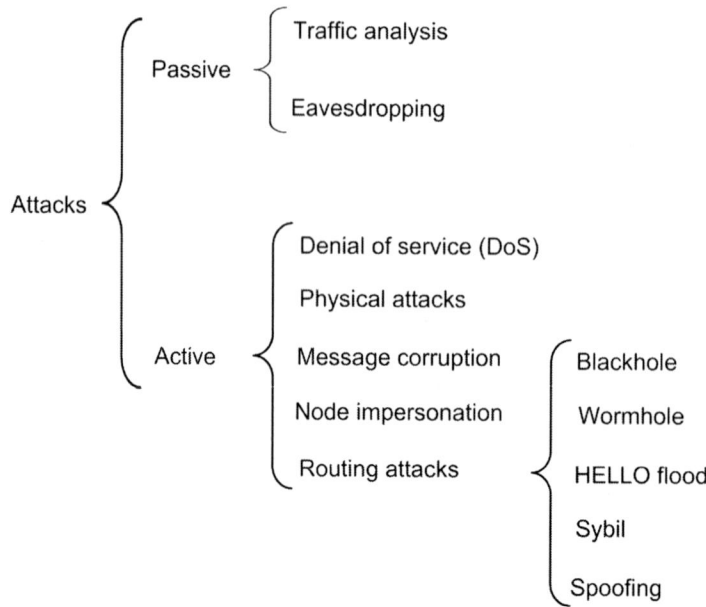

ther, an adversary could disable the sensor node by physically destroying the device. Moreover, the network can be disrupted if an attacker perturbs a compromised node.

Instead, the weaknesses of the medium access control (MAC) and of the routing protocols for wireless ad hoc networks can be exploited by adversaries to devise sophisticated attacks that can fall into two categories:

- *Resource exhaustion attacks*, such HELLO flood, in which the attacker floods the network with data packets in order to consume its resources (e.g., the network bandwidth) or node resources (e.g., its storage space).
- *Routing disturbance attacks*, such as blackhole and wormhole attacks, which attempt to change the route of the data packets.

For a good overview of the routing and denial of service (DoS) attacks on WSNs the reader can consult the papers of Karlof and Wagner (2003) and Wood and Stankovic (2002). It is important to mention that all these attacks can be easily

mounted, especially when the routing protocols are designed without any regard to security. In order to avoid these issues, the forthcoming protocols should be devised by integrating robust security solutions that take into consideration the highlighted constraints.

Security Techniques for WSNs

The sensor node devices are characterized as severely resource-constrained in terms of available power, memory, bandwidth and computational capability. These sensor-specific factors set several constraints on the security architecture. As only a fraction of the total memory may be used by the cryptographic algorithms, the security architecture demands these to be very lightweight with a judicious execution time.

Due to the limited bandwidth of the system, the extra overhead required in providing the security facility should not substantially degrade the global efficiency of the system. The sensor network topology, flat or hierarchical, is another feature which should be considered when devis-

Table 1. WSNs attacks and their corresponding security solutions

Attack	Solution
Unauthorized access	Asymmetric cryptography Random key distribution
Message leakage	Link/network encryption Access control
Message corruption	Digital signature Digital watermarking Keyed secure hash function (KSHA)
Denial of service (DoS)	Intrusion detection
Node compromising	Node revocation Tamper-proofing
Routing attacks	Secure routing protocols (SRPs)
Intrusion attacks	Intrusion detection Secure group communication

ing authentication schemes that must not generate too many overhead messages. Furthermore, the cryptographic functions and the keying material must reside and be executable efficiently within each node.

Research into WSN security is still in its infancy since a clear line of defense is not available (Karlof and Wagner, 2003). Several security solutions have been proposed for: protecting sensor communication links, access control, message authenticity and integrity, and intrusion detection. A particular attention has been given to develop secure routing protocols (Karlof and Wagner, 2003; Hu, Johnson, & Perrig, 2002; Hu, Perrig & Johnson, 2005) and efficient key management schemes, which serve as the fundamental requirement for data encryption and authentication. The threats for WSNs and potential security mechanisms are summarized in Table 1.

The forthcoming subsections focalize on the main security approaches for link layer encryption, key management, digital watermarking and intrusion detection employed in the pervasive healthcare environment.

Link Layer Encryption

Various security mechanisms have been proposed for protecting the sensor network's link layer communications, the bottom layer of the network protocol stack. Depending on the support used for encryption, these schemes can be broadly subdivided into: software encryption and hardware encryption schemes.

Software Encryption Schemes

One of the most popular software encryption scheme for WSNs is TinySec (Karlof, Sastry, & Wagner, 2004) which is an integrated component of the TinyOS (TinyOS, 2004) developed at the Berkeley University. It achieves link layer authenticated encryption, with only 10% of performance overhead, by encrypting data packets using a group key shared among sensor nodes followed by the calculation of the message authentication code (MAC) for the whole packet (including the header).

However, the scheme relies on a single key manually programmed into the sensor nodes before deployment. This shared key, distributed over the entire network, provides merely a baseline level of security. Consequently, if an adversary compromises (or capture) a single node or learns the secret key, it can gain access to all data packets in the network or can inject his own packets. This is the weakest point in TinySec since node capture has been proved to be a fairly easy process (Karlof, Sastry, & Wagner, 2004).

Halperin et al. (2008) proposed a zero-power authentication technique based on RC5 (Rivest, 2006) that allows an implantable medical device (IMD), i.e., a UHF RFID tag (Sample, Yeager, Powledge, & Smith, 2007), to verify that it is communicating only with the programmer devices used by practitioners to perform diagnostics and adjust therapy settings. The commercial programmers know a master key k_M while each IMD has an identification number *ID* and a specific key *k*

$=f(k_M, ID)$, where f is a cryptographically strong pseudorandom function. More precisely, the IMD implements a simple challenge-response protocol which involves the following steps:

- *Step 1*. The programmer transmits a request to authenticate to the Wireless Identification and Sensing Platform (WISP).
- *Step 2*. The WISP responds with its identity *ID* and a pseudorandom number *n*.
- *Step 3*. The programmer calculates the IMD specific key k and further returns the response $r=RC5(k, n)$ to WISP.
- *Step 4*. The WISP computes the same value and verifies the value it received from the programmer against its result.
- *Step 5*. Finally, the WISP informs the IMD that the programmer has been successfully authenticated.

This prototype could be used for bootstrapping stronger authentication techniques. The major drawback of this scheme is lack of scalability, i.e., for large distributed sensor networks a unique shared key may incur an unacceptable risk (Halperin et al., 2008).

Recently, elliptic curve cryptography (ECC) has evolved as a promising encryption algorithm since the size of ECC keys is much sorter. The procedures for encryption and decryption based on the elliptic curve are found in Algorithm 1.

There have been notable advances in ECC implementation for WSNs in recent years. For example, CodeBlue (Lorincz et al., 2004) has implemented the ECC using merely integer arithmetic. With this implementation public keys can be generated on MICA2 in 34 seconds whereas shared secrets can be distributed among nodes in the same period, using approximately 1 kilobyte of static memory and 24 kilobytes of ROM.

Uhsadel et al. (2007) propose an efficient implementation of ECC and Liu et al. (2008) developed TinyECC, an ECC library that offers elliptic curve arithmetic over prime fields and uses inline assembly code to increase the speed of critical operations. Lately, Szczechowiak et al. (2008) presented NanoECC, which is relatively fast compared with other existing ECC implementations, although it requires a lot of memory resources.

In (Tan, Wang, Zhong, & Li, 2008; Tan, Wang, Zhong, & Li, 2009) a protocol based on identity-based encryption (IBE) (Shamir, 1985) and elliptic curves, called IBE-Lite, is introduced. IBE-Lite shares two properties with conventional IBE, namely the ability to use an arbitrary string to generate a public key, and the ability to generate a public key separately from the corresponding secret key. The intuition behind is to let a sensor independently generate a public key on-the-fly using an arbitrary string. Thus, using this string the sensor can derive a public key to encrypt data and send it to the storage site; there is no corresponding secret key created. In fact, the sensor cannot create the secret key needed to decrypt the message. This secret key only allows the practitioner to decrypt messages encrypted by a sensor using the same string.

Although elliptic curve cryptography is feasible on WSNs, its energy requirements are still orders of magnitude higher compared to that of symmetric cryptosystems. Due to this reason, elliptic curve cryptography is more appropriate for securing infrequent critical operations, such as key establishment during the initial configuration of the network (Großschadl, 2006) or code updates (Krontiris & Dimitriou, 2006).

Hardware Encryption Schemes

Alternatively, one could utilize hardware encryption supported by the ChipCon 2420 ZigBee complaint RF Transceiver which is the most popular radio chip on wireless sensor nodes. For instance, Warren et al. (2005) implement Advanced Encryption Standard (AES) hardware encryption in ChipCon 2420 using 128-bit keys. The idea is to use one key per session while the

Algorithm 1. Elliptic curve cryptography

```
Input:  m, the message; y, the public key; h(), a cryptographic hash func-
tion; P,  the base point of the elliptic curve; n, a  random generated number
(the symmetric key).
Output: c, the chipertext.


1.    Encrypt m, E(m, r).
2.    Compute α = h(r) · y.
3.    Compute β = h(r) · P.
4.    Compute δ = n XOR f(α), where f(α) gives the x coordinate of α.
5.    Output the chipertext: c = < E(m, r), β, δ,>


Input: c, the chipertext; k, the secret key.
Output:  m, the message.
1.    Calculate k · β = k · h(r) · P = h(r) · y = α.
2.    Determine the x coordinate f(α).
3.    Derive the symmetric key n:  δ XOR f(α) = n XOR f(α) XOR f(α)=n.
4.    Apply n to E(m, r) to obtain m.
```

personal server shares the encryption key with all the sensors during the session configuration. The global key sharing approach may not be suitable in the healthcare context where the security and privacy of each patient's data must be ensured. In addition, the considerations highlighted by Naveen and David (2004) may further reduce the security of the proposed scheme.

Hardware encryption is also adopted by ALARM-NET (Wood et al., 2006). One limitation of the method is that it provides AES decryption only at the base station. As a consequence, the transmitted information cannot be accessed by the intermediate nodes. Another drawback is that the scheme is highly dependent on the specific hardware platform.

Key Management

Among the stable development and deployment of link layer security, more attention has been given to efficient and secures key management schemes which apply different ways to establish and distribute cryptographic keys among the nodes in the sensor network.

Depending on the topology of the WSN, there are four types of key management schemes which have been evaluated:

- For *hierarchical WSNs* in the presence of resourceful gateways:
  - trusted server schemes;
  - public key infrastructure (PKI) schemes;
- For large *distributed WSNs*:
  - key pre-distribution techniques;
  - autonomous key set-up schemes.

The trusted server scheme is a less costly alternative and consists in bootstrapping the key agreement between nodes. Trusted servers are employed In order to share a long-term secret with each client (Perrig. Szewczyk, Tygar, Wen, & Culler, 2002). Some argue that one cannot generally assume the existence of a trusted infrastructure and the trusted server might become a single point of failure. Furthermore, communication overhead should be taken into consideration and several schemes require time synchronization between the sinks and the sensor nodes.

In the key pre-distribution technique, three approaches have been studied for efficient distribution of the key to sensor nodes:

- probabilistic distribution which distributes the keys by choosing them randomly from a key pool;
- deterministic processes are applied in order to provide better key connectivity (i.e., the key pool and the key chains design);
- hybrid mechanisms, reported in (Donggang, Peng, & Wenliang, 2005; Wenliang, Jing, Yunghsiang, Pramod, Jonathan, & Aram, 2005), that utilize both probabilistic and deterministic approaches to achieve higher scalability and resiliency.

However, the key pre-distribution scheme faces a scalability problem where the number of keys has to increase with the network size.

Dutertre, Cheung and Levy (2004) have proposed a lightweight key management system by leveraging initial trust to set up the cryptographic keys in an autonomous fashion. Currently, this scheme is used to secure the local links by establishing pairwise keys among the neighbor nodes of the network.

A key establishment method to secure communications in WSNs has emerged to be biometrics (Cherukuri, Venkatasubramanian, & Gupta, 2003; Venkatasubramanian & Gupta, 2007). It asserts the use of the body itself as a means of managing cryptographic keys for symmetric cryptography. For sensors attached on the same body, they measure a previously agreed physiological value simultaneously and use this value to generate a pseudo-random number. Then it can be used to encrypt and decrypt the symmetric key in order to distribute it securely. The physiological value to be used should be chosen carefully, as it must exhibit proper time variance and randomness. In different case, the whole scheme can be vulnerable to brute force attacks. For instance, blood glucose, blood pressure or heart rate are not appropriate. On the other hand, ECG (electrocardiogram) has been shown to be appropriate as seed for a pseudo-random number generator (Bui & Hatzinakos, 2008).

However, an important requirement is to have precise time synchronization, so that sensors take their measurements at the same time and produce the same value. To do that, a time synchronization protocol is needed, using reference broadcasts. Such protocols have been shown to be susceptible to attacks (Manzo, Roosta, & Sastry, 2005) and securing them will require even more resources. Another disadvantage of this method is that only sensors in and on the body can measure the philological values, so it cannot be applied for securing the communication of other sensors in a more general architecture. In addition, this method assumes that there is a specific pre-defined biometric that all sensors can measure, which is not necessarily true.

In IBE-Lite (Tan, Wang, Zhong, & Li, 2008) the key management is simplified, since the patient can generate the secret key on-demand without keeping track of which cryptographic keys were used to encrypt the data. The only requirement is that the string used to describe the event is the same.

The main assumption of the work reported in (Čapkun, Hubaux, & Buttyán, 2003) is that when the nodes of an ad hoc network are close to each other they can communicate using a secure side channel, like wire or infrared communication. Thus, at this point no man in the middle attack, which would perturb the communication between them, is possible. An additional supposition in their scheme is that each node can generate cryptographic keys and verify signatures. For WSNs this type of approach involves both advantages and limitations. No central authority is needed, but each node in the network must generate and verify the public keys, which imply heavy computation.

Furthermore, the idea of joining mobile and static nodes in WSNs to establish secure communication between could be a successful approach.

Digital Watermarking

Due to the rising dependence on digital media and the unexpected expansion of the distribution opportunities over the Internet, digital watermarking techniques for data authentication are achieving significant importance.

Digital watermarking is a widespread information hiding technique, aimed to resolve different multimedia security issues (e.g., copyright protection, illegal distribution, broadcast monitoring and authentication) by embedding secret information (i.e., digital watermarks) into data contents (Cox & Miller, 2002). Watermarking techniques have been proposed for two types of artifacts:

- Static artifacts that consist of components which are not altered during their use, i.e., images (Acharya, Anand, Bhat, & Niranjan, 2001; Chao, Hsu, & Miaou, 2002; Zhou, Huang, & Lou, 2001), audio (Tsai, Chang, & Liu, 2003) and video (Wu, Knog, Yang, & Niu, 2008).
- Functional artifacts that must preserve their functional specifications and can be implemented at several level design (Wong, Feng, Kirovski, & Potkonjak, 2006).

Depending on the type of application to which a watermarking scheme is applied, digital watermarks can be subdivided in (Cox, Miller, & Bloom, 2000) *robust watermarks*, *semi-fragile watermarks* and *fragile watermarks*. *Robust watermarks* are devised to resist against "non-destructive" manipulations of the media or against a reasonable amount of time spent to remove them. Both these requirements, together with the fidelity of the watermarked media, change drastically the entire design of the watermarking schemes. On the other hand, *fragile watermarks* are designed

to fail when the media is inadequately tampered while *semi-fragile* watermarks can survive to some image processing operations which do not change the meaning of the media. Both watermarks are intended for integrity verification (authentication) of digital media and, in addition, they must be capable to detect and localize content's modifications.

Furthermore, watermarking schemes can be splitted according to how the cover media is manipulated during the insertion process into (Cox, Miller, & Bloom, 2000):

- Methods working in the *spatial domain*, that insert the watermark by modifying or replacing redundant components of the original data. The main issue of these methods is due to weakness against small data modification.
- Schemes operating in a *transform domain*, which represent the original content in a transformed domain where the embedding is performed. It is worthwhile to point out that, these schemes are more robust against a wide range of signal processing operations than those in the spatial domain, since the watermark is embedded in significant areas of the original content. Common examples are schemes based on the *frequency domain*, such as the Discrete Cosine Transform (DCT), the Discrete Fourier Transform (DFT) and the Discrete Wavelet Transform (DWT) or schemes based on the Singular Value Decomposition (SVD).

There are many watermarking schemes proposed for content authentication but only few of them focus on healthcare environments. Zhou, Huang and Lou (2001) present a watermarking method for verifying authenticity and integrity of digital mammography image. They used digital envelope as watermark and the least significant bit (LSB) of randomly chosen pixels of the mammogram is replaced by one bit of the digital envelope bit stream. In order to verify the integrity of the medical data, the most significant bits (MSB) of each pixel are used. Instead, Acharya, Anand, Bhat and Niranjan (2001) reduce storage and transmission overheads of the previous watermarking scheme by interleaving patient information with medical images.

Chao, Hsu and Miaou (2002) propose a discrete cosine transform (DCT) based data-hiding technique that is capable of hiding those EPR related data into a marked image. The information is embedded in the quantized DCT coefficients. The drawback of the above watermarking approaches is that the original medical image is distorted in a non-invertible manner. Therefore it is impossible for watermark decoder to recover the original image.

The first watermarking algorithms for sensors networks were proposed by Feng and Potkonjak (2003). The idea is to impose additional constraints during the sensing date acquisition and sensor data processing. These constraints, which correspond to the encrypted embedded signature, are chosen such that they provide optimal tradeoffs between the accuracy of the sensing process and the strength of the authorship proof. The first technique embeds the signature into the process of sensing data. The technique can be applied to each individual of nodes or to a properly selected collection of nodes. The signature can also be embedded in the way this collection of nodes is chosen. The second technique is to embed signature during data processing, either in sensor data or control data which leads to NP-complete problems and approximate solutions.

Intrusion Detection

In WSNs common security techniques, such as link layer encryption and digital watermarking, can be applied against outsider attacks, although these measures cannot eliminate them. Moreover, authentication and encryption, which both rely on trustworthy cooperation between mobile nodes,

are unable to guard the ad hoc network against inside attacks, i.e., attacks originating from compromised nodes (Ng, Sim, & Tan, 2006; Giani, Roosta, & Sastry, 2008). Due to these considerations, new techniques which deal with these security issues and act as second line of defense, have been proposed (Deng, Han, & Mishra, 2006; Krontiris, Dimitriou, & Giannetsos, 2008).

The system that screens the events which take place in a network or computer system in order to identify possible threats or violations of security policies is called *intrusion detection system* (IDS). In order to detect possible infringements of security policies, IDSs use several approaches from which we can mention:

- *Signature-based detection* (also called *pattern-based detection*) consists of matching the patterns (signatures) of knowing threats with the monitored events to detect security incidents.
- *Anomaly-based detection* compares the normal activity of the network with the occurred events to identify important deviations.
- *Protocol analysis detection* is similar to the previous method the only difference being the admissible profiles which represent the normal activity of the network protocols, instead of the network components. Thus, these detection methods are able to scan and understand the state of network, transport and applications protocols. The main problem of protocol analysis detection is that it needs many resources due to the complex analysis involved in checking the integrity of the communication protocols.

The majority of the research in intrusion detection relates to MANETs because WSNs have much sever resource constraints. For a survey of IDSs for MANETs the reader may consult (Mishra, Nadkarni & Patcha, 2004). Regarding the intrusion detection techniques developed specially for

WSNs, these are quite rare (Zhang & Lee, 2000; Zhang, Huang & Lee, 2003; Deng, Han, & Mishra, 2006; Krontiris, Dimitriou, & Giannetsos, 2008).

The earliest anomaly-based detection schemes for ad hoc networks were proposed in (Zhang & Lee, 2000; Zhang, Huang, & Lee, 2003). The basic idea is the distributed monitoring and cooperation among all nodes. Specifically, each node independently observes its neighborhood within its radio range looking for signs of intrusion. An IDS agent is attached to each node in order to keep track of internal activities of the node and packet communications within its local neighborhood.

In (Krontiris, Dimitriou & Giannetsos, 2008), an automated mechanism that identifies the source of an attack and generates an alarm to notify the network or the administrator so that appropriate preventive actions can take place is presented. To achieve this goal, the scheme makes use of autonomous and cooperative IDS agents. The approach organizes the cooperation of the agents according to the distributed nature of the events involved in the attacks, and, as a result, an agent needs to send information to other agents only when this information is necessary to detect the attack. The coordination mechanism organizes the message passing between the agents in such a way so that the distributed detection is equivalent to having all events processed in a central place.

Intrusion-tolerant Routing Protocol for Wireless Sensor Networks (INSENS) (Deng, Han & Mishra, 2006) has proved that it can securely and efficiently construct tree-structured routing for sensor networks. Specifically, INSENS creates forwarding tables at each sensor node to enable communication between nodes and a sink (base station). It minimizes computation, communication and bandwidth requirements at the sensor nodes at the expense of increased computation, communication and bandwidth requirements at the base station. INSENS does not rely on detecting intrusions, but rather tolerates intrusions by avoiding the malicious nodes. An important feature of the proposed approach is that while a malicious node may be able to compromise a small number of nodes in its vicinity, it cannot widespread the damage in the network.

FUTURE RESEARCH DIRECTIONS AND CONCLUSIONS

It appears that more research should be conducted on the security issues of healthcare applications delivered over WSNs especially in authorization (key establishment and trust setup), authentication (based on digital watermarking) and service availability. Regarding the security against DoS attack a wealth of research have been conducted on improving network security protocols' efficiency under resource constraint such as computation offloading via client puzzles.

Although these methods reduce the DoS attack's efficacy, they still leave WSNs vulnerable. A possible solution might be to use a resource-rich device to facilitate the communication between a sensor node and a sink, like the proposed RFID proxies mediate the communication between RFID readers and RFID tags (Rieback, Crispo, & Tanenbaum, 2005). The communication between the sensor node and the proxy (e.g., a smart phone or watch) could use lighter-weight symmetric encryption and authentication schemes, whereas the communication between the mediator and the external programmer could use more expensive asymmetric cryptographic techniques. Nevertheless, augmenting the number of devices and protocols involved increases the size of the overall system's trusted computing base, which might make the system harder to secure.

In this paper we have discussed the security issues that arise when integrating wireless sensor networks into health care systems. The viability and long-term success of WSNs depend upon addressing these security threats successfully. We investigated the existing solutions that can be employed while highlighting their limitations and advantages. Furthermore, the exiting intrusion detection approaches, needed for ensure integrity and reliability of the entire system, were explored. However, the resource-constraint nature of sensor nodes raises stringent challenges in embedding the multi-layer security solution. Therefore, more work and effort are needed in this area to facilitate the wider application of pervasive computing in the healthcare industry for the benefit of the entire population.

REFERENCES

Acharya, R., Anand, D., Bhat, S., & Niranjan, U. C. (2001). Compact storage of medical images with patient information. *IEEE Transactions on Information Technology in Biomedicine, 5*, 320–323. doi:10.1109/4233.966107

Agrawal, R., & Johnson, C. (2007). Securing electronic health records without impeding the flow of information. *International Journal of Medical Informatics, 76*(5-6), 471–479. doi:10.1016/j.ijmedinf.2006.09.015

Aziz, O., Lo, B., Pansiot, J., Atallah, L., Yang, G.-Z., & Darzi, A. (2008). From computers to ubiquitous computing by 2010: health care. *Philosophical Transactions of the Royal Society A: Mathematical, Physical and Engineering Sciences, 366*(1881), 3805-3811.

BioHealth: Security and Identity Management Standards in eHealth including Biometrics. Retrieved December 23, 2009, from http://biohealth.helmholtz-muenchen.de/

Bui, F. M., & Hatzinakos, D. (2008). Biometric methods for secure communications in body sensor networks: resource-efficient key management and signal-level data scrambling. *EURASIP Journal of Advance Signal Processsesing, 8*(2), 1–16. doi:10.1155/2008/529879

Čapkun, S., Hubaux, J., & Buttyán, L. (2003). Mobility helps security in ad hoc networks. In *Proceedings of the 4th ACM international Symposium on Mobile Ad Hoc Networking and Computing* (pp. 46-56). New York: ACM Press.

Chao, H. M., Hsu, C. M., & Miaou, S. G. (2002). A data-hiding technique with authentication, integration, and confidentiality for electronic patients records. *IEEE Transactions on Information Technology in Biomedicine, 6*, 46–53. doi:10.1109/4233.992161

Cherukuri, S., Venkatasubramanian, K. K., & Gupta, S. K. S. (2003). BioSec: A biometric based approach for securing communication in wireless networks of biosensors implanted in the human body. In *Proceedings of the 1st Workshop on Wireless Security and Privacy* (pp. 432-439).

Chevrollier, N., & Golmie, N. (2005). On the Use of Wireless Network Technologies in Healthcare Environments. In *Proceedings of the fifth IEEE Workshop on Applications and Services in Wireless Networks* (pp. 147-152).

Chhanabhai, P., & Holt, A. (2007). Consumers Are Ready to Accept the Transition to Online and Electronic Records if they can be assured of the Security Measures. *MedGenMed, 9*(1), 8-20. Retrieved December 23, 2009, from http://www.ncbi.nlm.nih.gov/pmc/articles/PMC1924980/?tool=pubmed

COM. (2004). Communication from the Commission to the Council, the European Parliament. *the European Economic and Social Committee and the Committee of the Regions: e-Health-making healthcare better for European citizens: an action plan for a European e-Health Area.* Retrieved December 23, 2009, from http://eur-lex.europa.eu/LexUriServ/LexUriServ.do?uri=CELEX:52004DC0356:ES:HTML

Cox, I. J., & Miller, M. L. (2002). The first 50 years of electronic watermarking. *EURASIP Journal on Applied Signal Processing, 2*, 126–132. doi:10.1155/S1110865702000525

Cox, I. J., Miller, M. L., & Bloom, J. A. (2000). *Digital Watermarking*. San Francisco: Morgan Kaufmann.

De Moor, G. J. E., & Claerhout, B. (2004). Privacy enhancing techniques in E-Health: an overview. In G. Demiris (Ed.), *Studies in Health Technology and Informatics: Vol. 106. eHealth: Current Status and Future Trends* (pp. 75-82). Netherlands: IOS Press.

Deng, J., Han, R., & Mishra, S. (2006). INSENS: Intrusion-tolerant routingn for wireless sensor networks. *Computer Communications, 29*, 216–230. doi:10.1016/j.comcom.2005.05.018

Donggang, L., Peng, N., & Wenliang, D. (2005). Group-based key predistribution in wireless sensor networks. In *Proceedings of the 4th ACM Workshop on Wireless Security* (pp. 11-20). New York: ACM Press.

Dutertre, B., Cheung, S., & Levy, J. (2004). *Lightweight key management in wireless sensor networks by leveraging initial trust*. Technical Report SRI-SDL-04-02, SRI International.

Falcão-Reis, F., Costa-Pereira, A., & Correia, M. E. (2008). Access and privacy rights using web security standards to increase patient empowerment. In L. Bos, B. Blobel, A. Marsh, & D. Carroll (Eds.), *Studies in Health Technology and Informatics: Vol. 137. Medical and Care Compunetics 5 (pp. 275-285)*. Netherlands: IOS Press.

Feng, J., & Potkonjak, M. (2003). Real-time watermarking techniques for sensor networks. *Proceedings of the Society for Photo-Instrumentation Engineers, 5020*(391), 391–402.

Fragopoulos, A., Gialelis, J., & Serpanos, D. (2009). Security Framework for Pervasive Healthcare Architectures Utilizing MPEG-21 IPMP Components. *International Journal of Telemedicine and Applications, 2009*, 1–9. doi:10.1155/2009/461560

Giani, A., Roosta, T., & Sastry, S. (2008). Integrity checker for wireless sensor networks in health care applications. In *Proceedings of the 2nd International Conference on Pervasive Computing Technologies for Healthcare* (pp. 135-138).

Großschadl, J. (2006). TinySA: A security architecture for wireless sensor networks. In *Proceedings of the 2nd International Conference on Emerging Networking Experiments and Technologies*.

Hadim, S., & Mohamed, N. (2006). Middleware Challenges and Approaches for Wireless Sensor Networks. *IEEE Distributed Systems Online, 7*.

Halperin, D., Heydt-Benjamin, T. S., Fu, K., Kohno, T., & Maisel, W. H. (2008). Security and Privacy for Implantable Medical Devices. *IEEE Pervasive Computing / IEEE Computer Society [and] IEEE Communications Society, 7*(1), 30–39. doi:10.1109/MPRV.2008.16

Halperin, D., Heydt-Benjamin, T. S., Ransford, B., Clark, S. S., Defend, B., Morgan, W., et al. (2008). Pacemakers and Implantable Cardiac Defibrilators: Software Radio Attacks and Zero-Power Defenses. In *Proceedings of IEEE Symposium on Security and Privacy* (pp. 129-142).

Hu, Y.-C., Johnson, D. B., & Perrig, A. (2002). SEAD: secure efficient distance vector routing for mobile wireless ad hoc networks. In *Proceedings of the 4th IEEE Workshop on Mobile Computing Systems and Applications* (pp. 3–13).

Hu, Y.-C., Perrig, A., & Johnson, D. B. (2002). Ariadne: a secure on-demand routing protocol for ad hoc networks. *Wireless Networks, 11*(1-2), 21–38. doi:10.1007/s11276-004-4744-y

Joshi, A., Finin, T., Kagal, L., Parker, J., & Patwardhan, A. (2008) Security policies and trust in ubiquitous computing. *Philosophical Transactions of the Royal Society A: Mathematical, Physical and Engineering Sciences, 366*(1881), 3769-3780.

Karl, H., & Willing, A. (2005). *Protocols and Architectures for Wireless Sensor Networks.* West Sussex, England: John Willy & Sons. doi:10.1002/0470095121

Karlof, C., Sastry, N., & Wagner, D. (2004). TinySec: A link layer security architecture for wireless sensor networks. In *Proceedings of the 2nd ACM Conference on Embedded Networked Sensor Systems* (162–175).

Karlof, C., & Wagner, D. (2003). Secure routing in wireless sensor networks: attacks and countermeasures. *Ad Hoc Networking, 1*(2-3), 293–315. doi:10.1016/S1570-8705(03)00008-8

Katsikas, S., Lopez, J., & Pernul, G. (2008). The challenge for security and privacy services in distributed health settings. In B. Blobel, P. Pharow, & M. Nerlich (Eds.), *Studies in Health Technology and Informatics: Vol. 134. eHealth: Combining Health Telematics, Telemedicine, Biomedical Engineering and Bioinformatics to the Edge-Global Experts Summit Textbook* (pp. 113-125). Netherlands: IOS Press.

Konstantas, D., Jones, V., & Herzog, R. (2002) MobiHealth-Innovative 2.5/3G mobile services and applications for health care. In *Proceedings of the IST Mobile and Wireless Telecommunications Summit.*

Krontiris, I., & Dimitriou, T. (2006). Authenticated in-network programming for wireless sensor networks. In *Proceedings of the 5th International Conference on AD- HOC Networks & Wireless* (pp. 390-403).

Krontiris, I., Dimitriou, T., & Giannetsos, T. (2008). LIDeA: A distributed lightweight intrusion detection architecture for sensor networks. In *Proceeding of the fourth International Conference on Security and Privacy for Communication.*

Liu, A., & Ning, P. (2008). TinyECC: A configurable library for elliptic curve cryptography in wireless sensor networks. In. *Proceedings of the International Conference on Information Processing in Sensor Networks, 1,* 245–256.

Lorincz, K., Malan, D. J., & Fulford-Jones, T. R. F., Nawoj. A., Clavel, A., Shnayder, V., Mainland, G., Welsh, M., & Moulton, S. (2004). Sensor networks for emergency response: challenges and opportunities. *IEEE Pervasive Computing / IEEE Computer Society [and] IEEE Communications Society, 3,* 16–23. doi:10.1109/MPRV.2004.18

Lupu, E., Dulay, N., Sloman, M., Sventek, J., Heeps, S., & Strowes, S. (2007). AMUSE: autonomic management of ubiquitous e-Health systems. *Concurrency and Computation, 20*(3), 277–295. doi:10.1002/cpe.1194

Malasri, K., & Wang, L. (2007). Addressing security in medical sensor networks. In *Proceedings of the 1st ACM SIGMOBILE International Workshop on Systems and networking support for healthcare and assisted living environments* (pp. 7-12). New York: ACM Press.

Manzo, M., Roosta, T., & Sastry, S. (2005). Time synchronization attacks in sensor networks. In *Proceedings of the 3rd ACM Workshop on Security of Ad Hoc and Sensor Networks* (pp. 107-116). New York: ACM Press.

Marti, R., Delgado, J., & Perramon, X. (2004). Network and Application Security in Mobile e-Health Applications. In L. Bos, B. Blobel, A. Marsh, & D. Carroll (Eds.), *Lecture Notes in Computer Science: Vol. 3090. Information Networking (pp. 995-1004).* Berlin/Heidelberg: Spriger-Verlag.

Mishra, A., Nadkarni, K., & Patcha, A. (2004). Intrusion detection in wireless ad hoc networks. *IEEE Wireless Communications, 11*, 48–60. doi:10.1109/MWC.2004.1269717

Naveen, S., & David, W. (2004). Security considerations for IEEE 802.15.4 networks. In *Proceedings of the ACM Workshop on Wireless Security* (pp. 32-42). New York: ACM Press.

Neves, P., Stachyra, M., & Rodrigues, J. (2008). Application of Wireless Sensor Networks to Healthcare Promotion. *Journal of Communications Software and Systems, 4*(3), 181–190.

Ng, H. S., Sim, M. L., & Tan, C. M. (2006). Security issues of wireless sensor networks in healthcare applications. *BT Technology Journal, 24*(2), 138–144. doi:10.1007/s10550-006-0051-8

Ng, J. W. P., Lo, B. P. L., Wells, O., Sloman, M., Toumazou, C., Peters, N., et al. (2004). *Ubiquitous Monitoring Environment for Wearable and Implantable Sensors (UbiMon).* Paper presented at UbiComp, Nottingham.

Penders, J., van de Molengraft, J., Brown, L., Grundlehner, B., Gyselinckx, B., & van Hoof, C. (2009). Potential and challenges of body area networks for personal health. In *Proceedings of the Annual International Conference of the IEEE Engineering in Medicine and Biology Society* (pp.6569-6572). IEEE Engineering in Medicine and Biology Society. Washington, DC: IEEE Press.

Perrig, A., Szewczyk, R., Tygar, J., Wen, V., & Culler, D. E. (2002). SPINS: security protocols for sensor networks. *Wireless Networks, 8*, 521–534. doi:10.1023/A:1016598314198

Raghavendra, C. S., Sivalingam, K. M., & Znati, T. (Eds.). (2004). *Wireless Sensor Networks.* Berlin, Heidelberg: Spriger-Verlag. doi:10.1007/b117506

Rieback, M., Crispo, B., & Tanenbaum, A. (2005). RFID Guardian: A Battery-Powered Mobile Device for RFID Privacy Management. In C. Boyd, J. M. G. Nieto (Eds.), Lecture Notes in Computer Science: *Vol. 3574. Information Security and Privacy* (pp. 184-194). Berlin/Heidelberg: Spriger-Verlag.

Rivest, R. L. (2006). The RC5 encryption algorithm. In B. Preneel (Eds.), *Lecuture Notes in Computer Science: Vol. 1008. Fast software encryption* (pp. 86-96). Berlin/Heidelberg: Springer-Verlag.

Sample, A. P., Yeager, D. J., Powledge, P. S., & Smith, J. R. (2007). Design of a passively-powered, programmable platform for UHF RFID systems. In *Proceedings of IEEE International Conference on RFID* (pp. 149-156).

Savastano, M., Hovsto, A., Pharow, P., & Blobel, B. (2008). Security, Safety, and Related Technology-The Triangle of eHealth Service Provision. In S. K. Andersen, G. O. Klein, S. Schulz, J. Aarts, & M. C. Mazzoleni (Eds.), *Studies in Health Technology and Informatics: Vol. 136. eHealth Beyond the Horizon-Get IT There* (pp. 709-714). Netherlands: IOS Press.

Shamir, A. (1985). Identity-based cryptosystems and signature schemes. In *Proceedings of CRYPTO on Advances in Cryptology* (pp. 47-53).

Stingl, C., & Slamanig, D. (2008). Privacy-enhancing methods for e-health applications: how to prevent statistical analyses and attacks. *International Journal of Business Intelligence and Data Mining, 3*(3), 236–254. doi:10.1504/IJBIDM.2008.022135

Stojmenovic, I., & Olariu, S. (2005). Data-centric protocols for Wireless Sensor Networks. In Stojmenovic, I. (Ed.), *Handbook of Sensor Networks* (pp. 417–456). Sussex, England: John Willy & Sons. doi:10.1002/047174414X.ch13

Szczechowiak, P., Oliveira, L. B., Scott, M., Collier, M., & Dahab, R. (2008). NanoECC: Testing the limits of elliptic curve cryptography in sensor networks. In R. Verdone (Ed.), *Lecture Notes in Computer Science: Vol. 4913. Wireless Sensor Networks* (pp. 305-320). Berlin/Heidelberg: Spriger-Verlag.

Tan, C. C., Wang, H., Zhong, S., & Li, Q. (2008). Body sensor network security: an identity-based cryptography approach. In *Proceedings of the first ACM conference on Wireless network security* (pp. 148-153). New York: ACM Press.

Tan, C. C., Wang, H., Zhong, S., & Li, Q. (2009). IBE-lite: A lightweight identity based cryptography for body sensor networks. *IEEE Transactions on Information Technology in Biomedicine, 13*(6), 926–932. doi:10.1109/TITB.2009.2033055

TinyOS project. (2004). Berkeley University. (n.d.). Retrieved December 23, 2009, from http://webs.cs.berkeley.edu/tos/

Tsai, H.-H., Cheng, J.-S., & Yu, P.-T. (2003). Audio Watermarking Based on HAS and Neural Networks in DCT domain. *EURASIP Journal on Applied Signal Processing*, (3): 252–263. doi:10.1155/S1110865703208027

Uhsadel, L., Poschmann, A., & Paar, C. (2007). Enabling Full-Size Public-Key Algorithms on 8-bit Sensor Nodes. In F. Stajano, C. Meadows, S. Capkun, & T. Moore (Eds.), *Lecture Notes in Computer science: Vol. 4572. Security and Privacy in Wireless Sensor Networks* (pp. 73-86). Berlin/Heidelberg: Spriger-Verlag.

Venkatasubramanian, K., & Gupta, S. K. S. (2007). Security for Pervasive Healthcare. In Y. Xiao (Eds.), *Security in Distributed, Grid, Mobile, and Pervasive Computing* (pp. 443-464). Berlin: Auerbach Publications, CRC Press.

Vogel, S., Hulsbusch, M., Hennig, T., Blazek, V., & Leonhardt, S. (2009). In-Ear Vital Signs Monitoring Using a Novel Microoptic Reflective Sensor. *IEEE Transactions on Information Technology in Biomedicine, 13*(6), 882–889. doi:10.1109/TITB.2009.2033268

Vouyioukas, D., Kambourakis, G., Maglogiannis, I., Rouskas, A., Kolias, C., & Gritzalis, S. (2008). Enabling the provision of secure web based m-health services utilizing XML based security models. *Journal Security and Communication Networks, 1*(5), 375–388. doi:10.1002/sec.46

Warren, S., Lebak, J., Yao, J., Creekmore, J., Milenkovic, A., & Jovanov, E. (2005) Interoperability and security in wireless body area network infrastructures. In *Proceedings of the 27th Annual International Conference of the IEEE Engineering in Medicine and Biology Society* (pp. 3837–3840).

Waterman, J., Curtis, D., Goraczko, M., Shih, E., Sarin, P., & Pino, E. (2005). (Scalable Medical AlertResponse Technology). In *Proceeding of Washington DC, American Medical Informatics Association* (pp. 1182–1183). Demonstration of SMART.

Wenliang, D., Jing, D., Yunghsiang, S. H., Pramod, K. V., Jonathan, K., & Aram, K. (2005). A pairwise key predistribution scheme for wireless sensor networks. *ACM Transactions on Information and System Security, 8*, 228–258. doi:10.1145/1065545.1065548

Wong, A. W., McDonagh, D., Omeni, O., Nunn, C., Hernandez-Silveira, M., & Burdett, A. J. (2009). Sensium: an ultra-low-power wireless body sensor network platform: design & application challenges. In *Proceedings of the Annual International Conference of the IEEE Engineering in Medicine and Biology Society* (pp.6576-6579). IEEE Engineering in Medicine and Biology Society. IEEE Press.

Wong, J. L., Feng, J., Kirovski, D., & Potkonjak, M. (2006). Security in Sensor Networks: Watermarking Techniques. In Raghavendra, C. S., Sivalingam, K. M., & Znati, T. (Eds.), *Wireless Sensor Networks* (pp. 305–323). Berlin, Heidelberg: Spriger-Verlag.

Wood, A., Virone, G., Doan, T., Cao, Q., Selavo, L., Wu, Y., et al. (2006). *ALARM-NET: Wireless sensor networks for assisted-living and residential monitoring*. Technical Report CS-2006-1, Department of Computer Science, University of Virginia. Retrieved December 23, 2009 from http://www.cs.virginia.edu/wsn/medical/about/ publications

Wood, A. D., & Stankovic, J. A. (2002). Denial of service in sensor networks. *IEEE Computer*, *35*(10), 54–62.

Wu, D., Kong, W., Yang, B., & Niu, X. (2008). A fast SVD based video watermarking algorithm compatible with MPEG2. *Standard Soft Computing-A Fusion of Foundations. Methodologies and Applications*, *13*(4), 375–382.

Zhang, Y., Huang, Y.-A., & Lee, W. (2003). Intrusion detection techniques for mobile wireless networks. *Wireless Networks*, *9*, 545–556. doi:10.1023/A:1024600519144

Zhang, Y., & Lee, W. (2000). Intrusion detection in wireless ad-hoc networks. In *Proceedings of the 6th Annual ACM International Conference on Mobile Computing and Networking* (pp. 275-283).

Zhao, F., & Guibas, L. (2004). *Wireless Sensor Networks: an information processing approach*. San Francisco: Morgan Kaufmann, Elsevier.

Zhou, X. Q., Huang, H. K., & Lou, S. L. (2001). Authenticity and integrity of digital mammography images. *IEEE Transactions on Medical Imaging*, *20*, 784–791. doi:10.1109/42.938246

ADDITIONAL READING

(n.d.). BioHealth: Security and Identity Management Standards in eHealth including [from http://biohealth.helmholtz-muenchen.de/]. *Biometrics*. Retrieved December 23, 2009.

Body Sensor Networks Conference (BSN 2009).(n.d.). Retrieved from http://bsn2009.org/bsn2009.html

Dishongh, T. J., & McGrath, M. (2009). *Wireless Sensor Networks for Healthcare Applications*. Norwood, MA: Artech House.

Fisher, C., & Gellersen, H. (2009). Location and Navigation Support for Emergency Responders: A Survey. *IEEE Pervasive Computing / IEEE Computer Society [and] IEEE Communications Society*, *9*(1), 38–47. doi:10.1109/MPRV.2009.91

Guizani, M., Du, X., Chen, H.-H., & Mueller, P. (Eds.). (2007). *Security in Wireless Mobile Ad Hoc and Sensor Networks (Special Issue)*. IEEE Wireless Communication Magazine.

Gyselinckx, B. Vullers, R. Hoof, C. V. Ryckaert, J. Yazicioglu, R.F. Fiorini, & P. Leonov, V. (2006). Human++: Emerging Technology for Body Area Networks. In *Proceedings of the IFIP International Conference on Very Large Scale Integration* (pp. 175 - 180). Washington, DC: IEEE Press.

Ilyas, M., & Dorf, R. C. (2003). *The Handbook of Ad Hoc Wireless Networks*. Boca Raton, FL: CRC Press.

International Conference on Electronic Health (eHealth, 2009).Retrieved from http://www.electronic-health.org/2009/index.shtml

International Workshop on Ubiquitous Body Sensor Networks (UBSN 2010). (n.d.). Retrieved from http://sites.google.com/site/ubsn2010/

Jovanov, E., Poon, C. C. Y., Yang, G.-Z., & Zhang, Y. T. (Eds.). (2009). Body Sensor Networks: From Theory to Emerging Applications [Special Issue]. *IEEE Transactions on Information Technology in Biomedicine, 13*(6)..doi:10.1109/TITB.2009.2034564

Katzenbeisser, S., & Petitcolas, F. A. P. (Eds.). (2000). *Information Hiding techniques for Steganography and Digital Watermarking*. London: Artech House.

Korhonen, I., & Bardram, J. E. (Eds.). (2006). Pervasive Healthcare (Special Section). *IEEE Transactions on Information Technology in Biomedicine, 8*(3). doi:.doi:10.1109/TITB.2004.835337

Mishra, A., & Nadkarni, K. M. (2003). Security in wireless ad hoc networks. In Ilyas, M., & Dorf, R. C. (Eds.), *The Handbook of Ad Hoc Wireless Networks* (pp. 30-1–30-49). Boca Raton, FL: CRC Press.

Papadimitratos, P., & Haas, Z. J. (2003). Securing Mobile Ad Hoc Networks. In M. Ilyas & R. C. Dorf (Eds.), *The Handbook of Ad Hoc Wireless Networks* (pp. 31-1 – 30-21). Boca Raton, FL: CRC Press.

Penders, J., Gyselinckx, B., Vullers, R., Rousseaux, O., Berekovic, M., & De Nil, M. (2007). HUMAN++: Emerging Technology for Body Area Networks. In de Micheli, G., Mir, S., & Reis, R. (Eds.), *VLSI-SoC: Research Trends in VLSI and Systems on Chip* (*Vol. 249*, pp. 377–397). Boston: Springer. doi:10.1007/978-0-387-74909-9_21

Reddy, A. M., Kumar, A. P., Janakiram, D., & Kumar, G. A. (2009). Wireless sensor network operating systems: a survey. *Int. J. Sen. Netw., 5*(4), 236–255. doi:10.1504/IJSNET.2009.027631

Sarrafzadeh, M., Kaiser, W., & Wu, W. (Eds.). (2009). *Wireless Health (Special Issue)*. IEEE Transactions on Information Technology in Biomedicine.

Schneier, B. (1996). *Applied cryptography*. San Francisco: John Wiley & Sons.

Shen, X., Kato, N., & Lin, X. (2010). Wireless technologies for E-healthcare [Special Issue]. *IEEE Wireless Communication Magazine., 17*(1), 1–111.

Shen, X., Zhang, Q., & Qiu, R.-C. (Eds.). (2007). *Wireless Sensor Networking (Special Issue)*. IEEE Wireless Communication Magazine.

Wu, S. X., & Banzhaf, W. (2010). The use of computational intelligence in intrusion detection systems: A review. *Applied Soft Computing, 10*(1), 1–35. doi:10.1016/j.asoc.2009.06.019

Zhou, D. (2003). Security issues in ad hoc networks. In Ilyas, M., & Dorf, R. C. (Eds.), *The Handbook of Ad Hoc Wireless Networks* (pp. 32-1–32-25). Boca Raton, FL: CRC Press.

KEY TERMS AND DEFINITIONS

Ad Hoc Network: consists of a group of mobile nodes (peers) which are able to communicate with each other without the intervention of an access point. Depending on their application, wireless ad hoc networks can be further classified into: mobile ad hoc networks (MANETs), wireless mesh networks (WMNs) and wireless sensor networks (WSNs)

Wireless Sensor Network (WSN): consists of many spatially distributed autonomous devices, called smart sensor nodes, which cooperatively screen the environmental or physical conditions at different locations

Authorization: refers to the access control mechanisms and to the ability of an entity to access shared resources.

Authentication: mechanisms that allow an entity to prove its identity to a remote user.

Data Integrity: refers to methods which assure that data transmitted between two parties has not been changed.

Digital Watermarking: is a widespread information hiding technique, aimed to resolve different multimedia security issues such as, copyright protection, illegal distribution, broadcast monitoring and authentication, by embedding secret information (i.e., digital watermarks) into data contents

Cryptography: is the since of hiding information. It consists of two main steps: encryption which converts data (i.e., plaintext) into unintelligible gibberish (i.e., ciphertext) through an encryption key, and decryption which performs the reverse operation using the corresponding decryption key. Depending on the cryptographic keys applied, cryptography can be split into: private (symmetric) cryptography which uses the same key to perform encryption/decryption, and public (asymmetric) cryptography that employs different keys to encrypt and decrypt data.

Digital Signature: is a cryptographic primitive that demonstrates the authenticity of a digital message or document.

Cryptographic Hash Function: is a function that takes arbitrary-length strings and compress them into shorter strings. In addition, this function it is "easy" to compute but "hard" to invert, i.e., collision resistant.

Elliptic Curve Cryptography (ECC): is a cryptographic method based on the algebraic structure of elliptic curves over finite fields. Cryptography is based on the intractability of certain mathematical problems. In case of ECC, it is presumed that finding the discrete logarithm of an elliptic curve element is computationally unfeasible.

Secure Routing Protocol: is a protocol suite which secures the communication in wireless ad hoc networks against routing attacks, i.e., the control plain attack, the blackhole attack, the wormhole attack, etc. The crucial idea is to establish trustworthy communications between the participating nodes by controlling the message integrity and confidentiality, i.e., through message authentication codes (MACs) or digital signatures hash chains.

Intrusion Detection System (IDS): is a system that screens the events which take place in a network or computer system in order to identify possible threats or violations of security policies.

Section 2
User–Centered Design of Assistive Technologies

Chapter 6
An Approach to Participative Personal Health Record System Development

Vasso Koufi
University of Piraeus, Greece

Flora Malamateniou
University of Piraeus, Greece

George Vassilacopoulos
University of Piraeus, Greece

ABSTRACT

Healthcare delivery is undergoing radical change in an attempt to meet increasing demands in the face of rising costs. Among the most intriguing concepts in this effort is shifting the focus of care management to patients by means of Personal Health Record (PHR) systems which can integrate care delivery across the continuum of services and also coordinate care across all settings. However, a number of organizational and behavioral issues can delay PHR adoption. This chapter presents a general approach to breaking down barriers that exist at the level of individual healthcare professionals and consumers. According to this approach, user participation in PHR system development is considered essential for achieving systems implementation success. Realizing a participative PHR system development, where users are full members of the development team, requires not only choosing an appropriate methodology but also organizing the participation process in a way that is tailored to the particular situation in order to achieve the desired results.

INTRODUCTION

Throughout their lives, individuals receive care in various healthcare organizations. This results in patient health data being scattered around disparate and geographically dispersed information systems hosted by different healthcare providers (Koufi and Vassilacopoulos, 2008; Tang, Ash, Bates, Overhage and Sands, 2006). The lack of interoperability among these systems impedes optimal care as it leads to unavailability of important information

DOI: 10.4018/978-1-60960-469-1.ch006

regarding patient health status when this is mostly needed (e.g. in case of an emergency).

Recently there has been a remarkable upsurge in activity surrounding the adoption of Personal Health Record (PHR) systems for patients (Tang, Ash, Bates, Overhage and Sands, 2006). A PHR is a consumer-centric approach to making comprehensive electronic health records (EHRs) available at the point of care while protecting patient privacy (Lauer, 2009). Unlike traditional EHRs which are based on the 'fetch and show' model, PHRs' architectures are based on the fundamental assumptions that the complete records are held on a central repository and that each patient retains authority over access to any portion of his/her record (Lauer, 2009; Wiljer, Urowitz, Apatu, DeLenardo, Eysenbach, Harth, Pai, Leonard, 2008). In essence, a PHR is a health record bank account which operates much like a checking account (Yasnoff, 2008). Instead of depositing money, healthcare providers deposit copies of the patients' new records after each care episode (which they must do at the patient's request under the Health Insurance Portability & Accountability Act, or HIPAA) (Yasnoff, 2008). Thus, an entire class of interoperability is eliminated since the system of storing and retrieving essential patient data is no longer fragmented. Hence, quality and safety of patient care is enhanced by providing patients and health professionals with relevant and timely information while ensuring protection and confidentiality of personal data.

Providing patients with access to their electronic health records offers great promise to improve patient health and satisfaction with their care, as well as to improve professional and organizational approaches to health care (Wiljer, Urowitz, Apatu, DeLenardo, Eysenbach, Harth, Pai and Leonard, 2008). In particular, much potential can be realized if cooperation among disparate healthcare organizations is expressed in terms of cross-organizational healthcare processes, where information support is provided by means of PHR systems. Under this process-oriented, patient-centric model, health systems can integrate care delivery across the continuum of services, from prevention to follow-up, and coordinate care across all settings. Thus, healthcare processes are supported in a more direct way, since tasks to be performed are actively delivered to the right persons at the right time with the necessary information and the application functions needed (Reichert & Dadam, 1998). Workflow technology provides an appropriate infrastructure to realize process-oriented PHR systems. It allows modeling the control and data flow within healthcare processes separately from the implementation of the application programs (Malamateniou & Vassilacopoulos, 2002). It supports the controlled exchange of information between them, it provides worklists to users and it invokes the application programs associated with work items from these lists.

Although many benefits have been identified, there are many questions about best practices for the implementation of PHR systems (Wiljer, Urowitz, Apatu, DeLenardo, Eysenbach, Harth, Pai and Leonard, 2008). As with EHR, a number of impediments to PHR adoption has been identified which is not limited to technical ones. In addition to the economic and technical challenges, organizational and behavioral issues can delay PHR adoption. Barriers exist both at the environmental level and at the level of individual consumers and healthcare professionals (Tang, Ash, Bates, Overhage and Sands, 2006). With regard to consumers, individual-level barriers are due to the concerns consistently ranked by them about security and privacy of PHR information (e.g. health, financial). Moreover, the development of a workflow-based PHR system poses problems not encountered in conventional information systems. It requires taking a horizontal, process-oriented view of each healthcare organization and undertaking the system's development process within the context of a process engineering life-cycle (Walter & Herrmann, 1998). This may provoke greater resistance from healthcare professionals as it involves making larger financial, sociocultural and political commitments (Berg & Toussaint, 2003). This chapter addresses these issues from a sociotechnical perspective and presents a workflow sociotechnical analysis that requires a continuous recognition of the interaction that is taking place between technical, economic, organisational and social factors when workflow systems are being designed and, afterwards, when they are being used by groups that need the data they can provide. In addition, an approach to developing an effective workflow-based PHR system is introduced that is built on the simple premise that by inviting users (e.g. consumers, healthcare professionals) to participate in the system development process, the likelihood of system success (often measured in terms of system usage or user information satisfaction) is increased as users are expected to develop positive attitudes toward the new system (Gulliksen, Goransson, Boivie, Blomkvist, Persson & Cajander, 2003; Baroudi, Olson & Ives, 1986; Hartwick & Barki, 1994; King, & Lee, 1991).

BACKGROUND

Workflow-Based PHR Systems: A Sociotechnical Approach

Today's health information systems are social systems that have a complicated interrelationship with technology; that is, they are inherently complex sociotechnical systems. In complex sociotechnical systems, behavior is not centered in individual actors or even in groups of actors but is distributed among actors and the information available in the environment (Berg, 1999). According to the Actor-network theory (ANT), which evolved from the work of Michel Callon (1991) and Bruno Latour (1992), actors, human and non-human, constitute a network where they assume identities according to prevailing strategies of interaction (Bardini, n.d.). Actors' identities and qualities are defined during negotiations between

representatives of human and non-human actants (Bardini, n.d.). In this perspective, "representation" is understood in its political dimension, as a process of delegation (Bardini, n.d.). The most important of these negotiations is "translation", a multifaceted interaction in which actors construct common definitions and meanings, define representativities and co-opt each other in the pursuit of individual and collective objectives (Bardini, n.d.). In the actor-network theory, both actors and actants share the scene in the reconstruction of the network of interactions leading to the stabilization of the system (Bardini, n.d.). The crucial difference between them is that only actors are able to put actants in circulation in the system (Bardini, n.d.).

Although, health information systems have multiple users they are rarely designed to support cooperative work-and almost certainly are not designed for flexibility or creativity. PHR systems have the potential to stimulate transformational changes in healthcare delivery by (Alberta Health Services, n.d):

- Enabling access to comprehensive real-time patient data for clinicians and administrators across various care settings and facilities.
- Providing clinicians with tools to improve their partnership and coordination across different care settings.
- Achieving a level of integration that will allow data to flow seamlessly across the health system to enable the required tools and capabilities.

To design effective PHR systems for complex, dynamic sociotechnical organizations requires that the designer understand how the organization works, the cultural context, and how people interact with available information (Effken, 2002). That is, developers of PHR systems must have a full understanding of individuals' and clinicians' mental models of healthcare processes and related workflows. Nowadays, workflow models for both providers and patients are poorly understood. For example, while informaticians have studied clinical workflow models in settings of care, they are rarely concerned with describing patient flow in the community and fitting the PHR into it.

On the other hand, healthcare consumers must understand and accept their roles and responsibilities related to their own healthcare. An individual's PHR can only be useful if the person understands the importance of maintaining and coordinating health-related documentation and activities with health care providers. Education on health management techniques can lead towards this end while development of PHR systems tailored to the consumers' needs and preferences (in terms of interface, technology and security issues), will further contribute in breaking down the barriers to PHR adoption by gaining higher user acceptance.

On these grounds, PHR system designers should take a sociotechnical approach to achieve an improved quality of life for users and not focus solely on achieving internal economic goals. When there is divergence between the views of designers and users there will almost certainly be problems when the system is implemented (Jeffcot, 2001; Berg, 2001). Systems design is never simple and there is always likely to be a degree of uncertainty in the decisions that are taken, with no guarantee that the right decisions are being made. Also, today's health information systems design is almost always taking place in situations which are in a state of change, often a rapid change. This can mean that systems design assumptions and plans have to be constantly reviewed. A successful system design has been achieved when a desired result is achieved with direct links between diagnosis, planning, design and use.

Successful system design is related to three different skills 'capability', 'competence', and 'coordination' (Mumford, 2000). Ideally both designers and users will have these although they make take different forms. If a sociotechnical approach is being used then an important capability will be the need to give internal and external users an improvement in aspects of their lives that they regard as important. Sociotechnical competence requires knowledge of how to achieve social and organizational as well as technical goals. Coordination is the third important sociotechnical concept in problem solving and is particularly relevant to the design and implementation of information technology, where designers and users must collaborate closely if systems are to succeed.

The right capabilities, competencies and coordination facilities are essential requirements for today's and tomorrow innovation, but other skills are required for successful systems design. Teamwork is also very important. Knowledge will need to be shared, strategies agreed and individual competencies used effectively. Lastly, motivation for both the group and the individual is essential. The systems designers and users must actively want to understand and solve the design problems and make a contribution to an effective workable system (Aaltonenm, Nurminen, Rejonen & Vuorenheimo, 2002). All aspects of good system design are dependent on knowledge. Success requires the ability to search for, analyze and synthesize relevant information and relate it to current and future needs. A sociotechnical approach would ensure that all groups have knowledge relevant to their own use of the system. Knowledge should lead to considered action and an ability to work well in potentially stressful situations (Berg, Langenberg, Berg & Kwakkernaat, 1998).

It must always be remembered that a sociotechnical approach requires the social to be given equal importance to the technical. A new technology can impact the very nature of the work being carried out to the point of imposing new requirements in the behaviors that are expected from users. Whether or not a technological innovation ends up yielding the intended results will in part depend on whether the behavioral requirements it imposes are compatible with the current culture or whether the current culture can be altered so as to become compatible with those requirements (Cabrera, Cabrera & Barajas, 2001). Aligning

Figure 1. Sociotechnical perspective of organizational design

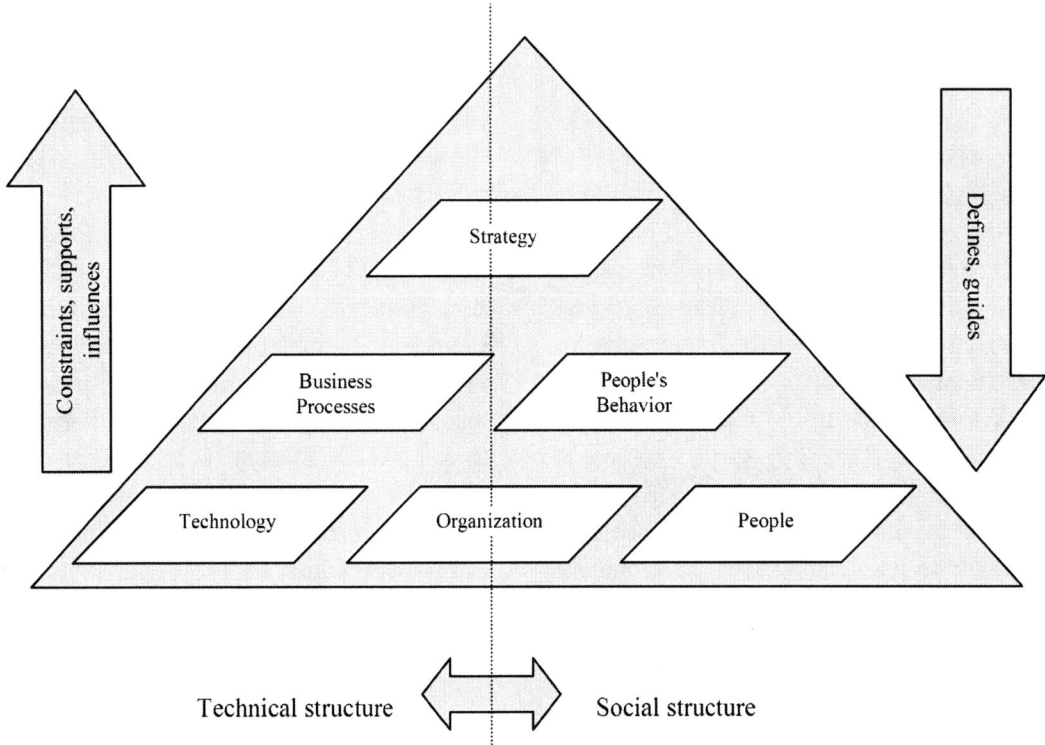

technology and culture is not an easy task, among other reasons because they both interact with other key organizational subsystems: the organization's formal structure and procedures, its processes and its strategic intent. Figure 1 shows these complex interconnections. Organizational effectiveness is considered to be a function of how well the social and the technical systems are designed with respect to one another and with respect to the demands of the outside market.

On these grounds, one approach to developing an effective workflow-based PHR system is to invite users to participate in the system development process. User participation has been strongly advocated by several studies as a way of ensuring that genuine user needs are satisfied and of gaining acceptance of a new system. The basic contention of these studies is that users who participate in the system development process will likely influence design and implementation deci-

sions in accordance with their needs and desires, resulting in a system they perceive useful and usable, and in an implementation strategy they perceive suitable for the particular situation. Thus, users are expected to develop positive attitudes toward the new system, increasing the likelihood of system success (often measured in terms of system usage or user information satisfaction).

A participative approach to PHR systems development implies that users are actually full members of the project team, so that they can exert constructive influence by instilling their knowledge and concern into the development process. Contrary to a traditional systems development process, where specialists make design and implementation decisions on the basis of users' experience (as this is expressed by users and perceived by specialists), participative development is concerned not only with making users' knowledge explicit (i.e., eliciting users' knowledge) but also with developing users' knowledge and producing new conceptions.

The aforementioned studies are mostly concerned with explaining the effect of user participation on system success. However, they do not address issues surrounding the realization of participation processes in the variety of systems development situations that occur in practice. This chapter focuses on a host of such issues with regard to PHR system development projects. In particular, this chapter discusses issues associated with user participation in PHR system development situations and presents an approach for effecting user participation. According to this approach, users are involved in system development process through a succession of collaborative workshops according to the Joint Application Development (JAD) methodology (Alexandrou, n.d.).

WORKFLOW-BASED PHR SYSTEMS

The main characteristics of healthcare processes are: (i) the processes are mostly cross-functional and highly complex, involving several people from different disciplines for their execution, (ii) process change takes place often due to a variety of factors including the introduction of new administrative procedures, medical approaches and technological developments, (iii) most of the activities in each process can only be partially automated as many trade-offs, decisions and actions must be performed by people and cannot be automated or even partially delegated to automated means, (iv) there is a large variety and amount of information exchanged within and between processes, (v) the quality and degree of collaboration and coordination among humans, and between humans and automated means play a crucial role in delivering high quality services to the patients and in containing costs, and (vi) process execution should conform to the security policy of each organization. These characteristics of healthcare processes make it highly advanta-

geous to develop workflow-based PHR systems so that to provide a flexible and automated basis, which enables collaborative, coordinative and secure execution of process activities that traditional Heath Information Systems or individual applications are unable to provide (Vassilacopoulos & Paraskevopoulou, 1997).

Moreover, the drive in healthcare to simultaneously reduce costs and improve quality has been forcing healthcare organizations to change their organizational structures and/or operational procedures focusing on the services patients need and on efficiently controlling the administration of these services (Staccini, Joubert, Quaranta, Fieschi & Fieschi, 2001). For example, the emerging online health management seeks to achieve more effective chronic disease management and higher quality in healthcare delivery by reducing unnecessary patient visits and treatments. Thus clinicians can devote more time to patients who truly need face-to-face care. Also, an online health management focus suggests a horizontal, process-view of healthcare organizations, requiring increased integration among functional units that will allow data to flow seamlessly across the health system to enable the required tools and capabilities (Vassilacopoulos & Paraskevopoulou, 1997; Alberta Health Services, n.d). This creates an impetus for the development of PHR systems that will support and serve healthcare orgnizations' business processes, in line with recent trends in information systems developments that exhibit a shift of attention from data to business processes, from hospital-centric to patient-centric care and from function-oriented systems to network-oriented systems of the networked economy (Davis, Morrell & McFaddin, 1999; Tang, Ash, Bates, Overhage & Sands, 2006; Alberta Health Services, n.d).

The transformative potential of PHR system can be realized by evolving PHR technology well beyond providing a consolidated patient record – in ways that make it more widely applicable and valuable to health systems. To this end, workflow technology can be used to develop

Figure 2. An overview of a workflow system development process

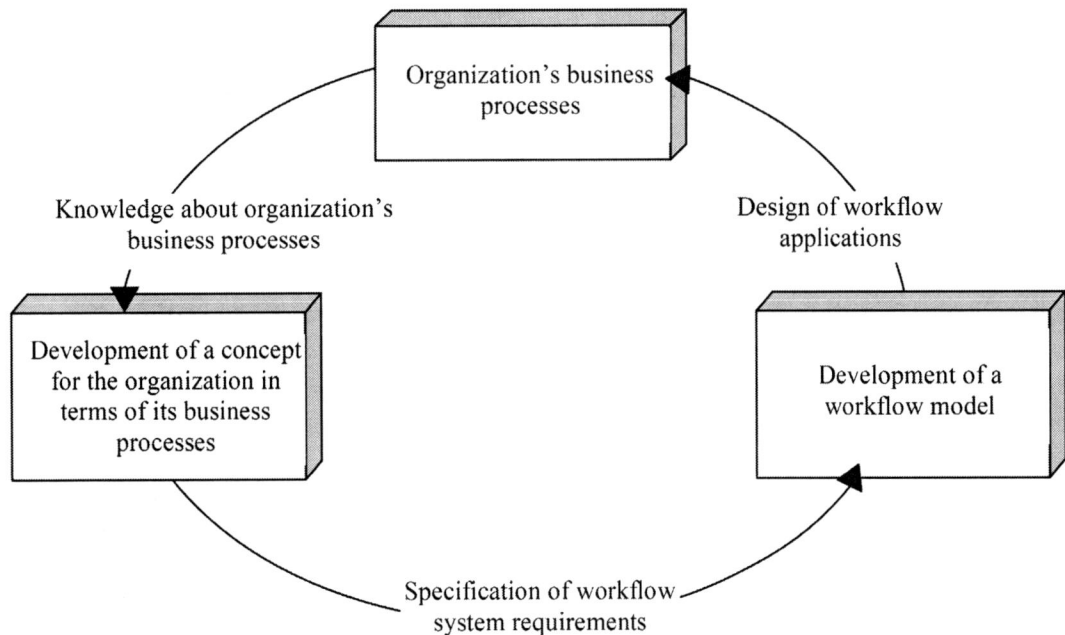

process-oriented PHR systems in an attempt to integrate care delivery across the continuum of services, from prevention to follow-up, and coordinate care across all settings. PHR systems development activities can be conducted in the context of larger process improvement or reengineering efforts (Graeber, 1997). This approach (where information systems development and business process change efforts are conducted concurrently) recognizes the fact that to introduce new technology to an organization can affect its processes and that to change a process can require alterations to the support technology. Hence, it aims at achieving the desirable fit between the business processes and the process-oriented PHR system that supports them through a convergence procedure requiring active user participation to arrive at feasible solutions based on compromise and consensus (Vassilacopoulos & Paraskevo-poulou, 1997). Thus, technology considerations are made during the process modeling activity. A high-level view of a process-oriented PHR system development approach is contained in Figure 2.

This managing of the relationship between the support technology and the organization is at the heart of a workflow system development process (Stohr & Zhao, 2001).

SOCIOTECHNICAL WORKFLOW SYSTEM ANALYSIS

Information Technology (IT) not only is important in implementing new processes, it also makes possible entirely new process designs. Therefore, IT should be considered both before and after process design. After a process design is envisioned, the focus should shift to IT implementation issues-supporting the new process with information from applications and databases.

To focus only on information and associated technologies as vehicles for process change is to overlook other factors that are at least as powerful, namely, organization structure and human resources policy. In fact, information and IT are rarely sufficient to bring about process changes, most of which are enabled by a combination of IT and organization/human resource changes (Kueng, 1998).

Because they have been a part of the enterprises for a much longer period that IT, organization structure and human resource policy are more familiar to managers as change tools. The great irony is that familiarity seems to have bred neglect, in part because the evangelists of reengineering are much more likely to lead the information services function than the human resources function. They undertake carefully managed projects, employing tested methodologies and strict timetables, to build new systems to enable processes that, because the human aspects of change are managed as afterthoughts, lead to significant human resource problems in implementation. If reengineering is to succeed, the human side cannot be left to manage itself (Martinsons, 1995). Organizational and human resource issues are more central than technology issues to the behavioral changes that must occur within a process.

Organizational enablers of reengineering fall into two categories: structure and culture (Davenport, 1995). Of the many kinds of structural changes that can facilitate new, process-oriented behaviors, one of the most powerful involves structuring process performance by teams.

Development teams should increasingly include consumers as well as representatives from all the functions involved in the development process. Moreover, most human beings seem to prefer jobs that include social interaction, and work teams provide opportunities for small talk, development of friendships and empathic reactions from other employees. However the social interactions of team members are not always positive. Particularly when teams are cross-functional, members may lack a shared culture, leading to conflict and misunderstanding. Therefore attention should be paid to cultural compatibility issues in selection of team members (Cabrera, Cabrera & Barajas, 2001).

Changes in organizational culture can facilitate new process designs. Most recent shifts in organizational culture have been in the direction of greater empowerment and participation in decision-making and more open, nonhierarchical communications. The resulting participative cultures, which have a structural side in flatter organizational hierarchies or broader spans of control, have been widely documented to lead to both higher productivity and greater employee satisfaction. In a reengineering context, these cultural changes are intended to empower process participants to make decisions about process operations (Davenport, 1995). Participative cultures may even lead to self-design of smaller, restricted processes by employee teams.

Human resource enablers of reengineering involve the way individual consumers and workers are skilled, motivated, compensated, evaluated, and so forth. New processes invariably involve new skills. Because reengineering often leads to both greater worker empowerment and a broader set of work tasks, the requisite new skills may involve both greater depth of job knowledge and greater breadth of task expertise. A variety of programs, including specific process training, and on-the-job-training, must be undertaken if the requisite skills are to be available when needed. Such skills as the use of information technology, detailed knowledge of the entire business process in which one works, and mastery of a wide variety of job tasks are all likely to be useful after reengineering.

Motivation levels of employees are another key determinant of process performance (Martinsons, 1995). The consensus model in studies of work organization suggests that work motivation derives from skill variety, completion of an entire task, task significance, autonomy, and feedback. Reengineering often involves establishing higher levels of these factors in new processes.

A FRAMEWORK FOR USER PARTICIPATION IN PHR SYSTEM DEVELOPMENT

User participation in an information system development project is often defined as the extent to which end-users or their representatives are engaged in activities related to system development (Gulliksen, Goransson, Boivie, Blomkvist, Persson & Cajander, 2003; Baroudi, Olson, & Ives, 1986; Hirschheim, 1985; Land & Hirschheim, 1983; Mumford, 1981; Mumford, 1983). For example, users may participate in planning the project, specifying information requirements, evaluating and approving the work done by analysts, designing the user interface, designing user training programs and defining the implementation strategy. For the most part, these activities involve both users and specialists. Thus, a prime requirement for a participative PHR system development project is to create an effective communication pattern of the user-specialist interaction (Hartwick & Barki, 1994; Hirschheim, 1985; King & Lee, 1991). However, since the interaction depends on the particular situation in which it occurs, it is also necessary to describe a framework for user participation that accommodates a variety of PHR system development situations of the real world.

User participation is often considered in relation to the stages of the project lifecycle defined for a particular situation (Gulliksen, Goransson, Boivie, Blomkvist, Persson & Cajander, 2003; Baroudi, Olson & Ives, 1986; Land & Hirschheim, 1983). The project lifecycle encompasses all the administrative, control and development activities to be performed during a project. Thus, the definition of a project lifecycle has implications for the *content* of a participation process. With regard to a district-wide PHR system development, the definition of project lifecycle is primarily affected by three interrelated factors: (i) the development scope defined by the health district (e.g. PC-based PHR system, Internet-based PHR system), (ii) the development strategy chosen (e.g.

vendor-developed, package-based system), and (iii) the development approach used by the system developers (e.g. structured lifecycle, prototyping).

As an example of the association between the project lifecycle and the content of the participation process, consider the case where a health district decides to contract with a software vendor for the development of a new PHR system. Then, user participation may occur in administrative and control stages such as project definition, tender preparation, evaluation of proposals, contract negotiation, and review and evaluation of deliverables, as well as in development stages such as requirements analysis, logical design, physical design and testing, and system's implementation and evaluation.

The *extent* (breadth and depth) of user participation in the project lifecycle specified for a particular situation varies with the district-wide participation policy on PHR system development. In turn, the policy may have been formulated through a compromise and a consensus with the users.

There is a broad array of both macro- and micro-level contextual/conditional factors that should be taken into account in defining a district-wide participation policy on PHR system development. Among these are included: the perceived value of user participation in achieving system's success, in enhancing opportunities for users to learn new skills, develop new capabilities and adopt innovative procedures, and in increasing intrinsic motivation of users through the assignment of greater authority or responsibility for the development of a system that they eventually have to operate; the assessed feasibility for conducting a user participation process in the particular social, organizational, management and technological context of the health district; and the estimated time and cost involved in a participative development with regard to the schedule and budget set for the project. Figure 3 shows the factors that set the framework for the content and extent of

Figure 3. A conceptualization of user participation in PHR system development

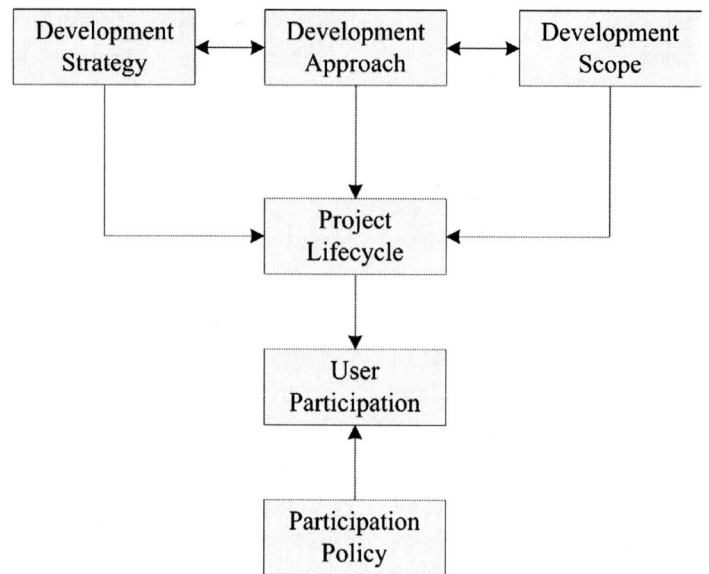

user participation in PHR system development situations.

AN APPROACH TO REALIZING USER PARTICIPATION IN PHR SYSTEM DEVELOPMENT

Despite the arguments in favor of participative systems development, achieving effective participation has proved a nontrivial matter in practice (Land & Hirschheim, 1983). Thus, once the health district comes to the conclusion that user participation in PHR system development is both needed and desirable, the challenge at hand is to realize the participation process in a way that is most suitable to the situation in which it is to take place. The approach described here was developed during a recent project concerned with designing and implementing a district-wide, workflow-based PHR system in the context of an e-prescription system, realized for the needs of the Greek social security system. In broad terms, the approach consists of the following stages:

1. Define the stages of the project lifecycle that is suitable to the particular situation (e.g., using a particular system development methodology).
2. Specify the extent and content of user participation with regard to the stages of the project lifecycle.
3. Define the functional subsystems to be supported by the workflow-based PHR system, disregarding organizational boundaries.
4. Identify user roles that are involved in each subsystem and select representatives of each role to take part in the participative PHR system development process.
5. Design and conduct a training program aiming at developing user representative capabilities for active participation.
6. Undertake the stages of the project lifecycle through user participation.
7. Monitor progress and response, and take control action as necessary.

This listing of stages is not intended to imply a once-through process or indeed a sequence. Stage 2 must follow stage 1 and stages 4 and 5 must follow stage 3, but stage 7 must be continuous during the participative development process and the control action necessary at any stage may involve significant iteration. Moreover stages 1 through 5 and stage 7 may also be undertaken through user participation at a higher level. For example, users may participate in the definition of the project lifecycle and in performing the monitor and control function.

In essence, the above approach focuses on defining the project lifecycle and on developing healthcare activities' description within a health district (e.g. services for elderly, clinical support services, primary care and community services) to specify the extent and content of user participation in system development (within the framework of the health district participation policy), and to define the user representatives (who are to take part in the participation process) and their training needs. To this end, the variety of health district functions and associated computer applications as well as the great diversity in skill, motivation and reaction to computers that characterize health district end-user population should also be taken into account (Anderson, Jay, Perry & Anderson, 1989; Mandell, 1987; Assimacopoulos, Elsig, Griesser & Scherrer, 1988).

In summary, the approach described above can be divided into three parts. The first part includes stages 1 through 5 which are concerned with preparing the user participation process; the second includes stage 6 which is concerned with system development through user participation; and, the third includes the monitoring and control function (stage 7) that is necessary in order to ensure that the participative process progresses as required.

Intuitively, the approach appears to have potential application in a variety of participative PHR development situations that occur in practice due to its adaptability to particular circumstances. Thus, it may also be used in conjunction with a systems development methodology/approach that encourages user participation as an integral part of the development process. The MERISE

methodology (Quang & Chartier-Kastler, 1991), the ETHICS methodology (Mumford, 1981; Mumford, 1983) and the prototyping approach (Alavi, 1984) are typical examples. More recently, iterative systems development approaches, such as Rational Unified Process (RUP) and eXtreme Programming are based to a large extent on active user participation (Pilemalm, Lindell, Hallberg, & Eriksson, 2007; Tattersall, 2002). In these development processes, users are involved actively in most phases such as the ones concerned with providing initial requirements, developing prototypes, assessing prototypes and providing more requirements and, finally, fully testing and accepting the resultant system. Hence, user participation contributes substantially to systems success as measured by its usage. On the other hand, participative development requires setting criteria for selecting appropriate user groups, planning for avoiding organizational operation disruptions and motivating users to participate through particular measures. All of these requirements deserve particular consideration in the sensitive healthcare environment and, hence, lie in the realm not only of the project managers but also of the healthcare providers.

While the methodology aims at setting the framework for conducting a participative PHR system development process effectively, it is not concerned with specifying how each stage should be undertaken or whether each stage is the responsibility of a specialist or a user or allocated to a user-specialist group. It is believed that these problems can be tackled most appropriately within the context of a particular health system by taking into account the relevant participation policy and the type of management and organizational style of its constituent healthcare organizations.

A CASE STUDY

To illustrate the participative perspective in a workflow-based PHR system development a case study in the e-prescribing domain will be described. E-prescribing work embraces a wide range of activities that may be divided into those directly pertaining to patient prescription procedures (e.g. perform medical examinations, reach diagnosis, decide therapeutic regime, issue prescription) and those pertaining to prescription administration (e.g. read drug formulary information). As these activities are interlinked and interdependent in a manifold manner, there is a need to provide appropriate computer support to activity execution and coordination in order to improve prescription services. The approach to participative PHR system development described above has been applied in this project.

For this particular situation, the project lifecycle was defined to be comprised of three stages: requirements analysis, system implementation and system validation. User participation in the stages of the project lifecycle was defined in terms of decision-making authority as consensus participation, for the first and the third stage, and consultative participation (decision making assigned to analysts) for the second stage.

The example described here draws on a process model that was developed to express the progress concerned with dispensing drugs which have been prescribed by physicians. This process affects the quality of service delivered to patients as it increases patient safety by eliminating illegible prescriptions and allowing for real-time safety checks and may involve substantial cost containment for the insurance organizations and/or the healthcare system. Due to the complexity of the domain knowledge about healthcare and healthcare delivery processes, active user participation in a healthcare system development process is particularly important.

Broadly, this process begins with a physician reaching a diagnosis and deciding the therapeutic regime, proceeds with issuing a prescription; and ends with dispensing prescription drugs to the patient. This is a highly complex, cross-functional process that concerns inpatient, outpatient and emergency cases, interacts with other processes and involves several people form different disciplines (e.g. physicians, nurses, pharmacists, health insurers). Figure 4 shows a high level view of the process using IBM MQSeries Workflow.

When developing technical systems than involve extensive human activity (i.e. socio-technical systems), it is crucial to understand the context and environment of system operation. This activity is greatly facilitated by active user participation as users possess the necessary domain knowledge. This implies that current difficulties, problems and needs for change are explicitly captured, in depth analyzed and incorporated into the modeling work. In this framework, one of the uses of the workflow model concerning the prescription process was to define the user roles responsible for undertaking the constituent activities according to job specification; user representatives in the system development process were elected by the users holding each role. Then, a training program for user representatives was carried out that included topics on the system development methods used in the project.

Each process activity comprising the workflow model was analyzed further, thus producing a model at a lower level of resolution, as required. In this way, a validated process model is produced upon which the relevant applications were mapped and compared for further system development. Process definition needs to be based on knowledge about and experience with both the work to be supported and the technical possibilities and limitations. Hence, user participation during process description was necessary in order to discover how work was really carried out and the resulting process model to describe the users' interpretations of their work and not some procedural or managerial view of it. Thus, a succession of collaborative workshops called JAD sessions was organized. These group sessions are managed by means of procedural rules. A number of sample JAD rules are illustrated in Table 1. By means of these sessions users were required to exert constructive influence

Figure 4. A high-level, simplified view of the e-prescription process

ReachDiagnosis   DecideTherapeuticRegime   IssuePrescription   DispensePrescriptionDrugs

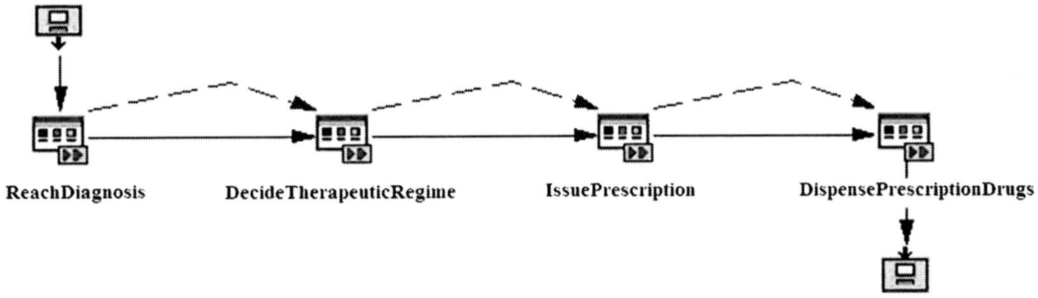

by instilling into the process modelling activity their knowledge and concern about the problem domain, the particular organizational context and existing information systems. Where perceived problems and objectives required change to the process the proposals were modelled and their likely implications were analyzed. The process model's validation was based on user responses about the desired process characteristics, within the constraints posed by the health district context and about the fit of these processes into an overall organisation of working practice.

The implementation of workflow technology intends to improve the prescription process by automating its execution as much as possible. The improvement will come because of the automation of the execution of the process. This is, once the workflow system was installed, the people working in the process will not have to worry about the sequencing of the process, the system will do. However, the workflow system forces people to work in a predefined manner by changing their existing work patterns and consequently provoking user resistance. Therefore, users were early involved in the workflow system's development. Involvement by users was seen as the most efficient method of determining what processes need to be altered and revised. In this way, users took more ownership of the process being developed and were more willing to understand and accept changes that they were instrumental in determining.

FUTURE RESEARCH DIRECTIONS

PHRs are increasingly recognized and used as a tool to address various challenges stemming from the scattered and incompatible personal health information that exists in each health care system. Although activity around PHR development and deployment has increased in recent years, a number of impediments exist that can delay PHR adoption. Some of them relate to individual healthcare professionals as well as consumer/patients. For PHR technology to improve care in the face of rising costs it must evolve well beyond providing a consolidated patient record—in ways that make it more widely applicable and valuable to health systems. To this end operators must harness information technology to tailor care more closely to the needs of both consumers/patients and healthcare professionals. Success in implementation of PHR systems that meet these requirements can only be achieved if users instill their knowledge and experience in the development process. In this chapter, a methodology has been proposed for the realization of a participative PHR system development, where users are full members of the development team. A potential limitation of the methodology is that it requires rigorous activities to be carried out and that it may involve a substantial time and cost overhead. This is an issue that has to be weighed against the potential benefits accrued from user participation before committing a participative approach to PHR

Table 1. Sample JAD Rules (Kettelhut, 1993)

1.	Select participants who have expert knowledge in their functional tasks.
2.	Select participants who represent their functional areas and who can make decisions during the meeting to commit their area to specifics of the design.
3.	Keep discussions limited to the scope of the meeting (use the agenda for control).
4.	Allow only one conversation at a time.
5.	Define issues so that the group arrives at a Yes or No answer (it is difficult to specify requirements that are in question).
6.	Encourage users to ask for anything they want.
7.	Use brainstorming to encourage alternative ideas and ensure that the process remains free of criticism.
8.	Work to build consensus in decisions that affect requirements or specific features of the system to be implemented.
9.	Encourage equality through voting mechanisms.
10.	Encourage equal participation.
11.	Where there is conflict, use voting or structural mechanisms to limit escalation (e.g. follow a ten-minute rule – if a discussion is at an impasse, document the subject as an open issue and move on)
12.	Take frequent breaks and require everyone to break together.
13.	Enforce attendance requirements.
14.	Limit observers to answering questions.
15.	Ensure content is provided by user attendees (the facilitator disclaims ownership of documents, screen designs, other presentation materials).

system development. Although the methodology seems intuitively appealing, its validity in a variety of real-world situations remains to be proved. In particular, its enforcement in the context of a wide spectrum of intra- and inter-organizational healthcare processes is certainly needed to reveal the methodology's potential strengths and weaknesses. Another task that suggests directions for future work and will be undertaken in the near future is concerned with the investigation of potential problems related to IT governance.

CONCLUSION

This chapter is addressing workflow-based PHR systems development from a sociotechnical perspective and illustrates the deep interrelation of technical and social aspects in the development process. The implementation of a workflow-based PHR system is a process of mutual transformation: the health district is affected by the coming of the new technology, but the technology is in turn inevitably affected by the specific organizational dynamics of which it becomes a part. User participation in PHR system development can be considered as a means towards improving the quality of design and implementation decisions, improving user skills in system utilization, developing user abilities to define their own information requirements and increasing user commitment to and acceptance of the resultant system. A methodology for conducting a participation process in the health district context has been described in this paper, preceded by an analysis of the participation concept.

REFERENCES

Aaltonen, S., Nurminen, M., Rejonen, P., & Vuorenheimo, J. (2002, August). *User-driven Implementation of Information Systems*. Paper presents at the 25th Information System Research Seminar in Scandinavia, Bautahol, Denmark.

Alavi, M. (1984). An Assessment of the Prototyping Approach to Information Systems Development. *Communications of the ACM, 27*, 556–563. doi:10.1145/358080.358095

Alberta Health Services. (n.d.). Engaging the Patient in Healthcare: An Overview of Personal Health Record Systems and Implications for Alberta, *White Paper*.

Alexandrou, M. (n.d.). *Joint Application Development (JAD) Methodology*. Retrieved August 16, 2009, from http://searchsoftwarequality.techtarget.com/sDefinition/0,sid92_gci820966,00.html

Anderson, J. G., Jay, S. J., Perry, J., & Anderson, M. (1989). Increasing Physician Use of Computerized Hospital Information System. In B. Barber, D. Cao, D. Qin, & G. Wagner (Eds), *Proccedings of the 6th World Conference on Medical Informatics*, North-Holland.

Assimacopoulos, A., Elsig, R. N., Griesser, V., & Scherrer, J. R. (1988). End User Training for Hospital Information Systems: Catching Up with Technology. In Bakker, A. R., Ball, M. J., Scherrer, J. R., & Willems, J. L. (Eds.), *Towards New Hospital Information Systems*. North-Holland.

Bardini, T. (n.d.). *What is Actor-Network Theory?* Retrieved March 20, 2010, from http://carbon.ucdenver.edu/~mryder/itc_data/ant_dff.html.

Baroudi, J. J., Olson, M. H., & Ives, B. (1986). *An Empirical Study of the Impact of User Involvement on System Usage and Information Satisfaction*.

Berg, M. (1999). Patient care information systems and health care work: a sociotechnical approach. *International Journal of Medical Informatics, 55*(2), 87–101. doi:10.1016/S1386-5056(99)00011-8

Berg, M. (2001). Implementing Information Systems in Health Care Organizations: Myths and Challenges. *International Journal of Medical Informatics, 64*(2-3), 143–156. doi:10.1016/S1386-5056(01)00200-3

Berg, M., Langenberg, C., Berg, I., & Kwakkernaat, J. (1998). Considerations for sociotechnical design: experiences with an electronic patient record in a clinical context. *International Journal of Medical Informatics, 52*(1-3), 243–251. doi:10.1016/S1386-5056(98)00143-9

Berg, M., & Toussaint, P. (2003). The mantra of modelling and the forgotten powers of paper: A sociotechnical view on the development of process-oriented ICT in healthcare. *International Journal of Medical Informatics, 69*(2-3), 223–234. doi:10.1016/S1386-5056(02)00178-8

Cabrera, A., Cabrera, E., & Barajas, S. (2001). The key role of organizational culture in a multi-system view of technology-driven change. *International Journal of Information Management, 21*(3), 245–261. doi:10.1016/S0268-4012(01)00013-5

Davenport, T. (1995). *Reengineering a business process*. Harvard Business School Case Studies.

Davis, J., Morrell, J., & McFaddin, G. (1999, November). *Workflow-based Lifecycle Modeling: A Paradigm for the Analysis and Architecture of Enterprise-wide-e-Health Applications*. Paper presented at OOPSLA Workshop on Objects, Workflow and the Virtual Enterprise. OOPSLA-99 Conference on Object-Oriented Programming, Systems, Languages and Applications, Denver, Colorando.

Effken, J. (2002). Different lenses, improved outcomes: a new approach to the analysis and design of healthcare information systems. *International Journal of Medical Informatics, 65*(1), 59–74. doi:10.1016/S1386-5056(02)00003-5

Graeber, S. (1997). *The Impact of Workflow Management Systems on the Design of Hospital Information Systems*. Paper presented at the American Medical Informatics Association (AMIA) Annual Fall Symposium, Vol. 856.

Gulliksen, J., Goransson, B., Boivie, I., Blomkvist, S., Persson, J., & Cajander, A. (2003). Key Principles for User-centred Systems Design. *Behaviour & Information Technology, 22*(6), 397–410. doi:10.1080/01449290310001624329

Hartwick, J., & Barki, H. (1994). Explaining the Role of User Participation in Information System Use. *Management Science, 40*, 440–465. doi:10.1287/mnsc.40.4.440

Hirschheim, R. A. (1985). User Experience with and Assessment of Participative Systems Design. *Management Information Systems Quarterly, 9*(3), 295–304. doi:10.2307/249230

Jeffcott, M. (2001, September) *Technology Alone Will Never Work: Understanding How Organisational Issues Contribute to User Neglect and Information Systems Failure in Healthcare.* Paper presented at the IT in Healthcare: Sociotechnical Approaches International Conference, Rotterdam, The Netherlands.

Kettelhut, M. C. (1993). JAD Methodology and Group Dynamics. *Information Systems Management, 10*, 46–53. doi:10.1080/10580539308906912

King, W. R., & Lee, T. H. (1991, January). *The Effects of User Participation on System Success: Toward a Contingency Theory of User Satisfaction.* Paper presented at the 12th International Conference on Information Systems, New York, USA.

Koufi, V., & Vassilacopoulos, G. (2008). *HDG Portal: A Grid Portal Application for Pervasive Access to Process-Based Healthcare Systems.* Paper presented at the 2nd International Conference in Pervasive Computing Technologies in Healthcare (PervasiveHealth'08), Tampere, Finland.

Kueng, P. (1998). *Impact of Workflow Systems on People, Task, and Structure: a Post-implementation Evaluation.* In A. Brown, D. Remenyi (Eds), *Proceedings of the Fifth European Conference on the Evaluation of Information Technology* (pp. 67-75) Reading University, UK.

Land, F. F., & Hirschheim, R. A. (1983). Participative Systems Design: Rationale, Tools, and Techniques. *Journal of Applied Systems Analysis, 10*, 327–338.

Lauer, G. (2009). *Health Record Banks Gaining Traction in Regional Projects.* Retrieved December 15, 2009, from http://www.ihealthbeat.org/features/2009/health-record-banks-gaining-traction-in-regional-projects.aspx

Malamateniou, F., & Vassilacopoulos, G. (2002). Developing a Virtual Patient Record as a Web-based Workflow System. In G. Surján, R. Engelbrecht & P. McNair (Eds), *Medical Informatics Europe: Vol. 90. Studies in Health Technology and Informatics 2002* (pp. 298-304). Amsterdam: IOS Press.

Mandell, S. F. (1987). Resistance to Computerization. *Journal of Medical Systems, 11*(4), 311–318. doi:10.1007/BF00994015

Martinsons, M. (1995). Radical Process Innovation Using Information Technology: The Theory, the Practice and the Future of Reengineering. *International Journal of Information Management, 15*(4), 253–269. doi:10.1016/0268-4012(95)00023-Z

Mumford, E. (1981). *Participative Systems Design: Structure and Method: Systems, Objectives, Solutions.* North-Holland.

Mumford, E. (1983). *Designing Participatively.* Manchester, UK: Manchester Business School.

Mumford, E. (2000). A Socio-Technical Approach to Systems Design. *Requirements Engineering, 5*(2), 125–133. doi:10.1007/PL00010345

Peimann, J. C. (1998). Modeling Hospital Information Systems with Petri Nets. *Methods of Information in Medicine, 27*, 17–22.

Pilemalm, S., Lindell, P., Hallberg, N., & Eriksson, H. (2007). Integrating the Rational Unified Process and participatory design for development of socio-technical systems: a user participative approach. *Design Studies, 28*, 263–288. doi:10.1016/j.destud.2007.02.009

Quang, P. T., & Chartier-Kastler, C. (1991). *Merise in Practice* (Avison, D. E., Trans.). Basingstoke: Macmillan.

Reichert, M., & Dadam, P. (1998, September). *Towards Process-oriented Hospital Information Systems: Some Insights into Requirements, Technical Challenges and Possible Solutions.* Paper presented at 43 Jahrestagung der GMDS (GMDS'98) (pp. 175-180), Bremmen, Germany.

Staccini, P., Joubert, M., Quaranta, J., Fieschi, D., & Fieschi, M. (2001). Modelling health care processes for eliciting user requirements: a way to link a quality paradigm and clinical information system design. *International Journal of Medical Informatics, 64*(2-3), 129–142. doi:10.1016/S1386-5056(01)00203-9

Stohr, E., & Zhao, L. (2001). Workflow Automation: Overview and Research Issues. *Information Systems Frontiers, 3*(3), 281–296. doi:10.1023/A:1011457324641

Tang, P. C., Ash, J. S., Bates, D. W., Overhage, J. M., & Sands, D. Z. (2006). Personal health records: definitions, benefits, and strategies for overcoming barriers to adoption. [JAMIA]. *Journal of the American Medical Informatics Association, 13*(2), 121–126. doi:10.1197/jamia.M2025

Tattersall, G. (2002). *Supporting Iterative Development Through Requirements Management.* Retrieved March 3 2010 from: http://www.ibm.com/developerworks/rational/library/2830.html.

Varadharajan, V. A. (1991). Petri Nat Model for System Design and Refinement. *Journal of Systems and Software, 15*, 239–250. doi:10.1016/0164-1212(91)90040-D

Vassilacopoulos, G., & Paraskevopoulou, E. (1997). A Process Model Basis for Evolving Hospital Information Systems. *Journal of Medical Systems, 21*(3), 141–153. doi:10.1023/A:1022808222057

Walter, T., & Herrmann, T. (1998). The Relevance of showcases for the participative improvement of business processes and workflow management. In R. Chatfiled, S. Kuhn & M. Muller (Eds), *Proceedings of the participatory design conference* (pp. 117-127). Seattle, WA, USA.

Wiljer, D., Urowitz, S., Apatu, E., DeLenardo, C., Eysenbach, G., & Harth, T. (2008). Patient accessible electronic health records: exploring recommendations for successful implementation strategies. *Journal of Medical Internet Research, 10*(4). doi:10.2196/jmir.1061

Wilson, B. (1984). *Systems: Concepts, Methodologies and Applications.* New York: Wiley.

Yasnoff, W. A. (2008). *Electronic Records are Key to Health-care Reform, BusinessWeek.*

ADDITIONAL READING

Andrews, D. C., & Leventhal, N. S. (1994). *Fusion: Integrating IE, CASE, and JAD: A Handbook for reengineering the Systems Organization.* Upper Saddle River, NJ: Yourdon Press.

Basson, G. (2009). Process-oriented Systems Paradigm for the Process Age. *BPMInstitute.org.* Retrieved December 27, 2009, from http://www.bpminstitute.org/articles/article/article/process-oriented-systems-paradigm-for-the-process-age.html.

Bizovi, K. E., Beckley, B. E., McDade, M. C., Adams, A. L., Lowe, R. A., Zechnich, A. D., & Hedges, J. R. (2002). The Effect of Computer-assisted Prescription Writing on Emergency Department Prescription Errors. *Academic Emergency Medicine, 9*(11), 1168–1175. doi:10.1111/j.1553-2712.2002.tb01572.x

Brennan, S., & Spours, A. (2000). Barriers to the Successful and Timely Implementation of Electronic Prescribing and Medicines Administration. *British Journal of Healthcare Computing and Information Management, 17*(8), 22–25.

Brennan, S., & Spours, A. (2003). Electronic Prescribing and Medicines Administration: Are We Overcoming the Barriers to Success? *British Journal of Healthcare Computing and Information Management, 20*(4), 19–22.

Casati, F., & Sham, M. C. (2002). Event-Based Interaction Management for Composite E-Services in eFlow. *Information Systems Frontiers, 4*(1), 19–31. doi:10.1023/A:1015374204227

Corley, S. T. (2003). Electronic Prescribing: A Review of Costs and Benefits. *Topics in Health Information Management, 24*(1), 29–38.

Dadam, P., & Reichert, M. (2000). *Towards a New Dimension in Clinical Information Processing.* Paper presented at Medical Informatics Europe Conference (pp. 295-301). Amsterdam: IOS Press.

Detmer, D., Bloomrosen, M., Raymond, B., & Tang, P. (2008). Integrated Personal Health Records: Transformative Tools for Consumer-Centric Care. *BMC Medical Informatics and Decision Making, 8,* 45. doi:10.1186/1472-6947-8-45

Dumas, M., van der Aalst, W., & ter Hofstede, A. (2005). *Process-aware Information Systems.* New York: Wiley. doi:10.1002/0471741442

eHealth Initiative. (2004). *Electronic Prescribing: Toward Maximum Value and Rapid Adoption.* Washington, DC.

Framinan, J. M., Parra, C. L., Montes, M., & Pérez, P. (2006). Collaborative Healthcare Process Modelling: A Case Study. In Camarinha-Matos, L. M., Afsarmanesh, H., & Ortiz, A. (Ed.), *Collaborative Networks and Their Breeding Environments, Vol. 186. IFIP TC5 WG 5.5 Sixth IFIP Working Conference on VIRTUAL ENTERPRISES* (pp. 395-402). Springer-Verlag.

Groen, P. J. (2008). Personal Health Record (PHR) Systems and Return on Investment (ROI). *Virtual Medical Worlds.* Retrieved December 25, 2009, from http://www.hoise.com/vmw/09/articles/vmw/LV-VM-01-09-1.html.

Groen, P. J., Goldstein, D., & Nasuti, J. (2007). *Personal Health Record (PHR) Systems: An evolving challenge to HER systems.* Retrieved December 8, 2009, from http://www.hoise.com/vmw/07/articles/vmw/LV-VM-08-07-26.html.

Hoffer, J. A., George, J. F., & Valacich, J. S. (2002). *Modern Systems Analysis and Design.* Upper Saddle River, NJ: Prentice Hall.

Holtzblatt, K., & Jones, S. (1993). Contextual Inquiry: A Participatory Technique for System Design. In Schuler, D., & Namioka, A. (Eds.), *Participatory design: principles and practices* (pp. 177–210). Mahwah, NJ: Lawrence Erlbaum.

Lafky, D. B., Tulu, B., & Horan, T. A. (2006). A User-driven Approach to Personal Health Records. *Communications of the Association for Information Systems, 17,* 46.

Lemos, R. (2001), Medical Privacy Gets CPR. *ZDNet.* Retrieved December 25, 2009, from http://www.zdnet.com/zdnn/stories/news/0,4586,2667243,00.html.

Muller, M. (1993). PICTIVE: Democratizing the Dynamics of the Design Session. In Schuler, D., & Namioka, A. (Eds.), *Participatory design: principles and practices* (pp. 211–237). Hillsdale, NJ: Lawrence Erlbaum.

Parviainen, P., Tihinen, M., Lormans, M., & van Solingen, R. (2005). Requirements Engineering: Dealing with the Complexity of Sociotechnical Systems Development. In Mate, J. L., & Silva, A. (Eds.), *Requirements Engineering for Sociotechnical Systems.* United Kingdom: Information Science Publishing.

Raisinghani, M. S., & Young, E. (2008). Personal Health Records: Key Adoption Issues and Implications for Management. *International Journal of Electronic Healthcare*, *4*(1), 67–77. doi:10.1504/IJEH.2008.018921

Shortliffe, E. (1999). The Evolution of Electronic Medical Records. *Academic Medicine: Journal of the Association of American Medical Colleges*, *74*(4), 414–419.

Siddiqi, J. (1996). Requirement Engineering: The Emerging Wisdom. *IEEE Software*, *13*(2), 15–19. doi:10.1109/MS.1996.506458

Soltys, R., & Crawford, A. (n.d.). *JAD for Business Plans and Designs*. TheFacilitator.com. Retrieved December 25, 2009, from http://www.thefacilitator.com/htdocs/article11.html

Sommerville, I., & Sawyer, P. (1997). *Requirements Engineering: A Good Practise Guide*. New York: John Wiley & Sons.

Sullivan, J. M. (1998). Process Modeling for Health Care Organizations. *College Review (Denver, Colo.)*, *15*(2), 85–103.

Teich, J. M., Merchia, P. R., Schmiz, J. L., Kuperman, G. J., Spurr, C. D., & Bates, D. W. (2000). Effects of Computerized Physician Order Entry on Prescribing Practices. *Archives of Internal Medicine*, *160*(18), 2741–2747. doi:10.1001/archinte.160.18.2741

U.S. Department of Health and Human Services. Personal Health Records and Personal Health Record Systems. (n.d.). *A Report Recommendation from the National Committee on Vital and Health Statistics*; Washington D.C.; Feb 2006.

Win, K. T., Susilo, W., & Mu, Y. (2006). Personal Health Record Systems and their security protection. *Journal of Medical Systems*, *30*, 309–315. doi:10.1007/s10916-006-9019-y

Zachman, J. (1987). A Framework for Information Systems Architecture. *IBM Systems Journal*, *26*(3), 276–292. doi:10.1147/sj.263.0276

KEY TERMS AND DEFINITIONS

Business Process: A collection of related, structured activities or tasks that produce a specific service or product (serve a particular goal) for a particular customer or customers.

Process-Based Healthcare System: A healthcare system where collaboration of individual caregivers and departments and coordination of their activities is achieved by means of processes.

Workflow Management System: A computer system that manages and defines a series of tasks within an organization to produce a final outcome or outcomes. Workflow Management Systems allow the definition of different workflows for different types of jobs or processes.

Personal Health Record (PHR): An electronic application through which individuals can access, manage and share their health information, and that of others for whom they are authorized, in a private, secure, and confidential environment.

Joint Application Development (JAD): A process used in the prototyping life cycle area of the Dynamic Systems Development Method (DSDM) to collect business requirements while developing new information systems for a company. JAD accelerates the design of information technology solutions as it uses customer involvement and group dynamics to accurately depict the user's view of the business need and to jointly develop a solution.

Systems Development Lifecycle: In systems engineering and software engineering, it is the process of creating or altering computer or information systems, and the models and methodologies that people use to develop these systems.

E-Prescribing System: A computer-based system that enables electronic transmission of prescriptions between health care professionals and mail order or retail pharmacies. An ePrescribing system allows health care professionals to check medication history, patient allergies, drug interactions, recommended dosage, payer covered drug lists, and much more to ensure that the medication prescribed is the safest and most effective choice for the patient. Pharmacies can also communicate with health care professionals through e-Prescribing systems.

Chapter 7

How Knowing Who, Where and When Can Change Health Care Delivery

William D. Kearns
University of South Florida, USA

James L. Fozard
University of South Florida, USA

Rosemarie S. Lamm
University of South Florida Polytechnic, USA

ABSTRACT

Everything that happens to a person during their lifetime happens in the context of place, and the movements made by the person through and within that place. Persons begin life with a birthplace; they remember exactly where they were when they first laid eyes on their true love, the street address of their first home, etc. New research suggests that changes in movement patterns which occur in home and public spaces may be significant indicators of declining mental and physical health. In this chapter the authors discuss efforts to measure natural human movement, present a novel technique that uses a referential grid system to study the relationship of movement to health changes. The authors then present several syndromes whose understanding may be increased by a more thorough analysis of movement. They conclude with a discussion of how location aware technologies can play a role in identifying problems and solutions in the design of living spaces for the elderly.

DOI: 10.4018/978-1-60960-469-1.ch007

INTRODUCTION: THE POTENTIAL OF ACTIVE LOCATION AWARE TECHNOLOGY IN HEALTH CARE

Locomotion is elemental to the definition of what it is to be human and to our understanding of what constitutes proper health. Disorders such as Parkinson's disease and other neurological maladies which restrict mobility are among the most feared of disorders because they cause such dire limitations in a person's activities. While a person in the later stages of a movement limiting disease may clearly evidence the disorder, the disorders may begin slowly and reveal themselves in subtle changes in movements which may not be apparent to the afflicted.

The main argument of the present chapter is that current location aware technology can be used to detect subtle changes in movement patterns in everyday living situations as well as in formal assessments of gait and balance. The Information so obtained can be used as an aid to diagnosis of movement disorders as well as a way of monitoring the effectiveness of interventions for them.

In this chapter we present information on emerging location aware technologies that show promise for detecting some forms of dementia. We then present several disorders whose early detection and diagnosis may be aided by location aware technologies. Finally we present to the reader a framework in which location aware technologies can augment existing care environments both in the home and in formal settings.

BACKGROUND

In Asia in 2000 fully 6% and in Europe 15.5% of the population was older than 65 years of age, percentages that are projected to grow at an accelerating rate (US Centers for Disease Control, 2003). The US fares a bit better than Europe at 12.4% due to sustained immigration of younger persons and their families. The swelling health-

care budget has forced governments to consider innovative technological approaches to mitigate rising healthcare costs. One innovation under study is to implement "smart house" technologies in the homes of persons who may be at risk of developing expensive chronic disorders or suffering the effects of their sequelae (Pavel et al., 2007). This strategy includes monitoring and evaluating behavioral changes (Harvey, Zhou, Keller, Rantz, & He, 2009) including the early detection of potentially expensive or lethal disorders, the delineation of high fall risk areas in the home through the study of resident traffic patterns (Wang, Skubic, & Zhu, 2009), or detecting falls and injuries rapidly and summoning prompt assistance in order to minimize recovery costs (Hamill, Young, Boger, & Mihailidis, 2009). In each case the intent is to improve care through improved surveillance and significantly reduce the likelihood that the resident will transit into an expensive formal care environment before it is absolutely necessary. A considerable body of mental and physical health evidence supports the practice of maintaining persons in their own homes vs. transferring them to formal care settings where they may be cut off from their social support networks (Mihailidis, Cockburn, et al. 2008; Demiris, Rantz, et al. 2004; Sixsmith 2000; Ni Scanaill, Carew, et al. 2006).

CHAPTER FOCUS: SPACE–THE CONTEXT FOR LIFE'S MOVEMENTS, MEMORIES AND GOALS

In our investigations we employ the movement ecology paradigm as the theoretical framework for studying human path tortuosity (the degree to which an elder's movement path deviates from a straight line) in dementia; it is a transactional analysis that links three features of an individual—their internal state, their navigational capacity and their motion capacity—with features of their external environment (Nathan et al., 2008 p.10954). Each change in the location of the individual, termed a "movement path", brings about a change in the person-environment dynamic that potentially alters any or all of the three components of the moving individual. In our work, the internal state, or "why move", is defined by the goal of traversing a common living space for a meal, getting to a sleeping area, or to engage in recreation. Navigational capacity, having the ability to execute "where to move", is differentially affected by the presence of dementia and by differences in the individual's cognitive abilities. Motion capacity, or knowing "how to move", applies to both persons who walk independently, with the aid of a walker, or who use a wheelchair. The movement ecology paradigm informs our understanding of dementia's effect on navigational capacity, as reflected in the shape of the movement paths elders make while traveling.

Dementia may affect movement paths in several ways; it might affect navigational capacity either by changing orientation or attention. However the determination of which influence is at play strictly from a study of the movement data alone is challenging. Luis and Brown (2007) summarize two lines of research theorizing why movements might change with cognitive impairment and dementia. One group of studies hypothesized that disordered spatial orientation was responsible for dementia related wandering (Snyder, Rupprecht, Pyrek, Brekhus, & Moss, 1978; Henderson, Mack, & Williams, 1989; de Leon, Potegal, & Gurland, 1984). An alternative hypothesis postulated that difficulty shifting attention—an executive function—was responsible for wandering (Ryan et al., 1995; Chiu et al., 2004; Passini, Rainville, Marchand, & Joanette, 1995). Both hypotheses are consistent with observations of higher movement path variability in elderly with clinical diagnoses of dementia, which may indicate impaired memory for waypoints required for successful navigation in familiar environments. At present no convincing evidence exists to refute either hypothesis, partly because researchers have included persons at different stages of dementia.

Another way dementia might affect path tortuosity is through motion capacity or "how to move". Stride to stride gait speed and length, measured when elders walk on prescribed paths, correlates negatively with cognitive performance measures, including the MMSE, in both normal aged and in persons with clinical diagnoses of dementia (Hausdorff, Rios, & Edelberg, 2001; Verghese et al., 2002). Standardized gait and balance assessments (SGB) include stride length, step length, support base, step time, swing time, stance time, single support time, double support time and average velocity measures (Jensen, Nyberg, Gustafson, & Lundin-Olsson, 2003; Rubenstein, 2006). Static balance assessment includes body sway measures recorded when standing on one or two legs with eyes open or closed; dynamic balance assessments are made while walking and performing an additional task such as talking on a cell phone. Recently researchers (Hausdorff et al., 2001; Verghese, Holtzer, Lipton, & Wang, 2009) have employed fractal analytic techniques to SGB thereby unveiling gait and balance variability information leading to improved fall prediction. Hausdorff and colleagues (Hausdorff et al., 2001) have found that increased stride time variability predicted heightened fall risk in community dwelling elders; stride time variability in this study also correlated negatively (-.47) with participants' MMSE scores.

In dementia, all three movement ecology paradigm hypotheses (why move, where to move and how to move) predict dementia will increase movement path tortuosity through its degenerative neurological effects on structures controlling motivation, navigational abilities, and skeletal muscle activity. When applied to the study of animal models of movement path tortuosity, the movement ecology paradigm has focused on four main factors; the ability or strength to orient towards a specific goal in space (Benhamou & Bovet, 1992), the distance at which an animal orients towards that goal (Goodwin, Bender, Contreras, Fahrig, & Wegner, 1999), the tendency for the animal to continue travelling in the direction it has been going (i.e. angular momentum) (McCulloch & Cain, 1989) and speed of travel (Codling, Plank, & Benhamou, 2008). An animal travels with a more tortuous path when any of orientation strength, orientation distance, angular momentum or speed decreases. Both disordered spatial orientation and shifting attention would affect the ability to consistently orient towards a spatial goal. Increased gait variability would decrease angular momentum. All of these factors individually or combined would result in more tortuous movement paths. Obtaining accurate spatial data requires accurate mapping of movement paths over long intervals in natural environments using sensor networks.

UNDERSTANDING MOVEMENT DISORDERS RELATED TO AGE AND DISEASE REQUIRES A QUALITY DESCRIPTION OF A PERSON'S LOCATION AND MOVEMENT IN SPACE

Within the US significant attention has been directed towards using inexpensive sensor technology to monitor the movement of individuals in homes and formal care settings. These technologies offer a number of benefits besides low cost which include wide availability and the existence of a considerable body of private sector expertise in their use. Indeed, many of these sensors are found in home security systems and at least one commercial smart home surveillance system employs a modified home security system and sensor technologies to keep an eye on the residents (Rowe, Lane, & Phipps, 2007). The inexpensive sensor technologies currently employed in home surveillance can provide key information about general health. For example a simple switch attached to the flush control of a standard toilet provides information about daily elimination, an indicator of general health. Similarly, passive infrared sensors located near bedroom entrances provide informa-

tion on when an individual arises and retires, but also about disturbances in sleep patterns which may affect general cognitive functioning (Adami, Hayes, Pavel, & Singer, 2005). Changes in sleep patterns may presage other health problems and may result in increased sedative and/or alcohol consumption; sleep deprivation is associated with an increased risk of traffic fatalities in the general population. Inexpensive sensors include passive infrared devices (PIR) (Suzuki, Murase, Tanaka, & Okazawa, 2007) which detect the presence of infrared energy emitted by the human body during normal thermogenesis. PIR systems yield binary (on/off) data similar to contact closures. These sensors can be "tuned" to admit IR from a specific direction thereby enabling detection of the presence of persons in a small region of a room or within a wide area. This feature enables multiple devices to be used in conjunction to get rudimentary data on direction and speed of travel as one sensor "hands off" the signal to the next sensor in the series as the resident passes by. A shortcoming of the PIR sensor is that detectable IR emissions do not differ reliably by individual making it impossible to differentiate among persons living in the same environments. Attempts have been made using PIR and mathematical models to study individuals based on patterns of sensor firings (Pavel, Hayes, Adami, Jimison, & Kaye, 2006). However these approaches have shown only modest success and depend on a consistent census in the dwelling being monitored. The introduction of a new resident renders the process of accurate differentiation impossible using only PIR based systems.

Radio frequency identification devices (RFID) in conjunction with PIR and contact switch closures offer a method to improve differentiation of individuals (Pavel et al., 2007) and improve localization. RFID is widely used in the commercial sector to manage inventory, prevent theft and to speed checkout lines. A miniaturized RFID "tag" includes a transponder which echoes an identification number whenever it is struck by radio waves of a specific frequency. Some versions of the tag are implantable in humans (Verichip) and have a 10 year lifespan inside the body but have raised some security concerns (Halamka, Juels, Stubblefield, & Westhues, 2006). The most commonly used RFID tags, termed "passive RFID", derive their power from a stationary reader less than a few meters from an individual which emits radio waves and listens for the echoed tag number. When used in conjunction with a network of PIR sensors it is possible to obtain data on an individual's location, rate and direction of travel. Using this approach Pavel, Hayes and colleagues have successfully studied movement variability in persons with Parkinson's syndrome (Pavel et al., 2007).

A second more capable but also more expensive form is "active RFID" which is used to manage wandering behavior in persons with dementia in assisted living facilities and nursing homes. Active RFID systems employ a powered electrical circuit which allows them to be far more sensitive to the presence of the tag (Weinstein, 2005). This approach has distinct advantages over passive RFID which can operate only at short ranges. A person wandering and intending to elope may deliberately charge an exit door, giving very short notice of their intentions to leave. A passive RFID system might not have sufficient time to respond to the rapid approach of the individual since it activates only when the individual is very close to the door at perhaps the last moment and so may fail to lock the door in time, prohibiting their departure. Active tags can be read by readers at distances measured in hundreds of meters and can be precisely tailored to lock an exit door when an individual is several meters away from it. Unfortunately active tags must be worn on the wrist, ankle or as a pendant and cannot be implanted. Implantation of powered RFID devices results in the attenuation of the radio signal generated by the devices, shortening their range from a few hundred meters to just a few meters. There are also questions related to teratogenicity of long term exposure to strong radio waves emanating

from an internal device and possible interference of active implanted RFID with other implanted devices such as pacemakers, however experience with low power active RFID devices has found them to be safe (Wyld, 2006). Most active RFID systems improve upon passive RFID through their extended transmission range (Weinstein, 2005). In general however they do not provide information about their location unless readers are placed in strategic locations and the signal strength received from the active RFID tag is used as an indication of the relative position of the tag to the readers (where greater signal strength equates to proximity to the reader). This strategy works provided the tag's signal strength remains constant over its lifetime, which cannot be guaranteed since signal strength is related to battery power levels and the tag's battery life varies as a function of how often it responds to probes for its identification number by the readers. A tag receiving infrequent probes may have its battery last 2 years, while a tag probed multiple times per second may exhaust its battery in just a few hours. An additional problem associated with attempting to triangulate tag position based on signal strength alone is the "multipath" problem which confronts RFID use in indoor environments. Multipath refers to the phenomenon of multiple radio reflections which originate from a source confounding the reliable location of the source of the radio signal (Fontana & Gunderson, 2002). Multipath problems loom large in buildings and vary as a function of the amount of reflective materials in the building's structure, the number of steel items such as desks and filing cabinets, stoves, tables and refrigerators.

In our work we focus on the measurement of people's location and movement inside structures in order to learn more about their health and cognitive function. One of our key areas of interest is the early detection of dementia. Dementia affects 6 million Americans (Alzheimer's Association, 2009) for Europeans the 2010 estimate is also 6 million which will grow to over 14 million by 2050 (Mura, Dartigues, & Berr, 2009). There is no known cure for dementia although early detection coupled with medications such as Aricept has shown some effectiveness in slowing the rate of decline (Geldmacher, 2004). Blood tests for dementia do not exist and differential diagnosis of Alzheimer's dementia from other varieties (vascular dementia and others) must be obtained postmortem. Behavioral symptoms such as memory loss, confusion, inability to perform common activities such as adding up a column of numbers typically eventuate in a neurological assessment being performed and a diagnosis rendered by a qualified professional. Unfortunately at that stage in the disorder, irreversible impairment is present and the best the individual can hope for is that the medication is effective and their condition does not degrade further.

A characteristic of 40-60% of persons with dementia is a tendency to wander, which is defined here as aimless locomotion coupled with confusion resulting in becoming lost in familiar locales (Algase, Moore, Vandeweerd, & Gavin-Dreschnack, 2007). Wandering places a significant strain on the caregiver who must be vigilant to the ever present likelihood that the person with dementia may wander away, become lost and perish. At last count there were in excess of 20 different definitions of wandering which included among other elements the determining of the intent of the wanderer, i.e. to go to unrealistic places such as to visit a dead relative (Algase, Moore, Gavin-Dreschnack, & VandeWeerd, 2007), making comprehensive study of the phenomenon rather difficult. In our studies we have focused on aimless movement as a key component of dementia and we assert that, when correctly measured, all walking, including that of normal individuals, contains a certain amount of "aimlessness" which increases proportionately with the severity of the dementia.

The measurement of aimless movement presupposes the existence of two elements: The first is a system capable of providing accurate positioning of an individual's location over extended observation intervals and second a means to quantify "aimlessness" in the movement pattern. Fortunately the first element exists in a specialized variant of active RFID known as Ultra Wideband RFID or UWB (Kearns, Algase, Moore, & Ahmed, 2008; Kearns & Moore, 2008). UWB is specifically designed for operation inside environments capable of producing multipath interference and renders tag locations to +/- 20cm or better. The tag dimensions and weight make it acceptable as a "wristwatch" to most elders and in practice we have observed battery life is about 2 years. Positional data can be rendered at up to 10/sec; however, we have determined that one update per.43 seconds is adequate to obtain accurate tracking information from our freely moving research participants.

Our research environment is the assisted living facility (ALF), which offers hotel services but no professional medical care to individuals needing assistance with one or more activities of daily living. The proportion of residents with diagnoses of dementia at our ALF partners' sites ranges up to 70%. To detect aimless movement we employ four UWB "readers", one each at four corners of an atrium connecting dormitory areas to a dining area and front porch (Kearns & Fozard, 2009; Kearns, Nams, & Fozard, In Press). Because the area is a conduit to important locations, research participants pass through the area frequently and provide a sample of their walking behavior. Hence our subjects generate thousands of paths for evaluation in the span of a single month.

The extraction of the aimless component (tortuosity) from the path data is performed using fractal mathematics, specifically "Fractal Dimension" (or Fractal D) (Nams, 2005; Nams, 1997-2001) which is a method for estimating the tortuosity of a path composed of X and Y coordinates. In its simplest form, Fractal D can vary from a value of 1 for a perfectly straight path requiring only 1 dimension (length) to describe it to a value of 2 which describes a path which is so chaotic that it covers the entirety of a 2 dimensional plane (i.e. Brownian motion). Hence Fractal D may vary continuously from a value of 1.0 to 2.0 according to the amount of the second dimension (width) that is required to describe the path. Using Fractal D we were able to obtain measures of path tortuosity for all subjects taking part in our study.

In a recently completed investigation of 25 elders monitored using UWB over a one month period, a significant negative association (Pearson r = -.44 probability = .02) was found between Fractal D path tortuosity and subjects' MMSE scores (Kearns, Nams, Craighead and Fozard, in review) supporting our working hypothesis that disordered movement predicted cognitive decline in elders. Figure 1 presents data from the tracks of two elders recorded for two hours at approximately the same time one with a diagnosis of dementia (top) and the other without (bottom). The differences in their paths are readily apparent. Further investigations will determine whether Fractal D calculations can be used as a proxy for conventional cognitive measures and allow the near realtime detection of dementia in its nascent stages.

While the application of Fractal D to the study of movement variability has shown promise for the early detection of dementia, it is likely that other physical and mental disorders may have unique movement characteristics, which make them amenable to study using the technology described above.

ISSUES AND PROBLEMS: NORMAL AGING, CHRONIC DISEASES AND GAIT, BALANCE AND FALLS

It is important for the reader to understand that not all changes in movement variability indicate the presence of disease processes. Many changes occur as a natural function of aging; however others coincide with the onset of disease processes. In this section we present an overview of changes in physiological function affecting locomotion which accompany normal aging, as well as introducing

several syndromes which might fruitfully be studied using location aware technology.

Normal Physical Changes in Aging Produce Changes in Gait

Normal biological aging is associated with diminished dynamic complexity in organ system function resulting in an impaired adaptability to environmental stressors. Normal physiological changes associated with aging result in slower reaction and movement times and gait, decreased muscle strength, endurance, and sensory perception—all changes that may increase the risk for falls and fractures.

Stable gait and balance are essential to maintaining equilibrium while moving and proprioception requires input from visual and vestibular brain regions with efferent control via the spinal cord and peripheral muscles. Systemic declines occur in persons over 50 years of age slowing reaction time and contributing to balance and gait disorders (Kenny, 2005, p132). These changes are not inevitable, however; there is a significant literature indicating that strength training, direct training in balance, e.g., Tai Chi, can reduce risk for falls and other problems associated with movement (Hurley et al., in press). Location aware technology which serves as a diagnostic indicator may also serve a second purpose by providing information on the effectiveness of the training interventions.

Clinical studies and research on preclinical changes in behavior of persons who develop dementia indicate that gait disturbances are the earliest signs of a progression toward clinically diagnosed dementia (Johnson, Storandt, Morris, & Galvin, 2009; Ramakers et al., 2007). Therefore a broader understanding of disordered movement in the context of normal aging and in chronic illness may improve the early detection of dementia and other syndromes. The early detection of clinically significant movement disorders can lessen the likelihood of catastrophic medical events result-

Figure 1. Raw location data for two subjects for 2 hours recorded beginning at 9 a.m. The top panel (a) reveals a subject (#10) with a highly variable paths resulting in a mean Fractal D of 1.62. The lower panel (b) shows a subject who followed relatively straighter paths (#13) and who had a mean Fractal D of 1.24. The subject in the upper frame had the 4th highest fractal D value of any subject and suffered a hip fracture from a fall, which occurred after the study's completion. Ovals denote the locations of sensors in the room

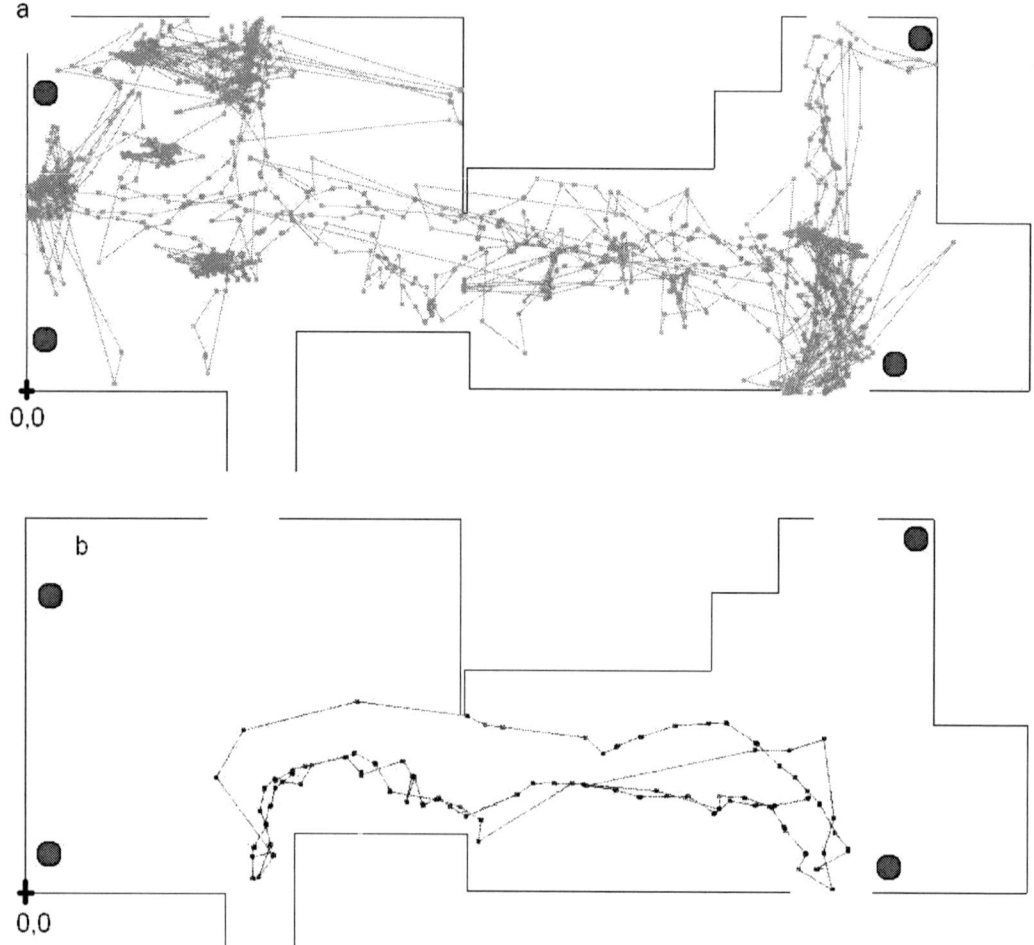

ing in disability. An evaluation of health status that examines gait changes, decreasing muscle strength and altered sensory perception is essential to improving care. Falls related to these physical changes are associated with high mortality and morbidity rates in the elderly population. Fall risks for cognitively impaired older persons are double those for normal elders (Kinney, 2005, p131).

Chronic Diseases Affect Mental Status and Movement Ability

Depression in the elderly is frequently overlooked in routine medical care. Depression results in limited activities and isolation of the individual. Cardiac disease and "metabolic syndrome" may cause vascular dementia, one of a class of dementing disorders which include Alzheimer's disease. Dementia as has previously been discussed is associated with gait changes, wandering behavior, confusion, and loss of physical ability to perform activities of daily living.

A detailed medical and life events history provides valuable information for establishing a diagnosis while computed tomography (CT) and magnetic resonance imaging (MRI) tests are valuable tools for assessing brain changes. When combined with neuropsychological testing they allow the establishment of a diagnosis with an intervention plan to mitigate injuries associated with gait changes, altered proprioception, confusion, wandering, and other movement disorders.

Diabetes Mellitus: The Most Devastating Disease Seen Today in Medicine Worldwide

Diabetes mellitus is a disease characterized by impaired output of the Islet cells of the pancreas, and/or resistance of end-organ receptors to the utilization of insulin. This results in muscle strength loss and atrophy, weakness of cardiac muscle, inability to metabolize lipids, and changed endothelial artery lining throughout the body. Alterations in cerebral, renal, cardiac, and peripheral vasculature occur resulting in impaired mental functioning, inability to walk, lethargy and visual deficits. (Lamm & Lamm, 2008). hypoglycemia is defined as abnormally low plasma glucose levels that may occur in diabetic individuals. During hypoglycemic episodes the brain stimulates hormonal and neuroendocrine responses to restore glucose to normal levels. Insulin is suppressed decreasing glucose uptake and utilization in peripheral tissues resulting in neuroglycopenic symptoms that include confusion, dizziness, convulsions and loss of consciousness. Diabetics may also exhibit tremors, palpitations, and loss of coordination and these symptoms may produce impaired mental functioning and gait disturbances. Research is needed to determine if the clinically described

movement changes associated with diabetes mellitus differentiate the disorder from dementia. The lessened ability to adapt to the environment begins a downward spiral of reduced activities and a corresponding increase in falls and injuries, and medical emergencies thereby isolating the afflicted from family and friends. We believe that the evaluation of elder movement should be included in assessment strategies with the intent of prevention of devastating injuries.

Coronary Artery Diseases

These include the abnormal conditions of arteriosclerosis, atherosclerosis, and arteritis of the coronary arteries (Osborn, Wraa, & Watson, 2010, p1159) which often cause peripheral vascular diseases such as stroke and arterial venous malformations. Stroke is defined as "a heterogeneous, neurological syndrome characterized by the gradual or rapid, nonconvulsive onset of neurological deficits that fit a known vascular territory and that last for 24 hours or more" (Hickey, 2010, p757) Strokes may result in the loss of physical ability to speak, ambulate and/or do self care thus producing limitations of activities.

Cardiovascular disease potentiates many physiological alterations of the heart and vascular system and changes in blood pressure. Blood pressure measurement provides information related to blood volume, cardiac output and peripheral vascular resistance. Hypertension indicates peak pressure exerted against the arteries during systole and residual pressure in diastole. Blood pressure measurement provides an index of the health of the cardiac system, and a warning when hypertension is detected. Hypertension is a robust risk factor for coronary heart disease indicating hypercholesterolemia, atherosclerosis and/or arteriosclerosis and treatment often includes medication, dietary alterations, and weight loss. Iatrogenesis often results from the side-effects of the anti-hypertensive drugs; patients often become lethargic, dizzy, hypotensive, and often experience diuresis. Iatrogenic patients may experience the loss of proprioception producing impaired coordination and an inability to ambulate. The altered proprioception and ensuing gait changes are a risk factor for falls and subsequent injuries. Early detection of the individual's motion may provide a model for early diagnosis and intervention. Recent research has shown that the skeletal muscles of hypertensives display lower muscle firing rates than normals suggesting that neurological changes affecting gait and balance in hypertensives may begin long before treatment starts and may thus be evaluated using gait detection algorithms (Krotish, Mitchell, Hirth & Shin 2010).

When the cardiac muscle does not receive sufficient blood flow, it becomes ischemic and irritable thus causing cardiac dysrhythmias which are slight irregularities in the heart rhythm resulting in impaired mental functioning as well as physical limitations. Hypertension is associated with "metabolic syndrome" often producing orthostatic or postprandial hypotension causing individuals to fall. Metabolic syndrome is a cluster of cardiovascular risk factors including the major components of dyslipidemia, hypertension, and insulin resistance. (Roth & Laurent-Bopp, 2004, p58) When individuals have three of five risk factors, they are prone to develop coronary heart disease. These risk factors include; hypertension, diabetes, obesity, high triglycerides, low HDL-c, and fasting glucose above 100 mg/dl. Individuals with these symptoms are more likely to develop coronary heart disease because of the increased sympathetic nervous system activation, and have an increased risk of arrhythmia, and increased sodium and water retention. These physiological changes cause generalized weakness, altered gait, and decreased sensory perception.

Parkinson's Disease

This is a movement disorder characterized by stiffness, rigidity, resting tremor and postural instability. This disease is a slowly progressive neurodegenerative disorder occurring when neurons in the substatia nigra die or become impaired. There is increased recognition of the importance of the "non-motor" features of Parkinson's Disease. These symptoms include reduced sense of smell, fatigue, disturbances in the autonomic nervous system, sleep disorders, anxiety and depression. As a consequence, biomarkers are very important in making early diagnosis of the disease. Brain imagery may be useful in establishing changes in the nondopaminergic regions of the brain. Movement disorder measurement related to fatigue and autonomic nervous system alterations may provide early diagnosis and intervention with neuroprotective therapies.

Dopamine reduction results in impaired transmission of information to areas of the brain that coordinate muscle function and movement. The individual's body responds to the declining levels of dopamine with short-stepped, shuffling gait, reduced arm swing, soft muffled speech patterns, reduced eye blinking, and frequency of swallowing. This pattern of response to the disease also produces instability and impaired ambulation, thus identification of symptoms might initiate early treatment.

Impaired ambulation is highly correlated with injury and postural instability and gait difficulty predict increased mortality risk (Lo, 2010). Individuals may also exhibit "freezing", being stuck in place when attempting to walk and retropulsion, a tendency to fall backwards. Walking with quick, small steps called festination may also promote impaired balance resulting in falls. Bradykinesia is a profound slowness of movement and loss of spontaneous autonomic movement preventing individuals from walking easily (Houghton, Hurtig, & Brandabur, 2008; Houghton et al., 2008). These physical impairments alter the ability to ambulate in a direct pathway, thus technological supervision of movement may assist in the prevention of falls and accidents. Considerable effort has been placed on early diagnosis of Parkinson's disease through the evaluation of stride time variability measures (Hausdorff, Rios & Edelberg, 2001)

Medications Which Often Result in Iatrogenesis

Medications may precipitate confusion, psychosis, and behavioral changes leading to iatrogenesis. Polypharmacy may result in pseudo-dementia as well as physical complications such as changed gait, and an inability to control body functions In order to prevent iatrogenesis, a complete evaluation of individual's medication regime, treatments and health status is performed. A physical exam including a neurological review of systems assists in establishing a relationship between symptoms and medical intervention. Studies of movement and changes in gait offer early recognition of instability leading to catastrophic physical events. Early intervention will prevent the need for placement of elders in long-term care and assisted living, promoting independent living while they age in place.

FUTURE RESEARCH DIRECTIONS: SAFE MOVEMENTS IN INDIVIDUAL AND CONGREGATE LIVING SETTINGS

The well documented desire of older persons to maintain their independence in their own home (Fozard & Kearns, 2006, Table 1) is complemented by policy makers' interest in using technology to reduce the costs of health care services provided in institutional settings. "Independence" requires the ability to move or be moved safely and effectively throughout different living spaces and to manipulate and operate the products and appliances that support the multiple activities carried out in the home. Both the common age related changes in gait and those associated with strokes as well as progressive diseases that affect gait can create challenges to maintaining independence—challenges

involving one or more of the three dimensions of movement, why, where and how to move. The normal age-related changes in gait relate most clearly to the 'how' dimension--relatively shorter strides taken in a wider stance--both adaptations in gait that result in greater stability while walking (Spirduso, 1995). Those associated with chronic and progressive diseases that involve gait vary with the disease as described earlier in the chapter.

The following sections describe the use of active location aware technology to increase the success of technology-based interventions designed to maintain independence. First, we discuss an extension of our ongoing research in AFL settings to improve safety of pedestrian movements in home settings. Second, we briefly describe the conceptual framework we currently employ in a 'smart' rehabilitation setting to use signals from active location aware technology for switching among networked technological devices and services that promote independent functioning. The technology can be extended to the home. Third we discuss some uses of active location aware technology for studying interactions between staff and patients in a rehabilitation setting and improving formal analyses of gait and balance.

Research to Improve Movement Safety in Home Settings

Active location aware technology can provide detailed monitoring of ordinary daily pedestrian movements in individual family homes and changes in those patterns over time. As with research using other location aware technologies, the goal is to identify typical patterns of movement near and on stairs, in bedroom, bath and kitchen and other living areas where accidents and falls are likely to occur. Changes in the typical patterns of movement that might result from changes in health status, e.g., a transient ischemic event or small stroke, medications and or accidents would be studied to determine their predictive value for future adverse events and ultimately personal or environmental interventions.

The justification for using active location aware technology is that the modal pattern of aging occurs and will continue to occur in existing individual homes with multiple occupants—homes that are not designed to be user-friendly for persons who have or who are developing limitations in personal mobility. Determining what 'user-friendly' means for individuals in specific homes is an idiosyncratic and complex process; the starting point for many planners are the building codes used for congregate living settings for elderly and wheel-chair bound persons. They do not apply to individual homes although Great Britain has introduced such a code for new private home construction. With some variations, such building codes typically include: a level entry to the principal entrance; an entrance door wide enough to allow wheelchair access; wide hallways; a bathroom on the entrance level or first habitable story; and a level or gently sloping approach from the parking space to the dwelling (Iwarsson, 2003). These architectural features may be supplemented by additional modifications in working and living spaces that support independent functioning for wheelchair-bound persons. Modifying existing individual housing stock along the lines of the building codes described is impractical, expensive and for most elderly persons, unnecessary.

Systematic efforts to customize specific modifications to existing homes to the unique individual needs of its aging occupants have been made in Europe and the United States mostly by occupational therapists. The most sophisticated of these grew out of a six-country study of housing used by elderly persons in Europe (Oswald et al., 2007). Data from this study, called ENABLE-AGE, included descriptions of the house, the health and functional capacities of its elderly occupants and observations of the occupants carrying out daily tasks. (Iwarsson, 2003 Fig. 4.3, p.98) lists 15 functional limitations including interpreting information, limitations in vision, hearing, balance,

reaching, use of mobility aids, extremes of weight, etc, and relates them to necessary modifications in the interior and exterior of the house. The instrument used by the expert observer is called the Housing Enabler; a self-administering version for use by the resident is called "Usability in my home." Iwarsson recommends that both versions be used in planning home modifications, partly to engage the interest and cooperation of the resident. A similar instrument, "Comprehensive Assessment and Solution Process for Aging Residents" (CASPAR) (Sanford, Pynoos, Tejral, & Browne, 2001) has been developed in the United States; it is specifically designed to actively involve the resident in decisions about home modifications. The importance of involving the resident in plans for home modification includes the observation by outside evaluators that, because of their familiarity with the home environment, the elderly resident may underestimate the difficulties of maneuvering through the home.

The home adaptations can take many forms depending on the structure of the home and the specific needs of the occupants. Grayson (1997) identifies three levels of complexity: I—no modification of existing physical, mechanical or electrical systems; II—replacing and adding to existing elements—widening doorways, installing grab bars, installing emergency alerting systems; and III—major time consuming alterations, e.g., replacing kitchen and bathroom fixtures, adjustable height cabinets and work surfaces.

Active location aware technology can supplement and broaden the observations and recommendations made by the expert observer and it provides a longer time frame for establishing patterns of movement as well as changes in those patterns after the modifications are made. When coupled with other technologies that identify hand and arm movements, information about approaches to and leaving sites where daily activities are performed can be obtained using machine based data to supplement information gained by expert observers.

The arguments for using active location aware technology as a tool for planning and evaluating home modifications apply equally to more established rehabilitation and training programs, e.g., stroke rehabilitation. Over a long period, three concerns with these programs have been raised and addressed in various ways: the duration of the rehabilitation program for elderly persons; the continuity of the benefits of the rehabilitation after the formal program ends (strength training that is an essential component of the rehabilitation may not be continued); and that the benefits of the formal training do not transfer to everyday tasks at home. Two approaches have been used to increase the verisimilitude of the rehabilitation programs. One was the creation of a day care setting for stroke rehabilitation (initially created by the Veterans Administration Extended Care Service). The idea was that the veteran would learn to apply the benefits of the daytime rehab services to the home setting better than would be the case if the patient resided in an institutional setting during the rehabilitation program (Fozard, 2000). Second, during the 1990s, several programs were created using lifelike situations that supplemented or replaced the traditional equipment used in rehabilitation. Spaces were created with mockups of entry doors to automobiles, ATMs, shopping and meal preparation settings. Although formal comparisons between the effectiveness of traditional and the newer settings are inconclusive, the usefulness of the high verisimilitude settings for increasing the confidence of the patient was evident (Fozard & Heikkinen, 1997).

Active Location Aware Technology in Networked Systems

Gerontechnology

Fozard (2005) identifies four health related goals of technology, three of which correspond closely to the major goals of public health—primary, secondary, and tertiary prevention. Location aware technology plays a role at all three levels. Prevention and engagement refers to technology that delays or prevents age-associated physiological and behavioral changes that restrict functioning. In housing, this includes long term support of health through creation and monitoring of safe environments, technology that facilitates the performance of ADLs and IADLs, and adaptability of housing to support the changing needs of people as they age. Active location aware technology can be used to evaluate the safety and use of furniture and appliances in a monitored living space. In congregate living situations it provides information about how residents use space and furnishings for social activities, hobbies, and interactions with fellow residents and staff.

Compensation and assistance refers to technology that compensates for common age associated losses in strength and mobility, sensory and perceptual function, and cognitive function. In living settings, interventions are designed to alter intensity and placement of sources of light or sound, reduce visual glare and masking noise and provide alternative sources of environmental information and the means to respond to it. The goals for persons with cognitive limitations relate to safety, communication, use of environmental information to compensate for memory loss, and assistance to caregivers. The roles of location aware technology include triggering lights, thermostats, alarm systems, controls on doors, etc.

Care support and organization refers to the use of technology either for self-care by elderly persons with existing functional limitations or for care provided by nonprofessional or professional caregivers. Examples include devices that lift and move physically disabled persons, machines that monitor and administer oral and injectable medications, and technology that provides behavioral and physiological information to remote—usually professional—caregivers. Location aware technology supports the monitoring of movements by persons with disabilities, the deployment and monitoring of robots and other devices that serve as surrogates to human caregivers.

Cutting across the other three is technology for enhancement and satisfaction—interactive communication, self adapting equipment, and simpler devices—that expand the range and depth of human activities related to comfort, vitality and productivity. Location aware technology facilitates communication with equipment and other people

The Health-Related Goals of Technology Can Be Met at Three Levels of Complexity

We distinguish between three levels of smart environments: clever, smart and wise smart living spaces. Location aware technology is plays a major role in defining these levels.

Clever living spaces refer to applications of single technological products—alarms, thermostats, sound activated switches—with no connections among them. Clever technologies meet the minimum goals of individual compensation interventions, e.g., warning signals, sound activated switches to turn on electric lights.

Smart living spaces refer to multiple networked applications with a common user interface; they meet requirements of many care type and some prevention oriented interventions. Remote controllers of window blinds, remote control of outside doors, etc. are examples.

Wise living spaces refer to multiple networked applications with possible remote management capabilities, which usually meet most requirements for prevention level interventions. Examples include interactive Bluetooth and other communication devices such as wearable sensors, handheld controls, etc.; technology that serves as a surrogate for human assistance for persons with functional limitations; technology that reinforces the acquisition and maintenance of healthy life styles; and technology to support behavioral therapeutic goals.

Chan and colleagues (Chan, Esteve, Escriba, & Campo, 2008 p.57, Fig. 1) identify four levels of technological complexity in a fully integrated (wise) system of consumer products, automated monitoring systems and automated therapeutic services: they include databases, data processing, customized software and decision algorithms. Active location aware technology is useful at all levels of complexity described. It can provide customizable information about the location of objects and appliances in the living space monitored as well as the changing locations of people moving within the area. Accordingly, it can provide direct information to other devices based on the location of the individuals wearing the transponders, thereby directly initiating or terminating the activity of the devices. A person who falls would provide location information about the "z" dimension (vertical) of transponder location that characterizes the fall. The implementation of any of the three levels of technology can be accomplished with Levels I and II of the home modification levels by (Grayson, 1997).

Other Uses of Active Location Aware Technology

The main advantage of active location aware technology over passive devices is its ability to uniquely relate location information of objects or persons wearing the transponders. The Ubisense RFID technology was developed for tracking location of "assets," e.g., the location of mobile equipment in a hospital, or the location of parts used in construction of complex pieces of equipment, e.g., airplanes or cars. The technology is also used in military training exercises showing the consequences of movements of soldiers in house to house combat in battle simulations.

One feature of Ubisense active location aware ultra-wideband technology is the wide range of sensitivity of the transponders. In earlier research using this equipment (Kearns et al., In Press) the location of the tag was determined approximately every 0.4 sec. However, it is possible to estimate tag location more than ten times per sec, thereby making it possible to track movements more precisely. Accordingly, we are currently comparing this technology against other conventional methods and equipment used to assess gait and balance. If comparable results occur, the equipment used to monitor everyday movements of residents in congregate living settings could also serve to perform the standard gait and balance assessments.

It is possible to monitor the movements of large numbers of people simultaneously using ultra-wideband RFID technology. This creates opportunities to study the locations and time course of interactions among residents in congregate living situations. If staff in the congregate living settings also wear transponders further opportunities are created for studying the location and time course of interactions between staff and residents, something of considerable interest to managers of Assisted Living Facilities. By the same token, it is possible to evaluate the use of furniture, and appliances placed in common spaces of congregate living settings. Analyses of hourly activity levels in two Assisted Living Facilities (Kearns, Nams, Fozard, 2010) show that activity increases around scheduled events such as meals and administration of medications by staff to residents, and decreases during other times of the day. Altering the arrangement and type of furniture and appliances in the common spaces may increase social interactions and amount of individual movement by residents, thereby potentially improving their mental health. Additional sensors would make it possible to remotely and unobtrusively monitor movements of residents in their bedrooms and baths, thereby serving as an alerting system for staff of possible falls or accidents.

CONCLUSION

In this chapter we have presented arguments and research to show how movement information can provide valuable insights into disorders and can broaden our understanding of their pathogenesis. We have focused not so much upon the gross amount of movement as we have the structure of the movement itself. By differentiating random from well ordered movement components we find significant relationships between spatial variability and disease that complements relationships observed between temporal variability and disease by other researchers such as Hausdorff and Verghese. The study of movement variability using sensor networks may provide fertile ground for the study of Diabetes Mellitus and other disorders which have movement changes as part of their symptomatology.

Finally the study of movement variability can provide direct benefits to elders who seek to remain independent by permitting close study of their home environment's impact on their behavior and will facilitate the systematic restructuring of it to create a more well adapted home with fewer risks and more beneficial features.

REFERENCES

Adami, A. M., Hayes, T. L., Pavel, M., & Singer, C. M. (2005). Detection and Classification of Movements in Bed using Load Cells: Engineering in Medicine and Biology Society, 2005. IEEE EMBS 2005. 27th Annual International Conference of the. *Engineering in Medicine and Biology Society, 2005. IEEE-EMBS 2005. 27th Annual International Conference of the* (pp. 589-592).

Algase, D., Moore, D., Gavin-Dreschnack, D., & VandeWeerd, C. (2007). Wandering Definitions and Terms. In Nelson, A., & Algase, D. L. (Eds.), *Evidence-Based Protocols for Managing Wandering Behaviors*. New York: Springer Publishing Company.

Algase, D., Moore, D., Vandeweerd, C., & Gavin-Dreschnack, D. J. (2007). Mapping the maze of terms and definitions in dementia-related wandering. *Aging & Mental Health, 11*(6), 686–698. doi:10.1080/13607860701366434

Alzheimer's Association. (2009). 2009 Alzheimer's disease facts and figures. *Alzheimer's & Dementia, 5*(3), 234–270. doi:10.1016/j.jalz.2009.03.001

Benhamou, S., & Bovet, P. (1992). Distinguishing between elementary orientation mechanisms by means of path analysis. *Animal Behaviour, 43,* 371–377. doi:10.1016/S0003-3472(05)80097-1

Chan, M., Esteve, D., Escriba, C., & Campo, E. (2008). A review of smart homes- present state and future challenges. *Computer Methods and Programs in Biomedicine, 91*(1), 55–81. doi:10.1016/j.cmpb.2008.02.001

Chiu, Y. C., Algase, D., Whall, A., Liang, J., Liu, H. C., & Lin, K. N. (2004). Getting lost: Directed attention and executive functions in early Alzheimer's disease patients. *Dementia and Geriatric Cognitive Disorders, 17*(3), 174–180. doi:10.1159/000076353

Codling, E. A., Plank, M. J., & Benhamou, S. (2008). Random walk models in biology. *Journal of the Royal Society, Interface.*.doi:10.1098/rsif.2008.0014

de Leon, M. J., Potegal, M., & Gurland, B. (1984). Wandering and parietal signs in senile dementia of Alzheimer's type. *Neuropsychobiology, 11*(3), 155–157. doi:10.1159/000118069

Demiris, G., Rantz, M. J., Aud, M. A., Marek, K. D., Tyrer, H. W., & Skubic, M. (2004). Older adults' attitudes towards and perceptions of smart home technologies: A pilot study. *Informatics for Health & Social Care, 29*(2), 87–94. doi:10.1080/14639230410001684387

Fontana, R. J., & Gunderson, S. J. (2002). Ultra-wideband precision asset location system: Ultra Wideband Systems and Technologies, 2002. Digest of Papers. 2002 IEEE Conference on. *Ultra Wideband Systems and Technologies, 2002. Digest of Papers. 2002 IEEE Conference on* (pp. 147-150).

Fozard, J. (2000). How ten years with ageless rats and college sophomores led to a thirty something career in geropsychology. In Birren, J. E., & Schroots, J. H. H. (Eds.), *History of Geropsychology through autobiography* (pp. 91–108). Washington, DC: American Psychological Assn. doi:10.1037/10367-008

Fozard, J. (2005). Impacts of technology on health and self esteem. *Gerontechnology (Valkenswaard), 4*(2), 63–76. doi:10.4017/gt.2005.04.02.002.00

Fozard, J., & Kearns, W. (2006). Persuasive GERONtechnology: Reaping Technology's Coaching Benefits at Older Age. W. In *Ijsselsteijn, Y. de Kort, C. Midden, B. Eggen, & E. van den HovenPersuasive Technology, 3962* (pp. 199–202). Berlin, Heidelberg: Springer-Verlag.

Fozard, J. L., & Heikkinen, E. (1997). Maintaining movement ability in old age. In Graafinans, J. A. M., Taipale, V., & Charness, N. E. (Eds.), *Gerontechnology: A sustainable investment in the future* (pp. 48–61). Amsterdam: IOS Press.

Geldmacher, D. S. (2004). Donepezil (Aricept) for treatment of Alzheimer's disease and other dementing conditions. *Expert Review of Neurotherapeutics, 4*(1), 5–16. doi:10.1586/14737175.4.1.5

Goodwin, B. J., Bender, D. J., Contreras, T. A., Fahrig, L., & Wegner, J. F. (1999). Testing for habitat detection distances using orientation data. *Oikos, 84*(1), 160–163. doi:10.2307/3546877

Grayson, J. P. (1997). Technology and home adaptations. Landspery S, & Hyde J (Eds), *Staying put: Adapting the places instead of the people* (pp. 55-74). Amityville, NY: Baywood.

Halamka, J., Juels, A., Stubblefield, A., & Westhues, J. (2006). The Security Implications of VeriChip Cloning. *Journal of the American Medical Informatics Association, 13*(6), 601–607. doi:10.1197/jamia.M2143

Hamill, M., Young, V., Boger, J., & Mihailidis, A. (2009). Development of an automated speech recognition interface for Personal Emergency Response Systems. *Journal of Neuroengineering and Rehabilitation, 6*, 26. doi:10.1186/1743-0003-6-26

Harvey, N., Zhou, Z., Keller, J. M., Rantz, M., & He, Z. (2009). Automated estimation of elder activity levels from anonymized video data. *Conference Proceedings;... Annual International Conference of the IEEE Engineering in Medicine and Biology Society. IEEE Engineering in Medicine and Biology Society. Conference, 1*, 7236–7239.

Hausdorff, J., Rios, D., & Edelberg, H. (2001). Gait variability and fall risk in community-living older adults: A 1-year prospective study. *Archives of Physical Medicine and Rehabilitation, 82*(8), 1050–1056. doi:10.1053/apmr.2001.24893

Henderson, V. W., Mack, W., & Williams, B. W. (1989). Spatial disorientation in Alzheimer's disease. *Archives of Neurology, 46*(4), 391–394.

Hickey, J. (2010). Caring for the Patient with Cerebrovascular Disorders. In Osborn, K., Wraa, C., & Watson, A. (Eds.), *Medical Surgical Nursing*. Boston: Pearson.

Houghton, D., Hurtig, H., & Brandabur, M. (2008). *Parkinson's Disease: Medications*. Miami, Florida: Parkinson's Disease Foundation.

Hurley, B. F., Hanson, E. D., & Sheaff, A. K. (in press). Strength Training as a Countermeasure to Age Related Disease. *Sports Medicine (Auckland, N.Z.)*.

Ihgb, Ramakers, Visser, P. J., Aalten, P., Boesten, J. H. M., Metsemakers, J. F. M., Jolles, J. et al. (2007). Symptoms of Preclinical Dementia in General Practice up to Five Years Before Dementia Diagnosis. *Dementia and Geriatric Cognitive Disorders, 24*(4), 300–306. doi:10.1159/000107594

Iwarsson, S. (2003). Assessing the fit between older people and their physical home environments: An occupational therapy research perspective. In Wahl WE, Scheidt RJ, & Windley PG (Eds), *Annual Review of Gerontology and Geriatrics. Focus on aging in context: socio-physical environments* (Vol. 23pp. 85-109). New York: Springer.

Jensen, J., Nyberg, L., Gustafson, Y., & Lundin-Olsson, L. (2003). Fall and injury prevention in residential care--effects in residents with higher and lower levels of cognition. *Journal of the American Geriatrics Society, 51*(5), 627–635. doi:10.1034/j.1600-0579.2003.00206.x

Johnson, D. K., Storandt, M., Morris, J. C., & Galvin, J. E. (2009). Longitudinal Study of the Transition From Healthy Aging to Alzheimer Disease. *Archives of Neurology, 66*(10), 1254–1259. doi:10.1001/archneurol.2009.158

Kearns, W., Algase, D., Moore, D., & Ahmed, S. (2008). Ultra wideband radio: A novel method for measuring wandering in persons with dementia. *Gerontechnology (Valkenswaard), 7*(1), 48–57. doi:10.4017/gt.2008.07.01.005.00

Kearns, W., & Fozard, J. L. (2009). Evaluation of Wandering by Residents in an Assisted Living Facility (ALF) using Ultra Wideband Radio RTLS. *The Journal of Nutrition, Health & Aging, 13*, S54.

Kearns, W., & Moore, D. (2008). RFID: A tool for measuring wandering in persons with dementia. A. Mihailidis, J. Boger, H. Kautz, & L. Normie (Eds.), *Technology and Aging: Selected Papers from the 2007 International Conference on Technology and Aging* (Vol. 21pp. 154-164). Amsterdam: IOS Press.

Kearns, W., Nams, V., & Fozard, J. (in press). Wireless fractal estimation of tortuosity in movement paths related to cognitive impairment in assisted living facility residents. *Methods of Information in Medicine*.

Kearns, W., Nams, V., Fozard, J., & Craighead, J. (In review). Path Tortuosity Predicts Dementia in Assisted Living Facility Residents. *Methods of Information in Medicine*.

Kenny, R. (2005). Mobility and Falls. In Johnson, M., Bengston, V., Coleman, P., & Kirkwood, T. (Eds.), *The Cambridge Handbook of Age and Ageing* (pp. 131–134). Cambridge, UK: Cambridge University Press. doi:10.1017/CBO9780511610714.012

Krotish, D., Mitchell, P., Hirth, V., & Shin, Y. J. (2010). The use of time-frequency analysis using electromyography and foot pressure distribution for the determination of gait disorders. *Proceedings of the 3rd International Congress on Gait & Mental Functions: The Interplay Between Walking, Behavior and Cognition*. Geneva: Kenes.

Lamm, R., & Lamm, E. (2008). *Aging and Technology. Dagstuhl Seminar on Assisted Living Systems*. LZI.

Luis, C. A., & Brown, L. M. (2007). Neuropsychological correlates of wanderers. In Nelson, A. L., & Algase, D. L. (Eds.), *Evidence-based protocols for managing wandering behaviors* (pp. 65–74). New York: Springer.

McCulloch, C. E., & Cain, M. L. (1989). Analyzing discrete movement data as a correlated random walk. *Ecology, 70*, 383–388. doi:10.2307/1937543

Mihailidis, A., Cockburn, A., Longley, C., & Boger, J. (2008). The acceptability of home monitoring technology among community-dwelling older adults and baby boomers. *Assistive Technology, 20*(1), 1–12. doi:10.1080/10400435.2008.10131927

Mura, T., Dartigues, J. F., & Berr, C. (2009). How many dementia cases in France and Europe? Alternative projections and scenarios 2010-2050. *European Journal of Neurology*.

Nams, V. (1997-2001). *Fractal computer program, version 3.16*. Web site: URL http://www.nsac.ns.ca/envsci/staff/vnams/Fractal.htm

Nams, V. O. (2005). Using animal movement paths to measure response to spatial scale. *Oecologia, 143*, 179–188. doi:10.1007/s00442-004-1804-z

Nathan, R., Getz, W. M., Revilla, E., Holyoak, M., Kadmon, R., & Saltz, D. (2008). A movement ecology paradigm for unifying organismal movement research. *Proceedings of the National Academy of Sciences of the United States of America, 105*(49), 19052–19059. doi:10.1073/pnas.0800375105

Ni Scanaill, C., Carew, S., Barralon, P., Noury, N., Lyons, D., & Lyons, G. M. (2006). A review of approaches to mobility telemonitoring of the elderly in their living environment. *Annals of Biomedical Engineering, 34*(4), 547–563. doi:10.1007/s10439-005-9068-2

Osborn, K., Wraa, C., & Watson, A. (2010). *Medical Surgical Nursing*. Boston: Pearson.

Oswald, F., Wahl, H. W., Schilling, O., Nygren, C., Fange, A., & Sixsmith, A. (2007). Relationships between housing and healthy aging in very old age. *The Gerontologist, 47*(1), 96–107.

Passini, R., Rainville, C., Marchand, N., & Joanette, Y. (1995). Wayfinding in dementia of the Alzheimer type: planning abilities. *Journal of Clinical and Experimental Neuropsychology, 17*(6), 820–832. doi:10.1080/01688639508402431

Pavel, M., Hayes, T., Tsay, I., Erdogmus, D., Paul, A., Larimer, N., et al. (2007). *Continuous assessment of gait velocity in Parkinson's disease from unobtrusive measurements: CNE '07*. 3rd International IEEE/EMBS Conference on Neural Engineering, 2007. 5/2/2007-5/5/2007 Hawaii, USA 700-703.

Pavel, M., Hayes, T. L., Adami, A., Jimison, H., & Kaye, J. (2006). Unobtrusive assessment of mobility. *Conference Proceedings;... Annual International Conference of the IEEE Engineering in Medicine and Biology Society. IEEE Engineering in Medicine and Biology Society. Conference, 1*, 6277–6280. doi:10.1109/IEMBS.2006.260301

Roth, E., & Laurent-Bopp, D. (2004). Challenges of treating dyslipidemia in patients with the metabolic syndrome. *American Journal for Nurse Practitioners, 8*(4), 58–66.

Rowe, M., Lane, S., & Phipps, C. (2007). CareWatch: A home monitoring system for use in homes of persons with cognitive impairment. *Topics in Geriatric Rehabilitation, 23*(1), 3.

Rubenstein, L. Z. (2006). Falls in older people: epidemiology, risk factors and strategies for prevention. *Age and Ageing, 35*(Suppl 2), ii37–ii41. doi:10.1093/ageing/afl084

Ryan, J. P., McGowan, J., McCaffrey, N., Ryan, G. T., Zandi, T., & Brannigan, G. G. (1995). Graphomotor perseveration and wandering in Alzheimer's disease. *Journal of Geriatric Psychiatry and Neurology, 8*(4), 209–212.

Sanford, J. A., Pynoos, J., Tejral, A., & Browne, A. (2001). Development of a Comprehensive Assessment for Delivery of Home Modifications. *Physical & Occupational Therapy in Geriatrics, 20*(2), 43–55.

Sixsmith, A. J. (2000). An evaluation of an intelligent home monitoring system. *Journal of Telemedicine and Telecare, 6*(2), 63–72. doi:10.1258/1357633001935059

Snyder, L., Rupprecht, P., Pyrek, J., Brekhus, S., & Moss, T. (1978). Wandering. *The Gerontologist, 18*(3), 272.

Spirduso, W. W. (1995). *Balance, Posture and Locomotion. In W. W. Spirduso Physical Dimensions of Aging*. Champaign, Illinois: Human Kinetics.

Suzuki, T, Murase, S, Tanaka, T. & Okazawa, T. (2007). New *approach for the early detection of dementia by recording in-house activities, 13*(1), 41-44.

US Centers for Disease Control. (2003). Public Health and Aging: Trends in Aging-United States and Worldwide. *Morbidity and Mortality Weekly Report, 52*(6), 101–106.

Verghese, J., Holtzer, R., Lipton, R. B., & Wang, C. (2009). Quantitative Gait Markers and Incident Fall Risk in Older Adults. *The Journals of Gerontology. Series A, Biological Sciences and Medical Sciences, 64A*(8), 896–901. doi:10.1093/gerona/glp033

Verghese, J., Lipton, R., Hall, C., Kuslansky, G., Katz, M., & Buschke, H. (2002). Abnormality of Gait as a Predictor of Non-Alzheimer's Dementia. *The New England Journal of Medicine, 347*(22), 1761–1768. doi:10.1056/NEJMoa020441

Wang, S., Skubic, M., & Zhu, Y. (2009). Activity density map dis-similarity comparison for eldercare monitoring. *Conference Proceedings;... Annual International Conference of the IEEE Engineering in Medicine and Biology Society. IEEE Engineering in Medicine and Biology Society. Conference, 1*, 7232–7235.

Weinstein, R. (2005). RFID: a technical overview and its application to the enterprise. *IT Professional.*

Wyld, D. (2006). RFID 101: the next big thing for management. *Management Research News, 29*(4), 154–173. doi:10.1108/01409170610665022

ADDITIONAL READING

Algase, D., & Struble, L. (1992). Wandering behavior: What, why, and how. *Geriatric Mental Health Nursing: Current and Future Challenges,* 61-74.

Algase, D. L., Moore, D. H., Vandeweerd, C., & Gavln-Dreschnack, D. J. (2007). Mapping the maze of terms and definitions in dementia-related wandering. *Aging & Mental Health, 11*(6), 686–698. doi:10.1080/13607860701366434

Algase, D. L., Son, G. R., Beattie, E., Song, J. A., Leitsch, S., & Yao, L. (2004). The interrelatedness of wandering and wayfinding in a community sample of persons with dementia. *Dementia and Geriatric Cognitive Disorders, 17*(3), 231–239. doi:10.1159/000076361

Bashshur, R., Reardon, T., & Shannon, G. (2000). Telemedicine: a new health care delivery system. *Annual Review of Public Health, 21*(1), 613–637. doi:10.1146/annurev.publhealth.21.1.613

Benhamou, S., & Bovet, P. (1992). Distinguishing between elementary orientation mechanisms by means of path analysis. *Animal Behaviour, 43,* 371–377. doi:10.1016/S0003-3472(05)80097-1

Chiu, Y. C., Algase, D., Whall, A., Liang, J., Liu, H. C., & Lin, K. N. (2004). Getting lost: Directed attention and executive functions in early Alzheimer's disease patients. *Dementia and Geriatric Cognitive Disorders, 17*(3), 174–180. doi:10.1159/000076353

Codling, E. A., Plank, M. J., & Benhamou, S. (2008). Random walk models in biology. *Journal of the Royal Society, Interface.*.doi:10.1098/rsif.2008.0014

Craighead, J. (in Press). Using Fractal Dimension to Assess Robot Operator Skill. Proceedings of the 2009 IEEE International Workshop on Safety, Security, and Rescue Robotics. (SSRR 2009).

de Leon, M. J., Potegal, M., & Gurland, B. (1984). Wandering and parietal signs in senile dementia of Alzheimer's type. *Neuropsychobiology, 11*(3), 155–157. doi:10.1159/000118069

Fozard, J. L., & Kearns, W. D. (2008). Communication technology changes how we age. *Gerontechnology (Valkenswaard), 7*(2), 106. doi:10.4017/gt.2008.07.02.043.00

Friedman, R. H., Stollerman, J. E., Mahoney, D. M., & Rozenblyum, L. (1997). The virtual visit: using telecommunications technology to take care of patients. *Journal of the American Medical Informatics Association, 4*(6), 413–425.

Goodwin, B. J., Bender, D. J., Contreras, T. A., Fahrig, L., & Wegner, J. F. (1999). Testing for habitat detection distances using orientation data. *Oikos, 84*(1), 160–163. doi:10.2307/3546877

Hausdorff, J., Rios, D., & Edelberg, H. (2001). Gait variability and fall risk in community-living older adults: A 1-year prospective study. *Archives of Physical Medicine and Rehabilitation, 82*(8), 1050–1056. doi:10.1053/apmr.2001.24893

Hausdorff, J. M. (2007). Gait dynamics, fractals and falls: Finding meaning in the stride-to-stride fluctuations of human walking. *Human Movement Science, 26*(4), 555–589. doi:10.1016/j.humov.2007.05.003

Henderson, V. W., Mack, W., & Williams, B. W. (1989). Spatial disorientation in Alzheimer's disease. *Archives of Neurology, 46*(4), 391–394.

Ihgb, Ramakers, Visser, P. J., Aalten, P., Boesten, J. H. M., Metsemakers, J. F. M., Jolles, J. et al. (2007). Symptoms of preclinical dementia in general practice up to five years before dementia diagnosis. *Dementia and Geriatric Cognitive Disorders, 24*(4), 300–306. doi:10.1159/000107594

Jensen, J., Nyberg, L., Gustafson, Y., & Lundin-Olsson, L. (2003). Fall and injury prevention in residential care--effects in residents with higher and lower levels of cognition. *Journal of the American Geriatrics Society, 51*(5), 627–635. doi:10.1034/j.1600-0579.2003.00206.x

Johnson, D. K., Storandt, M., Morris, J. C., & Galvin, J. E. (2009). Longitudinal study of the transition from healthy aging to Alzheimer disease. *Archives of Neurology, 66*(10), 1254–1259. doi:10.1001/archneurol.2009.158

Kearns, W., & Fozard, J. L. (2009). Evaluation of Wandering by Residents in an Assisted Living Facility (ALF) using Ultra Wideband Radio RTLS. *The Journal of Nutrition, Health & Aging, 13*, S54.

Kearns, W., Nams, V., & Fozard, J. (in press). Wireless fractal estimation of tortuosity in movement paths related to cognitive impairment in assisted living facility residents. *Methods of Information in Medicine.*

Kearns, W. D., Algase, D., Moore, D. H., & Ahmed, S. (2008). Ultra wideband radio: A novel method for measuring wandering in persons with dementia. *Gerontechnology (Valkenswaard), 7*(1), 48–57. doi:10.4017/gt.2008.07.01.005.00

Kearns, W. D., & Fozard, J. (2008). Locomotor variability assessment of the elderly using ultra wideband radio. *Telemedicine and E-Health, 14*(6), 611–620.

Kearns, W. D., & Fozard, J. L. (2007). Gerontechnology, international computer networks and ICT. *Gerontechnology (Valkenswaard), 6*(3), 135–146. doi:10.4017/gt.2007.06.03.003.00

Kirtley, C. (2006). *Clinical gait analysis: Theory and practice.* Churchill Livingstone.

Lamm, R., & Lamm, E. (2008). *Aging and Technology. Dagstuhl Seminar on Assisted Living Systems.* LZI.

Lesnoff-Caravaglia, G. (Ed.). (2007). *Gerontechnology: Growing old in a technological society.* Springfield, Ill: Charles C. Thomas.

Luis, C. A., & Brown, L. M. (2007). Neuropsychological correlates of wanderers. A. L. Nelson, & D. L. Algase (Eds.), *Evidence-based protocols for managing wandering behaviors* (pp. 65-74). New York: Springer.

McCulloch, C. E., & Cain, M. L. (1989). Analyzing discrete movement data as a correlated random walk. *Ecology, 70*, 383–388. doi:10.2307/1937543

Merory, J. R., Wittwer, J. E., Rowe, C. C., & Webster, K. E. (2007). Quantitative Gait Analysis in Patients With Dementia With Lewy Bodies and Alzheimer's Disease. *Gait & Posture, 26*(3), 414–419. doi:10.1016/j.gaitpost.2006.10.006

Nams, V. (1999). Fractal: A program to estimate fractal dimensions of animal movement paths. Available at http://www.nsac.ns.ca/es/vnams/fractal.htm

Nams, V. O. (2006). Improving accuracy and precision in estimating fractal dimension of animal movement paths. *Acta Biotheoretica, 54*, 1–11. doi:10.1007/s10441-006-5954-8

Nams, V. O., & Bourgeois, M. (2004). Fractal dimension measures habitat use at different spatial scales: an example with marten. *Canadian Journal of Zoology, 82*, 1738–1747. doi:10.1139/z04-167

Nathan, R., Getz, W. M., Revilla, E., Holyoak, M., Kadmon, R., & Saltz, D. (2008). A movement ecology paradigm for unifying organismal movement research. *Proceedings of the National Academy of Sciences of the United States of America, 105*(49), 19052–19059. doi:10.1073/pnas.0800375105

Nelson, A. L., & Algase, D. L. (2007). Appendix B. Measurement Tools for Wandering. Revised Algase Wandering Scale-Community Version. AL Nelson, & DL Algase (Eds.), *Evidence-based protocols for managing wandering behavior* (pp. 385-397). New York: Springer.

Passini, R., Rainville, C., Marchand, N., & Joanette, Y. (1995). Wayfinding in dementia of the Alzheimer type: planning abilities. *Journal of Clinical and Experimental Neuropsychology, 17*(6), 820–832. doi:10.1080/01688639508402431

Rubenstein, L. Z. (2006). Falls in older people: epidemiology, risk factors and strategies for prevention. *Age and Ageing, 35*(Suppl 2), ii37–ii41. doi:10.1093/ageing/afl084

Ryan, J. P., McGowan, J., McCaffrey, N., Ryan, G. T., Zandi, T., & Brannigan, G. G. (1995). Graphomotor perseveration and wandering in Alzheimer's disease. *Journal of Geriatric Psychiatry and Neurology, 8*(4), 209–212.

Sanders, A., Holtzer, R., Lipton, R., Hall, C., & Verghese, J. (2008). Egocentric and Exocentric Navigation Skills in Older Adults. *Journals of Gerontology Series A: Biological and Medical Sciences, 63*(12), 1356.

Sheridan, P. L., & Hausdorff, J. M. (2007). The Role of Higher-Level Cognitive Function in Gait: Executive Dysfunction Contributes to Fall Risk in Alzheimer's Disease. *Dementia and Geriatric Cognitive Disorders, 24*(2), 125–137. doi:10.1159/000105126

Snyder, L., Rupprecht, P., Pyrek, J., Brekhus, S., & Moss, T. (1978). Wandering. *The Gerontologist, 18*(3), 272.

Spirduso, W. W., Francis, K., & MacRae, P. (Eds.). (2005). *Physical dimensions of aging.* Champaign, Ill: Human Kinetics.

Verghese, J., Holtzer, R., Lipton, R. B., & Wang, C. (2009). Quantitative Gait Markers and Incident Fall Risk in Older Adults. *Journals of Gerontology Series A: Biological and Medical Sciences, 64A*(8), 896–901. doi:10.1093/gerona/glp033

Verghese, J., Lipton, R., Hall, C., Kuslansky, G., Katz, M., & Buschke, H. (2002). Abnormality of Gait as a Predictor of Non-Alzheimer's Dementia. *The New England Journal of Medicine, 347*(22), 1761–1768. doi:10.1056/NEJMoa020441

Yogev-Seligmann, G., Hausdorff, J. M., & Giladi, N. (2008). The role of executive function and attention in gait. *Movement Disorders, 23*(3), 329–342. doi:10.1002/mds.21720

KEY TERMS AND DEFINITIONS

Location-Aware Technology: Devices which differentially respond based on the user's position in space (i.e. Global Positioning Systems).

Fractal Dimension: Fractal Dimension (Fractal D) is used in movement ecology studies to characterize exploratory behavior in numerous species, and is employed to characterize elder path tortuosity. Values of Fractal D range from 1 where a path follows a perfectly straight line (requiring only a single dimension, length, to describe it) to 2 where the path is so tortuous (chaotic) that it completely covers the plane of movement and requires all of a second dimension (width) to describe it.

Independent Functioning: The ability to live independently in the leisure / recreation, home maintenance and personal care, and community participation domains.

Smart Living Environments: Domiciliary areas implemented with sensor and artificial intelligence capable of responding to the physical and psychological needs and desires of the residents

Chapter 8
Integrating Telehealth into the Organization's Work System

Joachim Jean-Jules
Université de Sherbrooke, Canada

Alain O. Villeneuve
Université de Sherbrooke, Canada

ABSTRACT

With increased use of telehealth to provide healthcare services, bringing telehealth technology out of experimental settings into real life settings, it is imperative to gain a deeper understanding of mechanisms underlying the assimilation of teleheath systems. Yet, there is little understanding of how information systems are assimilated by organizations, more work is then warranted to understand how telehealth can be integrated into administrative and clinical practices and to identify factors that may impinge onto telehealth integration. Borrowing from institutional, structural and organizational learning theories, the authors develop a multilevel model for understanding assimilation of telehealth systems. Their study addresses limitations of past work and will be helpful for guiding research and managerial actions while integrating telehealth in the workplace.

INTRODUCTION

Telehealth has emerged as a key strategy for providing healthcare services to underserved or difficult-to-serve populations and low-cost specialty services to areas where full-time staffing would be uneconomical. It is expected to provide many other benefits such as shortening the time-frame for decision-making related to diagnosis and treatment, cutting emergency transfer costs, reducing expenses for patient travel from remote regions to healthcare service points, reducing delays in providing healthcare, promoting continuous healthcare, and attracting and retaining clinicians in remote regions.

However, the experience with telehealth has not always been positive, for many reasons: lack of acceptance by physicians, poor-quality technology

DOI: 10.4018/978-1-60960-469-1.ch008

(e.g., low resolution video data), and premature funding termination (Bashur, Sanders and Shannon, 1997). Although some of these limitations have been resolved recently, additional problems have emerged such as legal issues pertaining to professional liability and cross-province licensing; safety guidelines and standards regarding interconnectivity and interoperability; and the privacy, security and confidentiality of individually identifiable health information (DHSS, 2001).

Despite these barriers, governments keep funding telehealth projects and programs. Motivated by the collective performance of such programs in terms of clinical value and technical feasibility, governments are trying to integrate telehealth into the mainstream clinical care system. This concern, which seems a priori to be related to management, is also technological in nature, given the central role of information technologies in telehealth projects. Incorporating telehealth into the health-care system means inserting telehealth systems into clinical and administrative routines and integrating them into the technological and information architecture.

As a result, integration calls for adjustments not only to healthcare organizations' administrative and clinical routines (Saga and Zmud, 1994) but also to their work systems and technological configurations (Chatterjee and Segars, 2001; Keen and McDonald, 2000; Cooper and Zmud, 1990; Kwon, 1987). Indeed, to be truly valuable, telehealth systems not only need be accepted but also must be smoothly assimilated (routinized and infused) into existing routines, as well as into clinical and administrative functions (Zmud and Apple, 1992; The Lewin Group, 2000). Many experts recognize that the most effective telehealth programs are those that are most seamlessly integrated into current clinical and business practice and that can operate on their own in the absence of outside funding (Akerman, 2000). Their success should be measured by the extent to which they

are no longer stand-alone applications (Grigsby, Schlenker, Kaehny, Shaughnessy and Sandberg, 1995).

Thus, the assimilation of telehealth systems may not be as smooth as we would wish, as The Lewin Group Report states: "Unlike most new technologies that diffuse smoothly into health care delivery, implementing telemedicine systems and teleconsultation in particular, often presents departures from standard means of health care delivery, administration and financing" (2000, p.21). Therefore, understanding the mechanisms whereby telehealth systems are assimilated and the factors that influence this process is a matter of vital importance in both theory and practice. Little is known, however, about the process of telehealth systems assimilation and the enabling and impeding factors since most studies to date have focused on user acceptance and adoption; little has been said on what happens after the initial adoption decision has been taken.

In addition to being understudied in the literature on information systems, this phenomenon suffers from a lack of theorization. Consequently, the aim of this chapter is twofold. First, it is intended to enrich our understanding of the process of technology assimilation by making both its dimensions and the underlying mechanisms more explicit. As well, it uses this understanding as a basis for identifying factors that could potentially influence assimilation. Thus, this chapter attempts to add to our knowledge of assimilation of large-scale information systems in healthcare settings. Telehealth constitutes a new field for experimentation involving information technologies. It also provides a new context of study, given the specificities of the healthcare milieu in terms of organization, culture and professional practices. Due to their highly complex nature, healthcare organizations allow us to extend, propose and test theories that go beyond our current understanding of information technology assimilation. Borrowing from institutional, structuration and social cognition theories, this work proposes a multilevel model of the determinants relevant for the assimilation of telehealth systems in healthcare organizations.

The chapter begins with a consideration of the nature of telehealth systems and the issues related to their deployment. It then establishes a reference framework and principles guiding the modeling of the phenomenon and undertakes the multilevel development of the conceptual model as such. The chapter concludes by considering the theoretical and practical contributions of the study and specifies future orientations.

THEORIZING STRATEGY

As indicated above, this study proposes to develop a model of the assimilation of telehealth systems. Such an undertaking can only have value if the model is anchored in theory and if the theories applied make it possible to take account of the issues associated with the assimilation of these systems and analyze them appropriately. This entails at least two things. First of all, particular attention should be paid to the conceptualization of telehealth systems in order to clarify their characteristics. As well, it is necessary to take into consideration, on one hand, these systems' cultural and computational aspects and, on the other, the effect of the social, historical and institutional contexts, and the way in which the systems are understood and used (Orlikowski and Iacono, 2001). By articulating the nature and role of these systems within their organizational and institutional contexts (Latour, 1987), we were able to identify the issues related to their assimilation and the theories likely to inform these issues, and thus ultimately to formulate, in a robust and logical way, a network of factors likely to influence assimilation.

UNDERSTANDING TELEHEALTH SYSTEMS

Traditional Conceptualization of Telehealth Systems

Given the centrality of information technology in telehealth, many studies in the field of information systems (IS) have investigated telehealth systems. A close examination of these studies revealed three salient streams, namely (1) user acceptance/ adoption of telehealth systems (Mitchell, Mitchell and Disney, 1996; Hu and Chau, 1999; Cohn and Goodenough, 2002); (2) the characteristics of these systems (McKee, Evans and Owens, 1996); and (3) the effectiveness of telehealth systems compared to conventional face-to-face delivery in different medical specialties (Picolo, Smolle, Argenziano, Wolf, Braun et al. 2000; Nordal, Moseng, Kvammen and Lochen, 2001; Bishop, O'Reilly, Daddox and Hutchinson, 2002).

In the IS literature on telehealth, the Technology Acceptance Model (TAM) is the most widely used model. The TAM is intended to be a theoretical model of the determinants of information technology acceptance that can explain the behavior of a fairly wide range of applications and user populations. It is based on the Theory of Reasoned Action (TRA) of which it is in fact a specialized version in that TAM ignores the subjective norm. Based on this model, the effective use of a system is determined by the intent to use, which in turn depends on attitude. Attitude is influenced by two intermediate variables: perceived usefulness, which denotes the degree to which individuals believe that using a given system could enhance their job performance at work; and ease of use, which denotes individuals' beliefs regarding the effort required to use a given system. Venkatesh and Davis (2000) extended this model to include new constructs related to social influence. Their extension arises out of the recognition that the original version of the TAM might be inappropriate to account for the acceptance of systems according to whether their use is voluntary or obligatory. This extension links up with the position of Thompson (1998), who found that the addition of appropriate measures related to social factors and motivation could enhance the TAM's predictive power. Echoing this point of view, Hu, Chau and Sheng (2000) studied the adoption of telehealth. They claimed that, to improve the TAM's explanatory power, they needed to add the following two constructs: the presence of a champion and technological support. Along the same lines, Croteau and Vieru (2002) combined the constructs of the TAM with those of technology diffusion theory to develop a model that they used to study factors that might influence the intentions of two groups of physicians to adopt telehealth technology. Similarly, Succi and Walter (1999) extended the TAM by incorporating a new construct related to professional status in order to study physicians' acceptance of telehealth.

The models and theories of IS performance presented above have contributed considerably to enriching our understanding of the dynamics related to the adoption, use, impact and, finally, success of information systems and technologies in organizations. Nevertheless, according to certain researchers, they are quite restrictive in view of certain hypotheses that they make and could be inappropriate for analyzing some classes of IS, the development of which requires complex technical and social choices (Iacono and Kling, 1988). In fact, the models and theories of IS success that we described in the previous sections are, in Kling and Scacchi's (1982) terms, discrete-entity models in the sense that they view and analyze IS as discrete entities; the social context in which the technology is developed and used and the history of the participating organizations are ignored. In discrete-entity models, the main impacts of a new technology are interpreted as a transposition of its technical attributes (quality of the system, quality of information, etc.) and its social attributes (better decisions). Thus, the system is examined in isolation from the operating

activities and work organization that it is intended to automate or enable (Kling and Scacchi, 1982), leading to the idea that these models are universally applicable. The popularity of these models is partly due to their simplicity, which makes it easy to grasp their reasoning. An analysis conducted with these models needs to focus on only the technical and economic characteristics of the new technology (Kling and Scacchi, 1982). The technical development of systems according to these models is based on two logics: substitution and incrementation (Kling and Scacchi, 1982). In the first case, to improve a system's processing capacity, it is sufficient to substitute another that has greater capacity; in the second case, an existing system may be expanded. From the perspective of these models, the causes of system failure are also easily identifiable discrete entities, such as lack of support from senior management, lack of interest by users, insufficient system capacity, etc.

Discrete-entity models define an ideal. As such, they bring together several conceptions of information systems and technologies, namely the vision of technology as a tool, the vision of technology as a proxy and finally the information-centered vision of technology (Orlikowski and Iacono, 2001).

The tool point of view is the most widespread conception of what technology is and means (Orlikowski and Iacono, 2001). According to this concept, an IS constitutes an artifact that is supposed to achieve the aim for which it was designed. Thus, the IS nature and functioning are perceived as technical phenomena; that is, they are defined, separable from other phenomena, fixed and subject to human control. As a tool, an IS may constitute a substitute for human work, a lever to increase productivity, a means of processing data and information, or finally, an element of social relations in the sense that we recognize that the introduction of new IS is likely to modify work processes, which can lead to a change in communication methods and means. Thinking of IS as tools has several implications. First of all, they constitute a resource whose use is independent of practices, the organization of work and the context in which the system is developed and used (Kling and Scacchi, 1982), since a well-designed tool should clearly indicate what it is intended to be used for. As well, the metaphor of the tool suggests that users have control and that they must be very careful to choose the most appropriate tools for the task or activity to be performed (Nardi and O'Day, 1999). In other words, there is presumably an explicit process of alignment between the task and the tool, and consequently the impact of an IS on individual performance due to the match between the task and the selected tool (task-technology fit) is the result of a decision process.

The proxy point of view assumes that the critical aspects of IS can be captured by indirect reflexive measures, which are often quantitative in nature, such as individual perceptions, the diffusion rate, incurred expenses, etc. (Orlikowski and Iacono, 2001). This conception incorporates the perception-centered perspective, with theories and models such as the TRA, the TAM, the theory of interpersonal behavior, etc. It includes the view of innovation centered on diffusion and the view that IS are an element of an organization's capital.

The information-centered view of technology is quite similar to the tool view. IS are viewed as technical artifacts, completely ignoring their social and organizational aspects. In this conception, capacities for information representation, storage, extraction and transmission are the only IS characteristics worthy of interest (Orlikowski and Iacono, 2001).

Discrete-entity models have the advantage of simplicity of analysis; they are able to explain the development and use of IS with which only a few actors within an organization interact. However, they have not succeeded in explaining the problems that organizations face with the design and implementation of IS and are of little use in explaining IS impact on individuals and organizations.

The Very Nature of Telehealth Systems

Telehealth systems are IS that use a bundle of technologies designed to remotely deliver healthcare services (disease management, home healthcare, long-term care, emergency medicine) and other health-related social services like tele-education. They are therefore extended systems that connect two or more organizations and several categories of actors from each one. Consideration of the social context is essential to ensure the successful deployment of such systems. An understanding of social relations, the division of labor, cultural factors and the history of technologies in these organizations also appears to be essential. In the case of information systems like those used in telehealth, there are numerous decisions and the technologies are too vast and complex to be grasped by any one person's cognitive capacity. As well, the decisions to acquire and deploy such systems are not generally at the discretion of a single member of the organization (Eveland and Tornatzky, 1990, p. 124). When the deployment of an information system requires complex organizational arrangements instead of individual decisions, as is the case with telehealth, the deployment is often the result of numerous decisions dictated by economic and social considerations that extend beyond simple managerial logic.

In addition to the organizational context, actors and history of the organization, an analysis of information systems and technologies should take account of the nature of the technologies underlying these systems. Telehealth systems are made up of a variety of technologies depending on the specialty in question, and whether the project focuses on telemonitoring, telemedicine or tele-education. There are therefore multiple telehealth applications deployed on the basis of varied technologies such as videoconferencing, medical imaging equipment such as Picture Archiving and Communications Systems (PACS), content entry devices, storage and extraction equipment (sounds, images, plans and alphanumeric data), etc. The distinctive characteristics of these diverse applications mean that they all require the implementation of infrastructure such as Quebec's health communication network (the RTSS), which permits data transmission, clinical data entry, the creation of multimedia databases, and communication among the various partner organizations. As such, telehealth systems include at least two of the three classes of information technology that can be found in healthcare organizations (Grémy and Bonnin, 1995).

In Class 1 technologies, the computer performs numerical or logical calculations without interacting with the user and without causing the user to lose any autonomy (Grémy and Bonnin, 1995). The partnership between human and machine can be subdivided into three successive steps: the user defines how the machine must function, the machine processes the instructions and provides the user with the results and new data, on the basis of which the user makes decisions (Grémy and Bonnin, 1995).

Class 2 technologies are designed to support clinical activities, reasoning and evaluation, and medical education. This class of technologies presupposes a high level of interaction with professionals since it represents an intrusion in their area of activity. Consequently, individuals may experience a certain loss of autonomy in terms of their control over time and in terms of the representation of the world that the system imposes on them. Reactions can range from fascination for some users to frustration for others (Grémy and Bonnin, 1995).

Class 3 technologies operate at a more collective level. They are linked to systems used in large institutions such as hospitals, where the challenge is to manage large volumes of information coming from varied sources and destined for different entities, departments or people. These systems have no separate existence; they are an integral part of the bureaucratic organization (Grémy and Bonnin, 1995).

Telehealth systems can combine technologies from all three classes, as needed. They are therefore composed of an assembly of heterogeneous equipment made up of intrinsically complex and independent components (Paré and Sicotte, 2004). For this reason, it appears more appropriate to use web models to attempt to grasp these IS and capture the complex social consequences associated with their deployment. Unlike discrete-entity models, web models allow one to make explicit the connections between a technological system and its political and social contexts (Kling and Scacchi, 1982). The web concept makes it clear that, even though the artifact is a central element of a technological system, it is just one element of an ensemble that also includes the components needed to apply the technical artifact to a given socioeconomic activity (Kling and Dutton, 1982; Illich, 1973). These components include commitment, additional resources such as training, qualified personnel, organizational arrangements, the compensation policy and system, in short everything that is necessary to foster the effective management and use of the system (Kling and Scacchi, 1982). One can then conceptualize IS as evolving systems embedded in a dynamic and complex social context (Orlikowski and Iacono, 2001) and thus examine how different social influences contribute to modeling the deployment of an IS and how different groups of users take ownership of it. Approaching telehealth IS with a web model also allows one to conceptualize them as structures in the sense that IS incorporate a set of rules and resources (Giddens, 2005/1987). These rules and resources are introduced by the designer during the design phase and are appropriated by users during their interactions with the system.

TELEHEALTH SYSTEM DEPLOYMENT: RELATED CONCERNS

Traditionally, computerization projects in the healthcare environment are analyzed at the organizational level, and concerns generally relate to the individual preferences of the professionals who influence the phenomenon in question. Nevertheless, given the organizational arrangements that the implementation of telehealth projects requires, the analysis of telehealth IS deployment needs to focus on several levels of analysis, including the healthcare system, for two reasons. First of all, the integration of telehealth into the healthcare system has the mission of mitigating the inadequacies of the conventional healthcare system, which it expands and complements. This conceptualization of the usefulness and potential of IS did not come out of nowhere and is not maintained by its own internal logic; rather, it is developed and supported by certain allegiances emerging from the social and economic maneuvers of society that it appeals to (Klecun-Dabrowska and Cornford, 2002). Secondly, the implementation of telehealth projects, and consequently of the IS that support them, requires complex institutional arrangements that involve different organizations and different units within a single organization. This complexity is increased by the fact that each of these organizations possesses specific clinical and organizational routines (Paré and Sicotte, 2004). For example, the telemedicine component of the National Infrastructure Initiative in Taipei brings together hospital centers that provide third-line care as well as university hospitals and regional hospitals providing second- and third-line care. Thus, in addition to extending the provision of care beyond geographical and temporal barriers, this program vertically integrates first-, second- and third-line care (Hu, Wei and Cheng, 2002). For all these reasons, the conventional analysis of individual factors must be taken to a higher level so that institutional influences can also be considered.

Telehealth projects in fact constitute a new way of providing healthcare services. Because of the institutional arrangements that these projects involve, these IS are likely to substantially change habits, rules and practices in the participating organizations, and thus in turn to influence the institutional environment into which they are inserted. For example, when interacting with a patient in a virtual context, a physician must learn new ways of feeling and seeing, which represents a real challenge from the point of view of learning (Hu et al., 2002).

Conditions that may potentially favor or disfavor the deployment of telehealth systems are some of the issues raised by the encounter of the healthcare system as an institution and telehealth projects as the expression of a new process of institutionalization. It is important to recognize that the healthcare system has sufficient weight to foster or constrain the implementation of telehealth projects and that the importance attributed to telehealth projects results from negotiations of meaning among social groups with divergent material interests. Moreover, telehealth systems are not neutral. They are able to influence the institutional environment as much as they are influenced by it. It should also be remembered that institutional weight does not nullify the role of the preferences and the power of social groups and individuals in isolation.

MODEL DEVELOPMENT

Theoretical Logic and Principles

The development of the model in figure 1 is based on three premises. The first considers that an organization is a social entity characterized by systems of activities and a permeable border (Daft, 1995) that includes individuals who interact within collectives such as dyads, groups, teams, etc. (Klein,

Dansereau and Hall, 1994). As a result, the organization is essentially multilevel in nature, and so are organizational phenomena (Rousseau, 1985). In fact, these phenomena possess the properties of dynamic systems, namely critical antecedents and processes and results that affect several levels of analysis within the organization (Chan, 1998). Although it is more complex and more difficult to apply, the decision to adopt a multilevel perspective has some specific advantages (Barley, 1990). The second premise relates to the phenomenon of assimilation. Routinization and infusion are two concepts borrowed from Cooper and Zmud's (1990) view of the IS implementation process, which comprises initiation, adoption, adaptation, acceptance, routinization and infusion. This model is inspired by Lewin's (1947) planned change model. Adaptation corresponds to the unfreezing phase, while acceptance, routinization and infusion correspond to the refreezing phase (Saga and Zmud, 1994). However, it is important to point out that researchers in this field soon moved away from the planned change model and began to view the IS implementation process as a dynamic process of mutual adaptation between the organization and the system (Leonard-Barton, 1988). Moving still further in this direction, Orlikowski (1993) and Orlikowski and Gash (1994) proposed the situated change model wherein change is significant but flexible and subtle. This transformation is primarily anchored in organizational routines, and secondarily in actors' practices. More specifically, it applies when the users of a technology must handle the exceptions, opportunities, contingencies and unexpected consequences related to their tasks (Barley, 1990). To sum up, researchers in this area recognize that technological innovations trigger changes in organizational routines (Barley, 1986; Tyre and Orlikowski, 1994), which have been found to be strongly associated with cognitive and personal changes (Barley, 1986; Orlikowski, 1993). Based on these insights, we consider that the assimilation of IS innovations is essentially a multilevel phenomenon that originates in individual and collective cognition (social cognition), before manifesting itself at the organizational level. The third premise considers that an organization is an open system. As such, the members of the organization also belong to other social systems. Ultimately, the conceptual model will be a multilevel model in the sense that it articulates the phenomenon we are interested in – assimilation – at several levels of analysis at the same time as it describes the relationships among dependent and independent variables located at different levels of analysis. Such an undertaking requires some guidelines.

To guide the multilevel modeling, we were mainly inspired by the work of Rousseau (1985), Klein et al. (1994), Chan (1998), Morgesson and Hofmann (1999) and Kozlowski and Klein (2000). Three major concerns became evident. The first was the necessity of properly laying the theoretical foundations for the model; the second concerns the necessity of adequately clarifying the levels of analysis to avoid flaws in reasoning; and the third refers to the necessity of specifying the sources of variability. These concerns are expressed in the following guidelines.

A theorization exercise must start by designating and defining the phenomenon of interest and the theoretical constructs used to conceptualize it, because they determine the levels and the connection processes that the theory or model must address (Kozlowski and Klein, 2000).

It is also indispensable to specify the hierarchical levels of interest that are relevant in the development of the theory or model. According to Kozlowski and Klein (2000), the process of specification must be sure to distinguish between formal and informal units. The importance of this distinction resides in the fact that problems can arise if one analyzes a phenomenon within certain formal units, when it is underpinned by informal organizational processes. Consequently, the levels and units of analysis must be coherent with the phenomenon of interest (Kozlowski and Klein, 2000). Rousseau (1985) recommends dis-

Figure 1.

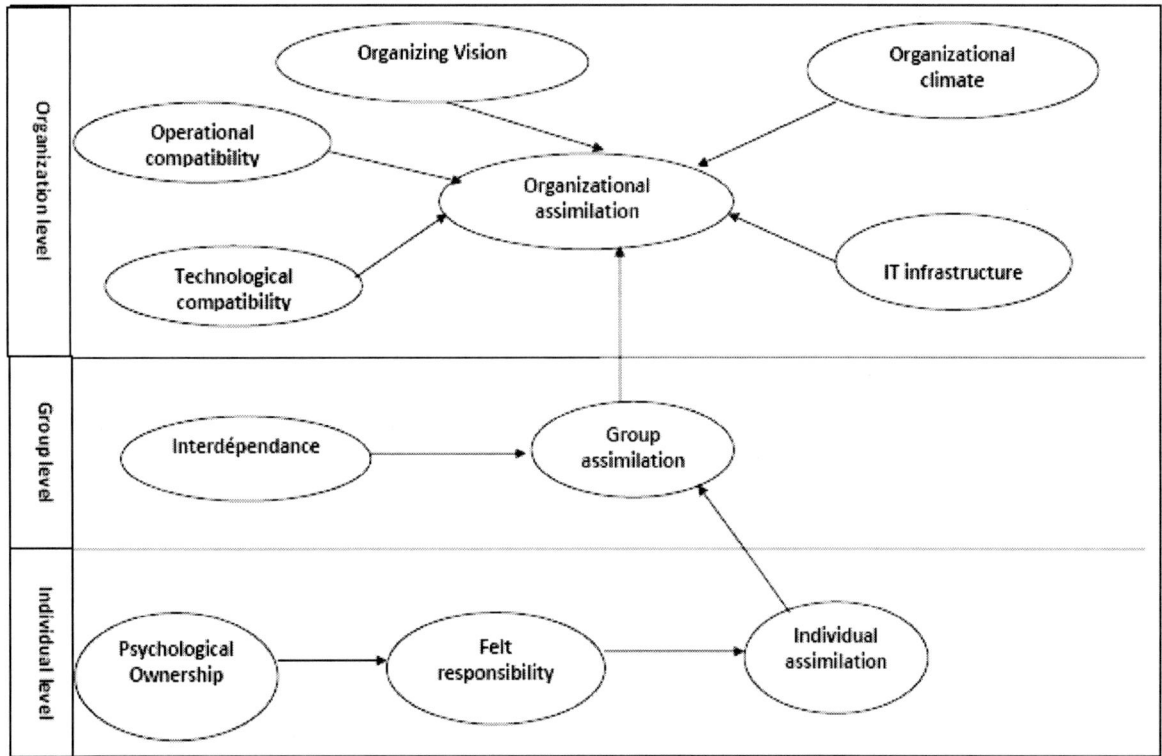

tinguishing between the reference, measurement and analysis levels. The reference level constitutes the focal level in the sense that it is at this level that generalizations are made. The measurement level corresponds to the unit directly associated with the data. The analysis level refers to the level at which statistical analyses are carried out. Serious validity problems can arise if the different levels are not appropriately identified and are involuntarily mixed up during the formulation of hypotheses, collection and analysis of data, and generalization of results (Rousseau, 1985). Rousseau recommends (1) explicitly defining the appropriate levels at which one can generalize; (2) specifying the functional relationships of constructs at the different levels; (3) considering the potential distortions associated with measuring the constructs at one level and then analyzing them at another; (4) defining the analysis levels coherently with the focal or reference level; and

(5) paying particular attention to the determination of the appropriate level for the dependent variable.

Given that multilevel models essentially aim to describe the phenomena that take place at one level and are generalizable to several levels, it is imperative to specify the formation of collective constructs by clarifying their structures and functions (Morgesson and Hofmann, 1999); this amounts to clarifying how the phenomena are interrelated at different levels (Kozlowski and Klein, 2000). Collective constructs refer to the abstractions used to conceptualize collective phenomena resulting from the collective action of individuals, groups, departments, organizations, institutions, etc. (Morgesson and Hofmann, 1999). Within these collectives, individuals and subgroups meet and interact within space-time. This interaction constitutes an event that is followed by other events, triggering a joint behavioral cycle or pattern defined as collective action. This structure allows collective phenomena to emerge from interactions at the micro level; these phenomena in turn have the capacity to influence subsequent interactions. In this sense, collective constructs are essentially dual. They result from the interactions among their components and become the context in which later interactions take place. Consequently, Morgesson and Hofmann (1999) recommend (1) clearly identifying these cycles of events that structure the collective phenomenon; (2) specifying the processes involved in the emergence of collective constructs while being sure to note which ones are associated with critical events; and (3) considering the context in which these collective constructs emerge, while paying particular attention to the influence it could have on their emergence and structure.

Collective processes can develop via contextual top-down processes or emergent bottom-up processes Kozlowski and Klein (2000). Top-down processes refer to the influence factors at one level have on lower levels. Conversely, bottom-up processes concern entities located at one level that emerges at higher levels. In the case of emergence, it is necessary to clarify whether composition or compilation is involved. Composition presupposes isomorphism and describes phenomena that are similar when they emerge at different levels (Kozlowski and Klein, 2000). These phenomena or constructs share the same content but are qualitatively different from one level to another (Chan, 1998). There are five types of composition model: additive, direct consensus, referent-shift consensus, dispersion and process (Chan, 1998, p. 235). Consequently, relations among the variables are supposed to be functionally similar at the different levels (Rousseau, 1985). Compilation describes phenomena that concern a common domain but are different when they emerge at different levels. In this case, by adopting a certain configuration, lower-level characteristics combine to form a higher-level property that is functionally equivalent to its constituent elements. In other words, the constructs occupy the same function at different

levels but are not structurally identical (Morgesson and Hofmann, 1999; Kozlowski and Klein, 2000). It also means that is mandatory for the theoretician or modeler to specify the construct's original and current levels (Kozlowski and Klein, 2000), because the construct level determines the measurement and analysis procedures to be used. Once the emergence process has been described and the nature or structure of the phenomena at different levels have been identified, Kozlowski and Klein (2000) recommend clarifying how the constructs and the phenomenon of interest are related at these different levels. The functional analysis of collective constructs may constitute an excellent means of linking constructs at different levels (Morgesson and Hofmann, 1999). Although the constructs' structures tend to differ from one level to the next, their functions usually do not. Functional analysis therefore appears to be a mechanism for integrating the constructs into a nomological network. Indeed, a type of process whereby a lower-level construct emerges to form a higher-level construct corresponds to each kind of functional relations among constructs (Chan, 1998). Finally, the sources of variability must be specified (Klein et al., 1994).

By applying these principles to the case that concerns us, we were able to develop the conceptual model in Figure 1, which shows the different forms of assimilation at the individual, group and organizational levels and the factors related to these three levels that may influence the process. In the following sections, we describe the construction of the model and discuss its various elements.

Assimilation

The concept of assimilation is defined in different ways in the literature, as Table 1 shows.

Inspired by these definitions, and especially the last one, we define organizational assimilation as a phenomenon that occurs after a technological innovation is implemented; it has two dimensions: routinization (or institutionalization) and infusion.

Table 1. Definitions of assimilation

Meyer and Goes, (1988)	An organizational process that (1) is set in motion when individual organization members first hear of an innovation's development, (2) can lead to the acquisition of the innovation and (3) sometimes to fruition in the innovation's full acceptance, utilization, and institutionalization (p.897).
Fichman and Kemerer, (1997)	Assimilation is defined as the process spanning from an organization's first awareness of an innovation to, potentially, acquisition and widespread deployment (p.1346)… and is best conceptualized as process of organizational learning wherein individuals and the organization as a whole acquire the knowledge and the skills necessary to effectively apply the technology (Attewell, 1992) (p.1345).
Purvis, Sambamurthy and Zmud, (2001) Chatterjee, Grewal and Sambamurthy, (2002)	Assimilation is defined as the extent to which the use of a technology diffuses accross organization work processes and becomes routinized in the activities associated with those processes (Cooper et Zmud, 1990; Tornatzky et Klein, 1982).

Routinization expresses the idea that an information system is inserted into the organization's practices in such a way that, over time, it ceases to be perceived as a novelty and starts to be taken for granted (Saga and Zmud, 1994; Ritti and Silver, 1986; Zucker, 1977). The term infusion is used when the system becomes so deeply embedded in the organizational routines that it configures the workplace architecture by contributing to linking different organizational elements such as roles, formal procedures and emergent routines (Cooper and Zmud, 1990; Kwon, 1987). Thus, routinization and infusion refer to the two organizational manifestations of assimilation. The focal or reference level of our study – that is, the level at which generalizations will be made – is the organization. The study, then, is limited to the organizational field. Since we are studying a multilevel phenomenon, its manifestations at the individual and group levels are also presented. By doing this, we plan to show the structure and function of the collective constructs of assimilation at each level, and reveal the processes of composition or compilation whereby the lower-level constructs contribute to organizational assimilation, defined in terms of routinization and infusion.

Individual assimilation or interpretation. At the individual level, we conceive of assimilation as resulting from an individual's engagement in a process of making sense when he or she is faced with the potential use of a technological innovation. In the course of this interpretative effort, individuals are engaged at three levels – emotional, behavioral and cognitive (Drazin, Glynn and Kazanjian, 1999; Kahn, 1990) – since interpretation requires individuals to explain by words or actions their understanding, no matter how embryonic, of the object, both to themselves and to other people (Crossan, Lane and White, 1999).

In the case that concerns us, the need for interpretation – for making sense of telehealth systems – is the result of two conjoined events, namely the nature of these systems and the fact that telehealth constitutes a new way of providing health services.

Telehealth systems are complex information systems, not only because of the institutional arrangements necessitated by their deployment but also because of their constituent technologies. For example, the wound care tele-assistance project set up by the Réseau universitaire intégré de santé (RUIS) de Sherbrooke (Sherbrooke integrated university health network) is deploying 73 tele-assistance technologies in 65 points of service. The deployment is expected to take place in eight phases, each of which has a planned preparation activity that includes at least the organization of new clinical services, the development of a deployment strategy for these new virtual clinics, etc. (RUIS de Sherbrooke, 2007). In fact, telehealth systems combine diverse technologies such as medical imaging, videoconferencing systems, etc., whose deployment requires frequent interventions to improve and adapt them, which means that the development and implementation of these systems becomes an ongoing process (Weick, 1990).

Because of the combination of technologies, the presence of such systems in the healthcare environment can cause unaccustomed problems of interpretation and sense-making for both managers and healthcare professionals (Weick, 1990). Since these technological innovations are exogenous to the organizational context, their introduction is likely to create a certain mismatch between the existing systems of meaning, legitimation and domination and the new requirements for day-to-day activities in the organizational context (Barley, 1986). These new technologies therefore affect the ability of members of the organizational context to reason about the structures making up telehealth systems; because technologies in general and new information technologies in particular lend themselves to interpretive flexibility (Weick, 1990) in the sense that they allow different possible and plausible interpretations by various social groups and may therefore be misunderstood, uncertain and complex (Pinch and Bijker, 1987; Weick, 1990; Orlikowski and Gash, 1994).

New technologies mean many things because they are simultaneously the source of stochastic events, continuous events, and abstract events. Complex systems composed of these three classes of events make both limited sense because so little is visible and so much is transient, and they make many different kinds of sense because the dense interactions that occur within them can be modeled in so many different ways. Because new technologies are equivocal, they require ongoing structuring and sensemaking if they are to be managed. (Weick, 1990, p. 2)

In addition, the meaning attributed to the technology may depend on a given actor's ability to access the system's schemas and artifacts, that is, the ability to reinterpret the schemas of the set of artifacts other than by means of the schemas already incorporated into these artifacts (Chae, 2002).

This interpretive flexibility is based on the fact that any information system comprises both information technology artifacts and schemas (Orlikowski and Iacono, 2001; Chae, 2002). Artifacts include tangible resources such as equipment and applications (Kling, 1987), intangible resources such as networking capacities and programming languages (Chae, 2002) and structural elements incorporated in the technologies (De Sanctis and Poole, 1994). Schemas refer to generalizable procedures that emerge from the context or from pre-existing institutions (Chae, 2002). In the context of implementation and use, they can refer to the installed base of the social organization of computerization (Kling and Iacono, 1989). Unlike resources, which are objective, schemas are essentially virtual:

Schemas can be inferred from an array of extant institutional arrangements and cognitive imageries which include an organization's (or group's, intra-organization's) structure and history; value systems, norms, organizational routines and informal procedures, individual and collective memory culture, and existing bodies or rules, laws and regulations. They are the source for enactment (Weick, 1990) of technology (Chae, 2002, p. 52).

The ambiguity introduced by telehealth systems is even stronger because in some cases the systems involved are extremely large: not only are numerous resources deployed on a large scale but many different entities are involved. For example, the wound care tele-assistance project includes 13 health and social services centers in three geographic regions of Quebec and anticipates mobilizing 90 resource nurses. Consequently, there are numerous and complex schemas, which, moreover, are embedded in multiple structures.

All of the above arguments highlight both the ambiguous nature of telehealth systems for actors and the need for these actors to make sense of the technologies underlying these systems so that they can use them and integrate them into their practices. Interpretation, the process of making sense, is essential to assimilation, since the way in which individuals interact with a technology depends on their interpretation of it (Orlikowski and Gash, 1994).

Based on their interpretations, actors develop a certain number of hypotheses and expectations that form their understanding of what the technology is and what it can be used for (Orlikowski and Gash, 1994). Thus, the process of interpretation or sense-making is ultimately applied to grasp the reasoning, the philosophy underlying the development of the system, or in other words, its spirit (De Sanctis and Poole, 1994). During the course of interpretation, individuals develop a kind of cognitive map (Porac, Thomas and Baden-Fuller, 1989), schema or frame in which language plays a central role by allowing the individual to start naming and explaining what had formerly been a matter of sensation or feeling (Crossan et al., 1999). This new meaning of technology concerns not only the nature of the information technology but also its applications and the consequences associated with their use in a given context (Orlikowski et Gash, 1994). It conditions the actors' actions: "… in this sense-making process, they develop particular assumptions, expectations, and knowledge of the technology, which serve to shape subsequent actions toward it" (Orlikowski and Gash, 1994, p. 175). Thus, sense-making is the principal generator of individual action with regard to innovation (Drazin et al., 1999).

Group assimilation. At the group level, we think of assimilation as an integration process during the course of which shared understandings are formed and mutual adjustments are made between individual interpretations. Social interaction in the form of dialogue and joint actions is indispensable to this integration (Morges-

son and Hofmann, 1999; Crossan et al., 1999; Lauriol, 1998), which continues the process of interpretation by giving it the status of a social activity that contributes to clarifying images and eventually creating shared understandings and meanings. By allowing the group to arrive at a common discourse and decide on a principle for action (Lauriol, 1998), integration helps to reduce the ambiguity surrounding innovation (Daft and Weick, 1987). Our conceptualization is similar to that of Hall and Loucks (1977) regarding individuals' levels of technology use over time. In the view of these authors, individuals first collect information about the technology so that they can make sense of it and prepare to use it. Later, they tend to move up to an increased level of use of the technology. To do this, they refine their understanding of both the technology and its various possible applications by interacting with it more, discussing their experiences with other people and, finally, coordinating their activities with those of other users. This last step is crucial in understanding technology assimilation since it constitutes the essence or engine of organization learning, of which routinization and infusion are the outcome. In fact, when users of a system must carry out interdependent activities using it, they need to confront their understandings of the system's nature and what it is meant to do. A shared understanding is indispensable to the coherence of collective action and may differ from one social group to another. The social cognition theory of knowledge creation teaches us that every social group, like every individual, is likely to develop common understandings – cultural and cognitive frames (Scott, 2001), also called technological frames (Orlikowski and Gash, 1994) – which are specific to itself. These frames develop due to the close relationships between group members resulting from the coordination of their activities (Schein, 1985; Strauss, 1978) and also due to the group's influence on its members through its specific system of meaning and norms (Porac et al., 1989; Gregory, 1983; Van Maanen and Schein,

1979). In short, the integration of individual interpretations into shared understandings of what telehealth systems are and what they should be used for establishes a consensus on the meaning of these systems within the reference group.

Organizational assimilation. At the organizational level, we claim that assimilation has two aspects: first a process of institutionalization or routinization, then a process of infusion. Routinization ensures that actions are specified, tasks are defined and the organizational mechanisms necessary for their achievement are set up (Crossan et al., 1999). Shared understandings lead to collective actions. Over time, the repetition and persistence of these collective actions define patterns of interaction and communication, which routinization tends to formalize. By coordinating their actions with those of others, users or groups of users construct new cognitive coordinations, memorize them and repeat them, transposing them to new situations until their use is perceived as normal, and using them more frequently, which means inserting them into the organization's routines. As well, coordination requires one to take into consideration the organizing principles for interaction, such as norms and rules, as well as the organizing principles for individuals, such as scripts and previous representations. Taking these principles into consideration contributes to institutionalizing (or routinizing) the use of the system, by reproducing or enacting structures, since these organizing principles may conflict with the group's sociocognitive orientations. When conflict occurs, it generates new cognitive configurations and thus is likely to lead to a renewed social representation of the system as a function of the social marking that characterizes it (Lauriol, 1998). Thus, as the organization advances in its understanding of the technology and its possibilities, it is likely to modify its work architecture, following a cumulative learning curve:

Each successive configuration builds on the functionality of the previous one, which parallels an incremental learning process as the technology's users gain experience and knowledge about the technology and technology-facilitated work tasks. (Saga and Zmud, 1994, p. 80)

According to these authors, this in-depth understanding and the change in work architecture that it induces cause users to (1) use more and more of the system's functionalities to execute a larger set of tasks; (2) use the system in a more integrated way to build links between sets of activities; (3) use the technology to perform activities that were not identifiable or feasible before the system was introduced. These three ways of using the system help to infuse it in the organization (Cooper and Zmud, 1987).

To sum up, we consider that assimilation occurs first by means of an individual interpretation process in which individuals succeed in making sense of the new technology, then developing new categories and new schemas and scripts that shape their representation of the system. Then, through a process of integration, the individuals interact and integrate their understandings in order to coordinate their activities. By doing this, they develop shared understandings or frames specific to their group. Over time, these frames are incorporated into routines, then infused into practices and beliefs until they endure within the organization even after the individuals who originated them have left.

The Emergence of Collective Assimilation Constructs

From the individual to the group: In the previous section, assimilation was viewed as a phenomenon that can be seen at different hierarchical levels of the organization: individual, group and organizational, with the individual as the level of origin. We can deduce at least two things from this: first, at these three levels, assimilation is defined as qualitatively distinct constructs; second, assimilation is manifested as an emergent phenomenon. In this regard, it is important to specify the nature of this emergence from the individual to the group and then on to the organization. Individuals interpret technological innovation within the framework of the organizational context. Individual cognitive frames, namely the expectations and hypotheses they develop regarding the technological innovation, are marked by social interactions with their colleagues who are also engaged in the interpretation effort. It is legitimate to consider that, through this interaction, individual scripts, schemas and semantic labels are pooled to develop shared understandings and a principle for action. In fact, when individuals face ambiguous situations, they start to seek the interpretations of other people who are experiencing the same thing (Swanson and Ramiller, 1997; Volkema, Farquhar and Bergmann, 1996). Through these interactions, schemas and individual categorizations are diffused throughout the reference group (Poole and DeSanctis., 1990). Interaction is undoubtedly the vehicle of this pooling, but common frames result primarily from the frequency of these interactions, which make up a cycle of events (Morgesson and Hoffman, 1999). A high level of interdependence among group members' activities increases the presence of such cycles and consequently the emergence of group assimilation. The collective construct may result from the composition or compilation of individual interpretations (Kozlowski and Klein, 2000). We opt for the first possibility, since assimilation at the individual and group levels involves cognitive processes that result in the generation of reference and categorization frames, etc. In other words, the constructs of individual and group assimilation are similar in function but different in structure. We also hypothesize that individuals act homogeneously within the group when they pool their individual reference frames (Klein et al., 1994), since it is difficult to distinguish between individual and group contributions in the creation of common frames (Drazin et al., 1999). Likewise, the group reflects the steps of individual assimilation in its approach,

namely the development of images, categories, a language, expectations and hypotheses, etc. In short, group assimilation and individual assimilation are functionally isomorphic, in that both constructs have the same meaning and share the same content and the same nomological network (Kozlowski and Klein, 2000). This leads to the following hypothesis:

Proposition 1: *Group assimilation results from intragroup consensus around individuals' assimilation.*

From the group to the organization: Routinization and infusion, the two manifestations of assimilation, are two essentially organizational phenomena and have no individual counterparts. Consequently, assimilation at the organizational level cannot occur on the basis of group assimilation. It is true that routinization results from the repetition of behavior patterns as a result of group consensus. Nevertheless, when one moves from the group level to that of the organization, the assimilation process becomes less fluid and incremental and more punctuated and disconnected (Crossan et al., 1999). Indeed, organizational assimilation usually entails modifications being made to existing systems and processes (Keen and McDonald, 2000; Chatterjee and Segars, 2001). Such modifications raise issues that extend beyond the field of social cognition. In particular, one might mention the inertia characterizing existing institutions, which results in the more punctuated nature of organizational assimilation mechanisms compared to the greater fluidity of the phenomenon at the individual and group levels (Crossan et al., 1999). Moreover, through routinization, the modified structures, systems and procedures provide a new context for interaction such that the representations of groups, and still more so of individuals, have less weight because they are embedded in the organization (Crossan et al., 1999).

Moreover, there are theoretical reasons for believing that the emergence of organizational assimilation, which involves hundreds of people, may be substantially different from assimilation at the group level, which may involve no more than five or six people. In a large organization, individuals only interact regularly with a subset of other employees, whereas they will end up interacting with most, if not all, of the other members in a group (Dawson, Gonzalez-Roma, Davis and West, 2008). Thus, organizational assimilation is probably a slower and more risky process and therefore is more sensitive to contextual factors. In fact, each social group within the organization (physicians, nurses, administrators, technicians) may well develop its own technological frames regarding telehealth systems for reasons as diverse as their specialty, occupation, ideology, etc. (Orlikowski and Gash, 1994; Weick, 1995). We can therefore imagine that, at the organizational level, assimilation results from a process of negotiation among the different frames specific to each group involved, with their divergent belief systems and interests (Drazin et al., 1999). In our view, there are two possibilities. First, the different groups' technological frames, that is to say, their expectations and hypotheses regarding the role of the technological innovation in business processes and its nature and use, may be irreconcilable. In that case, the implementation of the technological innovation will become a source of conflict (Orlikowski and Gash, 1994). On the other hand, when the different groups' frames are congruent (Orlikowski and Gash, 1994), an implicit and reasonable agreement may result concerning the nature, use and consequences of use of the technological innovation (Finney and Mitroff, 1986).

Cognitive frames of any kind guide how individuals or groups understand and act toward an organizational phenomenon. Frames give meaning to events, which then determine courses of action (Goffman, 1974). Thus, the frames specific to each group determine how that group inserts the use of the new technology into its practices. When the

different frames are mutually coherent, in the sense that they share a certain number of categories and contents (Orlikowski and Gash, 1994), one can imagine that these specific practices may combine to configure the insertion of the technological innovation into the organizational routines of which it will become an integral part. It is also possible to imagine that, as this use is institutionalized, it will become more widespread and more integrated and modifications may be made to the technological architecture to take into consideration the way in which various organizational elements such as roles, formal procedures and emergent routines will henceforth be connected (Cooper and Zmud, 1990; Kwon, 1987).

On the basis of the above discussion, we consider that organizational assimilation emerges from the compilation of the various frames specific to each social group. In other words, assimilation at the organizational level results not from the convergence of the technological frames of the various groups involved but instead from a combination of these frames in a particular configuration. Consequently, at the group and organization levels, the two constructs are qualitatively different even though they are functionally equivalent (Kozlowski and Klein, 2000). While group-level assimilation results in a consensus concerning the role and use of the technological innovation, organizational assimilation is reflected in the insertion of the innovation into organizational routines and subsequent changes to the administrative and technological infrastructure (Zmud and Apple, 1992). Thus, both constructs concern the same domain, but they are manifested in different ways at the two levels of analysis. This development leads us to formulate the following hypothesis:

Proposition 2: *Organizational assimilation results from a configuration of each group's specific assimilation.*

Antecedents of Assimilation

In the previous section, we established the relationship between the constructs of assimilation at different levels. In addition to the question of the structure of assimilation, which concerns the manifestations of the phenomenon at different levels, we also need to consider how the phenomenon functions and, in particular, to identify its antecedents at the different levels of analysis.

Individual Factors

Psychological Ownership for the Organization and Felt Responsibility

Psychological ownership defines a state in which individuals feel that an object belongs to them, in whole or in part (Beggan, 1992; Pierce, Rubenfeld and Morgan, 1991). This feeling may develop for either tangible or intangible objects (Isaacs, 1993; Pierce, Kostova and Dirks, 2001). Empirical studies have shown that individuals may experience feelings of possession toward their work (Beaglehole, 1932), their organization (Dirks, Cummings and Pierce, 1996), the practices of the organization (Kostova, 1998), and particular problems facing their organization (Pratt and Dutton, 2000). As well, psychological ownership of an organization denotes a psychological phenomenon whereby an employee develops feelings of ownership toward a target (Van Dyne and Pierce, 2004). This target may be any material or social object associated with the organization, such as particular problems or the technologies that contribute to solving them. Thus, psychological ownership is an attitude that includes both affective and cognitive components (Pierce et al., 2001). Three main mechanisms participate in the emergence of psychological ownership: control of the target or object for which ownership is felt; intimate knowledge of this target; and finally, self-investment in the target (Pierce et al., 2001).

Organizations give their members many opportunities to control, to varying degrees, differ-ent factors that then constitute potential targets of psychological ownership (Pierce et al., 2001; Hackman and Oldham, 1980). The greater the degree of autonomy inherent in a job, the greater the level of control required and, as well, the greater the probability that employees will develop a feeling of ownership toward certain targets of the organization (Pierce et al., 2001). In healthcare organizations in particular, professionals enjoy a very high degree of autonomy in their areas of expertise because of the complex tasks they have to perform. The low level of bureaucratic formalization and the decentralized decision-making power that characterize healthcare organizations are factors that favor high autonomy for healthcare professionals and, consequently, the likelihood that they will develop feelings of ownership for their work or for specific organizational problems related to it (Pierce et al., 2001).

Organizations also give their members opportunities to become more familiar with certain targets of psychological ownership. This intimate knowledge is fostered by the information given to employees concerning the organization's objectives and problems and, above all, by seniority in the organization. In turn, intimate knowledge favors the development of a feeling of ownership toward the organization or some of its targets (Pierce et al., 2001). The collegial nature of healthcare organizations means that professionals are constantly being informed and consulted about their institution's problems and objectives and often about those of other establishments in the same administrative region. In addition, these organizations are characterized by low employee turnover, given the structure of the sector. All of these factors contribute to the fact that healthcare professionals know their organizations very well and thus increase the probability that they will develop feelings of ownership toward some of its targets.

Finally, organizations give their members opportunities to invest themselves in different aspects of organizational life. This investment may relate to the individual's ideas, time, or physical and psychological energy (Pierce et al., 2001). The greater the investment, the greater the psychological ownership of the target (Pierce et al., 2001). The degree of investment depends on the characteristics of the activity. Non-routine activities, which require more discretion, mean that the people who perform them invest more of their ideas, their specific knowledge and their personal style (Pierce et al., 2001). These activities therefore favor the development of psychological ownership of the result of this self-investment. Now, one of the most important characteristics of healthcare institutions resides in the uniqueness and novelty of the problems they are called upon to solve. This is reflected in non-routine activities whose duration, content and characteristics are unpredictable. Indeed, executing these activities requires healthcare professionals to acquire information and knowledge through the social processes of discussion, reading and education, then to apply this knowledge to solving their patients' problems. It is therefore legitimate to think that such a working environment promotes the development of psychological ownership of targets such as certain organizational challenges, protocols or practices, etc.

When individuals who are members of an organization feel that they own it, they tend to believe they have certain rights such as being kept informed and influencing the organization's orientations, but they also tend to feel more accountable to it than individuals who do not share this feeling (Pierce et al., 1991; Kubzansky and Druskat, 1993; Rodgers and Freudlich, 1998). And it has been shown that the felt responsibility leads individuals to adopt behaviors that go beyond the requirements of their formal roles (Pearce and Gregersen, 1991).

The above discussion helps us to understand that healthcare organizations combine conditions that favor the development of psychological ownership of certain targets by their members. One of these targets could be telehealth, given

the fervor it has stirred up because of expectations that it will solve certain limitations hampering the current healthcare system. We also believe that the felt responsibility that results from psychological ownership is one of the factors that explains why individuals in these organizations engage themselves in three ways – emotionally, behaviorally and cognitively (Drazin et al., 1999; Kahn, 1990) – in the effort to understand what telehealth systems are and what they should be used for. We therefore hypothesize that there will be a positive relationship between psychological ownership and individual assimilation, but that this relationship will be mediated by the feeling of responsibility.

Proposition 3a: *Psychological ownership of the organization should have a positive impact on the individual assimilation of telehealth systems.*

Proposition 3b: *Felt responsibility will mediate the influence of psychological ownership of the organization on the individual assimilation of telehealth systems.*

Group Factors

Interdependence

One of the fundamental characteristics of organizations is the need for coordination. In addition to administrative prescriptions, coordination is the result of structural factors such as interdependence (Van De Ven, Delbecq and Koenig, 1976).

Interdependence expresses the extent to which the behavior of one member of a group affects that of the other members. In this research, the term group has a collective sense and designates any combination of individuals or work units that are interdependent and whose work is purposeful (Morgesson and Hoffman, 1999). The object in respect of which the group members perceive themselves to be interdependent determines the nature and degree of this interdependence. These objects may include the differentiation of roles, the distribution of competencies and resources, the operating processes and technologies supporting them, and how performance is compensated (Wageman, 1995, p. 146). Notwithstanding these different sources, a distinction must be established between task interdependence and goal interdependence (Mitchell and Silver, 1990).

Definitions of task interdependence (TI) are quite varied (Pearce et Gregersen, 1991). In some authors' view, TI designates to what extent the members of a group depend on one another to achieve their respective tasks due to the structural relations among group members (Van De Ven et al., 1976; Van der Vegt, Emans and van de Vliert, 1998; Thompson 1967). From this structural perspective, the patterns of interaction among group members vary depending on whether their interdependence is pooled, sequential or reciprocal (Thompson, 1967) or team interdependence (Van De Ven et al., 1976). Team interdependence is associated with the most complex form of interaction. Other researchers have defined TI as the degree of interaction among members due to the nature of the task (Shea and Guzzo, 1987; Campion, Medsker and Higgs, 1993). Ultimately, we consider that TI expresses the extent to which group members must exchange resources (information, advice and expertise) and coordinate their efforts to perform their tasks (Mitchell and Silver, 1990; Wageman, 1995).

Goal interdependence (GO) expresses the extent to which members perceive their respective goals as being related to those of the group and acknowledge one another as contributors to a common project (Deutsch, 1973, 1949).

The fact that healthcare organizations are considered to be professional bureaucracies (Mintzberg, 1981), in which professionals are given a great deal of autonomy, does not preclude the need for coordination, and therefore the interdependence. On the contrary, the structural changes that have occurred in these organizations in recent years tend to reinforce this need. In Quebec, for example, structural problems related to the accessibility, coordination and continuity of healthcare and services have led to the emergence of several solutions, including the integration of services through the creation of integrated health and social services networks. The goal, of course, is the complementary use of resources and expertise, with the aim of facilitating the ongoing provision of healthcare and services. Despite these changes, two modes of intervention appear to coexist in healthcare institutions: multidisciplinarity and interdisciplinarity, with the emphasis upon the former.

Multidisciplinarity refers to the juxtaposition of professionals who are working with the same user (D'Amour, Ferrada-Videla, San Martin Rodriguez and Beaulieu, 2005; Payette, 2001). Each aspect of the user's problem is handled by different professionals, who keep one another informed about the actions to be taken and the progression of results. In this way, they identify specific contributions, set rules for coordination and share information (Viens, 2006).

Interdisciplinarity, on the other hand, requires the integration of knowledge, expertise and specific contributions from each discipline in the process of solving complex problems (Payette, 2001). It presupposes a common goal and integrated practices. Thus, while multidisciplinarity is most appropriate for less complex needs (D'Amour, 2006), interdisciplinarity has proven to be more appropriate for complex cases (Payette, 2001). By necessitating convergent care, such cases create a situation of interdependence and partnership among stakeholders (Viens, 2006).

Despite their relative autonomy, then, stakeholders in healthcare organizations are not totally independent from one another. The nature of their interdependence varies based on the complexity of the care services they provide. In all cases, if this interdependence is to be operative, stakeholders must share common frames regarding the nature of the care, practices and technologies they need to mobilize. This is especially true in the case of telehealth, where information technologies play a pivotal role. On this basis, it is reasonable to make the following propositions:

Proposition 4a: *Task interdependence should have a positive impact on consensus building within different groups regarding what telehealth systems are and what they should be used for.*

Proposition 4b: *Goal interdependence should have a positive impact on consensus building within different groups regarding what telehealth systems are and what they should be used for.*

Organizational Factors

At the organizational level, in view of how assimilation is manifested, it may be influenced by specific organizational capacities and by the interaction between IS and the organization.

In the context of this study, the organizational capacities that appear most relevant to us are those associated with the technological and sociocognitive environments. The former refers primarily to the technological infrastructure's IT capacities and the latter to the organizational climate.

Regarding the interaction between the system and the organization, we essentially refer to compatibility between the technological innovation and the institutional system, on one hand, and the organization's existing technological systems, on the other.

IT Capacities

As indicated above, organizational assimilation implies that changes must potentially be made to the technological architecture to take account of how various organizational elements such as roles, formal procedures and emergent routines will henceforth be connected (Cooper and Zmud, 1990; Kwon, 1987). To support the emergence and implementation of such changes, the organization must possess IT capacities that cover both technological and organizational dimensions (Bharadwaj, Sambamurthy and Zmud, 1999). In

particular, the organization needs the capacity to maintain a close, ongoing partnership between the heads of business and IT processes. It also needs the capacity to mutually adjust operating and technological processes to maintain their efficiency and effectiveness and exploit the capacities of emerging IT (Bharadwaj et al., 1999). In order to possess these capacities, the organization must have a sufficiently flexible, integrated IT infrastructure; this is critically important (Broadbent and Weill, 1997), since it makes it possible to ensure continuous compatibility and interoperability between telehealth systems and the systems already in place in the organization (Kayworth, Chatterjee and Sambamurthy, 2001). Moreover, the wide variety of hardware, operating systems and development tools makes it more and more crucial to maintain an IT infrastructure that is sufficiently coherent to avoid fragmentation and lack of integration of the various systems. However, to ensure this cohesion between telehealth systems and the other information systems, networks and applications that are critical to the organization's mission, the technological infrastructure must have the necessary architecture. In fact, this integrated IT infrastructure must constitute a platform on which the organization's shared IT capacities are articulated (Weill, Subramani and Broadbent, 2002).

By IT infrastructure, we mean a shared organizational resource comprising physical elements such as technological artifacts and intellectual elements such as knowledge and know-how (Broadbent, Weill, Brien and Neo, 1996), all of which are kept in step by standards (Kayworth et al., 2001). The physical elements determine the infrastructure's IT capacities, namely its ability to combine the organization's resources in order to support their effectiveness (Amit and Shoemaker, 1993). As for the intellectual elements, they materialize in the relational and integration architectures required to exploit the IT capacities. Relational architecture is required to configure the operating modalities for IT capacities, while the function of integration architecture is to coordinate IT capacities in relation to the business capacities they are there to support (Sambamurthy and Zmud, 2000). The sophistication of the IT infrastructure has been found to have a significant influence on the assimilation of information technologies.

Ultimately, an organization that has the necessary capacities to maintain a close interrelationship between IT professionals and users of the IT and continually adjust the interface of its operating and technological processes, and whose technological infrastructure is flexible enough not only to allow these adjustments but to permit the exploitation of emerging technologies, provides favorable conditions for the routinization and infusion of a technological innovation. This leads to the following proposition:

Proposition 5: The presence of a flexible infrastructure that can integrate existing and emerging operating and technological processes should have a positive impact on the organizational assimilation of telehealth systems.

Organizational Climate

For the same reasons mentioned in the previous section, we believe that the work environment, and in particular the organizational climate, may constrain or promote the organizational assimilation of telehealth systems.

Organizational climate is defined as the individual perceptions concerning the most salient characteristics of the organizational context (Schneider, 1990). It therefore corresponds, unlike psychological climate, to patterns of meaning shared by the individual members of the organization with regard to certain characteristics of the organizational context (Tracey, Tannenbaum and Kavanagh, 1995). It results from the interaction among objective elements that are observable in the organizational context and the perceptual processes of individual members of the organization (Schneider, 1983). It is therefore theoretically possible to influence perception of the climate by

appropriately configuring the elements and processes of the organizational context (Kozlowski and Hults, 1987). As well, organizational climate is useful for understanding the normative response trends of members of the organization (Kozlowski and Hults, 1987). An overall conceptualization of organizational climate could prove somewhat irrelevant for studying a specific phenomenon (Kozlowski and Hults, 1987). Rather, the concept of organizational climate should be considered as a broad, multidimensional perceptual domain for which construct definition depends on the variable of interest (Schneider, 1985). Moreover, an organizational environment may have several climates depending on whether individuals attach specific meanings to separate sets of organizational events or factors (Schneider and Reichers, 1983). From this point of view, a work environment may be characterized by a climate of service, a climate of workplace safety or a climate of self-fulfillment (Mikkelsen and Gronhaug, 1999). Bearing this in mind, we shall consider only the dimensions of climate that appear to us to be most relevant to the routinization (or institutionalization) and infusion of telehealth systems.

The assimilation of telehealth systems derives its meaning from a long-term vision that views telehealth as a new way of organizing healthcare services that complements and extends existing systems. This perspective highlights at least two points: first, information and communication technologies are constantly changing. Consequently, one must plan for continual updates of both the telehealth systems as such and the other information systems in order to benefit from technological advances to improve the quality of patient care and cope with emerging needs. Secondly, this means that medical, administrative and IT staff members must constantly upgrade their skills since the institutionalization of a technological innovation entails that staff competencies must be developed and updated (Kozlowski and Hults, 1987). Furthermore, the structure of healthcare organizations is such that individuals may belong to one or more groups dedicated to specific activities, but they have to work with members of other groups to provide patient care (Dawson et al., 2008). When this reality is reinforced by well-thought-out integration strategies, as was the case with Quebec's health and social services networks, it can look like a climate of integration that fosters professional interdisciplinarity and cohesion among case managers, teams and departments, which then become institutionalized (Kozlowski and Hults, 1987). In our view, such a climate is favorable both to the routinization of telehealth systems and to their use in more extended and integrated ways, which leads to infusion (Zmud and Apple, 1992). It is therefore reasonable to think that if healthcare organizations implement strategies that reinforce learning, continuous upgrading and integration of their staff members' competencies, they could induce normative responses by their members that promote continuous upgrading of their skill level. An organizational climate that unites these three dimensions (learning, upgrading and integration of skills) could prove favorable to the assimilation of telehealth systems. This leads to the following proposition:

Proposition 6: An organizational climate that focuses on upgrading skills should have a positive impact on the organizational assimilation of telehealth systems.

Compatibility

Telehealth systems are not deployed in a vacuum, but in organizational contexts with well-established social structures such as practices, professional culture, technologies and other sociotechnical elements (Gosain, 2004). It is essential to consider the impact of these structural elements on the assimilation of telehealth IS, because studies have shown that they can either constitute barriers to IS implementation or facilitate it by providing the necessary infrastructure or strengthening the organization's absorptive capacity (Kling and Iacono, 1989; Chae and Poole, 2005). Similarly,

because of the organizational arrangements they require, telehealth IS have the capacity to structure the behaviors of the organizations involved. Thus, the deployment of a new system, especially a complex system like the ones supporting telehealth, not only triggers a process of mutual structuring among the host organizations and the system but may also raise the possibility of a mismatch (institutional misalignment) between the institutional regime of the organizations involved and the institutional logics conveyed by the technology (Gosain, 2004). It is therefore possible that conflicting structural components may come into contact. To explain this, one must remember two things: first, the healthcare community is characterized by a strong disciplinary tradition characterized by well-established values, norms and cultural and cognitive schemas that shape and guide the behaviors of members of the medical profession. This tradition develops and is maintained thanks to the activities and vigilance of a number of institutional agents such as the educational system, supervisory agencies, professional associations, etc. The elements of this tradition are instantiated in rules, work procedures, protocols and codes of ethics, and the technologies used in the sector tend to stabilize professional practice. Indeed, disciplines as bodies of knowledge preserve concepts, practices, and values that are employed in action (Pickering, 1995) Moreover, information systems are "complex social objects" (Kling and Scacchi, 1982) laden with intentionality (Chae and Poole, 2005). Because of the artifacts that compose them, IS form a unique combination of three kinds of agency: material, human and disciplinary (Chae and Poole, 2005; Pickering, 1995). Agency denotes the capacity of a person or an object to produce a particular result. Human agency refers primarily to individuals' reflexivity and ability to adjust their actions with the aim of achieving a defined goal, which may be a plan or intention (Chae and Poole, 2005). Material agency is physical or biological in nature. It is revealed in the actions of the specific powerful forces of certain generative mechanisms (Harre and Madden, 1975). Finally, disciplinary agency corresponds to the shaping and orientation of human action by cultural and conceptual systems (Pickering, 1995). In fact, in the development phase of a system, it goes through a "registration process" during which the dominant interests and the developers' responses to institutional pressures and their vision of the world are reflected in the system's functioning (Latour, 1992). In this sense, the people who develop telehealth systems have the opportunity to incorporate rules, functionalities and resources into them that are capable of structuring the users' interaction with the system.

The above discussion helps us to understand that the encounter between telehealth systems and the organization raises the problem of compatibility between the systems and the organization's operating infrastructure, on one hand, and the organization's technological infrastructure in the sense of software, hardware and IT management procedures, on the other. In the first case, we refer to operational compatibility, whereas the second corresponds to technological compatibility (Jones and Beatty, 1998).

We therefore believe that if telehealth systems are compatible with the existing technological infrastructure and operating procedures, this will facilitate the assimilation of these systems into the organizations involved in the telehealth project:

Proposition 7: Telehealth systems' compatibility with the organization's operating infrastructure will have a positive impact on their assimilation.

Proposition 8: Telehealth systems' compatibility with the organization's existing technological infrastructure will have a positive impact on their assimilation.

Organizing Vision

In the case of innovations like telehealth systems, institutional processes play a role from the outset of the diffusion of such systems and help to reduce the ambiguity surrounding them by proposing an organizing vision (Swanson and Ramiller, 1997). Since telehealth systems are essentially interorganizational in their application, their origin and rationale must be sought at the level of the organizational field (DiMaggio and Powell, 1983), which is made up of the various entities comprising the healthcare system. The organizing vision (OV) is created and developed at this level:

...an interorganizational community, comprised of a heterogeneous network of parties with a variety of material interest in an IS innovation, collectively creates and employs an organizing vision of the innovation that is central to decisions and actions affecting its development and diffusion. (Swanson and Ramiller, 1997, p. 459)

This makes it clear that, when the actors involved in telehealth projects must make sense of the system, they are not acting in a vacuum but also making use of the representations of other actors to develop their own, since the organization of which they are members is not isolated:

Instead it [organization] belongs to a complex community of organizations, the many members of which actively contemplate the new technology and ponder to varying degrees publicly what it means and where it is going. Thus much of what the sensemakers in the prospective adopter do is search and probe and engage the interpretations of others. (Swanson and Ramiller, 1997, pp. 459-460)

In other words, an essential part of actors' effort to interpret telehealth systems consists of inquiring about and evaluating the interpretations conveyed at the level of the organizational field. Indeed, telehealth projects can be very different from one another, which means that the systems use quite different technologies that have often not stabilized yet and are sometimes still in the prototyping phase (Klecun-Dabrowska and Cornford, 2002). The technologies used and users' understanding of them are incomplete and unstable (Rosenberg, 1994). In short, the components of these systems are not always well articulated and their implications may not be well understood (Swanson and Ramiller, 1997). In this context, the OV acts to formulate the spirit of the system in the sense of the philosophy underlying the artifact and the motives that led to its development (Chae, 2002). The OV is a meaning-making structure that actors make use of to understand the nature of telehealth systems and their roles in the social, technical and economic context (Klecun-Dabrowska and Cornford, 2002). In this way, the telehealth OV may remove, or at least reduce, the ambiguity characterizing telehealth systems and their possible applications:

An organizing vision arises to encode and provide the necessary interpretations and to give institutional coherence to initiatives that might otherwise be viewed as of limited relevance, even organizationally idiosyncratic [p. 460]... that provide important cognitive structures that shape thought relative to innovation involving innovation technologies. (Swanson and Ramiller, 1997, pp. 460 and 471)

By formulating expectations, hypotheses and knowledge regarding the key aspects of telehealth systems, the OV contributes to ensuring the congruence of the different groups of actors' technological frames (as discussed above) and may also align the institutional logics incorporated in the configuration of these systems with the organization's institutional regime (values, practices, norms, culture and technologies). When this happens, organizations experience less conflict in the implementation and use of new systems (Orlikowski and Gash, 1994). Thus, we believe that the following proposition applies:

Proposition 9a: A preeminent organizing vision should have a positive impact on the assimilation of telehealth systems.

The OV also provides a legitimation structure, which complements the meaning-making structure by considering in its discourse the aspects that justify the innovation. The discourse on the system's legitimacy uses technical and functional arguments, as well as political, organizational and business arguments (Klecun-Dabrowska and Cornford, 2002). This dimension of the OV endeavors to communicate not only the expected benefits of the innovation, but also its spirit, that is, the underlying philosophies and the reasons motivating its development (Chae, 2002). For example, by presenting telehealth as a solution to the health problems experienced by people in remote regions and by underserved groups, and to the problem of recruiting and keeping physicians in these regions, etc., the OV not only clarifies the benefits of telehealth but also ties in with society's concern for equity. By doing this, it emphasizes the importance of telehealth systems and strengthens the social norms and values that encourage and value their use (Orlikowski and Gash, 1994), and ensures that users take ownership of them. In turn, legitimacy favors the mobilization of the resources needed to move telehealth from the status of project to the status of current service, which involves changing practices and operating infrastructure so the telehealth system can be integrated. All of this leads us to think that an OV that formulates the rationale for telehealth systems in terms of existing values and social norms in the healthcare sector is likely to have a positive impact on the assimilation of telehealth systems by promoting the mobilization of the necessary resources. On this basis, we make the following proposition:

Proposition 9b: An OV that formulates the rationale for telehealth systems in terms of existing values and social norms in the healthcare sector should have a positive impact on the assimilation of telehealth systems.

CONCLUSION

This chapter has undertaken a multilevel modeling approach that clarifies the process of assimilation. Our theory development involved introspection concerning the technological artifact to ensure that this concept and the social and institutional context are at the core of the model. Moreover, the model is anchored in theory, and the theories mobilized here have enabled us to take into account the issues associated with information system assimilation and to analyze them appropriately.

This chapter developed a theoretical perspective that enables us to gain a better understanding of the assimilation of information systems, based on their nature and the problems associated with their development. In this way, this chapter contributes to research in this area by emphasizing the necessity of anchoring the theorization process in the characteristics of the technological artifact and of the social and institutional context in which these systems are applied. Moreover, earlier work on the organizational assimilation of information technologies (Zmud and Apple, 1992; Saga and Zmud, 1994; Fichman and Kemerer, 1997/1999; Meyer and Goes, 1998; Purvis et al., 2001; Gallivan, 2001; Chatterjee et al., 2002) has certainly enriched our knowledge of this phenomenon. Nevertheless, the fact that these studies considered assimilation as an exclusively organizational phenomenon has undoubtedly overshadoweded more micro or meso explanations that could enrich our understanding still more. In particular, these studies are silent about the structure and functions of the assimilation constructs. Unlike those prior studies, our model proposes a detailed account of the assimilation process by clarifying both the structure (Kozlowski and Klein, 2000) and the functional relationships of the phenomenon (Morgesson and Hofmann, 1999). Put simply, the model accounts for how individual, group and organization characteristics interact to structure assimilation. Briefly, the adoption of a multilevel perspective resulted in a more comprehensive understanding of how the assimilation process unfolds across levels in organizations.

Our study also has implications for practice. In particular, it points to the importance of examining assimilation within the continuum of IS phenomena surrounding the deployment of telehealth systems. As such, it helps understand why managerial actions intended to facilitate the assimilation process should be employed as early as the adoption phase. For instance, issues related to the systems' compatibility with the organization's work infrastructure should be managed during the development phase. Briefly, even though routinization and infusion are post-implementation behaviors, factors that are likely to influence them should be taken into consideration before systems are acquired. Moreover, by making explicit the functional relationships at the individual, group and organizational levels, this work highlights the range of managerial interventions required to secure the IS assimilation and consequently the telehealth systems' effectiveness. In addition, beyond the policy level, the model provides a better understanding of the locus of authority for each specific managerial intervention. In so doing, it will help to enhance the effectiveness of managerial actions and smooth the IS governance aspects of telehealth systems.

FUTURE WORK

The next step in our agenda is to test the model in an empirical, real-life setting. In addition to testing the model, this will allow us to identify additional contributing factors so we can better understand the assimilation of telehealth systems into the workplace.

REFERENCES

Ackerman, M. (3 May). *Personnal Interview. Lister Hill National Center for Biomedical Communications of the NLM.*

Amit, R., & Schoemaker, P. J. H. (1993). Strategic assets and organizational rent. *Strategic Management Journal, 14*(1), 33. doi:10.1002/smj.4250140105

Barley, S. R. (1986). Technology as an Occasion for Structuring: Evidence from Observations of CT Scanners and the Social Order of Radiology Departments. *Administrative Science Quarterly, 31*(1), 78. doi:10.2307/2392767

Barley, S. R. (1990). The Alignment Of Technology And Structure Through Roles And. *Administrative Science Quarterly, 35*(1), 61. doi:10.2307/2393551

Bashshur, R. L., Sanders, J., & Shannon, G. W. (1997). *Telemedicine: Theory and practice.* Springfield: Charles Thomas.

Beaglehole, E. (1932). *A Study in Social Psychology.* New York: Mcmillan.

Beggan, J. K. (1992). On the Social Nature of Nonsocial Perception: The Mere Ownership Effect. *Journal of Personality and Social Psychology, 62*(2), 229. doi:10.1037/0022-3514.62.2.229

Bharadwaj, A., Sambamurthy, V., & Zmud, R. W. (1999). IT Capabilities: Theoretical Perspectives and Operationalization. *Proceedings of the Twentieth International Conference on Informations Systems, Charlotte, NC.*

Bishop, J. E., O'Reilly, R. L., Daddox, K., & Hutchinson, K. (2002). Client Satisfaction in a faisability Study Comparing face-to-face Interviews with Telepsychiatry. *Journal of Telemedicine and Telecare, 8*(4). doi:10.1258/135763302320272185

Broadbent, M., & Weill, P. (1997). Management by Maxim: How Business and IT Managers Can Create IT Infrastructures. *Sloan Management Review, 38*(3), 77.

Broadbent, M., Weill, P., Brien, T., & Neo, B.-S. (1996). Firm context and pattern of IT infrastructure capability. *The International Conference on Information Systems.*

Campion, M. A., Medsker, G. J., & Higgs, A. C. (1993). Relations between work group characteristics and effectiveness: Implications for designing effective work groups. *Personnel Psychology, 46*(4), 823. doi:10.1111/j.1744-6570.1993.tb01571.x

Chae, B. (2002). *Understanding information systems as social institutions: Dynamic institutional theory.* Unpublished doctoral dissertation, Texas A&M University, Texas, USA

Chae, B., & Poole, M. S. (2005). The surface of emergence in systems development: agency, institutions, and large-scale information systems. *European Journal of Information Systems, 14,* 19–36. doi:10.1057/palgrave.ejis.3000519

Chan, D. (1998). Functional relations among constructs in the same content domain at different levels of analysis: A typology of composition models. *The Journal of Applied Psychology, 83*(2), 234. doi:10.1037/0021-9010.83.2.234

Chatterjee, D., Grewal, R., & Sambamurthy, V. (2002). Shaping up for e-commerce: Institutional enablers of the organizational assimilation of web technologies. *Management Information Systems Quarterly, 26*(2), 65. doi:10.2307/4132321

Chatterjee, D., & Segars, A. H. (2001). Transformation of the Enterprise through E-Business: An Overview of Contemporary Practices and Trends. *Report to the Advanced Practices Council of the Society for Information Management,* (July).

Cohn, J. R., & Goodenough, B. (2002). Health Professionals Attitudes to Videoconferencing in Pediatric Heathcare. *Journal of Telemedicine and Telecare, 8*(5). doi:10.1258/135763302760314243

Cooper, R. B., & Zmud, R. W. (1990). Information Technology Implementation Research: A Technological Diffusion Approach. *Management Science, 36*(2), 123. doi:10.1287/mnsc.36.2.123

Crossan, M. M., Lane, H. W., & White, R. E. (1999). An organizational learning framework: From intuition to institution. Academy of Management. *Academy of Management Review, 24*(3), 522. doi:10.2307/259140

Croteau, A.-M., & Vieru, D. (2002). *Telemedicine Adoption by Different Group of Physicians*. Proceedings of the 35th Hawaii International Conference on System Sciences IEEE.

D'Amour, D. (Centre Mont-Royal, Montréal, 2006). *Collaboration interprofessionnelle: Bien saisir les enjeux. Colloque: L'Interdisciplinarité, Défi Ou Déni.*

D'Amour, D., Ferrada-Videla, M., San Martin Rodriguez, F., & Beaulieu, M. D. (2005). The conceptual basis for interprofessional collaboration: Core concepts and theoretical frameworks. *Journal of Interprofessional Care, 1*(Supplement), 116–131. doi:10.1080/13561820500082529

Daft, R., & Weick, K. E. (1984). Toward a Model of Organizations as Interpretation Systems. *Academy of Management Review, 9*, 284–295. doi:10.2307/258441

Daft, R. L. (1995). *Organization Theory and Design* (5th ed.). Minneapolis: West Publishing Co.

Dawson, J. F., Gonzalez-Roma, V., Davis, A., & West, M. A. (2008). Organizational climate and climate strength in UK hospitals. *European Journal of Work and Organizational Psychology, 17*(1), 89. doi:10.1080/13594320601046664

DeSanctis, G., & Poole, M. S. (1994). Capturing the Complexity in Advanced Technology Use: Adaptive Structuration Theory. *Organization Science, 5*(2), 121–147. doi:10.1287/orsc.5.2.121

Deutsch, M. (1949). An experimental study of cooperation and competition upon group process. *Human Relations, 2*, 199–231. doi:10.1177/001872674900200301

Deutsch, M. (1973). *The resolution of conflict: Constructive and destructive process.* New Haven, CT: Yale University Press.

DHSS. (2001). *Report to Congress on Telemedicine*: Secretary of Health and Human Services.

DiMaggio, P. J., & Powell, W. W. (1983). The Iron Cage Revisited: Institutional Isomorphism and Collective Rationality in Organizational Fields. *American Sociological Review, 48*(2), 147–160. doi:10.2307/2095101

Dirks, K. T., Cummings, L. L., & Pierce, J. L. (1996). Psychological ownership in organizations: Conditions under which individuals promote and resist change. In Woodman, R. W., & Pasmore, A. W. (Eds.), *Research in organizational change and development* (*Vol. 9*, pp. 1–23). Greenwich, CT: JAI Press.

Drazin, R., Glynn, M. A., & Kazanjian, R. K. (1999). Multilevel theorizing about creativity in organizations: A sensemaking perspective. *Academy of Management. Academy of Management Review, 24*(2), 286. doi:10.2307/259083

Eveland, J. D., & Tornatzky, L. (1990). The Deployment of Technology. In In Tornatzky, L., & Fleischer, M. (Eds.), *The Processes of Technological Innovation*. Lexington: Lexington Books.

Fichman, R. G., & Kemerer, C. F. (1997). The assimilation of software process innovations: An organizational learning perspective. *Management Science, 43*(10), 1345. doi:10.1287/mnsc.43.10.1345

Fichman, R. G., & Kemerer, C. F. (1999). The illusory diffusion of innovation: An examination of assimilation gaps. *Information Systems Research, 10*(3), 255. doi:10.1287/isre.10.3.255

Finney, M., & Mitroff, I. I. (1986). Strategic Plans Failures: The organization as its own worst enemy. *The Thinking Organization* (317-335). San Francisco: Jossey-Bass.

Gallivan, M. J. (2001). Organizational adoption and assimilation of complex technological innovations: Development and application of a new framework. *The Data Base for Advances in Information Systems, 32*(3), 51.

Giddens, A. (2005). *La Constitution de la Société: éléments de la théorie de la structuration (traduit de l'anglais par Michel Audet)*. Paris: Quadridge PUF (1ère édition).

Goffman, I. (1974). *Frame Analysis*. New York: Harper & Row.

Gosain, S. (2004). Enterprise Information Systems as Objects and Carriers of Institutional Forces: The New Iron Cage. *Journal of the Association for Information Systems, 5*(4), 151–182.

Gregory, K. L. (1983). Native-View Paradigms: Multiple ultures and culture conflicts in organization. *Administrative Science Quarterly, 28*(3), 359–376. doi:10.2307/2392247

Grémy, F., & Bonnin, M. (1995). Evaluation of Automatic Health Informations Systems. What and How? E. In Van Gennip, et J. Talmon (Eds.), *Assessment and Evaluation of Information Technologies in Medicine*. Amsterdam: IOS Press.

Grigsby, J., Schlenker, R., Kaehny, M. M., Shaughnessy, P. W., & Sandberg, E. J. (1995). Analytic framework for evaluation of telemedicine. *Telemedicine Journal, 1*(1), 31–39.

Hackman, J. R., & Oldham, G. R. (1975). Development of the Job Diagnostic Survey. *The Journal of Applied Psychology, 60*(2), 159–170. doi:10.1037/h0076546

Hall, G., & Loucks, S. (1977). A developmentla Model for Determining Wether the Treatment is Actually Implemented. *American Educational Research Journal, 14*(3), 263–276.

Harre, R., & Madden, E. H. (1975). *Causal Powers: A Theory of Natural Necessity*. Oxford: Blackwell.

Hu, P., & Chau, P. (1999). Physician acceptance of telemedicine technology: an empirical investigation. *Topics in Health Information Management, 19*(4), 20–35.

Hu, P. J., Chau, P. Y. K., & Sheng, O. L. (2000). Investigation of factors affecting healthcare organization's adoption of telemedicine technology. *Proceedings of the 33rd Hawaii International Conference on System Sciences*.

Hu, P. J.-H., Wei, C.-P., & Cheng, T.-H. (2002). Investigating Telemedicine Developments in Taiwan: Implications for Telemedicine Program. *Proceedings of the 35th Hawaii International Conference on System Sciences*.

Illich, I. (1973). *Tools for conviviality*. New York: Harper and Row.

Isaacs, S. (1933). *Social Development in Young Children*. London: Routledge and Kegan Paul.

Jones, M. C., & Beatty, R. C. (1998). Towards the development of measures of perceived benefits and compatibility of EDI: a comparative assessment of competing first order factor models. *European Journal of Information Systems, 7*(3), 210–220. doi:10.1057/palgrave.ejis.3000299

Kahn, W. A. (1990). Psychological Conditions of Personal Engagement and Disengagement at Work. *Academy of Management Journal, 33*(4), 692. doi:10.2307/256287

Kayworth, T. R., Chatterjee, D., & Sambamurthy, V. (2001). Theoretical justification for IT infrastructure investments. *Information Resources Management Journal, 14*(3), 5.

Keen, P., & McDonald, M. (2000). *The eProcess Edge: Creating Customer Value and Business Wealth in Internet Era*. Berkeley, CA: McGraw Hill.

Klecun-Dabrowska, E., & Cornford, T. (2002). *The Organizing Vision of Telehealth*. Gdansk, Poland: ECIS.

Klein, K. J., Dansereau, F., & Hall, R. J. (1994). Levels issues in theory development, data collection, and analysis. *Academy of Management. Academy of Management Review, 19*(2), 195. doi:10.2307/258703

Kling, R. (1987). Defining the Boundaries of Computing Accross Complex Organizations. In Bolland, R., & Hirscheim, R. A. (Eds.), *Critical Issues in Information Systems Research.* London: John Wiley.

Kling, R., & Dutton, W. H. (1982). The computer package, dynamic complexity. In J. N. Danziger, D. W. H., R. Kling, & K. L. Kraemer (eds) *Computers and Politics: High Technolgy in American Local Governments.* (p.22-50). New York: Columbia University Press.

Kling, R., & Iacono, C. (1989). The Institutional Character of Computerized Information System. *Office Technology & People, 1*(1), 24–43.

Kling, R., & Scacchi, W. (1982). The Web of Computing: Computer technology as Social Organization. *Advances in Computers,* (21), 1-90.

Kostova, T. (1998). Quality of inter-unit relationships in MNEs as a source of competitive advantage. M. Hitt, J. Ricart, & R. Nixon (Eds.), *New Managerial Mindsets: Organizational transformation and strategy implementation.* Chichester, UK: Wiley.

Kozlowski, S. W. J., & Hults, B. M. (1987). An Exploration of Climates for Technical Updating and Performance. *Personnel Psychology, 40*, 539–563. doi:10.1111/j.1744-6570.1987.tb00614.x

Kozlowski, S. W. J., & Klein, J. K. (2000). A Multilevel Approach to Theory and Research in Organizations: Contextual, Temporal, and Emergent Process. In J. K. Klein, & S. W. J. Kozlowski (eds.), *Multilevel Theory, Research, and Methods in Organizations* (3-90). San Francisco: Jossey-Bass.

Kubzansky, P. E., & Druskat, V. U. (1993). Psychological sense of ownership in the workplace: Conceptualisation and measurement. *Paper Presented at the Annual Meeting of the American Psychological Association, Toronto, Canada.*

Kwon, T. H. (1987). *A Study of the Influence of Communication Network on MIS Institutionalization.* Unpublished doctoral dissertation, The University of North Carolina at Chapel Hill, United States -- North Carolina.

Latour, B. (1992). The sociology of a few mundane artifacts. B. In Bijker, and J. Law (eds.), *Shaping Technology/Building Society Studies in Socio-technological Change* (135-150). Cambridge, MA: MIT Press.

Lauriol, J. (1998). Les représentations sociales dans la décision. In H. Laroche, et J-P. Nioche (dir.), *Repenser la stratégie.* France: Vuibert.

Leonard-Barton, D. (1988). Implementation as mutual adaptation of technology and organization. *Research Policy, 17*(5), 251–267. doi:10.1016/0048-7333(88)90006-6

Lewin, K. (1947). Frontiers in Group Dynamics: Concept, Method and Reality in Social Science; Social Equilibra and Social Change. *Human Relations, 1*(5).

McKee, J. J., Evans, N. E., & Owens, F. J. (1996). Digital Transmission of 12-Lead Electrocadiograms and Duplex Speech in the Telephone Bandwith. *Journal of Telemedicine and Telecare, 2*(1). doi:10.1258/1357633961929150

Meyer, A. D., & Goes, J. B. (1988). Organizational Assimilation of Innovations: A Multilevel Contextual Analysis. *Academy of Management Journal, 31*(4). doi:10.2307/256344

Mikkelsen, A., & Gronhaug, K. (1999). Measuring Organizational Learning Climate. *Review of Public Personnel Administration, 19*(4), 31. doi:10.1177/0734371X9901900404

Mintzberg, H. (1981). Organiser l'entreprise: Prêt-à-porter ou sur mesure? *Harvard, L'Expansion,* (été), 9-23.

Mitchell, B. R., Mitchell, J. G., & Disney, A. P. (1996). User adoption Issues in Renal Telemedicine. *Journal of Telemedicine and Telecare, 2*(2). doi:10.1258/1357633961929835

Mitchell, T. R., & Silver, W. S. (1990). Individual and Group Goals When Workers Are Interdependent. *The Journal of Applied Psychology, 75*(2), 185. doi:10.1037/0021-9010.75.2.185

Morgeson, F. P., & Hofmann, D. A. (1999). The structure and function of collective constructs: Implications for multilevel research and theory development. *Academy of Management. Academy of Management Review, 24*(2), 249. doi:10.2307/259081

Nardi, B. A., & O'Day, V. L. (1999). *Information Ecologies: Using Technologies with Heart.* Cambridge, MA: MIT Press.

Nordal, E. J., Moseng, D., Kvammen, B., & Lochen, M. (2001). A Comparative Study of Teleconsultation versus Face-to-Face Consultations. *Journal of Telemedicine and Telecare, 7*(5). doi:10.1258/1357633011936507

Orlikowski, W. J. (1993). Learning from notes: Organizational issues in groupware implementation. *The Information Society, 9*(3), 237. doi:10.1080/01972243.1993.9960143

Orlikowski, W. J., & Gash, D. C. (1994). Technological frames: making sense of information technology in organizations. *ACM Transactions on Information Systems, 12*(2), 174–207. doi:10.1145/196734.196745

Orlikowski, W. J., & Iacono, C. S. (2001). Research commentary: Desperately seeking "IT" in IT research - A call to theorizing the IT artifact. *Information Systems Research, 12*(2), 121. doi:10.1287/isre.12.2.121.9700

Paré, G., & Sicotte, C. (2004). Les technologies de l'information et la transformation de l'offre de soins. *Cahier Du GReSI,* (04-04).

Payette, M. (2001). Interdisciplinarité: Clarification des concepts. *Interaction, 5*(1).

Pearce, J. L., & Gregersen, H. B. (1991). Task Interdependence and Extrarole Behavior: A Test of the Mediating Effects of Felt Responsibility. *The Journal of Applied Psychology, 76*(6), 838. doi:10.1037/0021-9010.76.6.838

Pickering, A. (1995). *The Mangle of Practice.* Chicago: The University of Chicago Press.

Picolo, D., Smolle, D., Argenziano, G., Wolf, I. H., Braun, R., & Cerroni, L. (2000). Teledermoscopy: Results of a Multicentre Study on 43 Pigmented Skin Lesions. *Journal of Telemedicine and Telecare, 6*(3). doi:10.1258/1357633001935202

Pierce, J. L., Kostova, T., & Dirks, K. T. (2001). Toward a theory of psychological ownership in organizations. *Academy of Management. Academy of Management Review, 26*(2), 298. doi:10.2307/259124

Pierce, J. L., Rubenfeld, S. A., & Morgan, S. (1991). Employee Ownership: A Conceptual Model of Process and Effects. *Academy of Management. Academy of Management Review, 16*(1), 121. doi:10.2307/258609

Pinch, T., & Bijker, W. (1987). The social connstruction of facts and artifacts. W. In Bijker, T. Hughes and T. Pinch (eds.), *The Social Construction of Technological Systems* (159-187). Cambridge, MA: MIT Press.

Poole, M. S., & DeSanctis, G. (1990). Understanding the Use of Group Decision Support Systems: The Theory of Adaptive Structuration. In Fulk and Steinfield (eds), *Organizations and Communication Technology.* (173-193). Newbury Park, CA: Sage Publications.

Porac, J. F., Thomas, H., & Baden-Fuller, C. (1989). Competitive groups as cognitive communities: The case of Scottish knitwear manufacturers. *Journal of Management Studies, 26*(4), 397–416. doi:10.1111/j.1467-6486.1989.tb00736.x

Pratt, M. G., & Dutton, J. E. (2000). Owning up or opting out: The roles of identity and emotions in issue of ownership. In N. Ashkanasy, C. Hartel, & W. Zerbe (eds.), *Emotions in the workplace: Research, theory, and practice* (103-129). New York: Quorum.

Purvis, R. L., Sambamurthy, V., & Zmud, R. (2001). The assimilation of knowledge platforms in organizations: An empirical investigation. *Organization Science, 12*(2), 117. doi:10.1287/orsc.12.2.117.10115

Ritti, R., & Silver, J. (1986). Early Processes of Institutionalization: The Dramaturgy of Exchange in Interoganizational Relations. *Administrative Science Quarterly, 31*, 25–42. doi:10.2307/2392764

Robinson, D. F., Savage, Gr. T., & Campbell, K. S. (2003). Organizational Learning, Diffusion of Innovation, and International Collaboration in Telemedicine. *Health Care Management Review, 28*(1), 68.

Rodgers, L., & Freundlich, F. (1998). *Employee Ownership Report*. Oakland, CA: National Center for Employee Ownership.

Rosemberg, N. (1994). *Exploring the Black Box: Technology, Economics and History*. Cambridge, UK: Cambridge University Press. doi:10.1017/CBO9780511582554

Rousseau, D. M. (1985). Issues of Level in Organizational Research: Multi-Level and Cross-Level Perspectives. In Cummings, L. L., & Staw, B. M. (Eds.), *Research in Organizational Behavior (Vol. 7)*. Greenwich, CT: JAI Press.

Ruis de Sherbrooke. (2007). La téléassistance en soins de plaies, orientée vers une amélioration continue de la qualité des soins. *Manuel D'Organisation De Projet,* 1-63.

Saga, V., & Zmud, R. (1994). The nature and determinants of information technology acceptance, routinization and infusion. In Levine. L. (ed.), *Diffusion, Transfer, and Implementation of Information Technology* (67-68). Noth-Holland, Amsterdam.

Sambamurthy, V., & Zmud, R. W. (2000). Research commentary: The organizing logic for an enterprise's IT activities in the digital era - A prognosis of practice and a call for research. *Information Systems Research, 11*(2), 105. doi:10.1287/isre.11.2.105.11780

Schein, E. (1985). *Organizational Culture and Leadership*. San Francisco: Jossey-Bass.

Schneider, B. (1990). The Climate for Service: An application of the climate construct. In *Social and Behavioral Science Series., Organizational Climate and Culture*. San Francisco: Jossey-Bass.

Schneider, B., & Reichers, A. E. (1983). On the Etiology of Climates. *Personnel Psychology, 36*(1), 19–39. doi:10.1111/j.1744-6570.1983.tb00500.x

Scott, W. R. (2001). *Institutions and Organizations* (2nd ed.). Thousand Oaks, CA: Sage Publications.

Shea, G. P., & Guzzo, R. A. (1987). Groups as human resources. G.R. Ferris and K.M. Rowland (eds.), *Research in personnel and human resources management* (Vol. 5) (323-356). Greenwich, CT: JAI Press.

Strauss, A. (1978). A Social World Perspective. *Studies in Symbolic Interaction, 4*, 171–190.

Succi, M. J., & Walter, Z. D. (1999). Theory of user acceptance of information technologies: An examination of health care professionals. *32nd Hawaii International Conference on System Sciences* IEEE Computer Society.

Swanson, B. E., & Ramiller, N. C. (1997). The Organizing Vision in Information Systems Innovation. *Organization Science, 8*(5), 458. doi:10.1287/orsc.8.5.458

The Lewin Group. (2000). *Assessment of Approaches to Evaluating Telemedicine. Final report prepared for the Office of the Assistant Secretary for Planning and Evaluation, of.* Department of Health and Human Services.

Thompson, J. D. (1967). *Organizations in action.* New York: McGraw-Hill.

Tornatzky, L., & Klein, K. J. (1982). Innovation Characteristics and Innovation-Implementation: A Meta-Analysis of Findings. *IEEE Transactions on Engineering Management, 29*(1), 28–45.

Tracey, J. B., Tannenbaum, S. I., & Kavanagh, M. J. (1995). Applying Trained Skills on the Job: The Importance of the Work Environment. *The Journal of Applied Psychology, 80*(2), 239–252. doi:10.1037/0021-9010.80.2.239

Tyre, M. J., & Orlikowski, W. J. (1994). Windows of opportunity: Temporal patterns of technological adaptation in organizations. *Organization Science, 5*(1), 98. doi:10.1287/orsc.5.1.98

Van De Ven, A. H., Delbecq, A. L., & Koenig, R. J. (1976). Determinants of coordination modes within organizations. *American Sociological Review, 41*, 322–338. doi:10.2307/2094477

Van der Vegt, G., Emans, B., & Van de Vliert, E. (1998). Motivating Effects of Task and Outcome Interdependence in Work Teams. *Group & Organization Management, 23*(2), 124. doi:10.1177/1059601198232003

Van Dyne, L., & Pierce, J. L. (2004). Psychological ownership and feelings of possession: three field studies predicting employee attitudes and organizational citizenship behavior. *Journal of Organizational Behavior, 25*(4), 439. doi:10.1002/job.249

Van Maanen, J., & Schein, E. (1979). Toward a theory of organizational socialization. *Research in Organizational Behavior, 1*, 209–264.

Venkatesh, V., & Davis, F. D. (2000). A theoretical extension of the Technology Acceptance Model: Four longitudinal field studies. *Management Science, 46*(2), 186–204. doi:10.1287/mnsc.46.2.186.11926

Viens, N. (2006). L'interdisciplinarité dans un CHU: Vers une approche contingente de soins. *Institut D'Adminatation Publique Du Québec.*

Volkema, R. J., Farquhar, K., & Bergmann, T. J. (1996). Third-party sensemaking in interpersonal conflicts at work: A theoretical framework. *Human Relations, 49*(11), 1437. doi:10.1177/001872679604901104

Wageman, R. (1995). Interdependence and Group Effectiveness. *Administrative Science Quarterly, 40*(1), 145. doi:10.2307/2393703

Weick, K. (1990). The vulnerable system: an analysis of the Tenerife Air disaster. *Journal of Management, ▪▪▪*, 16.

Weill, P., Subramani, M., & Broadbent, M. (2002). Building IT infrastructure for strategic agility. *MIT Sloan Management Review, 44*(1), 57.

Zmud, W. R., & Apple, L. E. (1992). Measuring Technology Incorporation/Infusion. *Journal of Product Innovation Management,* (9): 148–155. doi:10.1016/0737-6782(92)90006-X

Zucker, L. (1977). The Role of Institutionalization in Cultural Persistence. *American Sociological Review, 42*(5), 726–743. doi:10.2307/2094862

ADDITIONAL READING

Armstrong, C. P., & Sambamurthy, V. (1999). Information technology assimilation in firms: The influence of senior leadership and IT infrastructure. *Information Systems Research, 10*(4), 304–327. doi:10.1287/isre.10.4.304

Bolloju, N., & Turban, E. (2007). Organizational assimilation of Web services technology: A research framework. *Journal of Organizational Computing and Electronic Commerce, 17*(1), 29–52.

Harnett, B. (2008). Creating telehealth networks from existing infrastructures. *Studies in Health Technology and Informatics, 131*, 55–65.

Jennet, P., Yeo, M., Pauls, M., & Graham, J. (2003). Organizational readiness for telemedicine: implications for success and failure. *Journal of Telemedicine and Telecare, 9*(suppl. 2), 27–30. doi:10.1258/135763303322596183

Jennett, P., Bates, J., Healy, T., Ho, K., Kazanjian, A., & Woollard, R. (2003). A readiness model for telehealth is it possible to pre-determine how prepared communities are to implement telehealth? *Studies in Health Technology and Informatics, 97*, 51–55.

Jennett, P. A., Gagnon, M. P., & Brandstadt, H. K. (2005). Preparing for success: readiness models for rural telehealth. *Journal of Postgraduate Medicine, 51*(4), 279–285.

Jennett, P. A., Watson, M. M., & Watanabe, M. (2000). The potential effects of telehealth on the canadian health workforce: Where is the evidence? *Cyberpsychology & Behavior, 3*(6), 917–923. doi:10.1089/109493100452174

Lewis, L. F., Bajwa, D., & Pervan, G. (2004). An empirical assessment of the assimilation patterns and the benefits of collaborative information technologies. *Journal of Computer Information Systems*, (Summer): 16–26.

Liang, H., Saraf, N., Hu, Q., & Xue, Y. (2007). Assimilation of enterprise systems: The effect of institutional pressures and the mediating role of top management. *Management Information Systems Quarterly, 31*(1), 59–87.

May, C., Harrison, R., MacFarlane, A., Williams, T., Mair, F., & Wallace, P. (2003). Why do telemedicine systems fail to normalize as stable models of service delivery? *Journal of Telemedicine and Telecare, 9*(suppl. 1), 25–26. doi:10.1258/135763303322196222

McCartt, A. T., & Rohrbaugh, J. (1995). Managerial openness to change and the introduction of GDSS: Explaining initial success and failure in decision conferencing. *Organization Science, 6*(5), 569–584. doi:10.1287/orsc.6.5.569

Nash, M. G., & Gremillion, C. (2004). Globalization impacts the healthcare organization of the 21st century. Demanding new *ways to market product lines successfully. Nursing Administration Quarterly, 28*(2), 86–91.

Riva, G. (2000). From Telehealth to E-Health: Internet and Distributed Virtual Reality in Health Care. *Cyberpsychology & Behavior, 3*(6), 989–998. doi:10.1089/109493100452255

Robinson, D. F., Savage, G. T., & Campbell, K. S. (2003). Organizational learning, diffusion of innovation and international collaboration in telemedicine. *Health Care Management Review, 28*(1), 68–78.

Siddiquee, N. A. (2008). E-Government and Innovations in Service Delivery: The Malaysian Experience. *International Journal of Public Administration, 31*(7), 797–815. doi:10.1080/01900690802153053

Smith, R. (2004). Access to Healthcare via Telehealth: Experiences from the Pacific. *Perspectives on Global Development and Technology, 3*(1/2), 197–211. doi:10.1023/B:PERG.0000047195.65038.6a

Teo, H. H., Wang, X., Wei, K. K., Sia, C. L., & Lee, M. K. O. (2005). Organizational learning capacity and attitude toward complex technological innovations: An empirical study. *Journal of the American Society for Information Science and Technology, 57*(2), 264–279. doi:10.1002/asi.20275

Weaver, L., & Spence, D. (2000). Application of business case analysis in planning a province-wide telehealth network in Alberta. *Journal of Telemedicine and Telecare, 6*(suppl 1), 87–89. doi:10.1258/1357633001934267

Weinstein, R. S., Lopez, A. M., Krupinski, E. A., Beinar, S. J., Holcomb, M., McNeely, R. A., et al. (2008). Integrating telemedicine and telehealth: Putting it all together. In R. Latifi (ed), *Current principles and practices of telemedicine and e-Health*, 23-38. Amsterdam:IOS Press.

KEY TERMS AND DEFINITIONS

Telehealth: Healthcare services using information and communications technology such as tele-education, teleconsultation and teletraining, etc.

Routinization: the incorporation of an IS into the organization's work system in such a way that over time the IS ceases to be perceived as a novelty and starts to be taken for granted.

Infusion: an information system's embededness into the organization's procedures and work Architectures.

Top-Down Processes: address the influence of macro levels such as organizational or group characteristics on micro levels such as individuals.

Bottom-Up Processes: describe phenomena that have their theoretical origin at a lower level but have emergent properties at higher levels.

Composition Process: describes phenomena that are essentially the same as they emerge across levels.

Compilation Process: describes phenomena that comprise a common domain but are distinctively different as they across levels.

Chapter 9
Acceptance of Ambient Assisted Living Solutions in Everyday Life

Annette Spellerberg
University of Kaiserslautern, Germany

Lynn Schelisch
University of Kaiserslautern, Germany

ABSTRACT

The aim of "Ambient Assisted Living" -devices is to increase comfort and safety and to provide support for elderly people in their homes. In a housing estate in Kaiserslautern, Germany, a touch screen tablet-PC called PAUL (Personal Assistive Unit for Living), numerous sensors and an EIB/KNX-Bus were installed in 20 apartments. Within the framework of the project "Assisted Living", Urban Sociologists from the University of Kaiserslautern analyzed the elderly people's experiences and acceptance of the implemented home automation devices, especially of the tablet-PC over a period of two years of usage. Besides technical aspects social issues like community building are focused in the project. The main results of the project will be presented in the chapter.

INTRODUCTION

In aging societies, most elderly people wish to stay in their self-chosen-environment as long as possible, even if they experience a growing loss in quality of life and health problems. At the same time, the traditional system of care for the elderly ceases and the costs for professional care constantly grow. As a consequence, new social and technical solutions enabling elderly people to live independently as long as possible have to be developed.

Ambient Assisted Living (AAL) is seen as a promising contribution. But until now it is not clear which technological concepts and which single devices are of use for elderly people and are accepted at the same time. Apart from pilot projects AAL-technology is not prevalent in senior households. Housing companies and scientists who conducted pilot projects often experience

DOI: 10.4018/978-1-60960-469-1.ch009

disappointments, because the needs of elderly people are not considered adequately.

Therefore, the objective of the project "Assisted Living" is to directly involve the target group into the development process of an Ambient Assisted Living system. In the German city of Kaiserslautern a housing estate was equipped with scores of technical solutions from the field of home automation which aim to assist elderly people. The original project "Assisted Living" was conducted until March 2009 by the Institute of Automatic Control (Prof. Dr. Lothar Litz and Dipl.-Ing. Martin Floeck) and the Research Area for Urban Sociology (Prof. Dr. Annette Spellerberg, Dipl.-Soz. Jonas Grauel and Dipl.-Ing. Lynn Schelisch) at the University of Kaiserslautern. The project was funded by the Ministry of Finance of Rhineland-Palatinate and the housing societies BauAG Kaiserslautern, Gemeindliche Siedlungs-Gesellschaft Neuwied mbH and Gemeinnützige Baugenossenschaft Speyer eG. We would like to thank our partners for their kind support.

The impact and success of all technological features implemented in the project in Kaiserslautern were assessed by sociologists: To gather feedback about elderly people's experiences and acceptance of the technical devices, as well as to find out how technology supports their everyday life, the tenants were interviewed ahead of and while using the new technical devices two months after moving in and again one and a half year later. By bringing in the user perspective, potential improvements can be pointed out.

However, the vision of AAL in this project is not purely technologically oriented. Living in the social community with neighbors and preserving this integration are as well considered crucial factors for a high standard of living, regardless of the health situation. Hence, all technological development is accompanied by sociological research and support, helping to build a good community spirit.

The aim of this paper is to present the most important outcomes of the social research regarding the technological aspects of the project. First, we will shortly describe the applied concept and then we will present the experiences and habits of elderly people using the technical devices implemented in the housing estate in Kaiserslautern. Concluding, we suggest some new pathways AAL-projects should take.

BACKGROUND

Technical solutions facilitating independent living have not become accepted very well yet. There are various reasons: they are often intricately to use, are unattractive, appear stigmatizing, require a lot of technology expertise, and in particular, are too expensive (Meyer & Schulze, 2008; Mollenkopf & Kaspar, 2004; Mollenkopf, Oswald & Wahl 2007). In addition, there is also a great deal of restraint on the part of the landlords from the housing industry to invest in technical solutions.

A new batch can yet be expected, namely for four reasons: First, regarding energy costs, which suggest optimal heating, especially in tight pensions, and require intelligent sensors. Second, due to health reasons, because the health risks grow with higher life expectancy. Prevention, security and care itself, may be supported by technology and telemedicine. Third, the technical equipment regarding home appliances and the media is getting more advanced. The technical competence of the elderly is increasing. Therefore, fourthly, it is likely that technical solutions to facilitate independent living are accepted, if they are affordable (BIS & DZFA, 2002; Research Institute for Gerontology, 2006).

There are very wide-ranging approaches for technical solutions for living, which are known under the heading of "smart home", "smart neighborhood" and Multimedia-Services. In about 60 pilot projects across the EU smart-home concepts with so-called ambient technology is tested. In this case, ambient means a technological environment which is intelligent, but not necessarily

Figure 1. The housing estate in Kaiserslautern

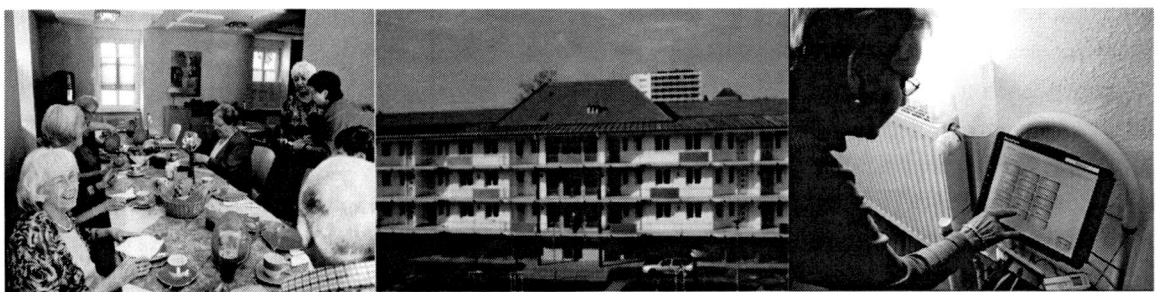

noticeable, and adapts to the daily lives of users. This includes networks of various switches and sensors in the homes and also special equipment for video phone, tele-health-monitoring, terminal for house control, emergency calls with services, central switches that turn off certain power sockets or community portals. These solutions require BUS-systems in the homes, or more recently, wireless and cable connections. The vast majority of the pilot projects represent laboratories, model homes or research houses. Only in nine out of the mentioned 60 projects technology is used in everyday life of elderly people in their private homes (Meyer & Schulze, 2008) – one of it being the project presented in the following.

"ASSISTED LIVING" IN KAISERSLAUTERN

The Housing Estate and its Residents

In the city of Kaiserslautern the construction of a housing estate with 20 barrier-free apartments was completed in November 2007 by a local housing society (BauAG Kaiserslautern). Besides 16 two-room apartments and two three-room apartments, a one-family house, a guest apartment and a recreation room belong to the building. It is located near the city center of Kaiserslautern and is integrated in a good infrastructure (several doctors, a farmer's market, shopping facilities and a park). The apartments are reached via an access balcony, which also serves as a place of communication for the residents. Many tenants have set up plants, tables and chairs in front of their entrances.

The housing society selected the tenants according to their interest in the housing community and in the use of technology. At the last survey, 25 residents lived in 19 households. The housing estate initially was planned as multigenerational housing, yet a thorough intermix with people of all ages could not be reached: most of the residents are aged over 60 years, but the tenants also include a number of middle-aged adults and a young family with three children. 17 of the 22 adult residents are female.

The majority of the residents (16 out of 21 interviewed) state, that they have health problems, including one third, which is restricted because of their health status and cannot participate in all (outside) activities. According to the tenants, there have been "four emergencies" since the move in. Despite the relatively high number of people with health problems, four fifths of the respondents mentioned to leave the house every day and can maintain moderate mobility.

Computers and the Internet can be regarded as key technologies for a variety of modern technological applications (Mollenkopf & Kaspar, 2004) and are hence good criteria for technology expertise. More than half of the interviewed tenants use computers or have done so in the past (for example at work). 12 of the 21 interviewed tenants currently own and use a computer, including four of them who have bought a computer only since moving into the apartment. Almost half of the tenants over 60 years of age own a computer. Accordingly, for the present age structure, the technology expertise of residents is disproportionately high. In recent surveys, the fraction of the computer and Internet users above 60 years of age composed between 10% and 20% (Doh & Kaspar, 2006; Korupp & Szydlik, 2005; Grauel & Spellerberg, 2007).

The computer course, which was organized by the tenants in the recreation room, is primarily attended by the ones who have a new computer. Most of the residents own a mobile phone and two thirds use it regularly. Also, more than half of the residents above 60 years of age use mobile phones. In case of problems and questions regarding technical issues, all residents know whom to ask for help, in most cases family members, but also work colleagues and neighbors.

The aim of the project is to not only promote a technical assistance, but also foster social integration through an active community and integration in the neighborhood. Therefore, emphasis is placed on community building in addition to the technical concept of the project. The project is accompanied by a community building process, moderated by the Research Area for Urban Sociology, whose aim is to achieve an active community and its involvement in the surrounding neighborhood. At monthly tenants meetings, the residents discuss the house rules, arrange joint activities in the recreation room and come up with ideas how the technical concept may be developed further.

Already a few weeks after moving in, the residents formed a community: they organize a café on Tuesdays as well as excursions, watch TV together and take care of each other. Trust is built through the community building process, which is essential to the further utilization of the technical potential in the apartments: For example, emergency calls can be sent to neighbors who can be trusted and who have a key to the apartment. In addition a so called district manager ("Quartiers-

manager") is involved in the process and brings ideas to involve the tenants in the surrounding neighborhood.

Technical Concept of the Project

All apartments are equipped with an EIB/KNX-Bus, several sensors to detect activity of the tenant (e.g. motion detectors, indication of water usage) and the touch screen tablet-PC called "PAUL" (Personal Assistive Unit for Living) which is core element of the AAL environment and was developed by the Institute of Automatic Control (Brinkmann, Floeck & Litz, 2008). There is a door camera, which shows the picture of visitors in front of the building, including a visitor's register. When leaving the apartment, a LED-light indicates open windows and a switch offers the possibility to turn off certain plugs (e.g. the oven plug). All lights and shutters in the apartment can be remote controlled. The front door can be opened by an automatic door key (transponder).

With this equipment, multiple functions in the areas of comfort, safety and security can be covered. For example the plug switch and the open window indication enhance safety, while the door camera offers protection against tricksters and the remote-controlled shutters improve comfort. Additionally, PAUL offers the possibility to access specific internet sites, a choice of music, certain radio stations and TV channels and includes an alarm clock. Other functions like PAUL-to-PAUL communication or memory training games will be implemented in a later phase.

Next to comfort, safety and security, health issues are also aspired to be covered in the future. Therefore, an approach to detect critical situations like downfalls (inactivity based alarm generation system) was developed by the Institute of Automatic Control (Floeck & Litz 2009) and implemented in some of the apartments as tests. Further information on this approach, see below.

Figure 2. Main Menu of PAUL

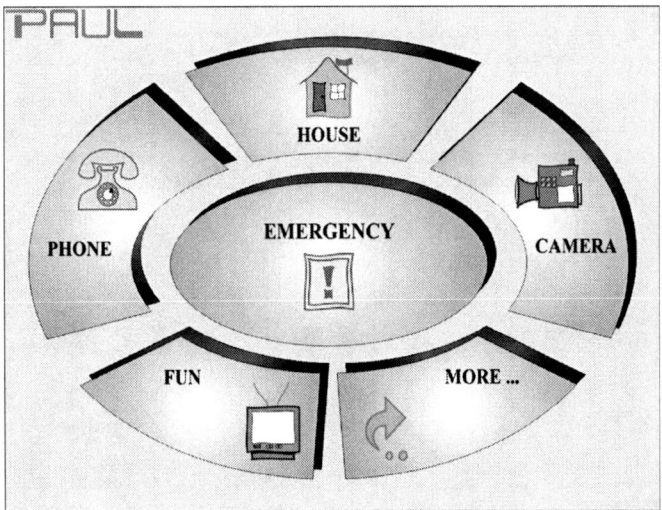

Personal Assistive Unit for Living

All the described functions in the fields of comfort, safety, security and entertainment can be operated via PAUL's touch screen: The tenants can monitor the state of the apartment, control the automation devices and access additional functions in the fields of communication and entertainment. There is one PAUL in each apartment. The aim of its user interface (Figure 2) is to make the handling as easy as possible for elderly people.

A menu with up to three layers was chosen. Large buttons and symbols ensure good perceptibility (Figure 3). To find out whether the user interface is suitable for the target group of senior citizens, a test was carried out in June of 2007 (Grauel & Spellerberg, 2008). Senior citizens were asked to perform different tasks (for example, "Please close all shutters" or "Play a music piece"). As the aim was to test if PAUL is intuitively to understand, no introduction to the operation was given. The test persons were then asked about their impressions. Seven of the eight test persons were able to complete the tasks without any problems. For them, the user interface is well designed. The symbols were judged to be intuitively to understand and nice to look at, the

fonts were assessed readable; also colors and contrast between symbols, buttons and background were judged as good.

Unlike the switches on the wall, all shutters in the apartment can be operated via PAUL individually. Because the usability should be as simple as possible, no external or on-screen-keyboard is used. To keep the handling intuitive, the internet options of PAUL are limited to a selection of information websites like weather forecast, bus schedule, theater and cinema programs, news ticker and so on.

Current features of PAUL (state of October 2009):

- control of technical devices in the apartment (shutters, lights, opening of the front door)
- operation of the door camera, including the visitor's register, showing guests the tenants have missed
- LED-indication for open windows
- switch to turn off certain plugs
- Internet access to certain websites (e.g. housing society, City of Kaiserslautern, theater, movie theater, weather, news, bus timetable, Deutsche Bahn)

Figure 3. Submenu for house features

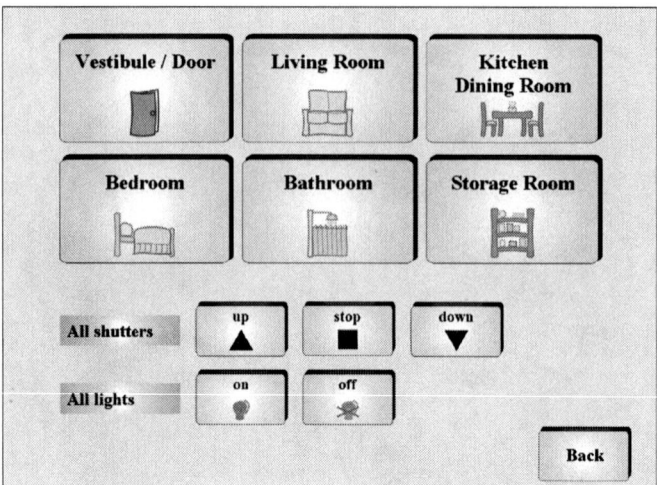

- choice of music
- reception of certain radio stations
- alarm clock
- clock
- picture gallery with pictures of the tenants (since summer 2008)
- TV channels (since fall 2009)
- server for collecting the signals from the sensors (see Figure 4).

The possibility of calling the telephone helpline of a medical provider (MD Medicus) using the "Help"-button was phased out after several months of testing. The residents could not relate to the anonymous service and although it was free of charge, they feared cost. By switching it off, their concern was reduced to accidentally press the button. Also the shopping list and memo function were removed, since there was no way to print the notes.

PAUL: EXPERIENCES IN EVERYDAY LIFE

The project aimed at evaluation of the requirements, experiences and acceptance of technical solutions. Therefore, the project is supervised by social research in order to determine the perspective of the users. The results of the concomitant research were directly taken into account for the ongoing development of PAUL.

A first evaluation of PAUL, which mainly focused on its usability, took place in May 2007, when a model apartment was completed. However the results have restricted validity only as all test persons (7, between 60 and 76 years of age) were "normally aging" persons without any specific health impairments and had an above-average technical competence for their age, too.

Two months after implementing the technical devices in all apartments (February 2008) and again eight months later (October 2008) the residents were questioned about their experiences and usage of the tablet-PC and the other home automation devices. The initial interview was carried out in a face-to-face situation, supplemented by a participant observation. 19 people were interviewed. The latest survey was carried out in October 2009, nearly two years after the tenant's moving in. 18 of 19 households (21 of 25 people) were reached.

This latest survey focused on the evaluation, whether and to which extend the acceptance and

Figure 4. Footprint of an apartment with sensors

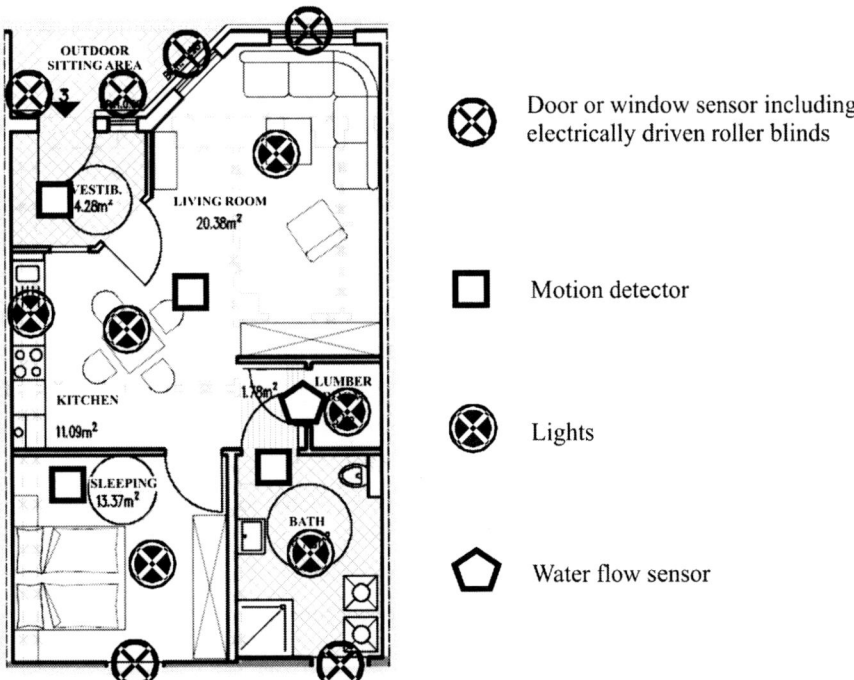

appropriation of AAL technology changed after two years of use, and also how the tenants value the technological devices, the apartment itself, the living environment and the neighborhood. The survey was conducted using guideline-based interviews. In addition, 16 people were observed while using PAUL. We would like to thank Mr. Guido Höffner, Director of the housing society BauAG Kaiserslautern for the kind support and the Stiftung Gesundheitsfürsorge as well as the Ministry of Finance, Rhineland-Palatinate, Germany for financing the tenant survey.

This chapter mainly contains the results of the third survey and focuses on the usage and acceptance of the technology used in the apartments. Comparisons with the survey in February 2008 can be made to a limited extent only, as not all tenants participated in both surveys: Two tenants have only participated in the survey in February 2008, five only in the one in October 2009.

Usability and Location of PAUL

The majority of residents got accustomed operating PAUL. Except for two interviewees, all observed manage to operate PAUL without any problems. 14 out of 16 residents quickly find the options on the menu bar and handle the tasks with ease. An elderly woman, most likely suffering from incipient dementia, is not able to operate any functions of PAUL by herself – even though she was able doing so during the first survey one and a half year earlier. Another younger, physically impaired woman, has to repeatedly tap on the screen (she uses the finger) until the corresponding action is executed. She frequently misses the right spot and needs time to select the correct menu, but can cope without outside help. She does not mention how often she uses PAUL.

The fact that PAUL is operated with ease by most of the tenants also corresponds to the statements of some interviewees that PAUL would not react quickly enough to their commands:

"Ich komme damit gut zurecht, doch. Wirklich. Ich bin manchmal ein bisschen zu schnell." (I'm getting along with it well. Really. I'm sometimes a bit too fast.)

In the survey in February 2008 all interviewees, except for one man suffering from dementia, were able to control PAUL independently. As in the survey of 2008, the recent results ratify the presumption of the survey of 2007 (Grauel & Spellerberg, 2008), that elderly people without mental disorders can utilize PAUL's user interface well, whereas it might be too complicated for forgetful persons.

All apartments are equipped with two power stations for PAUL, one in the bedroom and another in the combined kitchen and living room area. PAUL can be carried from one station to the other. Thereby it should be ensured that some functions are not devalued and the risk of a power-breakdown is at least minimized. In the majority of visited households (13 out of 18) PAUL is installed in the living room, the place where the tenants spend most of their time during the day. The number of households having PAUL in the living has even increased since the last survey. In only one sixth of the households PAUL is situated permanently in the bedroom. One tenant uses PAUL both in the bedroom and living room. Many respondents refuse to install PAUL in the sleeping room, as they find the ventilation noise distracting or are afraid of radiation.

Use of Different Features of PAUL

Frequency of Use

Two-thirds of the surveyed tenants (14 out of 20) use PAUL on a daily basis, whereas the intensity of use varies. The attribute of using PAUL daily was also assigned, if the interviewees mentioned to use the door camera each time (even if the door bell would not ring every day). Five tenants state they would use PAUL "every now and then" or

"sometimes". Amongst them is one who claims to use PAUL every now and then, however, the observation showed, that she cannot handle PAUL. Another tenant has deactivated the device at present: Although she indicates to use PAUL "sometimes" she is currently assigned as (the only) nonuser, especially as she had PAUL disconnected in the last survey as well.

Four interviewees indicate that they use some features of PAUL "for fun", without wanting to utilize a particular technical device or looking for specific information in the Internet. All of them are counted among the group of daily users.

"Die Bilder, ja, die habe ich mir schon öfters angeguckt, ja. Das ist halt wenn ich mal so sonntags, wenn kein Wetter ist und ich habe Langeweile, dann gucke ich mir so die Bilder an. Das ist ganz schön." (The pictures, yes, I have already looked at then several times, yes. That's when the weather is not so good on Sundays and I am bored, then I look at the pictures. That's quite nice.).

For some of the respondents the technical equipment does not (yet) play a very important role, but they see the technical support to be important once they get older.

Door Camera, Door Opener and Visitor's Register

16 out of 19 interviewees mention to look at the door camera at least from time to time when the door bell rings. However, only half of them use the door camera every time. Another four do not specify how frequently they use the camera. Despite the woman who has disconnected PAUL, another two residents state, that they never use the door camera.

It is possible to open the front door via a switch on the regular interphone or by PAUL. Four users of the door camera indicate explicitly that they open the front door with PAUL. It is likely, that more of those using the door camera to see who is in front the door, also use PAUL to open the door.

Out of the 15 respondents who mention the use of the visitor's register, 13 actually use this function. Two do not use it, including the one having PAUL deactivated. Among the users of the register there are three tenants who do not always look at the door camera and the person who never looks at the door camera.

PAUL's functions door camera and the visitor's register are the most important features for four tenants each.

Interviewer: „Und die schauen Sie auch an die Besucherliste?"

Mann: „Ja, das ist ja das Wichtigste vom Ganzen."

(Interviewer: And you also look at the visitor's register?

Man: Yes, that's the most important of it all.).

Electric Shutters

Six tenants mention the electric shutters to be the most important technical device in the apartment. 14 out of 18 state to actuate the shutters via PAUL at least occasionally. Four do not use this option. The possibility to adjust the shutters individually via PAUL is the reason for six tenants to use PAUL instead of the switches on the wall. In addition, three interviewees mention the possibility to leave the shutters ajar or rather to bring the shutter to stop at any point when operated by PAUL as an advantage. Due to the fact, that the shutters can be controlled individually via PAUL, this option is primarily used in summer:

"(...) Da muss ich ihnen sagen, im Sommer brauche ich den PAUL. Ich habe ja da keinen Balkon drüber und das heißt, da ist volle Pulle Sonne und dann muss ich ja diesen Rollladen öfter mal runter machen, den [Rollladen] brauche ich nicht so, aber den da und da brauche ich den PAUL dazu. Nämlich wenn ich den Knopf dort betätige, gehen beide runter und dann habe ich ja dunkel." *(I have to tell you, in summer I need PAUL. I don't have a balcony above and that means there's a lot of sun and then I have to close the shutters. I don't need this (shutter), but that one and I need PAUL for it. Because when I use the switch over there, both go down and then it's dark.).*

One person states, that she operates the shutters by using PAUL only in the living room, as this is the place PAUL is located. Most likely other tenants also act that way.

Picture Gallery

The picture gallery includes pictures of the tenants' conjoint activities. 12 out of 15 interviewees state to look at the gallery from time to time, including the one who cannot handle PAUL. Another one only looks at the pictures with guests. Three tenants mention, that the pictures could be updated more often.

Frau: Bilder natürlich, unser Lieblings-Dingens. Die Bilder von unseren Ausflügen, da kann man verschiedene Sachen ansehen.

Interviewer: Die gucken sie sich auch regelmäßig an?

Frau: Naja, nun habe ich alle schon so oft gesehen.

(Women: Pictures, of course, our favorite thingy. The pictures of our trips, you can see different things.

Interviewer: Do you look at them regularly?

Woman: Well, I've seen all of them so many times.)

Internet

Just over the half of the respondents (11 out of 21) visit PAUL's selected internet pages, including five out of twelve tenants owning a computer. Six out of nine not using an own computer take a look at the web pages via PAUL. Three tenants – all female and over 75 years of age – neither own a computer nor use the Internet via PAUL. One tenant mentions the small font as the reason for not using the Internet via PAUL. In other cases, the selected web pages are not considered as "the Internet", as the access is limited.

"Wo ich gucke ist Internet, aber da auch nur, was gibt es im Kino, weil er ist für mich auch relativ mühsam, sagen wir doch schon zeitintensiv, bis ich was..., weil ich keine Tastatur habe, ich kann ja nichts aufrufen, ich kann nur das verwenden was vorgegeben ist, das ist sehr eingeschränkt." *(I look at the Internet, but only in the movies, because it is relatively difficult for me, let's say time consuming, until I..., because I don't have a keyboard, I can't access anything, I can only use what is given which is very limited.).*

The most popular web page is the weather forecast (8 of 11), followed by internet portals of newspapers and newscasts (7 of 11). Other internet pages are less frequently used: magazines (3), movies / theater (3), BauAG (2) and Deutsche Bahn (1). Three respondents say they only access the weather page; one person only visits the news pages. For one tenant, reading the news via PAUL is less convenient than holding a newspaper. For another tenant this is only an option in case of being bedridden:
„Die Rheinpfalz. Na die kriege ich morgens im Briefkasten, dann lese ich sie nicht hier [über PAUL]. Aber wenn man krank ist und liegt im Bett, kann man sie hier auch lesen. Das ist gar nicht so schlecht." *(The Rheinpfalz [local newspaper]. Well, I get it in my mailbox every morning, then I don't read it here [via Paul]. But if you're sick*

and lying in bed, you can also read it here. That's not so bad.).

Radio and Music

Eight out of 20 respondents mention to listen to the radio via PAUL from time to time. The possibility of listening to the selected pieces of music is only used by one tenant. 14 state not to use this function. One tenant would listen to the radio and music pieces, if the sound could be turned on louder. In most cases, the reason for not using the functions is the fact, that the tenants own another radio receiver or a hi-fi system, respectively:

„(...) Aber ich habe ja einen Fernseher und habe eine Stereoanlage, da brauche ich ja nicht die Musik und den PAUL für das." *(But I have a TV-set and a stereo system, then I don't need the music and PAUL for it.).*

Some also mention that the selected choice of music is not diversified enough:

"Musik höre ich [über PAUL] nicht. Das ist auch immer dasselbe." *(I don't hear music [via Paul]. That's always the same.).*

Light Control

Six out of 18 respondents say they control the light in the apartment occasionally by using PAUL, yet no one uses PAUL for this function regularly. Twelve never use the light control. An explanation is only given in one case, why this function is operated via PAUL that rarely: the tenant prefers to turn off and on the lights by using the switch at the wall:

"(...) Licht an und aus, das mache ich lieber alles noch selbst. Das ist wenn man es mal nicht mehr so kann. Also da brauche ich den PAUL nicht dazu für Licht an und aus oder Tür auf und zu,

das mache ich noch selbst." (Light on and off, I still prefer to do everything by myself. That's when you can't do it anymore. I don't need PAUL for light on and off or door open or close, I do it by myself.).

TV

Only a few weeks before the survey took place in October 2009, the TV function at PAUL was activated. It is possible to receive certain TV channels, if a corresponding cable is attached to PAUL. There is a cable connection (socket) for receiving TV channels in all living areas (living room, bedroom and third room, if existing). However, during the interviews it became apparent, that at least three tenants had not noticed so far, that PAUL includes a TV.

Only two tenants point out to watch TV using PAUL, though in one case it does not become clear how often. One tenant uses the TV function on a regular basis (several times a week) in her bedroom, in case she cannot fall asleep.

"Ja. Ich gucke ab und zu im Schlafzimmer, weil ich schlafe so schlecht ein und dann hilft das manchmal." (Yes. I sometimes watch in the bedroom, because I fall asleep so badly and then sometimes it helps.).

Another three tenants mention that they would use the TV function in future, in case they become bedridden and partly have already connected the cable.

„Ja, der [Fernseher an PAUL] ist angeschlossen [...], ich brauche es ja jetzt nicht, aber ich rechne damit, wenn ich mal ein paar Tage im Bett liegen würde..., es ist ja nur so ein kleines Bild, aber es würde vielleicht ganz angenehm sein. [...] Das ist jetzt alles gerichtet, wenn ich mal ein paar Tage im Bett liegen sollte, dass ich mir das anschließen kann. (...) ich nutze ihn jetzt nicht, aber es ist beruhigend, ach, dann könnte ich ihn benutzen."

(Yes, the [television at PAUL] is connected [...], I don't need it now, but I reckon that when I have to lie in bed for a couple of days..., it's only a small screen, but it might be quite pleasant. [...] It's now ready if I have to lie in bed a couple of days, that I can connect it then. (...) I don't use it now, but it's comforting to know, I could use it then.).

The fact that the screen of PAUL is too small is mentioned as an explanation for not using the TV function. Many tenants have modern flat screen TVs.

Alarm Clock

Only one out of 21 respondents state to set the alarm clock at PAUL. Ten say they make no use of it. Another ten do not comment on the alarm; however one can emanate from the fact that no one of them used the alarm in the last survey, that they still do not use it.

Important Technical Features

Not all residents were asked about which technical features in the apartment are particularly important to them, and also some respondents could not give a precise answer. Besides, all answers were given spontaneously. Therefore, at this point, only a set of opinions can be given, about the importance of technology in their homes. Nine of 14 respondents mentioned one or more technical features which are particularly important. The most frequent (6 responses) are the electric shutters, although is it not clear in every case, whether the responses apply to automatic shutters in general, or specifically those controlled by PAUL. Next follow the door camera (4), and the visitor's register (2). In the course of the interview a couple mentioned that the door camera and the visitor's register were most important to them. The light control, the radio and the picture gallery were mentioned once each. Other answers include the electric door openers in the hallway as well as the low heating costs.

„Also mir ist besonders wichtig, dass ich weiß wer vor meiner Haustür steht, ja, wen ich rein lassen kann, ob jemand da war wenn ich nicht gerade zu Hause war, war das wichtig jetzt. Und das ist mir eigentlich wirklich das Allerwichtigste. (...)" (Well, to me it is very important, that I know who is at my front door, yes, who I can let in, if someone was there when I was not at home, that's important now. And that's really most important to me).

Future Add-On Functions of Paul

It is aimed to install additional features to PAUL for tenants, who ask for further functions. During the process of the project, the residents were asked for further ideas. At the time of the interviews in October 2009 two new functions – an inactivity based alarm generation system and an in house communication system – were tested in some apartments. The tenants were also asked about their stance on both systems and whether they would like to have them implemented or not.

Inactivity Based Alarm Generation

Next to comfort, safety and security, health issues are also aspired to be covered in future. Therefore, an approach to detect critical situations like downfalls was developed by the Institute of Automatic Control (Floeck and Litz, 2009). Starting in October 2009, a methodology for deriving alarms in cases of unexpected inactivity in senior citizens' homes was implemented in some of the tenant's apartments. Instead of sensors worn on the body, a state of the art home automation installation is chosen as technical base. The incoming signals are interpreted as human activity leading to activity profiles. For a straightforward alarm generation a new type of profile based on inactivity patterns is defined. Their advantages are used to establish an alarm generation con-

cept. If a person is in the apartment, but there is no activity for a certain period of time, PAUL is able to send out a telephone call automatically to the tenant's apartment. Reacting, the person can easily clarify false alarms. If nobody answers, PAUL initiates a telephone chain, according to the tenants declaration, e.g. to neighbors, relatives or an emergency center, asking for help. To get the information needed to create the activity profiles, activities like movements, the usage of PAUL, light switches and water are registered on the tablet-PC. For research purposes, to develop appropriate software, data is transferred to the Technical University. For a detailed description of this approach see (Floeck and Litz, 2009b).

A total of 17 respondents (out of 18) indicate that the inactivity based alarm generation is a good system. Even without being asked, two tenants mention the alarm generation to be an important function which should be implemented as soon as possible. Eight of the supporters, including two couples, restrict however, that they do not see the system as useful for themselves, but for other – solitarily living – people. Only one younger tenant is afraid of surveillance and thus is against the alarm generation. The other tenants do not mention fears because of surveillance or heteronomy. Nevertheless, some of the tenants question, if the system will work. During the interviews the concept of the inactivity detection had to be explained to four residents.

Although one respondent is skeptical about whether and how the inactivity based alarm generation exactly works, she sees advantages over other emergency detection systems, if the emergency transmission goes to the neighbors, who have access to the apartment. In her opinion, the advantage lies in the fact that the person in need does not have to actively call for help, but the call is sent automatically.

Communication via Paul

The application to communicate via PAUL-to-PAUL within the housing estate was in the test stage during the interviews. 13 out of 21 respondents would use this option and see special benefits, for example to make arrangements for grocery shopping.

"Das fände ich ganz klasse, also das fände ich drückt dem Ganzen noch einmal einen anderen Stempel auf. Wenn ich mir überlege, jemand geht samstags morgens Brötchen holen und schickt schnell über PAUL: „Ich gehe Brötchen holen, wer will was?" Oder, keine Ahnung. Ich glaube, das kommt ganz gut an, das wäre wirklich so ein ganz großes Ding, wenn das mal klappen würde." (I think this would be very great, I think that would leave another mark on the whole thing. When I think about someone going to get rolls on Saturday morning and quickly leaving a message on PAUL: "I'm going to get rolls. Who wants something?" Or, I don't know. I think that would go down well, that would be really a big thing, if that would work out.).

Three tenants are not fully positive about the idea, but would possibly test the function. Four tenants are quite skeptical and would rather not use the function. One resident would definitely not us the application, as she rather talks to people face-to-face.

„Möchte ich eigentlich nicht, ich meine, wenn ich mich mit jemanden unterhalten will, dann will ich ihn angucken, von Person zu Person, also nicht über Computer, das muss ich nicht haben." (I don't really want that, I mean, if I want to talk to someone, then I want to look at him, from face to face, not via a computer, I don't have to have that.).

All of the ones, not wanting or rather not wanting to use the communication via PAUL are 63 years old or younger. During the interviews two respondents mentioned that they are skeptical whether the communication will work.

Suggestions for Improving Paul

The tenants did not express a lot of suggestions for the improvement of PAUL. This could be due to the fact that their imagination is limited in how to construct new technologies. But the suggestions in the recent survey are little more diversified than those in February 2008. When asked, suggestions for improvements and / or requests for additional features of PAUL were mentioned by only half of the respondents. These were: games (3), keyboard (2), possibility to open windows via PAUL (2), emergency call (2), improved audio output (2), brain calisthenics (1), drug plan (1), in house communication via PAUL (1), voice entry (1), and WLAN (1). For some users the diameter of the touch screen is undersized to watch TV. Three tenants complain about the noise (humming) of PAUL. This is also the reason for one tenant, having PAUL removed from the bedroom:

"Ich habe ihn eigentlich hier raus gestellt, weil er mir im Schlafzimmer zu laut war. (...) Das Geräusch, das konnte ich nicht haben." (I actually took it out here, because it was too loud for me in my bedroom. (...) The noise, I could not stand that.).

Types of Acquirement

In general, PAUL is highly accepted and after almost two years of using, PAUL is integrated in most of the tenants' everyday life. However, the interviews and the observations showed that the tenants use PAUL in different ways. The process of acquirement is not homogeneous. There are tenants who show no or only little interest in technology, but use certain features of PAUL (shutters, door camera). Others show an intense acquirement and use (almost) all functions. Concerning the degree of interest in new technology, the number of used tasks and the frequency of utilization, the tenants can be assigned to three different types of use: creative acquirement, pragmatically use and disuse. For a more detailed description see (Grauel et al., 2008).

The tenants belonging to the type of "creative acquirement" are especially technophile. For acquisition they apply the trial-and-error method in an independent and creative manner. They use the majority of the offered functions including the internet-feature. Furthermore they propose additional options for use. For this group, PAUL is a valuable contribution to their everyday life, as it offers diversion, it is convenient and new actions can be learned. Nine out of 21 users are assigned to this type, six women and three men.

The tenants matching the type of "pragmatically use" apply only some selected tasks which he or she judges to the best advantage, such as the door camera or the remote-controlled shutters. These persons do not use the other functions regularly. This group also judges PAUL as a surplus but the enthusiasm is considerably lower than in the first group. Ten out of 21 users are assigned to this type, six women and two men.

The ideal type of "disuse" does not use PAUL at all or solely to show it to visitors. So PAUL is of little importance to this group. Two female tenants match this group.

Since the survey in February 2008 some classifications of the tenants' acquirement have changed: One former nonuser is now added to the type of creative acquirement. Her PAUL was defective and could not be used in the first survey, but is now used very frequently and diverse. One man, formerly matched to the type of pragmatically use now uses a couple of more functions and thus could be added to the group of creative acquirement, however, he still does not use the Internet via PAUL. A woman who was formerly assigned to the type of pragmatically use, cannot operate PAUL anymore due to health impairment and is thus belongs to the type of disuse. Two tenants (one male and one female) have changed

from creative acquirement to pragmatically use, as they now use fewer functions, both including the Internet. The woman has bought a new computer (her first one) and obviously finds it more attractive than PAUL. The man does not use the alarm clock, the Internet and the radio anymore. A total of five of the 16 tenants, who have participated in both surveys (February 2008 and October 2009), have changed their acquirement type: two use PAUL more diverse, three less.

Further Use of Home Automation

Besides the questions about the usage of PAUL, the tenants were also asked about the other installed home automation devices. The LED-indication for open windows is stated as useful by most tenants. Almost two thirds (12 out of 19) of the tenants take a look at the LED-indication for open windows every time they leave the apartment and react accordingly. Another four notice the light, but leave the windows open. Despite the fact that half of the surveyed residents (11 out of 21) state to use the switch to unplug certain plugs, only two households (3 persons) actually do so every time they leave the house. Two residents actuate the switch every night before bedtime, nine when leaving the house for a longer period of time, e.g. for several days. For some tenants, the switch is considered needless because no necessity to turn off plugs during absence is seen; others unplug all devices manually after using and thus feel safe. The two devices have gained importance over time: more people now look at the LED light and actuate the power switch, than one and a half years earlier.

The smoke detectors were scarcely noticed by the tenants and were considered as nothing special. However, 15 out of 17 interviewed tenants reply on demand, that the smoke detectors in the apartments are very good and important to them. Three of them explicitly specify that they provide security. The automatic door key for the front door is being used by all but two surveyed tenants. The transponder is not stated as a necessity, but as a convenient amenity, which is used also by the ones who are not physically impaired. Several tenants feel disturbed by the ceiling light in the corridor, which is attached to a motion detector and apparently switches on more often than desired. 11 out of 18 households have already switched off the automatic light or plan on doing so in the near future.

Comparison: Use of PAUL in the Course of Time

A comparison of the number of users in the recent survey (October 2009) to the first one in February 2008 is not always possible in detail, as for some functions there are only a small number of statements. As not all features were implemented in the first survey, an evaluation of the change of use was not possible for the TV and the picture gallery. A comparison of the users of the light control is not possible, due to the little number of users in February 2008. In addition, some tenants were not able to use all functions in February 2008 because they were malfunctioning, but operated well during the recent survey (e.g. radio and door camera).

There are statements on the general use of PAUL for all three survey periods (February 2008, October 2008 and October 2009) of 14 tenants. Of these, twelve used PAUL in all survey periods. One stated to use PAUL "sometimes" or "rarely", respectively in all interviews. The one having PAUL disconnected in October 2009 also had him off power in October 2008 and rarely used the device in February 2008. Thus, within this group of 14 there were no significant changes in usage. The remaining residents did not participate in either survey period, so comparisons are not possible.

Altogether, the number of statements of actual users of the light control (+5), the electric shutter (+3), the radio (+2) and the door camera (+1) have increased. This might also be due to a greater number of respondents in the recent survey, and the fact that the tenants were explicitly asked about the functions more often. The total number of users of the alarm clock (-2) and Internet users (-1) have decreased. Although the total number of users of the internet has only decreased by one from February 2008 until October 2009 (12 to 11 users), there has been a great hidden change, as four former users no longer use PAUL's Internet.

If a closer look is taken to only those tenants, who have mentioning the devices in both surveys, one gets a slightly different outcome. In this case, none of the functions have gained users in total, while the compositions of the users of the door camera and the electric shutters have not changed at all. The Internet (-4), radio (-3), music (-2) and alarm clock (-2) forfeit users. It becomes evident that the functions have been integrated differently into the tenants' everyday life.

In brackets: number of tenants, mentioning the devices in both surveys.

Importance of Technology in every Day Use

17 tenants were asked whether they have the feeling that they can handle technical devices more assuredly than before they moved into the housing estate. While for four tenants it may be presumed from their answers only, just one gave a clear positive response. She explicitly specifies that she can handle technical devises more assuredly, as she now is more interested in technology. She retired shortly before moving in and recently bought a new laptop:

Interviewer: Und dass Sie sich jetzt einen Laptop angeschafft haben, haben Sie das Gefühl, dass Sie überhaupt seit Sie hier wohnen mit Technik besser umgehen können?

Frau: Ja, das interessiert mich jetzt mehr. Genau. Ja.

Table 1. Use of selected devices over the course of time (total times mentioned)

	February 2008		October 2009		change of use
	used	**(mentioned)**	**used**	**(mentioned)**	
door camera	15	(17)	16	(19)	+1
Internet	12	(18)	11	(21)	−1
electric shutters	11	(16)	14	(18)	+3
light control	1	(5)	6	(18)	+5
radio	6	(13)	8	(20)	+2

Table 2. Change of Users of selected devices over the course of time

	users Feb 08/Oct 09	change of users	change of non-users	change of users (total)
door camera (15)	14/14	+1	+1	—
Internet (15)	11/7	—	+4	−4
electric shutters (13)	10/10	—	—	—
alarm clock (7)	3/1	—	+2	−2
radio (7)	6/3	—	+3	−3
music (5)	2/0	—	+2	−2

(Interviewer: And now that you've bought a laptop, do you have the feeling that you can deal better with technology since you live here?

Woman: Yes, I'm now interested more in that. Exactly. Yes.).

Two say they now feel more assure or have learned more about technical approach. However, they justify this by saying that one constantly learns. Altogether twice as many respondents do not feel more assure operating the devices, than people saying they do. Different responses were given as reasons. Some say that the devices in the apartments were nothing special, that they could be operated intuitively and hence the learning effect is low. Others state that they have "always" handled technical devices with ease and therefore nothing changed.

„Ich habe davor alles gemacht, nein. Außer dem PAUL da jetzt, aber das ist ja nichts, nur da drauf

drücken und so, das ist ja keine Technik." (I've done everything before, no. Besides PAUL, but that's nothing, just pressing on it and so on, that's not technology.).

One tenant mentions her lack of interest in technology as a reason:

„Nein, nicht wirklich, weil ich halt mich nicht interessiere. Ich sage es wie es ist, es interessiert mich nicht. Ich interessiere mich für viele Sachen, aber ich brauch es auch nicht." (No, not really, because I'm not interested. I tell it like it is, I'm not interested. I'm interested in many things, but don't I need it.).

The majority of respondents indicate on demand, that the technical devices in the apartment currently help them in everyday life (12 out of 18).

The electric shutters, the elevator/accessibility, the automatic door openers, the central switch for light, the transponder and PAUL in general were mentioned as examples. Another four interviewees do not see a benefit in the devices yet, but in future in case they will be impaired somehow:

„Ja, also ich denke, wie gesagt, ich bräuchte es jetzt noch nicht. Aber es ist doch auch gut wenn man es braucht, dass man es dann kann. " (Yes, I think, as I said, I don't need it yet. But it's also good when you need it, that then you can do it.).

During the interview almost all respondents mentioned that they feel at home in the housing estate. Two thirds of the interviewees (13 out of 21) say that the technical devices play a role that they feel at home in the housing estate, six deny this, and two do not give a precise answer.

„ (...) nachdem ich hier eingezogen bin und habe gesehen was hier los ist an Technik, muss ich sagen, es ist eine Bereicherung. " (After I moved in here and saw what's going on with regard to technology, I must say it is an asset.).

As technical reasons for feeling at home, the electric shutters and light control, the automatic door opener and "security" were mentioned as examples. For some tenants the devices are on one hand some kind of compensation for age-related physical limitations and on the other hand they promote to the sense of security. For three tenants the technology is an easement in everyday life, yet it does not contribute to the fact that they feel at home.

The results of the surveys show, that all tenants feel at home in the apartment complex. However, in this context, technology does not play a determining role. Almost all responds concerning technical devices as reasons for "feeling at home" were given on demand only. Just one woman mentioned technology as a reason by herself. For the tenants, the implemented technical devices do not represent "technology", as they would think of technology being complicated and can only be understood using a manual. Instead, the

features are inconspicuously integrated into their everyday life and adopted playfully. The decisive factors for feeling at home are primarily the community, respectively the fact of not being alone (anymore) and the matter of fact that the tenants feel comfortable in their apartments and in the building, which again is predominantly due to the barrier-free design and the good quality of the apartments. Two thirds of the respondents call the house their (new) home. Furthermore, the tenants also judge the surrounding neighborhood (location within the city and the shops nearby) as being good.

FUTURE RESEARCH DIRECTIONS

Overall we can say that PAUL and the other home automation devices certainly contribute to the tenants' coping in everyday life and to the positive feeling of living. Unanswered remains how the handling and the use of technology change with the state of health, in particular mental limitations of age-related dementia. To what extend the implemented automation components, apart from the other components, can actually contribute to a longer, self-determined life in an own home cannot yet be answered. Home automation features and PAUL may be supplements, which increase comfort, security and information further. Whether they contribute effectively and independently to a conventionally-equipped home designed according to elderly persons' requirements to enable a longer life in their own homes still remains questionable, since the contribution for the physical impaired is small. The facilitation of everyday life as well as safety, entertainment and information aspects might allow for a quality enhancement rather than a temporal extension of independent living. The automatic generation of alarms using inactivity patterns, which is currently under development, would be a milestone in order to increase the sense of security for independent living of elderly people for the elderly themselves and their relatives.

PAUL does not yet provide communication channels to keep in touch with people already known. This may soon be reached by the implementation of the in house communication via PAUL. In addition, PAUL does not yet offer opportunities to get in touch with new people, as known from the many Web 2.0 communities and social software applications. Theoretically it is possible to display and use a keyboard, however, due to data protection and virus reasons the Internet was not fully opened up yet. Intuitively usable information technologies may, indeed, contribute to a further closure of the "digital divide" between young and old (Korupp & Szydlik, 2005).

Besides technical solutions it is still necessary to find specific forms of service organizations which fit into the professional care institutions. To reach broader acceptance and new steps towards a socio-technical support system it will be necessary to continue developing technology and accompanying service packages in close contact with the target group.

PAUL has now reached a level of development, in which it would be realizable practically and commercially. In the first phase of the Assisted-Living project, which started late 2007, PAUL was used by the residents of a housing estate in Kaiserslautern in their daily lives. It is now in a second phase, to expand the AAL-concept to older housing stock with the help of meanwhile fully developed wireless technologies.

CONCLUSION

In the project "Assisted Living" several home automation devices were implemented into apartments of elderly people. The described home automation concept offers many useful features which can be controlled by the single device, called PAUL. After two years of usage it becomes evident that the tenants do not have any problems with the usage of PAUL. Most of them have integrated PAUL and the other technological features in the apartment, which are important to them, well into their everyday life. Especially the use of the functions door camera, electric shutters and visitor's register became normal actions for the residents. However, different types of acquirement can be pointed out. It becomes apparent that the features of PAUL are used more by tenants, in case the features are not present otherwise in the apartment, or if they offer benefits other conventional devices do not offer (e.g. individual control of shutters, quick check of weather forecast and news on the Internet). Radio, music, alarm clock and television can usually be operated as well on other devices, which offer a better sound quality, more variety and a bigger screen than PAUL.

The tenants in Kaiserslautern are very satisfied with their living conditions. The main reasons are the suitable apartments that guarantee mobility and access to inner city infrastructure. Another important reason is the lively neighborhood with good personal relationships, high level of engagement and leisure activities. Living in the social community with neighbors and preserving this integration are as well considered crucial factors for a high standard of living, regardless of the health situation. Also the advanced technology including automatic lights, transponders to open the entrance door, low costs for energy and access balconies are positively evaluated. The usage of the touch screen-PC PAUL is less important for high satisfaction. For most it is seen as a convenient amenity, not a necessity. This might change, however, when the inactivity based alarm generation is implemented in all apartments and emergencies can be noticed more quickly. But nevertheless the advanced technology and PAUL are main topic in neighborhood talks. It is easier to talk about PAUL than about illnesses, grandchildren or family topics. One can assume that this fact also leads to a more frequent use of PAUL. And it is clearly noticeable that the feeling of being part of a scientific project, contributes to the satisfaction of the residents. In this sense technology is an important and positive factor for a newly composed neighborhood that grows together.

REFERENCES

BIS Berliner Institut für Sozialforschung. DZFA Deutsches Zentrum für Alternsforschung (Ed.) (2002). *Technik im Alltag von Senioren. Arbeitsbericht zur vertiefenden Auswertung der sentha-Repräsentativerhebung.* Heidelberg

Brinkmann, M., Floeck, M., & Litz, L. (2008). Concept and Design of an AAL home monitoring system based on a personal computerized assistive unit. In Mühlhäuser, M., Ferscha, A., & Aitenbichler, E. (Eds.), *Constructing Ambient Intelligence: AmI 2007 Workshops* (pp. 218–227). Berlin: Springer. doi:10.1007/978-3-540-85379-4_27

Doh, M., & Kaspar, R. (2006). Entwicklung und Determinanten der Internetdiffusion bei älteren Menschen. In Hagenah, J., & Meulemann, H. (Eds.), *Sozialer Wandel und Mediennutzung in der Bundesrepublik Deutschland* (pp. 139–156). Münster, Germany: LIT.

Floeck, M., & Litz, L. (2008). Lange selbstbestimmt leben mit geeigneter Hausautomatisierung und einem persönlichen technischen Assistenten. *Ambient Assisted Living, 1. Deutscher Kongress mit Ausstellung, 30.1.-1.2.2008.* (pp. S. 287 – 290). Berlin.

Floeck, M., & Litz, L. (2009). Inactivity Patterns and Alarm Generation in Senior Citizens' Houses. In *Proceedings of the European Control Conference (ECC) 2009, Budapest,* 26 August 2009.

Grauel, J., & Spellerberg, A. (2007). Akzeptanz neuer Wohntechniken für ein selbständiges Leben im Alter – Erklärung anhand sozialstruktureller Merkmale, Technikkompetenz und Technikeinstellungen. *Zeitschrift für Sozialreform, 53*(2), 191–215.

Grauel, J., & Spellerberg, A. (2008). Wohnen mit Zukunft - Soziologische Begleitforschung zu Assisted Living-Projekten. In E. Maier & P. Roux (Ed.), *Seniorengerechte Schnittstellen zur Technik: Zusammenfassung der Beiträge zum Usability Day VI, 16. Mai 2008* (pp. 36-43). Lengerich: Pabst Science Publishers.

Grauel, J., Spellerberg, A., Leschke, B., & Schelisch, L. (2008). Acceptance of Assisted Living Solutions. In R. Anderl, B. Arich-Gerz & R. Schmiede (Ed.), *Technologies of Globalization. Intenational Conference.* October 2008 (pp. 328-343). Darmstadt.

Korupp, S., & Szydlik, M. (2005). Causes and Trends of the Digital Divide. *European Sociological Review, 4,* 409–422. doi:10.1093/esr/jci030

Meyer, S., & Schulze, E. (2008). *Smart Home für ältere Menschen. Handbuch für die Praxis.* Berlin: Berliner Institut für Sozialforschung GmbH.

Mollenkopf, H., & Kaspar, R. (2004). Technisierte Umwelten als Handlungs- und Erlebensraeume aelterer Menschen. In Backes, G., Clemens, W., & Kuenemund, H. (Eds.), *Lebensformen und Lebensführung im Alter* (pp. 193–221). Wiesbaden: Verlag für Sozialwissenschaften.

Mollenkopf, H., Oswald, F., & Wahl, H.-W. (2007). Neue Personen-Umwelt-Konstellationen im Alter: Befunde und Perspektiven zu Wohnen, außerhäuslicher Mobilität und Technik. In Wahl, H.-W., & Mollenkopf, H. (Eds.), *Alternsforschung am Beginn des 21. Jahrhunderts: Alterns- und Lebenslaufkonzeptionen im deutschsprachigen Raum* (pp. 361–380). Berlin: AKA Verlag.

ADDITIONAL READING

Anliker, U., Ward, J. A., & Lukoicz, P. (2004). Impact of monitoring technology in assisted living: Outcome pilot. *Transactions On Information Technology in Biomedicine, 10*(1), 192–198.

Dalal, S., Alwan, M., Seifrafi, R., Kell, S., & Brown, D. (2005). *A Rule-Based Approach to the Analysis of Elders' Activity Data: Detection of Health and Possible Emergency Conditions.* Paper presented at the AAAI Fall Symposium.

Enste, P., Heinze, R., Hilbert, J., Naegele, G., & Schneiders, K. (2006). *Wohnen im Alter: Seniorenwirtschaft in Deutschland.* Dortmund: Forschungsgesellschaft für Gerontologie.

Floeck, M. & Litz, L. (2007). Ageing in Place: Supporting Senior Citizens' Independence with Ambient Assistive Living Technology. *mst|news* 6, 34-35.

Floeck, M., & Litz, L. (2008). Lange selbstbestimmt leben mit geeigneter Hausautomatisierung und einem persönlichen technischen Assistenten. *Ambient Assisted Living, 1. Deutscher Kongress mit Ausstellung, 30.1.-1.2.2008.* Berlin.

Friesdorf, W., & Heine, A. (Eds.). (2007). *Sentha. Seniorengerechte Technik im häuslichen Alltag.* Berlin: Springer Verlag. doi:10.1007/978-3-540-32818-6

Grauel, J., & Spellerberg, A. (2008). Attitudes and Requirements of Elderly People Towards Assisted Living Solutions. In Mühlhäuser, M., Ferscha, A., & Aitenbichler, E. (Eds.), *Constructing Ambient Intelligence. AmI 2007 Workshops Darmstadt, Revised Papers* (pp. 197–206). Berlin, Heidelberg: Springer Verlag.

Grauel, J., & Spellerberg, A. (2008). Soziologische Forschung im Kontext von Assisted Living. *Ambient Assisted Living, 1. Deutscher Kongress mit Ausstellung, 30.1.-1.2.2008* (pp. S. 73 – 78). Berlin: VDE Verlag.

Grauel, J., Spellerberg, A., & Schelisch, L. (2009). Ambient Assisted Living – ein erster Schritt in Richtung eines technisch-sozialen Assistenzsystems für ältere Menschen. *Hallesche Beiträge zu den Gesundheits- und Pflegewissenschaften,* 8(39), 5-19.

Hadidi, T., & Noury, N. (2009). A Predictive Analysis of the Night-Day Activities Level of Older Patient in a Health Smart Home. In *Proceedings of the 7th International Conference on Smart Homes and Health Telematics (ICOST '09)* (pp. 290-293). Berlin: Springer-Verlag.

Heinze, R., & Ley, C. (2009). *Vernetztes Wohnen: Ausbreitung, Akzeptanz und nachhaltige Geschäftsmodelle.* Bochum: InWIS. Retrieved March 30, 2010, from http://www.sowi.rub.de/mam/content/heinze/heinze/abschlussbericht_vernetzteswohnen.pdf

Jakobs, E. M., Lehnen, K., & Ziefle, M. (2008). *Alter und Technik. Studie zu Technikkonzepten, Techniknutzung und Technikbewertung älterer Menschen.* Aachen: Apprimus Verlag.

Kasper, R., Becker, S., & Mollenkopf, H. (2002). *Technik im Alltag von Senioren - Arbeitsbericht zu vertiefenden Auswertungen der BIS-Repräsentativerhebung (sentha: Senioren und Technik).* Heidelberg: BIS.

Krämer, S. (2005). Wohnen und Wohnen im Alter – heute. In Stiftung, W. (Ed.), *Wohnen im Alter* (pp. 40–68). Stuttgart: Karl Krämer Verlag.

Meyer, S., Böhm, U., & Röhrig, A. (2003). *Smart Home - Smart Aging. Akzeptanz und Anforderungen der Generation 50+. Vierter Smart Home Survey des BIS.* Berlin: BIS.

Oswald, F. (2002). Wohnbedingungen und Wohnbedürfnisse im Alter. In Schlag, B., & Megel, K. (Eds.), *Mobilität und gesellschaftliche Partizipation im Alter* (pp. 97–115). Stuttgart: Kohlhammer Verlag.

Schelisch, L., & Spellerberg, A. (2009, January). *Ein Dreivierteljahr mit PAUL: Assisted Living in Kaiserslautern.* Paper presented at the 2. German AAL- Congress, Berlin. VDE e.V. (Ed.). (2008). *VDE-Positionspapier Ambient Assisted Living. Intelligente Assistenz-Systeme im Dienst für eine reife Gesellschaft.* Frankfurt/M.: VDE.

Virone, G., & Sixsmith, A. (2008). Monitoring activity patterns and trends of older adults. In *Proceedings of the International Conference of the IEEE Engineering in Medicine and Biology Society* (pp. 2071-2074). Vancouver Canada: IEEE Engineering in Medicine and Biology Society

KEY TERMS AND DEFINITIONS

Ambient Assisted Living: Ambient Assisted Living (AAL) in general terms comprises of different methods, concepts, technical devices, products, and/or services which provide support in daily living and enhance the quality of living for people in all phases of life. An ambient environment is intelligent, but not necessarily noticeable and adapts to the daily lives of users.. In this study, AAL was deployed as technical assistance in elderly people's homes and also included a social environment to secure independent living.

Habitation in Advanced Age: When in course of life, requirements and demands of one's home change due to the ageing process, elderly people have different possibilities for living to choose from besides "regular" houses or apartments, for example barrier-free or handicapped accessible apartments, retirement homes, nursing homes, etc. Most elderly people wish to stay in their self-chosen-environment as long as possible. The needs of older people regarding their living and are based not only on structural and spatial aspects, but also relate to the social embedding and an attractive environment.

Research on the Elderly: Research on the elderly includes analyzing the standard of living, quality of life, activities of daily living and social behavior of people older than 60 years.

Research on Acceptance and Usability: Users are often not involved in the development process when new technologies are implemented. This often leads to a lower acceptance rate or non-use. In the field of AAL, housing companies and scientists who conduct pilot projects often experience disappointments, because the needs of elderly people were not considered adequately. To reach the acceptance of technology, it is necessary to consider e.g. the needs of elderly people regarding technical devices, costs and fear of surveillance. Research on acceptance and usability is necessary to clarify which technological concepts and which single devices are of use for elderly people and are accepted at the same time.

Section 3
Applications for Assisted Living

Chapter 10
Iterative User Involvement in Ambient Assisted Living Research and Development Processes:
Does It Really Make a Difference?

Sonja Müller
empirica, Germany

Ingo Meyer
empirica, Germany

Ilse Bierhoff
Stichting Smart Homes, The Netherlands

Sarah Delaney
Work Research Centre, Ireland

Andrew Sixsmith
Simon Fraser University, Canada

Sandra Sproll
University of Stuttgart, Germany

ABSTRACT

This chapter is based on results from the European research project SOPRANO which is developing supportive environments for older people based on the concept of Ambient Assisted Living (AAL).

The project adapts and applies Experience and Application Research (E&AR) methods involving active participation of older users throughout an iterative development and design process. Innovative participatory methods enable developers to thoroughly focus on the users when defining the system requirements, generating design solutions and evaluating these design solutions in both lab and real life settings.

The example chosen to best demonstrate how the character and detail of user ideas changed in the different stages of the R&D process is the development of an exercise support system applying an avatar showing the exercises on the TV in the home of an older person.

DOI: 10.4018/978-1-60960-469-1.ch010

INTRODUCTION

For the analysis and processing of user ideas a conceptual framework was developed that was applied in each of the development cycles in the project after the requirements elicitation process. This was crucial as every cycle of user interaction involved older end users in four countries (Germany, Spain, the Netherlands and United Kingdom), generating a large amount of feedback that could be contradictory in nature as well as providing consistent themes.

The chapter reviews of the importance of user involvement during the development process of AAL systems in general and exercise support in particular. After an introduction to the topic the chapter outlines results from the first phase of user involvement, where users significantly contributed to the requirements collection for the system. The conceptual framework that was applied during the system development process together with older people is then described. Results are presented from two user involvement cycles regarding the development of an exercise support system. The process by which ideas changed in each stage of the cycle, and how user ideas were processed and analysed in the development of the system is discussed. The chapter concludes with a critical review and next steps.

BACKGROUND: FROM INDEPENDENCE TO USER INVOLVEMENT

The SOPRANO (Service-oriented Programmable Smart Environments for Older Europeans) project is an EU project funded under the 6th Framework Programme developing supportive environments for older people based on the concept of "AAL", using pervasive ICTs to enable older people to live independently in their own homes.

The concept of "independent living" is very much at the core of the research and development carried out in SOPRANO and in similar projects in the field of AAL. The concept is increasingly used in policy addressing demographic ageing, social integration of older people as well as health and social care provision, reflecting the desire of older people to live independently in their own homes (Sixsmith, 1986; Gattuso, 1996; Moore, 2000). Despite its experiential and policy significance, it should be noted that the term "independent living" in itself is a high-level concept or an aggregation of a multitude of factors reaching down to the level of the individual and related to a fundamental question: "What is important for me to lead a good life (in old age)?" There is also evidence that this concept, particularly in relation to older people, is understood rather poorly today (Sixsmith, 1986; Secker et al, 2003). Few have asked what the term means, or what its constituent parts are. Some deconstruction of the term is therefore in order to better understand the role of user involvement in SOPRANO.

"Independent living" can be understood as the desire to lead one's life and at the same time avoid dependence. Such dependence can take different forms according to the area of life that is concerned. For the purpose of this deconstruction, we assume four such areas:

- **Social Interaction:** maintaining social contacts without becoming a burden on others, including family members, friends and neighbours.
- **Economic Welfare:** bearing the expenses of daily living (rent, shopping, travelling etc.) alone or together with a partner.
- **Mental Wellbeing:** possessing the necessary mental capabilities to carry out activities such as planning a holiday, remembering appointments and phone numbers, orientating oneself in the streets etc.
- **Bodily Wellbeing:** possessing the necessary physical capabilities to carry out activities such as shopping, washing, cleaning etc.

What all these four areas have in common – and which in turn can be considered a characteristic of the concept of "independent living" – is that they take the form of a continuum between undue or unwanted dependence on the one hand and acceptable or desired support on the other. While most people wish to avoid being a burden on others, they will usually aim to maintain a certain level of meaningful social contacts with people that are important in her or his life. In a similar manner, a certain amount of financial support from friends or relatives may be considered acceptable by many if, for example, given freely. In the case of mental and bodily wellbeing, acceptance of impairment occurs as well as denial, and a person accepting the loss of physical capabilities may well accept support through assistive devices. The exact form this continuum takes depends on the individual and his or her lifestyle, as formed by intrinsic and extrinsic factors.

Within health and social policy the focus has so far much been on dependence caused by mental and physical impairments associated with advanced age, concentrating on older peoples' capabilities to carry out activities of daily living. This instrumental approach is commonly reflected within the needs-based policies and practices of health and social care service providers, in which the major task is to meet individuals functional needs through the provision of (often equally functional) care (Bland, 1999; Tanner, 2003). While this kind of approach is important, its shortcomings in terms of supporting active living and respecting self-determination are recognised by care practitioners[1] and within the SOPRANO project.

In the RTD context the shortcomings of an overly instrumental approach to care provision are also apparent in a technology-push or problem-oriented mindset that tends to superimpose technological solutions on older people, formal and informal carers and care provider organisations based on the assumption that this meets their needs and solves their problems. Apart from neglecting most of what has been said above about independence being an individual fact or perception, this technology-push paradigm is neither user-driven nor likely to be successful in the long run, failing to capture the essential idea of independence in later life.

What is required is a more interactive and creative RTD approach that is driven by the people who will be the target groups of the applications and services to be developed and allows them to formulate their needs and ideas of appropriate help and support vis-à-vis technology and service developers. These in turn can take up those ideas, comment on them, suggest improvements and finally identify and develop technical effective solutions. This dialogue (e.g. a focus group) will usually be moderated (since user and developers are known to speak different "languages") and iterative (to allow for step-wise improvement), factually taking the form of a negotiation between user needs on the one hand and feasibility (technical, economical) on the other. With a view to a full RTD cycle, user involvement as it is understood here is continuous from the earliest stages of conceptualisation, via the definition of services up to the design of devices and user interfaces.

Reviewing EU-funded RTD in the past decade since the beginning of the 5th Framework Programme in 1998 it can be seen that user involvement has increasingly turned from lip-service to a reality, not least due to ever more concrete requirements being included in the programme descriptions. Nevertheless, criticisms remain and indeed the research agendas of most projects are still formulated long before users are involved in the process, which often happens only after first mock-ups or prototypes have been developed (Kubitschke & Meyer 2007).

PROCESS MODEL OF HUMAN-CENTRED DESIGN

According to ISO 9241 Ergonomics of human system interaction – Part 210: Human-centred

219

design processes for interactive systems – human-centred design is an approach to interactive system development. The approach aims to make systems usable focussing on the user's experience by applying human factors and usability knowledge: Effectiveness and efficiency, improves human well-being, user satisfaction, accessibility and sustainability of interactive systems should be enhanced. Systems designed using human-centred methods are particularly easier to understand, improve usability and user experience, reduce discomfort and stress and enhance quality.

The ISO 9241-210 suggests several principles to be followed in the design process: First of all, in order to get a clear and explicit understanding of users, tasks and environments, people who will use the system as well as stakeholder groups should be identified. People reflecting the characteristics, capabilities and experience of the later users should be involved throughout design and development, because they have valuable knowledge about the context of use. Appropriate representatives make sure that user requirements can be identified for inclusion in the system development. Iteration is necessary in order to minimize the risk that the system fails to meet the user requirements. Therefore, the requirements specification is refined iteratively by using scenarios, mock-ups and prototypes to obtain user feedback. The system should be designed for the totality of user's experience; that means all aspects of usability, desirability, but also support, training, branding and emotional aspects. User feedback is fundamental in human-centred design, in order to accurately fulfil user needs. User evaluation should take place both with preliminary scenarios to be fed back progressively into refined solutions and also as part of final acceptance of the product. Human-centred design teams should reflect skill areas like human factors, usability accessibility, human-computer interaction, user research, systems (hardware/software-) engineering, user interface design, marketing and sales, technical support, user management and so on,

in order to benefit from a multi-perspective and multi-disciplinary approach.

For projects following the human-centred design approach, four design activities are suggested in the ISO 9241-210 (Figure 1):

- Understand and specify the context of use
- Specify the user requirements
- Produce design solutions
- Evaluate

First of all, it is important to understand and specify the context in which the system will be used. Therefore, information on the current context is gathered and analysed in order to understand and specify the context for the future system. Deficiencies and baseline levels of performance and satisfaction should be worked out. In this step all relevant user groups are identified and their characteristics (e.g. knowledge, skills, experience, physical attributes, habits, preferences and capabilities) are analysed in order to achieve accessibility and suitable products. User characteristics are usually determined by gathering data through interviews and/or user profile questionnaires (Mayhew, 1999). Moreover, the tasks the users are to perform and the environment(s) in which the system is to be used have to be analysed.

The next step is the specification of user requirements. User needs and requirements should be identified, taking into account the context of use. User requirements are more specific than needs in that they exist only in a certain domain. In the domain of ICT, user requirements are specified user needs targeted towards a specific product or system. While user needs are connected to individuals, user requirements are requirements of individuals for a product or system. These requirements provide the basis for the design and evaluation of system to meet the user requirements. Their fulfilment and updating should be ensured during the life of the project. Kotanya and Sommerville (1998) distinguish between several different types of requirements:

Figure 1. Illustration of human-centred design activities as defined in ISO 9241-210

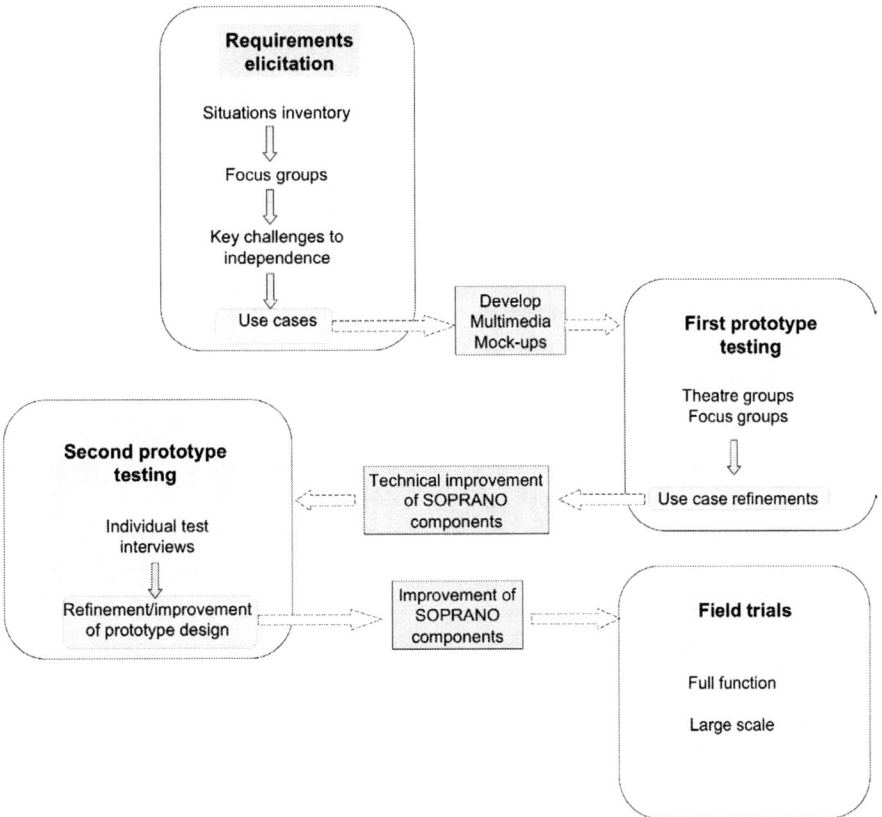

- Very general requirements: set out in broad terms what the system should do; e.g. "The system shall maintain records of all library materials including books, serials, newspapers and magazines, video and audio tapes, reports, collections of transparencies, computer disks and CD-ROMs".
- Functional requirements: define part of the system's functionality; e.g. "The system shall allow users to search for an item by title, author, or ISBN".
- Implementation requirements: state how the system must be implemented; e.g. "The system's user interface shall be implemented using a World-Wide-Web browser"
- Performance requirements: specify a minimum acceptable performance for the system; e.g. "The system shall support at least 20 transactions per second".

- Usability requirements: specify required usability aspects for the system; e.g. "The system facilities which are available to public users shall be demonstrable in 10 minutes or less".

In the literature several methods are recommended to be used in the requirement analysis, which were taken into account in SOPRANO. Well-established methods to learn more about requirements are interviews and questionnaires (Mayhew, 1999, Nielsen, 1993). Both involve asking user a set of questions and recording their answers. Many aspects can best be studied by simply asking the users, especially about issues relating to users´ subjective satisfaction and possible anxieties (Nielsen, 1993). Moreover, interviews and questionnaires are also useful for studying how the users use the system and what features they like or dislike. Focus groups are another popular method to collect requirements (Caplan, 1990; Goldman & McDonald, 1987; Greenbaum, 1988, O'Donnell et al. 1991). In focus groups, about six to nine users identify issues over period of about two hours. The focus group is run by a moderator who is responsible for maintaining the focus on whatever issues are of interest. Focus groups often bring out users´ spontaneous reactions and ideas through the interaction between the participants (Nielson, 1993). Another central method also used in SOPRANO is the creation of scenarios of use or use cases (Mayhew, 1999; Nielson, 1993; Vredenburg et al. 2002). The idea is to cut down on the complexity by describing possible uses of envisioned future systems according to the characteristics of an individual user under specified circumstances (Carroll & Rosson, 1992). Contextual Analysis (Beyer & Holtzblatt, 1998) is most appropriate when a set of functions is identified and methods of presenting problems and needs in the natural environment need to be understood.

In the next step of the human-centred design process design solutions are produced by drawing on the description of the context of user, the results of baseline evaluations and state-of-the-art and the experience and knowledge of the participants. The ISO 9241-210 suggest several principles to achieve a positive user experience: suitability for the tasks and learning, self-descriptiveness, conformity with user expectations, controllability, error tolerance and suitability for individualization (cf. ISO 9241-110). The focus should be on designing the interaction between human and system including issues of modality and the choice of media. Interaction design includes objects required for completion of tasks, the information architectures and sequences and timing. When designing user interfaces standards on displays, dialogue principles, menus, presentation of information, user guidance and accessibility guidelines should be considered. Following these principles, in SOPRANO particular emphasis was placed on

making the design solutions more concrete by using scenarios, simulation, mock-ups and other forms of prototypes. This allowed the researchers to explore the preferred system design as identified by users. Several iterations altering the design solutions based on user evaluation and user feedback make it possible to incorporate feedback early in the design process (cf. ISO 9241-210; Mayhew, 1999). Thereby, costs and benefits of any recommendation should be evaluated. Wixon and Wilson (1997) provide approaches to summarizing data. Interferential statistical analysis is often not appropriate in an engineering environment, because the sample size is usually too small and other criteria (e.g. random sampling) are not met. A more sophisticated way of summarizing data is, for example, an impact analysis table in order to weight the relative severity of identified problems. Criteria that facilitate summarizing data across all users could be the number of times a problem was experienced, the number of user experiencing a problem or the number of errors of all types of a particular task. For drawing conclusions and formulated recommendations Wixon and Wilson (1997) assign a severity ranking, an assessment of impact, alternative solutions, a recommended solution, costs of implementation and recommended actions to fulfil recommendations. In SOPRANO a three-step analytical framework was developed to this end (cf. paragraph "Analytical framework for processing ideas developed by potential end users"). Hence, the design solution is communicated to those responsible for the implementation.

In the last step of the human-centred design process the system is evaluated. Prototypes of different level of detail are the objects of the user assessment, for example in the early stages, a mock-up of the interaction through simulated tasks. Later in development, it could be assessed whether usability objectives have been met in the intended context by user testing. One form of user based testing is field trial validation in real world environments using field reports, performance data, satisfaction surveys, reports of health impacts and user observation. Long term performance data and reports about health effects through long-term monitoring provide valuable information, since some effects of living with an interactive system are not recognisable until it has been used for a period of time or until critical incidents happen. Expert evaluation could be applied to complement user testing in a cost effective way.

DEVELOPING A SUPPORT SYSTEM FOR EXERCISING AT HOME TOGETHER WITH OLDER END USERS

In order to be able to develop, implement and test a technical system that supports independent living of older people and to avoid the shortcomings of an overly functional approach, SOPRANO follows an iterative Experience and Application Research (E&AR) approach that actively involves users from an early stage and meets the requirements of a user-developer dialogue or negotiation as formulated above. A schematic overview of the process is provided in the figure below and it will be described in more detail using an example in the remainder of this text.

The SOPRANO E&AR approach comprises four instances of active user involvement and starts with the elicitation of basic service requirements. On the basis of an inventory of situations that can threaten the independence of older people, focus groups were carried out with the aim to formulate a list of key challenges to independence that was in turn used to formulate the first version of the SOPRANO use cases. Multimedia mock-ups and theatre plays were developed to show the use cases to users in the course of the first prototype tests. Outcomes of these tests were used to refine the use cases, based on which the user-facing components of SOPRANO were improved. The improved components were the subjects of the second prototype tests that led to a further improvement of the component design. The last step will be a field

trial where the system will be installed and tested in laboratory and home settings (cf. Figure 2).

Keeping Healthy and Active as One of the Key Challenges for Independent Living

Involving older end users in the creative innovation process at a very early stage of the research poses significant challenges to the whole research process since the creativeness of older end users needs to be supported and encouraged. Applying state of the art methods can for example be too tedious, standard questionnaires might not be understood by everyone, or expecting new ideas to be understood might be too challenging. Thus, suitable methods needed to be applied in order to help older people to contribute to the design process and to support older people to think creatively, without constraining their ideas within existing solutions. To facilitate this, a "tool" was constructed and applied using the metaphor of a Guardian Angel. Metaphors are useful in supporting potential users to generate completely novel ideas (Rosson & Carroll, 2002). The Guardian Angel metaphor helped to generate user driven ideas without being biased through explicit assumptions about what is possible with technology. It also helped the researchers to discuss possible supports and solutions to challenges faced by older people without referring to technological concepts at the outset, and to allow for freedom in first coming up with ideas before any discussion of potential (technical) support. The "Guardian Angel" could help in every imaginable way and was applied in focus groups with older people during the requirements elicitation process and during the process of design idea generation and evaluation.

In the course of the requirements elicitation in the first cycle of user involvement, keeping healthy and active was mentioned as one of the key challenges to independent living. The relative importance of physical fitness is also supported

Figure 2. Iterative development process in the SOPRANO project

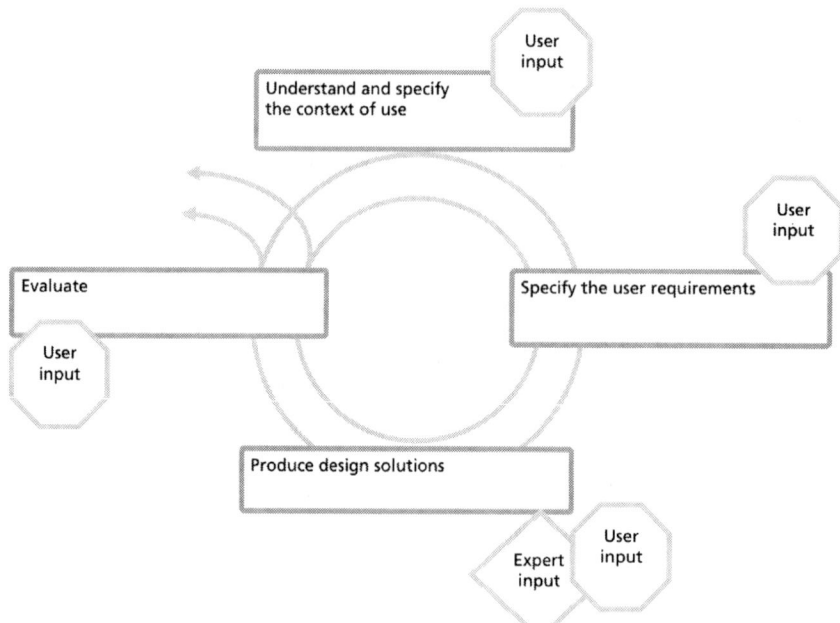

by other research. Rogers et al (1998) found that limitations in gross motor movements caused by e.g. knee or back problems or a more general loss of strength can significantly limit the ability to walk or bend over or to carry heavy items. Limitations in fine motor movements have an influence on activities such as writing, opening bottles or bags and so on. Difficulties with balance caused e.g. by loss of equilibrium or problems in coordination of movements strongly influence the capability to go up and down steps or ladders, getting in and out of vehicles or rising from a chair or a sofa. A decrease of the ability to maintain balance is also often associated with in increased risk of falling. These limited abilities as a consequence can severely limit the independence and quality of life. In this context, recent evidence on the effectiveness of exercises suggests that some form of conducting exercises can help to increase body strength and help maintain balance (Singh 2002) and in turn may help to better perform different activities of daily living and also prevent falls.

Regular exercising can produce improvements in muscle strength (de Carvalho Bastone & Filho, 2004) and as a consequence increase the ability to do simple activities such as getting up from a chair or climbing stairs (Skelton & McLaughlin, 1996). It has also a positive impact on the ability to do more complex activities of daily life, such as bathing or preparing a meal (Rogers et. al 1998; Penninx et. al 2001). Physical activity has also been shown to have positive effects on psychological well-being (Mather et al, 2002; Ruuskanen & Ruoppila, 1995) and significantly increase the quality of life of an older person.

For these reasons we will use a SOPRANO use case focusing on the support of physical exercises by means of a digital avatar to illustrate the project's iterative development approach.

SOPRANO Exercise Use Case

The use case addresses older people who have to do physical exercises prescribed by a physician or therapist (e.g. after a stay in hospital) and are basically capable of carrying out these exercises on their own after they were shown to them a couple of times.

A support system along with the necessary peripherals is installed and operated by a care provider organisation (CPO). The system is configured by the CPO so that the avatar on the TV can demonstrate the prescribed exercises to the older person. Whenever the exercises are due, the system will remind the user and, when he has given his consent, the exercises will be displayed on the TV for the user to follow them. During the first time, a carer from the care provider organisation will be present to introduce the user to the new procedure. Depending on the scenario, a feedback loop can be integrated in the procedure. In that case, the user will be recorded by video while doing the exercises and the video will be reviewed by the care provider organisation or a therapist at regular intervals to see if the exercises are done correctly. Via the system, the reviewing specialist can give feedback to the user that will be displayed the next time he does the exercises.

One of the main questions for this use case was the choice of the most suitable and usable interface because the interface between the user and a device is critical in determining acceptance by the user (Adlam & Orpwood 2003). Research evidence from e.g. the Ofcom Consumer Panel (2006) for example reveals that attitudes of older people (55+) towards PCs/the internet are very different to (digital) TV. Digital TV was regarded as accessible and mainstream, even by those who did not regard themselves as technically minded, whereas attitudes towards computers or the Internet were much more polarised. This is supported by Noe et.al. (2009) stating that older people often regard the user-interface-concept of computers as too complex and that they experience the TV as easier. Following these key advantages the TV was chosen as the main interaction device for the older users when conducting exercises at home. Another design decision that was taken at

the beginning of the project was to use the help of an avatar when conducting exercises.

Several recent studies (Ortiz et al, 2007; Kim, 2004) have concluded that conversational avatars are a good tool for obtaining more natural communication with a user. This is especially important for older people, because they are less familiar with new technologies than younger generations. Some of the conclusions that these studies have obtained are as follows:

- Conversational avatars allow social interaction with the computer. Prendinger et al. (2005) concluded that users interact in a natural way with the computer and they expect that computers act in the same way with them. The final proposal of their work recommends providing personality features and voice synthesis to the interface in order to improve the human computer interaction.
- Improve the reliability and credibility about the system. Koda & Maes (1996) found that a computer interface with face, eyes, body or voice improve reliability and credibility.
- Improve the commitment of the user. Kim (2004) carried out evaluations that demonstrated that students' perception in eLearning applications improves with the personification of a virtual tutor.
- Drive the user eye. User attention can be driven to key points with the use of an avatar.

Despite these important benefits, the use of avatars within AAL systems has been very limited. Moreover, using an avatar as tutoring system for physical exercises represents a completely new approach for this kind of environments.

Several aspects of this use case make it ideal to illustrate the methodology used in the Soprano project. First of all it addresses a key challenge mentioned by end users, informal carers and formal carers. On the other hand users also provided the research team with comments and concerns that should be taken into account. Thirdly from a technical point of view the use of the avatar is challenging and also evidence from user research exists that shows positive results when using avatars. These pre-conditions provide an ideal background to exploit the potential of the E&AR methodology, since refining this use case required an intensive and creative iterative process between developers and users.

As the use case could not be defined in detail at the requirement elicitation phase, this meant that some risks needed to be taken in the initial design. Preliminary design decisions, for instance to start developing an avatar, had to be taken at this rather early stage in order to allow the technical designers to start the development of the system architecture. To make sure that these design choices did not influence the user's ideas, innovative methods such as interactive drama presentations were used in order to support older end users to develop their own design ideas. This could however mean that these additional design ideas from the users would have an effect on the preliminary design choices that were made by the technical team.

ANALYTICAL FRAMEWORK FOR PROCESSING IDEAS DEVELOPED BY POTENTIAL END USERS

As described above, the research in the SOPRANO project follows an Experience and Application Research approach (European Commission, 2004). One major objective of this approach is the active involvement of older people at all stages of system design and development in order to meet the special needs of older users. This is crucial since it is nearly impossible to specify all requirements and needs in advance when applying a user-centred approach to technology development (Rosson & Carroll, 2002).

Based on the Human-Centred Design Process (according to ISO 9241-210, cf. Figure 1) the project goes beyond the state-of-the-art process by involving potential users also in defining functionality and interaction design in order to make sure that design solutions are based on the mindsets, experiences and mental models of the target group. In a standardised Human-Centred Design Process user input is required in the first two steps, in the specification of the context of use and the specification of user and organisational requirements, followed by the development of prototypes by experts. Usually experts define which functions and services are integrated and how the user should interact with the device or system. The user participates again in evaluating the prototypes based on the conceptual design ideas of the (technical) experts. As a consequence, in the state-of-the-art approach the initial design ideas are often not based on the mindsets, experiences and mental models of the users, but on the mindsets of the experts who develop the system.

In SOPRANO, instead of having experts responsible for the development of prototypes, a more user-centred design process was applied that involves users throughout the whole design process. The idea was that it is not the user who responds to the ideas of experts, but experts should base the development on the ideas of older people and their carers and respond to their input. Thus, the objective of the Experience and Application Research approach is to modify the state-of-the-art process of user-based design by enlarging the impact of potential users by involving them in every phase of system development. Following this approach also means implementing an iterative research process as described above.

By involving the future users in every cycle of the system development and evaluation, a lot of user input and feedback was generated during the project duration that had to be evaluated by the researchers. In the very first phase of the requirement analysis researchers together with older people identified key challenges to independence in several focus groups. Requirements and needs from older people were transformed into use cases. In the following phases, user input was transformed into prototypes of different levels of detail: In the first prototype testing users generated ideas how to refine the use cases and also evaluated the solution presented in the multimedia prototypes or in a theatre presentation. In this phase, researchers had to decide which user input would be integrated in the next cycle of prototype testing in order to design the system interaction. In the second phase of prototype testing, user input was gathered in individual sessions where single components of the system were tested and evaluated by the future users. The researchers had to identify user feedback and valuable ideas for improvements regarding the usability and acceptability of a component. The analysed user input of this phase was directly implemented into the close-to-final system that will be tested in demonstration homes and in real environments. Again, user feedback is gathered regarding acceptability and usefulness of the system in daily life. The evaluation of the feedback in the field trials is crucial to assess system benefits for older people.

The iterative process and the involvement of future users in every cycle of the project lead to a considerable amount of user data that was progressed according to a structured framework with pre-defined criteria for assessment.

The researchers applied a conceptual framework where user input and feedback was evaluated in three steps: In the first step the importance of the user input for SOPRANO was assessed, in the second step the cross-cultural validity was assessed, in order to fulfil the pan-European perspective of SOPRANO. The analysis at these two stages was mainly performed by researchers who either were responsible for the user involvement or represent the interests of the older users. If the input passed these evaluation steps, it was checked for its technical feasibility in the third step. In the feasibility analysis the expertise of the technical partners of the project was essential. Therefore,

they played a dominant role at this stage of evaluation. The overall methodology of evaluation was aligned to a qualitative research approach.

Assessment of the Importance of the User Input

First of all, the user input of every test site, i.e. every participating country was assessed for its value for the overall system development:

- If there were many users supporting an idea or assessment of an idea, its estimated value for SOPRANO was discussed by experts. These experts were partners with expertise in working with older people as well as in the AAL context, e.g. the user organisations, psychologists and researchers in the AAL field. An idea was considered to be important if implementation of the idea was likely to improve perceived usefulness, usability and acceptability of the system and its components. The idea was discussed against the background of the scientific knowledge in AAL, gerontology and usability engineering.

- If there were only few users supporting an idea or assessment of an idea, it had to be checked whether these users belong to a specific subgroup of the target group. It could be the case that only a few users from the respective subgroup were involved in the session, but the requirements of the subgroup were relevant for SOPRANO (e.g. modification of red/green buttons for colour-blind people). If the issue was assessed to be relevant for a subgroup of the target group, it was also checked for its value.

- In order to follow a qualitative approach, ideas that only a few users came up with, but seem to have a great impact, were also checked for their value. The dashed arrow in Figure 3 symbolises this function. If there were excellent ideas with significant impact, they were considered in the further development, even if they were mentioned by only few users.

Process

The results of the sessions with users constituted the input for the evaluation of importance. Results could be quantitative and qualitative data from questionnaires, transcripts of sessions, video tapes, templates with the users' quotes and observations by moderators, and other reports.

These data were screened for input of users and potentially important observations by the moderators and user representatives. Then, the screened and structured results were discussed shortly after the sessions by moderators, usability experts, user organisations and researchers in gerontology and AAL.

Criteria for the assessment of importance were the impact on acceptability, perceived usefulness and usability, design and ease of use of the SOPRANO system.

- Acceptability: Cost, Trustworthiness (reliability, safety, confidentiality), Compatibility (technology fit to personal life), Stigma, Concern/Hope, Attitude towards usage
- Perceived usefulness
- Usability, Design, Ease of use: Effectiveness, Efficiency, Satisfaction, Control over usage, Transparency of system behaviour, Aesthetics and Appearance

User input that was considered to be important and valuable for the system was further progressed in the next step of expert evaluation.

Cross-Cultural Analysis of User Input

In this analysis it was checked whether the important input is valid for only one country or in more than one country (Figure 3) in order to follow the pan-European approach of SOPRANO. Test sites were Spain, the Netherlands, Germany, and the UK. These countries represent different regions of Europe and thereby different cultural aspects. In the cross-cultural analysis the same experts were involved like in the first step, but focusing on cultural comparison.

- If the user input came up in several countries, one could assume that it was valid from a pan-European perspective. Then, the user input fulfilled the requirements to be an appropriate system for Europe in general. It could be forwarded to the third step of evaluation, the feasibility analysis.
- If the user input came up in only one country, country-specific particularities could be the reason. It was checked, if the input was also valid for other countries. Cultural differences had to be clarified by comparing the results. If the user input was specific for a country, this was documented, e.g. in order to explain future results of the field trials in the respective country and in order to understand differences. But the aim of SOPRANO is to develop a system appropriate for Europe in general. Therefore, it was important to implement ideas that were valid in more than one country.
- If the user input came up in only one country, but was rated to be also valid for other European countries by the experts of several test sites, it was also forwarded to the next step of assessment. The dashed arrow symbolises in Figure 3 this procedure.

Figure 3. Conceptual framework: Assessment of importance and cross-cultural analysis and feasibility analysis performed by experts in user research

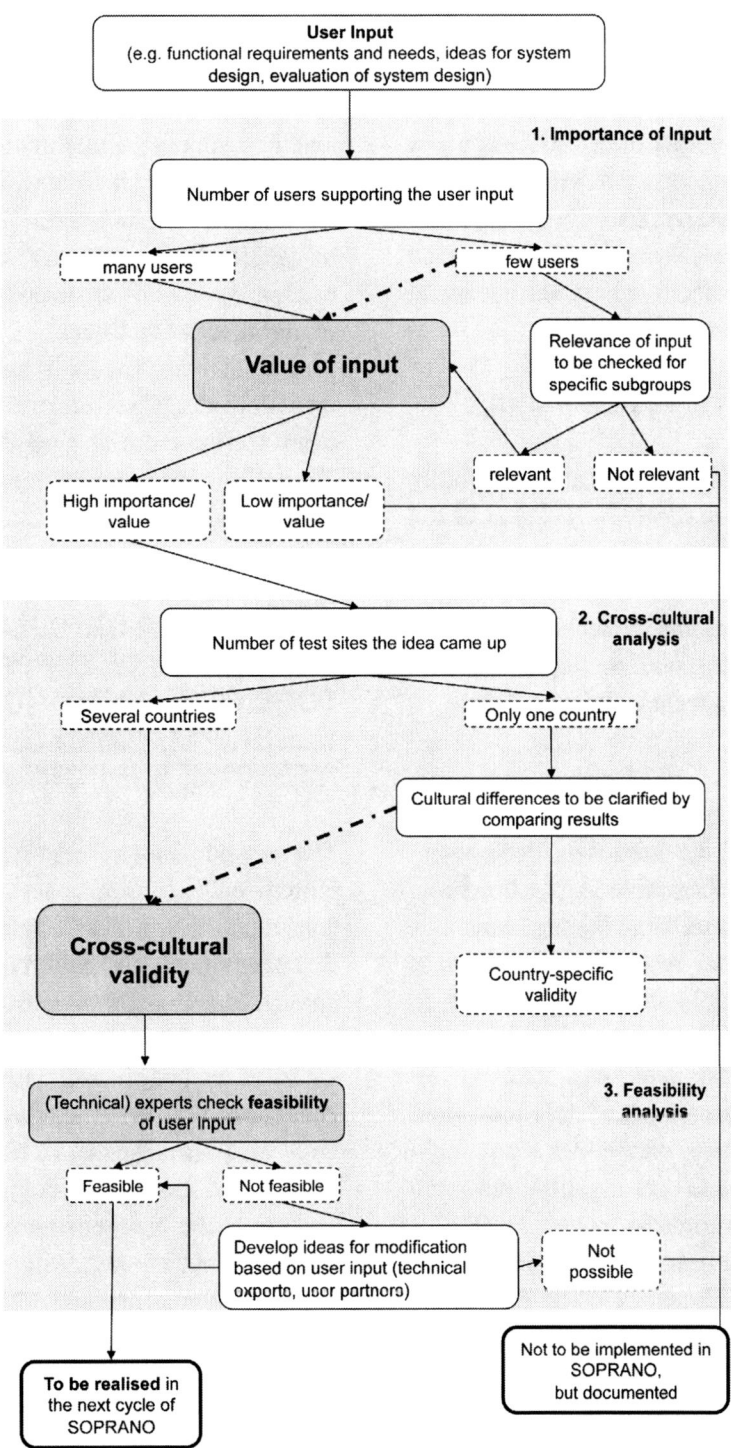

Process

The collection of important ideas and important feedback was discussed by experts from several test sites regarding its cross-cultural validity. In every cycle of the iterative process representatives of the different European regions took part in the analysis. The output of this process was a collection of important input that was valid from a pan-European perspective. User input that passed the cross-cultural analysis was further processed in the feasibility analysis where the technical partners were consulted.

Feasibility Analysis of User Input

The next step was the assessment of feasibility of relevant, important ideas. In this step of the evaluation technical developers of the project came into play. The user representatives introduced the collection of ideas and the technical partners checked whether they could be implemented or not (Figure 3) from a technical point of view.

- If the functional requirements and ideas were feasible, they were realised in the next cycle of the iterative development process. This alternative shows the direct influence of future users the best way.
- If the functional requirements and ideas were not feasible, modifications had to be developed in order to meet the users´ requirements the best way. Feasible alternatives to the proposed solutions were worked out. Based on the user input, technical partners and user organisations were involved in this process.
- If neither the original user input was feasible nor modifications were reasonable or feasible, it was not implemented, but documented.

Process

Input for the feasibility analysis was the collection of important input that was assessed for its cross-cultural validity by technical experts from the test sites.

The user representatives introduced the ideas and the rationale behind them and the respective technical experts checked whether the idea could be integrated in the system. In the development of modifications, technical experts as well as user partners were involved in order to meet the requirement of the users.

Outputs of the feasibility analysis were requirements and ideas that were rated as important, valid from a cross-cultural perspective and feasible. These ideas and requirements were implemented in the next cycle of the system development.

DESIGN IDEA GENERATION FOR EXERCISE SUPPORT TOGETHER WITH AND FOR OLDER PEOPLE IN NEED OF EXERCISE SUPPORT AT HOME

The second phase of user research after the requirements elicitation phase aimed at generating conceptual design ideas together with older users. Theatre methods and multimedia mock-ups were applied to help older people developing creative design ideas for the exercise support system.

24 older people were involved in the idea generation process for an exercise support system, 16 in focus groups where a multimedia mock-up was applied and 8 older people in a theatre group.

One of the main challenges of early user involvement during the design phase of a system was that potential users should create design ideas and evaluate a system that does not yet exist. The development of suitable methods encouraging potential end users to create innovative design ideas was thus crucial at this stage.

Theatre Methods

Theatre methods are an innovative approach to supporting the process of design idea generation and were used in combination with the Guardian Angel approach in a structured and moderated Focus Design Discussion (FDD). In the FDD the moderator encouraged the participants to develop their own ideas towards the exercise solution.

Theatre Methods allowed the visualisation of a situation in a very natural and immediate way, which made it easier to imagine and to remember a certain situation. A discussion could therefore be stimulated, even with participants with little or no technical knowledge. Plays were very suitable for activating memories and emotions of the users (Bortz & Döring, 1995). For example, the older people were able to make suggestions and interact with the actors to directly input into the use case scenario. It was also seen as very flexible, because suggestions by the participants could be enacted and experienced in real-time. It greatly helped people participating in the creative process of idea generation and was seen as providing many insights in a complex situation. The theatre method represented a very realistic situation, because the session allowed quite complex scenarios to be enacted, where mock-ups can only include rather basic details. Therefore, the theatre method allowed very quick iterations and was very flexible to the users´ input. The older users were highly motivated to take part in discussions concerning the SOPRANO functionality. The theatre method was a very effective method for generating conceptual ideas in the research team and revealed lively and fruitful discussions about possible design solutions. The data from the theatre session allowed a lot of improvements to be made to the skeleton of the initial use case.

It is also worthwhile mentioning that users enjoyed the session, had much fun and laughed a lot. They found the method to be useful which is confirmed by the observation that they were really engaged and enthusiastic. Moreover the participation in the theatre method sparked their interest in the future development of the exercise system which was somewhat contrary to the results from the first iteration cycle where feedback about the exercise support system was rather restrained: They were interested in the real set-up of the system and the conditions of purchase.

Multimedia Mock-Up

The multimedia mock-up is an animated video play of the use case that could be shown either on a TV screen or on the screen of a computer. Its goal was to present the key challenges that were the basis for the development of the SOPRANO use cases to the actual users involved in the project visually, in order to help them visualise the problem scenarios and to help them in the design idea generation. The scenarios were developed in the four languages (English, German, Dutch, and Spanish) that are spoken by the participants in the user sessions.

The mock-up started with a side-view presentation of a prototype SOPRANO house from where the moderator could start playing the use cases in two different modes: (a) in a scene-by-scene mode, where there is a pause after each scene and the moderator needs to explicitly move on the next scene, thus enabling discussion among the session participants; and (b) in a video mode, where the specific scenario plays continuously until its end, thus being suitable for use during a demonstration.

Similar to the theatre plays, the mock-up was used to first demonstrate a problem situation that occurs in daily life (e.g. the need to do rehabilitation exercises after a surgery or long hospital stay). This stimulated a discussion in which participants were asked to produce their own ideas on how to best address the problem from their point of view. In contrast to the theatre approach, the participants` input could not be incorporated as rapidly and flexibly. Therefore, two or three prepared alternative solutions were presented via multimedia mock-ups afterwards. The participants were shown a variety of design solutions and asked to decide on one design solution.

The application of the multimedia mock-up, while not as flexible as a theatre play, turned out to be a very effective approach for the generation of design ideas together with older end users. It was observed that after the introduction people had various ideas and showing the alternatives resulted in an additional discussion. Applying multimedia mock-ups at this stage of development is an effective means to encourage users to bring in their own ideas in relation to different functionalities and modalities of the system under development. However, testing usability and ease of use was only possible to a limited extent due to missing interactivity of the system at this stage.

Resulting Use Case Refinements

User input from this second phase of user research was used to refine the original exercise use case developed in the requirements elicitation phase at the very first beginning of the research. Use case refinements for the exercise support system were tremendously.

Older people from all countries involved in the research confirmed that recovering from injuries and the need to do exercises is a common need among older people. Many of the interviewees had to do some exercises at home after a hospital stay and others described when they had to help a member of the family to recover from an operation.

Most surprisingly and on the contrary to the results from the first stage of user involvement, the overall usefulness and acceptance of a technical exercising support system was rated very positively by the involved end users.

More than 3/4 of end users involved stated that overall it would be advantageous to use the exercise solution. Nearly all participants (85%) thought that older people living alone would benefit most from the "exercise" solution.

However, although the exercise use case was evaluated by potential older end users, the main focus of this phase in the development process was to generate design ideas together with older people that support the technical developers in improving and further developing the system. A range of more detailed user requirements and design ideas was developed and included in the refinement of the exercise use case.

People for example expressed that personal visits from a physiotherapist were still required. This was not part of the original use case and led to a change of the use case originated by older end users. User research also revealed that the pace of prompts is very important and needs to be geared to the pace of the user both in terms of speech synthesis and timing of exercise programme.

As a result from work with users during the first phase of user research, permanent video recording of the person performing the exercises was a component of the use case. This was implemented in the use case because older end users expressed the need for some quality control when conducting the exercises. However, during the next step in the development process where multimedia mock-ups and theatre groups were used to help people visualise the system, permanent video recording was not seen as very useful for the purpose of controlling the exercises and the use case was changed accordingly. However, since quality control was still seen as crucial by older end users, the system will monitor the movements of the user while a physiotherapist watches remotely (although likely to be on an occasional basis). This also allows for the requirement of receiving direct feedback.

Another functionality that was not considered during the initial phase of user research was to include a weekly exercise schedule showing all the exercise to be conducted by the user in the menu of the system (Figure 4).

Another additional design idea developed by the users and included in the refined use case was the possibility of the exercise support system to

Figure 4. Example showing how user ideas were further processed

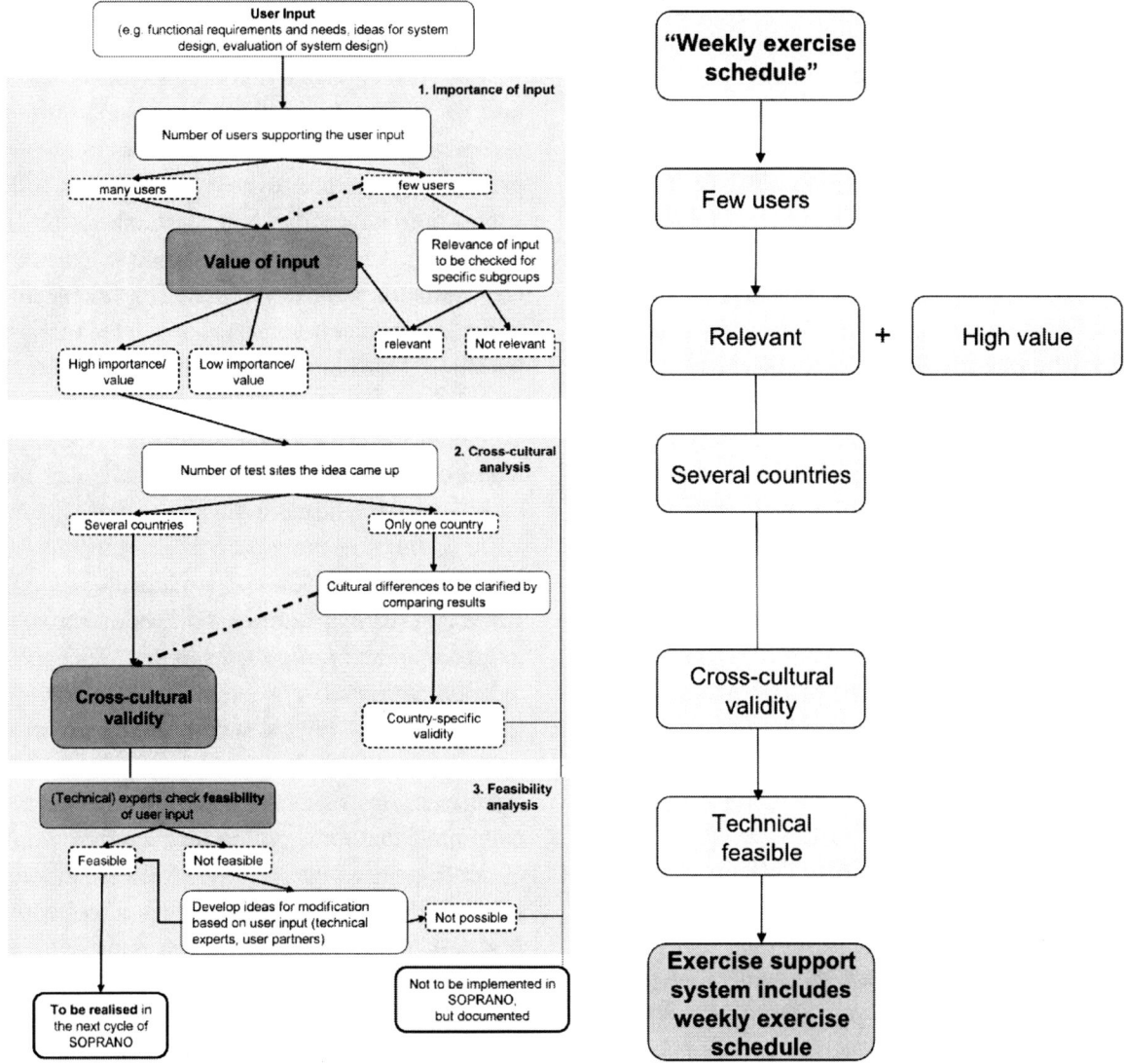

play background music or read audio books. This idea was developed against the background that users were concerned that the exercises at home could be boring and the recordings could help to maintain motivation.

Again, the possibility to give feedback into the system was stressed by the users. Users developed very concrete ideas how this could be realised and explained e.g. that a questionnaire should be implemented collecting feedback from the user after the exercises. This was seen as very

valuable by the researchers and as a consequence, the exercise support system will collect feedback from the user after each exercise session. For this purpose, a brief survey after the exercise will allow the user to report the effects, including negative ones such as pain. In that case the care provider organisation will be alerted to contact the user and, if necessary, adapt the exercises accordingly.

Also, some more concrete design ideas towards the avatar were developed by users. Although the avatar was not prototyped during the phase of system development users expressed some design requirements in relation to the avatar. One of the most important requirements was that the avatar should be personalisable and that the tone has to be empathic to the situation of the person, but at the same time be firm in terms of clearly defining the need for doing the exercises. This "tone" was very important to the look and feel of the avatar or interface- meaning that the emotional quality of this has to be right if it is to engage the person.

For this use case, also a personal assessment of the person and her/his needs was seen as essential. It is important that the person's living environment is assessed along with any assessment of their physical and mental abilities if the intervention is to be effective. Therefore this needs to be done by a rehabilitation professional prior to the use of the system or by some kind of remote evaluation of the site. Also, the positioning of the TV is crucial, especially if the assisted person is performing exercises- so this has to be determined when the system is installed.

TESTING PROTOTYPES OF COMPONENTS OF THE EXERCISE SUPPORT SYSTEM

The next step in the development of an exercise support system was the prototyping of the different components of the system, giving the users the opportunity to interact with the system for the very first time. While the previous user interaction cycles aimed at eliciting user requirements, generating and evaluating design ideas with potential end users of the system, this interaction cycle aimed at testing real component prototypes of the system with end users for the very first time to help technical designers to improve the prototype components and overall system.

Components were tested in single interviews and the tests were embedded in a use case scenario in order to stimulate user feedback, to support the user to imagine the situation with the components

coming into play, and to make the tests more lively and interactive, thus facilitating evaluation of the components to be tested.

Each test applied a mixture of scenario based task execution, observation, user walk-through and questionnaires. The system response was provided by the prototype component. In order to ensure comparability of the tests across the different sites, detailed implementation schemes and test protocols were developed. The first section of the test protocols consisted of a list of research questions (for instance: testing of graphical design, look & feel in general icon comprehensibility, and acceptability of the avatar) that could be used as a checklist by the researchers to make sure that every issue was discussed with the participant.

In the tests of the prototype exercise support system, about half of the test participants explicitly stated that seeing exercises motivated them to be more active and to do the exercises. This refers to being reminded to do exercises and also to the fact that, as one person stated, seeing exercises by an avatar makes believe that one is not alone doing exercises. However, some interviewees also mentioned that for a gymnastic class they would prefer to go to a club because of the social interaction and the opportunity to meet other people. It seems that doing exercises at home with an avatar, if the person is already quite active, is a good complement to existing sports and exercise activities. Where people are not self-motivated to do exercises, it appears to be good way to increase motivation to do some exercises at home. The results from the components tests also confirmed research from previous activities that revealed that staying active is one of the most important things in order to live an independent life.

The overall look and feel of the avatar (Figure 5) was well-received by users and needed no major revision. Although some suggestions for improvements were made, it was generally felt that the details of the avatar such as gender, hair colour etc are not relevant since one has to focus on the exercises and not on the avatar itself. This

Figure 5. The SOPRANO avatar

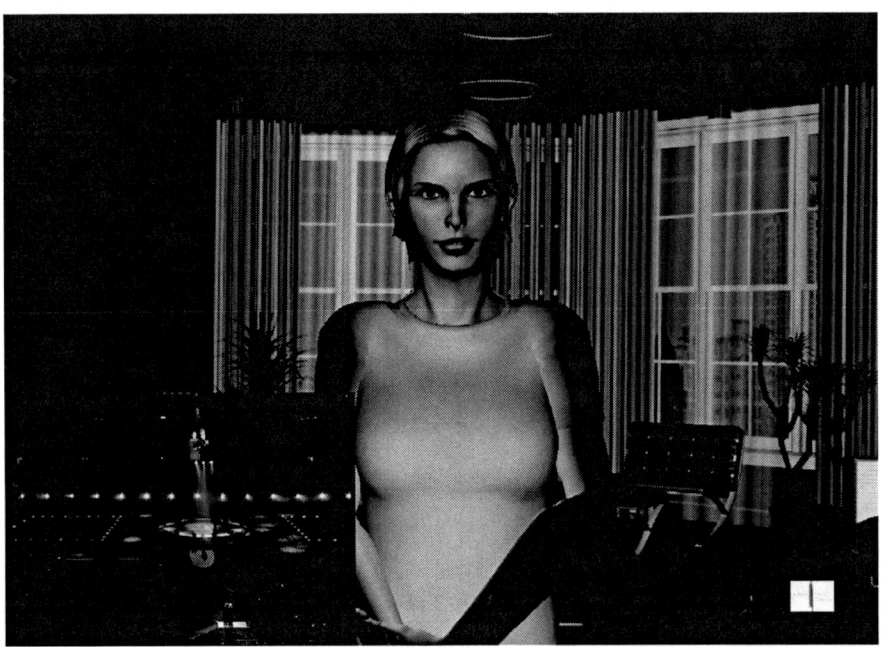

is contrary to the results from the previous phase of user interaction where users stressed the importance of a personalisable avatar. Surprisingly, only two out of 18 test participants said that they would prefer a real person showing the exercises.

One of the possible reasons why people accept the avatar as exercise guide is that it reduces the complexity of the exercises and focuses on the most important things without distracting the users with many details that a real person might show. One user even mentioned that with an avatar he would not feel like being in a competition as compared to a real (older) person showing the exercises and definitely preferred the avatar to a real person.

In general, users like the system and the design. They thought that the system was useful and the avatar was a motivation to do exercises at home. In most cases users did not have a problem recognising the avatar as a tutor and they followed its movements. Even in some cases where the verbal instructions and the movements of the avatar where not in concordance, people

followed the movements, which shows the power of using a visual guide to explain certain activities (Figure 6). Almost all test participants followed the avatar movements rather than listening to the verbal instructions. However, when asked people commented that the additional voice explaining the exercises is appreciated. There seems to be a difference between observation results and self-assessment of the users. Since previous phases of user involvement and also usability guidelines clearly reveal that addressing two senses is crucial, it was decided to support users in doing exercises by showing with the avatar and verbally explaining the exercises.

The research shows that using an avatar as an interface to guide the exercise worked very well. All test participants were able to follow the movements of the avatar, without any explanation or guidance from the researchers. The avatar seems to reduce the complexity of the exercise movements to its key elements without distracting people with irrelevant details. Test participants

Figure 6. User conducting exercises with the help of an avatar

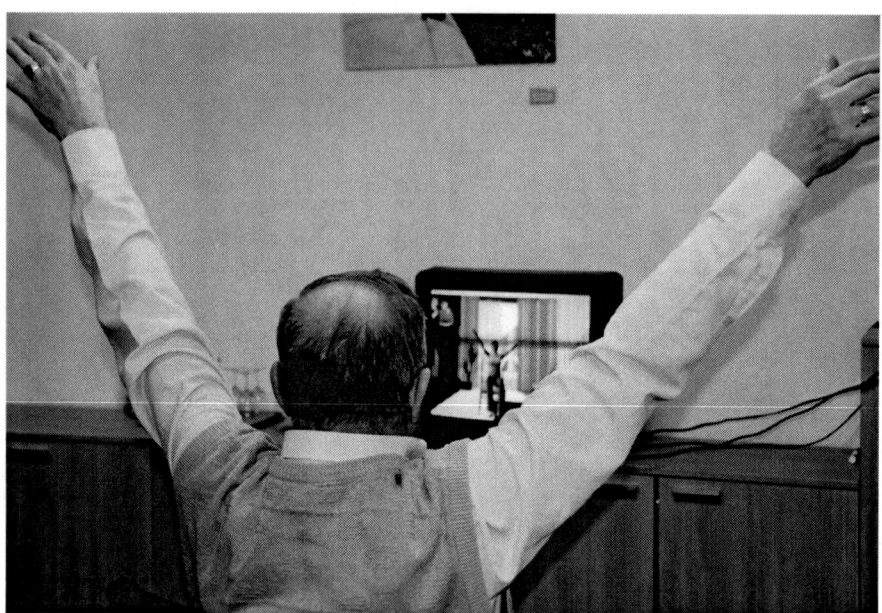

seem to have no problems accepting the avatar as a guide for doing the exercises.

The tone of the voice seems clear for many participants but some expressed the need to control the volume of the voice. As a design conclusion, this should be individually customisable.

However, during the avatar component tests some participants also expressed the requirement that the avatar should count the repetitions of an exercise verbally since they would then feel more comfortable and in more control. This was assessed as being of high importance for the further development of the system and the avatar itself. However, since the avatar already verbally explains the exercises it was seen as difficult to also let the avatar verbally count the repetitions of an exercise. Thus, the researchers looked for an alternative implementation equally addressing the underlying user need. As a consequence, the counting of the exercises will be displayed on the screen. Implementation of an exercise counter was not part of the original use case as derived from the first and second phase of user involvement. It is thus a good example of how user ideas

where further considered during iterative system development (Figure 7).

CRITICAL REVIEW AND CONCLUSIONS

Actively involving users in several stages of the development process makes a real difference and leads to usable and acceptable prototypes. As the example of the development of a technical system to support exercises at home illustrates, older users can significantly contribute to the concrete design of a technological support system. Ideas created by users become more and more explicit over time and users are more able to raise significant issues about the system functionalities and usability, even at rather early prototype stages. The methodologies developed and applied in the project thus clearly present an important advance in AAL research.

However, involving users from the very beginning of system development and at several stages of the development process clearly poses some

Figure 7. Example showing how user ideas were further processed during the second phase of prototype testing

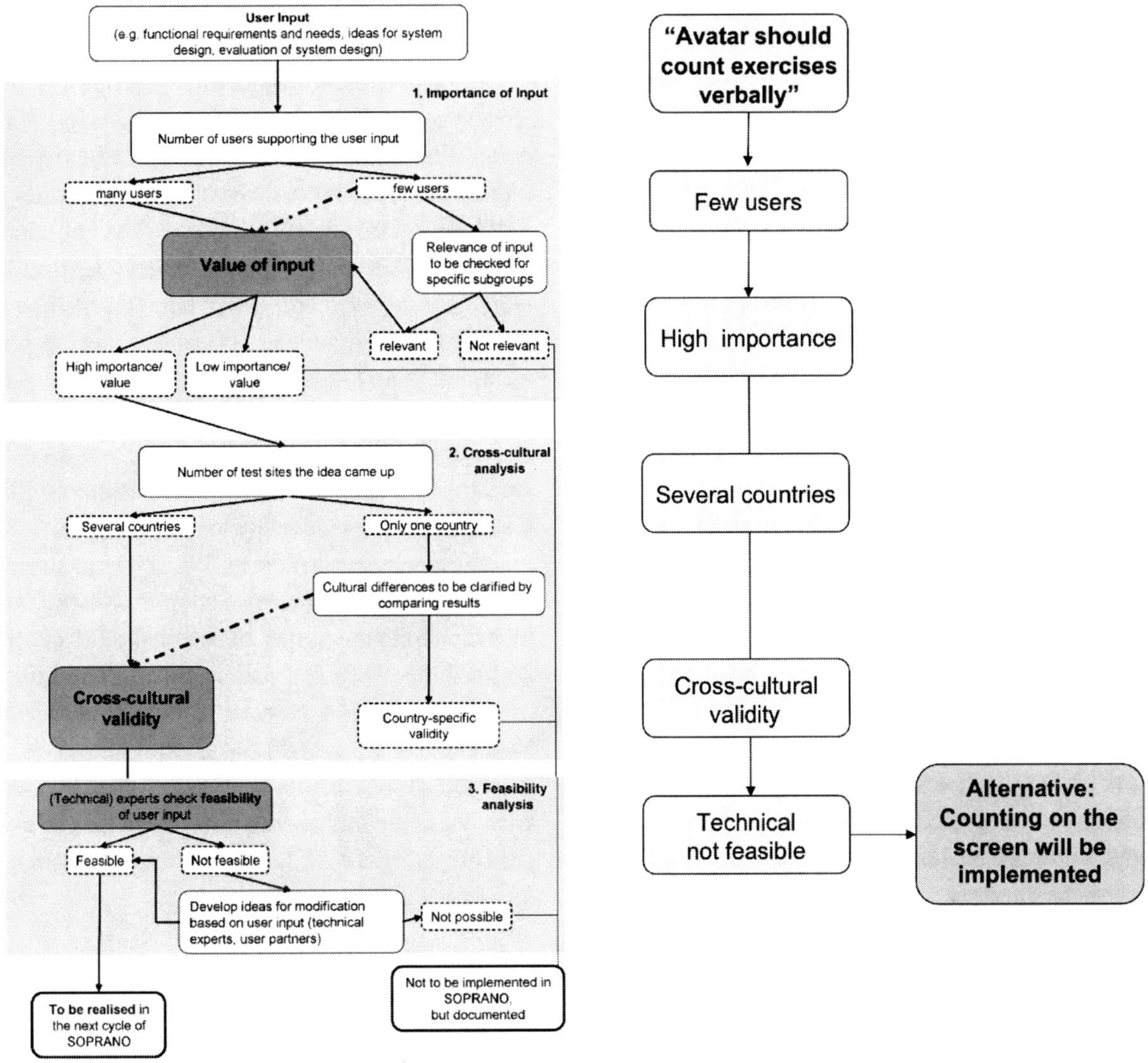

significant challenges and can sometimes also lead to contradictory results. Thus, an effective mix of suitable methods needs to be applied that take into account the different levels of system maturity during the development process and that are appropriate for each stage of the development process. Theatre methods that were applied in the project with the objective to generate conceptual design ideas are for example a very effective means to support older end users visualising the use of

the technology and providing interactive feedback. Participants seem to find it easy to come up with a range of design ideas and did so with enthusiasm. Interactive methods help the researchers to gather a lot of input from their envisaged target group and one can conclude that theatre groups are a very valuable means for working with older people in a technical context.

In addition to this, the organisation of four cycles of user involvement within a given timeframe of 40 months clearly poses significant challenges on the cooperation between researchers investigating requirements and design ideas together with end users and the technical developers. Strong cooperation between the two groups is an indispensable precondition for the success of the project. This makes it possible to combine knowledge at every moment in the process and is not sequential. For instance, experts are not the only ones who can introduce creativity. Users can also give creative solutions, although maybe on a different level of abstraction.

Although the users were the main focus, technological development is a balancing act between thoroughly and iteratively investigating user ideas and requirements on the one hand and proceeding with the technical developments within limited timeframes on the other. This at some stages of the project resulted in the necessity to anticipate user ideas in order to process technical development. However, as long as the users have, through the application of appropriate methods, the possibility to bring in their own design ideas and as long as the system development is open enough to be revised in order to take into account and implement (design) ideas coming from the users the approach of "real user involvement" is not affected. It must however be emphasised that iterative involvement of users and consequently iterative system and technology involvement requires much more resources than the usual technology-push developments.

Crucial to the meaningful incorporation of user input is the development of an analytical framework that helps to structure the input from the users and provides a decision guideline on how to process user ideas. The issue here is that different users have different priorities, contexts and living environments and thus different requirements for a support system, so that development of ideas is inevitably influenced by very individual circumstances.

In the next and final phase of the user involvement and system development process the system will be evaluated in two different ways. Firstly the system will be tested in its full functionality in demonstration homes in three European cities (Eindhoven, Newham and San Sebastian). This means that in addition to the exercise support system all use cases that were developed in the project will be installed and evaluated by older end users. Altogether 300 end users (older people, professional and family carers) will have the chance to explore and evaluate the system in guided exploration tours and focus groups. In addition to this, in depth usability test will again be conducted in order to also further improve usability aspects of system components that have not been thoroughly tested in the previous development stages.

Moreover, parts of the SOPRANO functionalities, including the exercise support system, will be installed in the homes of selected older people and will be evaluated under real-life conditions over a period of 4 months in field trials in the Netherlands, Spain and the United Kingdom. It is expected that results from the large scale field trials will help addressing the current lack of evidence to support AAL large scale implementations (Sixsmith, 2008).

ACKNOWLEDGMENT

SOPRANO (http://www.soprano-ip.org/) is an Integrated Project funded under the EU's FP6 IST programme Thematic Priority: 6.2.2: Ambient Assisted Living for the Ageing Society (IST – 2006 – 045212). The authors acknowledge the input and role of the SOPRANO consortium and would also like to thank the many people who volunteered in the various stages of user research described in this paper.

REFERENCES

Adlam, T. D., & Orpwood, R. D. (2003). Technology, Autonomy and Cognitive Disability. In *Proceedings of The 2nd International Workshop on Ubiquitous Computing for Pervasive Healthcare Applications (UbiHealth '03)*, Seattle, WA.

Beyer, H., & Holtzblatt, K. (1998). *Contextual Design: Defining Customer-Centered Systems.* San Francisco: Morgan Kaufmann.

Bland, R. (1999). Independence, privacy and risk: two contrasting approaches to residential care for older people. *Ageing and Society, 19*(5), 539–560. doi:10.1017/S0144686X99007497

Bortz, J., & Döring, N. (1995). *Forschungsmethoden und Evaluation.* Berlin: Springer.

Caplan, S. (1990). Using focus groups methodology for economic design. *Ergonomics, 33*, 527–533. doi:10.1080/00140139008927160

Carroll, J. M., & Rosson, M. B. (1992). Getting around the task-artifact cycle: How to make claims and design by scenario. *ACM Transactions on Information Systems, 10*, 181–212. doi:10.1145/146802.146834

De Carvalho Bastone, A., & Filho, W. J. (2004). Effect of an exercise program on functional performance of institutionalized elderly. *Journal of Rehabilitation Research and Development, 41*(5), 659–668. doi:10.1682/JRRD.2003.01.0014

European Commission. (2004). *ISTAG Report on Experience and Application Research- Involving Users in the Development of Ambient Intelligence.* Luxembourg: Office for Official Publications of the European Communities.

Gattuso, S. (1996). The meaning of home for older women in rural Australia. *Australian Journal on Ageing, 4*(15), 172–176. doi:10.1111/j.1741-6612.1996.tb00024.x

Gineste, Y. Pellissier & Humanitude, J. (2007). *Comprendre la vieillesse, prendre soin des Hommes vieux.* Paris: Armand Colin.

Goldman, A. E., & McDonald, S. S. (1987). *The Group Depth Interview: Principles and Practice.* Upper Saddle River, NJ: Prentice Hall.

Greenbaum, T. L. (1988). *The Practical Handbook and Guide to Focus Group Research.* Lexington, MA: D.C. Heath & Co.

International Organization for Standardization. ISO/*FDIS 9241-110. Ergonomics of human-system interaction -- Part 110: Dialogue principles.* International Organization for Standardization. ISO/*FDIS 9241-210. Ergonomics of human-system interaction -- Part 210: Human-centred design for interactive systems.* Retrieved December 28, 2009, from http://www.iso.org/iso/catalogue_detail.htm?csnumber=52075.

Kim, Y. (2004). *Pedagogical agents as learning companions: the effects of agent affect and gender on student learning, interest, self-efficacy, and agent persona.* PhD thesis, Tallahassee, USA.

Koda, T., & Maes, P. (1996). Agents with faces: The effects of personification of agents. *5th IEEE International Workshop on Robot and Human Communication*, Tsukuba, Japan.

Kotonya, G., & Sommerville, I. (1998). *Requirements Engineering - Processes and Techniques.* Chichester, UK: John Wiley & Sons Inc.

Kubitschke, L., & Meyer, I. (2007). WING - Watching IST Innovation and Knowledge. *Impact Analysis in the Domain of eInclusion – Final Report.* Bonn, Brussels.

Mather, A. S., Rodriguez, C., Guthrie, M. F., McHarg, A. M., Reid, I. C., & McMurdo, M. E. T. (2002). Effects of exercise on depressive symptoms in older adults with poorly responsive depressive disorder. *The British Journal of Psychiatry, 180*, 411–415. doi:10.1192/bjp.180.5.411

Mayhew, D. J. (1999). *The usability engineering lifecycle*. San Francisco: Morgan Kaufmann.

Moore, J. (2000). Placing home in context. *Journal of Environmental Psychology, 20,* 207–217. doi:10.1006/jevp.2000.0178

Nielson, J. (1993). *Usability Engineering*. New York: Academic Press.

Noe, B., et al. (2009). Home Centric ICT Services for the Ageing Society. In *Ambient Assisted Living 2*, German AAL-Congress, Conference Proceeding, Berlin, Germany, January 27-28, 2009.

O'Donnell, P. J., Scobie, G., & Baxter, I. (1991). The use of focus groups as an evaluation technique in HCI. In Diaper, D. & Hammond, N. (Eds.). *People and Computers VI*, 211-224. Cambridge, UK: Cambridge University Press.

Ortiz, M. P. C. A., Oyarzun, D., Yanguas, J. J., Buiza, C., González, M. F., & Etxeberria, I. (2007). Elderly Users in Ambient Intelligence: Does an Avatar Improve the Interaction? *Proceedings of 9th ERCIM Workshop 'User Interfaces For All'*, pp. 99-114.

Penninx, B. W., Messier, S. P., Rejeski, W. J., Williamson, J. D., DiBari, M., & Cavazzini, C. (2001). Physical exercise and the prevention of disability in activities of daily living in older persons with osteoarthritis. *Archives of Internal Medicine, 161*(19), 2309–2316. doi:10.1001/archinte.161.19.2309

Prendinger, H., Ma, C., Yingzi, J., Nakasone, A., & Ishizuka, M. (2005). Understanding the effect of life-like interface agents through users' eye movements. *Proceedings of the 7th international conference on Multimodal interfaces* (pp. 108-115), New York: ACM Press.

Rogers, W. A., Meyer, B., Walker, N., & Fisk, A. D. (1998). Functional Limitations to Daily Living Tasks in the Aged: A focus Group Analysis. *Human Factors. The Journal of the human factors and ergonomics society, 40 (1)*, 111-125.

Rosson, M. B., & Carroll, J. M. (2002). *Usability Engineering. Scenario-Based Development of Human-Computer Interaction.* San Francisco: Morgan Kaufmann Publishers.

Ruuskanen, J. M., & Ruoppila, I. (1995). Physical activity and psychological well-being among people aged 65 to 84 years. *Age and Ageing, 24*(4), 292–296. doi:10.1093/ageing/24.4.292

Secker, J., Hill, R., Villeneau, L., & Parkman, S. (2003). Promoting independence: but promoting what and how. *Ageing and Society, 23*(3), 375–391. doi:10.1017/S0144686X03001193

Singh, M. A. F. (2002). Exercise Come of Age: Rationale and Recommendations for a Geriatric Exercise Prescription. *Journal of Gerontology: Medical Sciences, 57*(5), 262–282.

Sixsmith, A. (1986). Independence and home in later life. In Phillipson, C., Bernard, M. & Strang, P. (Eds.), *Dependency and interdependency in old age- theoretical perspectives and policy alternatives* (pp. 338- 347). London, Croom Helm in association with The British Society of Gerontology.

Sixsmith, A. (2008). *Ambient technologies: developing user-driven approaches to research and development.* Paper presented at the Gerontological Society of America 61st Annual Scientific Meeting, Gaylord National Resort and Convention Center. *MD Medical Newsmagazine*, (November): 21–25.

Skelton, D. A., & McLaughlin, A. W. (1996). Training Functional Ability in Old Age. *Physiotherapy, 82*(3), 159–167. doi:10.1016/S0031-9406(05)66916-7

Tanner, D. (2003). Older people and access to care. *British Journal of Social Work, 33*(4), 499–515. doi:10.1093/bjsw/33.4.499

Vredenburg, K., Isensee, S., & Righi, C. (2002). *User-centred design.* Upper Saddle River, NJ: Prentice Hall.

Wixon, D., & Wilson, C. (1997). The Usability Engineering Framework for Product Design and Evaluation . In Helander, M., Landauer, T. K., & Prabhu, P. (Eds.), *Handbook of Human-Computer Interaction*. Englewood Cliffs, N.J.: Elsevier Science.

ADDITIONAL READING

Aarts, E., & Encarnação, J. L. (2005). Into Ambient Intelligence . In Aarts, E., & Encarnaçao, J. (Eds.), *True Visions: Tales on the Realization of Ambient Intelligence (pp.)*. New York: Springer.

Berg, R. L., & Cassells, J. S. (1990). *The second fifty years: Promoting health and preventing disability*. Washington, DC: National Academy Press.

Bonder, B. R., & Wagner, M. B. (2001). *Functional performance in older adults*. Philadelphia: F.A. Davis.

Branfield, F., & Beresford, P. (2006). *Making user involvement work- Supporting service user networking and knowledge*. York: Joseph Rowntree Foundation.

Bunce, D. J., Barrowclough, A., & Morris, I. (1996). The moderating influence of physical fitness on age gradients in vigilance and serial choice responding tasks. *Psychology and Aging*, *11*, 671–682. doi:10.1037/0882-7974.11.4.671

Carter, N. D., Kannus, P., & Khan, K. M. (2001). Exercise in the Prevention of Falls in Older People: A Systematic Literature Review Examining the Rationale and the Evidence. *Sports Medicine (Auckland, N.Z.)*, *31*(6), 427–438. doi:10.2165/00007256-200131060-00003

Davis, F., Bagozzi, R., & Warshaw, P. (1989). User acceptance of computer technology: A comparison of two theoretical models. *Management Science*, *35*, 982–1003. doi:10.1287/mnsc.35.8.982

Heckhausen, J. (2005). Psychological approaches to human development. In Johnson, M. L., Bengtson, V. L., Coleman, P. G., & Kirkwood, T. B. L. (Eds.), *The Cambridge Handbook of Age and Ageing*. Cambridge, New York: CUP. doi:10.1017/CBO9780511610714.017

Keil, M., & Beranek, P.M. &, B.R. (1995). Usefulness and ease of use: Field study evidence regarding task considerations. *Decision Support Systems*, *13*, 75–91. doi:10.1016/0167-9236(94)E0032-M

Machate, J. (2003). Von der Idee zum Produkt- mit Benutzern gestalten . In Machate, J., & Burmester, M. (Eds.), *User Interface Tuning. Benutzungsschnittstellen menschlich gestalten* (pp. 83–96). Frankfurt: Software & Support Verlag GmbH.

Mueller, S., & Sixsmith, A. (2008). *User requirements for Ambient Assisted Living: Some evidence from the SOPRANO project*. Paper at the 6th International Conference of the International Society for Gerontechnology/, Pisa, Tuscany, Italy, June 4-7.

Newell, A. F., Carmichael, A., Morgan, M., & Dickinson, A. (2006). The use of theatre in requirements gathering and usability studies. *Interacting with Computers*, *18*, 996–1011. doi:10.1016/j.intcom.2006.05.003

O'Donnell, P. J., Scobie, G., & Baxter, I. (1991). The use of focus groups as an evaluation technique in HCI . In Diaper, D., & Hammond, N. (Eds.), *People and Computers VI* (pp. 211–224). Cambridge, UK: Cambridge University Press.

Porteus, J., & Brownsell, S. (2000). *Using Telecare. Exploring Technologies for Independent Living for Older People*. Brigthon, UK: Pavilion Publishing.

Prensky, M. (2001). Digital Natives, Digital Immigrants, Part II: Do They Really Think Differently? *Horizon*, *9*(6).

Rogers, W. A., Mayhorn, C. B., & Fisk, A. D. (2004). Technology in everyday life for older adults . In Burdick, D. C., & Kwon, S. (Eds.), *Gerotechnology: Research and Practice in Technology and Ageing*. New York: Springer Publishing Company.

Scialfa, C. T., Ho, G., & Laberge, J. (2004). Perceptual aspects of gerotechnology . In Burdick, D. C., & Kwon, S. (Eds.), *Gerotechnology. Research and practice in technology and ageing*. New York: Springer Publishing Company.

Sixsmith, A., Hine, N., Neild, I., Clarke, N., Brown, S., & Garner, P. (2007). Monitoring the well-being of older people. *Topics in Geriatric Rehabilitation., 23*(1), 9–23.

Small, G., & Vorgan, G. (2009). *iBrain. Wie die neue Medienwelt Gehirn und Seele unserer Kinder verändert*. Stuttgart, Kreuz Verlag.

KEY TERMS AND DEFINITIONS

Ambient Assisted Living (AAL): "AAL refers intelligent systems of assistance for a better, healthier and safer life in the preferred living environment and covers concepts, products and services that interlink and improve new technologies and the social environment. It aims at enhancing the quality of life (the physical, mental and social well-being) for everyone (with a focus on elder persons) in all stages of their life". (AALIANCE (2009). Ambient Assisted Living Roadmap, p. 6)

Conversational avatar: Conversational avatars are virtual characters that simulate or replicate human behaviour. A large deal of research has been carried out on this topic in the last decades and as a result has been applied in many scenarios: Films, computer games, TV, Internet etc. Avatars have succeeded in achieving high degrees of realism in the graphical design, facial gestures, synchronisation with speech synthesizers and emotional expression.

Experience & Application Research: The concept of E&AR was developed in 2004 by the Information Society Technologies Advisory Group. E&AR asks for research, development and design by, with and for users. It also requests research into methods and tools that enable this. This approach is crucial to the development of human-centred ambient intelligent systems.

Focused Design Discussion: User ideas for system design can be effectively discussed in Focus Design Discussions (FDD). A FDD is a structured and moderated group discussion with a trained and skilled moderator. By using open-ended questions interaction is promoted and the participants´ perspectives and experiences are explored to generate qualitative data. The moderator encourages the participants with target-oriented questions to develop their own ideas or to give feedback to presented solutions and helps the participants to keep the focused aspects in mind. Thereby, the moderator follows an agenda, pays attention to the equality of participants and visualises results (Bortz & Döring, 1995, p.293 f). A factor the success of a FDD is a reliable and relaxed group atmosphere where people are willing to open their minds and be creative. One central aspect of the FDD is the use of metaphors. The "Guardian Angel metaphor" helps to generate user-driven ideas without being biased through explicit assumptions about what is possible with technology.

Guardian Angel Approach: The Guardian Angel is to be understood as a personification of the technical system under development. The idea is introduced so as not to have to explain exactly how information is gathered in the home or exactly how information is given. Users are able to overcome implicit or explicit assumptions about what is possible with technology they are familiar with. The Guardian Angel is not limited to any constraints. This approach enables to collect needs and wishes of older people in the area of the presented situations.

Multimedia Mock-up: A multimedia mock-up can be an online tool which the moderator of a focus group can use to visually demonstrate the different use cases to potential end users of an AAL system.

Theatre Method: Scenario Based Dramas or Theatre Methods are able to portray a situation in a very naturalistic and more immediate manner which makes it easier to imagine and remember a scene. Plays are very suitable for activating memories and emotions of spectators (Bortz & Döring 1995), an aspect which is an advantage in the work with older people. Theatre plays offer the possibility to enact a kind of play between users and experts and to include prototypes into the play. Also, theatre plays give a good basis for semi-structured interviewing.

ENDNOTE

[1]   A more in-depth analysis of new approaches to care provision is beyond the scope of the present text. Increasing activity in this field can be found in countries such as France, Belgium, Switzerland, Germany and Canada. The "Philosophie de soin de l'Humanitude" developed by Yves Gineste in France particularly for the care of people with dementia can be mentioned as an example (Gineste 2007).

Chapter 11

Wearable Systems for Monitoring Mobility Related Activities:
From Technology to Application for Healthcare Services

Wiebren Zijlstra
University Medical Center Groningen, The Netherlands

Clemens Becker
Robert Bosch Gesellschaft für medizinische Forschung, Germany

Klaus Pfeiffer
Robert Bosch Gesellschaft für medizinische Forschung, Germany

ABSTRACT

Monitoring the performance of daily life mobility related activities, such as rising from a chair, standing and walking may be used to support healthcare services. This chapter identifies available wearable motion-sensing technology; its (potential) clinical application for mobility assessment and monitoring; and it addresses the need to assess user perspectives on wearable monitoring systems. Given the basic requirements for application under real-life conditions, this chapter emphasizes methods based on single sensor locations. A number of relevant clinical applications in specific older populations are discussed; i.e. (risk-) assessment, evaluation of changes in functioning, and monitoring as an essential part of exercise-based interventions. Since the application of mobility monitoring as part of existing healthcare services for older populations is rather limited, this chapter ends with issues that need to be addressed to effectively implement techniques for mobility monitoring in healthcare.

DOI: 10.4018/978-1-60960-469-1.ch011

INTRODUCTION

One of the major challenges in health care is the ability to timely initiate interventions that prevent loss of functional abilities and maintain or improve quality of life. The individual capacity for safe locomotion is a major indicator for independent functioning in older people. However, within the growing population of older people, safe and independent mobility can be at risk due to age-related diseases such as osteo-arthritis, Parkinson's or Alzheimer's disease, and stroke. In addition, older people may become inactive and develop frailty without overt pathology. The latter increases the incidence and impact of falls which are a major threat for health related quality of life in older people (Skelton and Todd 2004).

In the next decades, Europe will face a sharp increase, in both relative as well as absolute terms, in the number of older adults. This development is a result of an increasing number of older adults and an average ageing of the population. In 2008, less than 15% of the Dutch population was aged 65 or older; by 2040 this percentage will have increased and reached its peak at approximately 26% (CBS, 2009). Estimates of ageing in other European countries, such as Germany and Italy, are even higher (Eurostat, 2008). The demographic trend towards an ageing society poses social as well as economic challenges. While the demands on health care services are steadily increasing, the (relative) number of persons to give care and to finance health care decreases. Thus, there is a need to adapt health care services. New technologies may aid in providing solutions.

Effective interventions are needed to maintain functioning and prevent the loss of independent mobility in older people. Wearable technology for monitoring the performance of daily life mobility related activities, such as lying, rising from a chair, standing and walking may be used to support interventions, which aim to maintain or restore independent mobility. However, at present the routine-use of movement monitoring for the

clinical management of care in older populations is limited. Therefore, this chapter aims to identify the potential relevance of wearable systems for monitoring mobility for exercise-based interventions and healthcare services by addressing: available wearable motion sensing technology and its application in methods for mobility assessment and monitoring; clinical applications of mobility monitoring; user perspectives on mobility monitoring; and present shortcomings that prevent an effective implementation of wearable solutions for mobility monitoring in health care services.

AVAILABLE WEARABLE TECHNOLOGY FOR MONITORING HUMAN MOVEMENTS

A general principle underlying studies of human movements is to consider the human body as a set of rigid bodies (e.g. foot, shank, or thigh), interconnected by joints (e.g. ankle, or knee). Human movement analyses thus require measuring the kinematics of one or more body segments, e.g. by a camera-based system for position measurements or by different motion sensors. The resulting kinematic data are input into further analyses. Depending on research aims, measurements may be simple (e.g. head or trunk position to study walking distance and speed), or highly complex (e.g. full-body measurements to study inter-segmental dynamics). Recent developments in the miniaturization of movement sensors and measurement technology have opened the way for wearable motion sensing technology (Bonato 2005) and the ambulatory assessment of mobility related activities (e.g. Aminian & Najafi 2004, Zijlstra & Aminian 2007). The recent advances even allow full-body ambulatory measurements by motion sensors. However, since monitoring techniques need to be applied over long durations and under real-life conditions, a number of feasibility criteria should be taken into account. These criteria encompass technical criteria (e.g.

the degree to which energy consumption limits the use of multiple sensors) as well as criteria which relate to user acceptance (e.g. the methods need to be non-obtrusive and easy-to-use). The latter aspects will be addressed in a subsequent section, in this section an a-priori choice will be made which facilitates technical and practical feasibility; namely a focus on single-sensor approaches to monitoring mobility. The next sub-sections give a short evaluation of available sensors, signal analysis aspects, and methods for mobility assessment and monitoring. The latter subsection will primarily address current possibilities and limitations of methods using single sensor locations, such as on trunk or leg segments.

Wearable Movement Sensors

Goniometers can be used to directly measure changes in joint angle. Regardless of sensor type, the basic principle consists of attaching the two axes of the goniometer to the proximal and distal segments of a joint and measuring the angle between these two axes. Drawbacks of using goniometers are sensor attachments which may hinder habitual movement, limited accuracy, and vulnerability of the sensors.

Accelerometers measure accelerations of body segments. Piezo-electric type accelerometers measure accelerations only. They are mainly used for quantifying activity related accelerations. Other accelerometers, i.e. (piezo)resistive or capacitive type accelerometers, measure accelerations (a) and the effect of gravitation (g). In the absence of movement, they can be used to calculate the inclination of the sensor with respect to the vertical. Thus, by attaching accelerometers on one or more body segments (e.g. trunk, thigh, and shank), the resistive type can be used to detect body postures at rest (e.g. standing, sitting, and lying). During activities, movements of body segments induce inertial acceleration, and a variable gravitational component depending on the change of segment inclination with respect to the vertical axis. Both

acceleration components are superimposed and their separation is necessary for a proper analysis of the movement.

Miniature gyroscopes are sensitive to angular velocity. Although their use for analyzing human movements is still rather new, gyroscopes are promising since they allow the direct measurement of segment rotations around joints. Unlike resistive type of accelerometers, there is no influence of gravitation on the signal measured by gyroscopes. The gyroscope can be attached to any part of a body segment: as long as its axis is parallel to the measured axis, the angular rotation is still the same along this segment. Rotation angles can be estimated from angular velocity by simple numeric integration. However, due to integration drift, it is problematic to estimate absolute angles from angular velocity data.

Earth magnetic field sensors or magnetometers measure changes in the orientation of a body segment relative to the magnetic North. Earth magnetic field sensors can be used to determine segment orientation around the vertical axis. Hence, they provide information that cannot be determined from accelerometers or by the integration of gyroscope signals. However, a disadvantage of magnetometers is their sensitivity to nearby ferromagnetic materials (e.g. iron) and magnetic fields other than that of the earth magnetic field (e.g. electro-magnetic fields produced by a TV screen).

Pressure sensors or foot switches attached to the shoe or foot sole can be used to detect contact of the foot with the ground. These sensors allow the identification of different movement phases during walking (i.e. swing, stance and bipedal stance phases), or they can provide pressure distribution of the foot during stance phases. These techniques allow the measurement of longer periods of walking with many subsequent stride cycles.

A **barometric pressure sensor** technically is not a movement sensor, but its sensitivity to air pressure can be used to estimate movement characteristics. Changes in altitude are reflected in a different air pressure, thus changes in the height of a body segment can be estimated from the measured pressure signal.

Use of a **Global Position System (GPS)** offers the possibility to locate (changes in) the position of body segments. However, the system can only be used outside and the accuracy of determining position is limited to ca. 0.3 m. The latter accuracy can be improved by use of so called differential GPS (dGPS).

At present, the most relevant movement sensors for use in wearable systems for mobility monitoring are (resistive type) accelerometers, gyroscopes and foot switches. Sometimes combinations of sensors are used (i.e. hybrid sensing) to overcome limitations of specific sensor types and therewith obtain optimal kinematic data of body segments. A well-known example of such a hybrid sensor consists of a combination of three-dimensional accelerometers, gyroscopes and earth-magnetic field sensors.

Analysis of Data from Motion Sensors

Unlike conventional camera-based methods for movement analyses, most motion sensors do not provide information about position of body segments, therefore the use of these sensors requires intelligent signal processing and appropriate methods to obtain relevant movement parameters. Advanced signal processing is necessary to extract relevant information from movement sensors. To begin with, appropriate signal processing methods are required in order to estimate body kinematics with an acceptable accuracy. Often the data analysis requires that kinematic data are transformed from a local to an inertial (i.e. gravity- or earth-oriented) reference frame. Accelerometers and gyroscopes measure within a local frame of reference, and the orientation of this local reference frame depends on the orientation of the body segment to which the sensor is attached. To transform the sensor data from a local segment oriented reference frame to an inertial reference frame requires knowledge of sensor orientation in space. This orientation can be estimated using data from different sensor types and adequate signal processing algorithms. For example, it has recently been demonstrated that the use of hybrid sensors, consisting of accelerometers, gyroscopes and magnetometers, and signal processing algorithms using a Kalman filter allows for an accurate sensor-based analysis of movements in an inertial frame of reference (e.g. see Luinge & Veltink 2005, Roetenberg et al. 2005). Another recent development is the possibility to combine hybrid sensors for analyzing movements of body segments and GPS for overall changes in position (e.g. Terrier & Schutz 2005).

Since the kinematics of body segments are task dependent, the analysis of time varying properties of segment kinematics requires methods that vary in dependence of the specific movement task (e.g. sit-to-stand, standing, or walking). In addition, the choice for signal processing of sensor data depends on the specific goal of the measurements. Not all analyses of human activities need a complete description of the movements of all body segments. The same activity, for example gait, may be analyzed differently depending on whether overall measures (e.g. duration of walking and estimated walking distance) or specific measures (e.g. gait variability, joint rotations) are required. As will be seen in the next section, data acquisition and signal analyses can be simplified if a-priori knowledge of a specific movement is available.

Methods for Mobility Assessment and Monitoring

Sensor-based assessments of mobility related activities can target both quantitative and qualitative aspects of movement performance. To quantify movement performance requires methods to detect specific postures, activities, or events from data measured by motion sensors. The qualitative analysis of mobility related activities requires algorithms, which extract relevant biomechanical parameters of movement performance from sensor data. As will be seen in the next sub-sections, a wide variety of different sensor configurations (i.e. the specific type of sensors and the location of sensors on body segments) has been used to extract quantitative and qualitative parameters of movement performance.

The detection of frequency and duration of specific body postures and activities from sensor signals, in the literature often indicated as *"Activity Monitoring"*, is at the heart of any method which aims to monitor mobility over long durations. The underlying principle for the detection of different postures is that during static conditions (e.g. lying, sitting or standing) the orientation of body segments can be determined from the static component in the measured acceleration signal. Thus, it is possible to deduce whether a person is standing, sitting or lying from the orientation of leg and trunk segments. Using (video-based) observations as a reference, several papers have demonstrated the validity of discerning different postures and activities based on accelerometers on trunk and leg segments (e.g. Bussmann et al. 1995, Veltink et al. 1996, Aminian et al. 1999). A sensitivity and specificity higher than 90% has been reported for the detection of different postures and activities based on multiple sensors. However, it should be noted that available validation studies typically are based on data-sets which have been obtained under conditions which are different from activity patterns in daily life. Whereas the first activity monitoring studies were all based on the use of sensors on multiple body segments (mostly trunk and leg), recent studies have shown possibilities to obtain similar information about frequency and duration of activities based on single sensor approaches. For example, based on the detection of transitions between postures by a hybrid sensor which combines a two-dimensional (2D) accelerometer and a gyroscope on the ventral thorax (Najafi et al. 2003) or based on a 3D ac-

celerometer at the dorsal side of the lower trunk (Dijkstra et al. 2008, Dijkstra et al. 2010) postures and activities can be detected.

Fall detection can be considered a special case within activity monitoring. Sensor-based fall detectors are highly relevant as the basis for reliable fall reports and automatic fall alarm systems. The advantage of sensor-based fall alarm systems over existing alarm systems is that in the event of a serious fall, the alarm can be triggered automatically. Thus, services can be initiated immediately even if a person is unable to trigger an alarm manually, or otherwise call for help. The available literature on sensor-based fall detection methods presents different approaches, which most often are based on accelerometers at body locations such as head, trunk, or wrist (e.g. Lindemann et al. 2005, Noury et al. 2006, Karantonis et al. 2006, Zhang et al. 2006, Bourke et al. 2007, Kangas et al. 2008). However, at present, there is little published information about the real-life validity of sensor-based fall detectors. The validity of fall detection methods is determined by their sensitivity to falls (i.e., "Does the method detect all falls?") and specificity (i.e., "Does the method correctly classify those situation where no falls occurred?"). The available studies often have followed a validation approach in which the sensitivity and specificity of fall detection algorithms are determined based on data measured in healthy subjects who simulate different type of falls. Although this approach is an essential first step, the real validation should come from real-life falls obtained in the target populations for applying a fall detection method.

In the last decades a steadily increasing number of papers report the use of sensor-based methods for a *qualitative analysis of the performance of mobility related activities* such as standing, walking, sit-to-stand movement (e.g. see Zijlstra & Aminian 2007). A considerable part of these papers are based on measurements at a single sensor location. The latter simplifies the procedures for data-acquisition, and is possible when a-priori knowledge exists about the characteristics of the movements to be measured. For example, many studies are based on measuring the kinematics of the lower trunk at a position close to the body's centre of mass, which during static standing conditions is located within the pelvis at the level of the second sacral vertebrae. The subsequent data-analyses and interpretations are then based on the assumption that the measured kinematics are similar to the movement patterns of the body's centre of mass.

A conventional approach to determine *postural stability during standing* is to analyze how well a subject is able to maintain his body position without changing the base of support. Data measured by a force plate under both feet allows for an analysis of the changes in centre of pressure position under the feet. Often these analyses are based on measures of the amplitude and frequency content of changes in the centre of pressure. During quiet standing conditions, the accelerations of the body's centre of mass are proportional to the changes in centre of pressure (Winter 1995). Thus, accelerations measured at the height of the body's center of mass should yield similar information about postural stability as the data measured by a force plate. The latter assumption seems to be confirmed by accelerometry based studies of trunk sway during different standing conditions (e.g. Mayagoitia et al. 2002, Moe-Nilssen & Helbostad 2002). In addition to accelerometry-based approaches, the use of gyroscopes to measure trunk rotations during standing has shown to be sensitive for difference in postural stability (e.g. Allum et al. 2005).

Spatio-temporal gait parameters such as walking speed, step length and frequency, duration of swing and stance phases can be determined from sensors on leg or trunk segments. Hausdorff et al. (1995) used foot switches to measure (the variability of) temporal gait parameters. Aminian et al. (2002) used gyroscopes on shank and thigh segments of both legs in combination with a geometrical model of the leg to estimate spatial

parameters in addition to temporal gait parameters. Based on knowledge of the mechanical determinants of trunk movements during walking (i.e. inverted pendulum characteristics (see Zijlstra & Hof 1997, Zijlstra & Hof 2003)), Zijlstra (2004) estimated spatio-temporal gait parameters using 3D accelerometry at a lower trunk position close to the body's centre of mass. Sabatini et al. (2005) used knowledge of specific constraints for human walking (i.e. repeated stance phases where the foot has no forward velocity) to overcome typical limitations of sensors and determine spatio-temporal gait parameters from a 2D hybrid sensor on the foot. When more than one sensor location is used, the basic spatio-temporal gait parameters can be complemented with additional parameters which depend on the exact sensor configurations (e.g. joint kinematics (Dejnabadi et al. 2005, 2006), trunk angles (Zijlstra et al. 2007), or joint dynamics (Zijlstra & Bisseling 2004).

Performance of the *Sit-to-Stand (STS) transfer* requires the ability to maintain balance while producing enough muscle force to raise the body's centre of mass from a seated to a standing position (e.g. see Schenkman et al. 1999, Ploutz-Snyder et al. 2002, Lindemann et al. 2003). Recent studies demonstrated that hybrid sensors can be used to obtain *temporal measures of STS* (e.g. Najafi et al. 2002), and estimations of *the power to lift the body's center of mass* during the STS movement (Zijlstra et al. 2010). Usually, the latter analyses of muscle power are restricted to a laboratory-based approach using cycle- or rowing-ergometers, or opto-electronic camera systems and force plates. However, based on laboratory validations, the recent study demonstrated that motion sensors can be used to obtain measures of muscle strength and power during the Sit-to-Stand (STS) movement in young and older (70+) subjects.

To summarize this section: the present literature indicates the availability of wearable technology and suitable methods for assessment of relevant quantitative and qualitative aspects of mobility related activities. As a general rule, the use of hybrid sensors and complex sensor configurations on the body offer better analytical solutions. However, even complex configurations of multiple hybrid sensors are limited with regard to the analysis of (changes in) position of body segments in relation to the support surface or objects in the environment. Furthermore, practical considerations may necessitate the choice for as few sensors as possible. It should be noted that the wealth of sensor-based approaches to mobility assessment and monitoring has not yet resulted in a standardization of procedures for data-acquisition, data-analysis and the validation of assessment methods.

EMERGING HEALTHCARE SERVICES BASED ON MOBILITY MONITORING

The World Health Organization's International Classification of Functioning (i.e. the ICF-model (see references)) presents a framework for studying the effects of disease and health conditions on human functioning. The model indicates that insight in the underlying mechanisms of functional decline requires insight in the complex relationships between body functions (e.g. joint flexibility, muscle force), activities (e.g. gait & balance capacity), and actual movement behavior in daily life. The ICF model underlines the need of assessing both *capacity* ("What a person can do under standardized conditions") and *performance* ("What a person really does in his or her daily life"). During daily life a person may use specific assistive devices and services (facilitators), or vice versa may encounter specific problems (barriers) in his or her personal situation. Thus, capacity and performance measures yield different information and the ICF model very clearly indicates the need to assess capacity and to monitor the performance of mobility related activities in real-life.

The ICF model is widely used as a framework for clinical research, but the model does not specify how capacity and performance should be measured. At present, the extent to which the ICF model is systematically used as part of the daily work routines of those disciplines which address impaired motor functioning and mobility seems rather limited. One reason for this situation is that tools to systematically address capacity and performance aspects of mobility have not been available for application in clinical practice. The tools which are based on wearable technology, as described in the preceding section, are based on recent developments, and there still is the need to resolve many issues before these new tools may become a standard part of clinical routine. First of all, an undisputed evidence-base is needed for the clinical relevance of monitoring based health-care services, and secondly the monitoring approaches need to be acceptable to the potential users. Thus, it is of paramount importance to not only have technical solutions available, it is also necessary to evaluate the clinical validity of tools for mobility assessment and monitoring, and to assess and incorporate user perspectives in the development of monitoring-based health-care services.

The next sub-sections will address some of the issues relating to clinical relevance by focusing on aspects of current clinical practice and the potential contribution of mobility monitoring techniques in new health care services. Examples will be given in relation to different conditions, which may lead to mobility impairments. This section will be followed by a next section, which specifically addresses the user perspective on wearable technology.

Current Clinical Practice

When aiming to provide optimal care to a patient, health-care professionals are typically confronted with a number of recurrent issues; e.g. the need to diagnose certain conditions, the need to evaluate outcome of an intervention, and the need to predict the risk of future adverse events. All these issues require decisions, which are based on adequate assessment tools. The quality of available tools for clinical assessment varies strongly between different clinical disciplines, and at present the clinical fields, which address (potential) mobility problems in different populations still need to further develop assessment tools of acceptable quality.

At present, the clinical assessment of mobility related activities mainly encompasses the use of field tests, observational methods, and self-report instruments. Rarely are objective quantitative methods used as part of the routine clinical assessments. The available clinical instruments that are used can be disease specific or generic, but generally, there are serious limitations to their use. For example, at present, there is little information to give evidence-based recommendations for specific existing field tests for balance and mobility in frail older persons (see the Prevention of Falls Network (www.ProFaNE.eu.org) and see Gates et al. 2008). Although many conventional clinical tests for balance and mobility (such as the Timed Up & Go (TUG), or Berg Balance Scale (BBS)) are easy-to-use, and hence allow for integration in clinical practice, they do have serious disadvantages. Most of the present field tests lack a conceptual fundament for balance assessment (e.g. Huxham et al. 2001); the scores which result from these tests are usually based on observation and simple time measures (e.g. time one one-leg, time required for standing up from a chair walking 3m, turning walking back and sitting down); and at present there is only limited evidence for the clinical validity of these measures for diagnosis, prognosis, or outcome evaluation.

Similarly, there are serious limitations to the use of self-report methods (such as diaries, questionnaires, or interviews) for obtaining information about the quantity of mobility related activities in daily life. Recalling physical activity is a complex cognitive task and the available self-report instruments vary in their cognitive demands. Older adults in particular may have memory and recall skill limitations, and generally people tend to overestimate their physical activity levels. In addition, the methods do not give a detailed profile of type, duration, frequency, and intensity of the most common daily physical activities. Although out-of-home activities, such as leisure time and sportive activities can be assessed by questionnaire, it is hard to assess non-exercise activities with thermogenesis (NEATs). In older people, more than 70% of physical activities occur at home and this should be included in an appropriate analysis. Particularly in sedentary frail older people, self-reports are insensitive to (small) changes in patterns of physical activity.

Currently, the available figures about the incidence of falls primarily depend on oral reports of the subjects themselves or their proxies. Thus, also the evaluation of fall prevention methods, in terms of a reduction in number of falls, depends on subjective reports. These reports can be biased, for example due to difficulties in defining a fall, not-remembering a fall, or due to the cognitive status of the subject who fell (e.g. see Zecevic et al. 2006, Hauer et al. 2006). In addition, the circumstances of a fall and the fall characteristics are seldom reported in a structured manner (Zecevic 2007). The lack of objective fall data seriously hampers the development and evaluation of effective fall prevention programs.

Potential Contribution of Mobility Monitoring to New Health Care Services

A large number of studies have demonstrated the potential clinical relevance of sensor-based mobility assessment and monitoring in older people (e.g. see Zijlstra & Aminian 2007). The shortlist of available sensor-based methods in the previous section clearly indicates that a variety of clinically relevant applications seem possible. However, at present there are no standardized sensor-based clinical tests for the assessment of balance and mobility. Furthermore, a recent systematic review (de Bruin et al. 2008) indicates that the majority of available studies, which have used wearable systems for monitoring mobility related activities in older populations have merely addressed the technical validity of monitoring methods. The number of studies that actually applied monitoring methods over long durations in support of clinical goals was (very) limited. Thus, the review unfortunately demonstrates that there is still the need to develop evidence-based applications of the available monitoring technology.

At present, a number of clinically relevant applications of monitoring techniques can be identified. First of all, a generic aspect of exercise-based interventions in different target groups is setting (individual) *target levels for physical activity.* To control whether target levels are reached (or not) requires appropriate monitoring information. These can be obtained by different monitoring techniques. Second, the *quality of care to specific patient groups* with mobility problems may be improved based on the systematic use of monitoring techniques. Third, the use of monitoring techniques can be used to identify persons with *an increased risk of falling*. Fourth, when a high fall risk has been established, reliable *fall detection methods* may be used to automatically detect a fall and initiate alarm services when necessary. These four examples of clinically relevant application of monitoring techniques will be elaborated in the next subsections.

Mobility Monitoring to Support Interventions Aiming to Stimulate Physical Activity

An increasing body of evidence demonstrates the importance of physical activity for general health in older adults (e.g. see position stand by the American College of Sports Medicine (ACSM), 2009). Regular physical activity has proven to be effective in the primary and secondary prevention of several chronic conditions and is linked to a reduction in all-cause mortality (e.g. U.S. Department of Health and Human Services

1996, Warburton et al. 2006). In addition, regular physical activity can enhance musculoskeletal fitness (Warburton et al. 2001, 2001), and cognitive functioning (Kramer et al. 2006, Hillman et al. 2008) which both are major prerequisites for functional autonomy. Physical inactivity, on the other hand, is associated with premature death and specific chronic diseases such as cardiovascular disease, colon cancer, and non-insulin dependent diabetes (Warburton et al. 2006). It is widely recognized that, in western societies, many older adults do not achieve sufficient levels of physical activity according to guidelines by the ACSM and the American Heart Association (cf. Nelson et al. 2007, Haskell et al. 2007). However, most of the present knowledge about daily physical activity patterns has been obtained through self-report based methods, and there still is a lack of objective data about physical activity in different older populations.

Recent data collected on 7 consecutive days by a body-fixed sensor in community-dwelling older adults demonstrate that on average the older persons spent ca. 5 hours in an upright position (i.e. standing and walking), the average cumulative walking time was approximately 1.5 hours. However, a strong inter-individual, and intra-individual day-to-day variability was observed (Nicolai et al. 2010). Monitoring variables such as cumulative walking and standing time can be used as a robust indicator of overall physical activity. This allows for self-management or remote counseling of older adults and specific patients groups as part of exercise-based interventions. Particularly when more specific information about qualitative aspects of movement performance can be monitored it will be possible to initiate remotely supervised exercise-programs (e.g. see Hermens & Vollenbroek-Hutten 2008). An individual personal coaching based on objective monitoring data might be used to optimize levels of performance. In specific patient groups, monitoring might also prove to be useful for the early detection of clinical deterioration and the management of chronic diseases.

Mobility Monitoring to Support Interventions in Specific Patient Groups

In several ways, the monitoring of quantitative and qualitative aspects of mobility related activities in patients with impaired mobility is likely to result in a better disease management and counseling. Not only can patients be monitored to see whether target levels for physical activity are reached (cf. preceding sub-section), monitoring may also contribute to a better diagnosis, prognosis, and evaluation of treatment effects. Thus, the treatment and guidance can be tuned to the individual needs of a patient. The following examples demonstrate potential clinical applications in specific diseases with a high prevalence, severe mobility problems, and considerable associated medical costs:

- *Arthrosis:* A very common age-associated problem is hip or knee arthrosis. In these conditions, the early course of the disease usually consists of pharmaceutical and/ or exercise-based treatment. In the more advanced stages, hip or knee replacement are the most common treatment options to regain pain relief, functional improvement and normal participation levels. Recent studies demonstrated systematic improvements in gait parameters (van den Akker-Scheek et al. 2007), and a poor relationship between self-reported and performance-based measures of physical functioning in patients after total hip arthroplasty (van den Akker-Scheek et al. 2008). Thus, the use of mobility monitoring seems ideally suited to document physical activity patterns and the treatment response of the patients in an objective and valid manner. The monitoring can demonstrate the improvement in walking distances and duration after the application of pain treatment as well as the

treatment response to an operative procedure. Although Morlock et al. (2001) used an ambulatory system to investigate the duration and frequency of every day activities in total hip patients, mobility monitoring has, to our knowledge, not yet been used to systematically document treatment effects in patients with arthrosis.

- *Chronic Obstructive Pulmonary Disease (COPD)*: COPD refers to chronic lung conditions in which the airways become narrowed; i.e. chronic bronchitis and emphysema. This results in a limited air flow to and from the lungs causing a shortness of breath and, thus, a limited capacity for physical activities. The disease usually is progressively getting worse over time. Medication can improve lung function and reduce the risk of pulmonary inflammations and thus enhance exercise tolerance. In addition it has been demonstrated that pulmonary rehabilitation can enhance exercise tolerance, improve symptoms and reduce exacerbations. Increasing exercise tolerance and the quantity of daily life physical activities is of crucial importance for COPD patients, because it has been shown that regular physical activity reduces hospital admissions and mortality (Garcia-Aymerich et al. 2006). A recent monitoring-based study confirmed that physical activity indeed is reduced in COPD patients (Pitta et al 2005). A subsequent study then showed that whereas pulmonary rehabilitation can improve exercise capacity, muscle force, and functional status after 3 months of rehabilitation, the improvements in daily life physical activities were first demonstrated after 6 months (Pitta et al. 2008). The latter finding demonstrates the need to develop effective strategies to enhance daily life physical activities in COPD patients. It can be expected that mobility monitoring could be used to support such strategies and thus enhance functioning and life-expectancy in COPD.

- *Parkinson's Disease (PD)*: This neuro-degenerative disease is common, its prevalence in the population above 65 is approximately 1-2 percent. Due to the increasing percentage of old people as part of the total population, its prevalence is increasing. Disease progression is mainly characterized by increasing postural instability, balance problems, and mobility impairment (cf. Hoehn & Yahr 2001), which also lead to an increased risk for falls and fall related injuries. In addition, PD patients suffer from symptoms such as a slowing of movement (bradykinesia) and tremors. Particularly in the later stages of the disease, additional difficulties may arise like emotional problems and cognitive deficits. The early stages of PD can be treated effectively with medication, but, after some years many patients develop disease related problems that can no longer fully be treated by medication. In these later stages, additional therapeutic strategies, such as deep brain stimulation may be initiated (Fahn, 2010).

During the early course of the disease, mobility monitoring can be used to document the effect of the medication on movement patterns, and to reach an optimal individual dosage of medication. This is highly relevant since the numbers of patient visits with the specialist usually are few and brief. The observed movement performance during these visits is not necessarily representative for movement performance in daily life. Thus, remote monitoring might lead to modifications in pharmacological treatment, which else would not have been possible. Due to the specific patho-physiology of PD, patients may profit from external information, which facilitates their movements. Provided that adequate algorithms and actuators are available, mobility monitoring in PD may be used as a foundation for initiating feedback-based interventions, or auditory and/or visual cues that facilitate movement performance. Anecdotal evidence and some studies indicate that PD patients do profit from such interventions. Recently, these possible treatment strategies have been addressed in research projects financed by the European Commission (e.g. see www.rescueproject.org, www.sensaction-aal.eu). In later stages of the disease, PD patients may develop motor problems such as hyperkinesias, freezing or off-periods that are intermittent and cannot be documented during the visit. Here, the movement monitoring allows the development of patient profiles to document changes due to the course of the disease or the changes in treatment. In addition, monitoring may be used to detect gait arrhythmia, which indicates an increased risk of falling that should be discussed with the patient and care-givers.

Identification of Persons at an Increased Risk for Falls

Regarding fall risk, a decreased gait speed (e.g. Lamb 2009), an increased variability in temporal gait parameters such as stride duration (e.g. Hausdorff 1997, 2001), variability in lower trunk accelerations (Moe-Nilssen & Helbostad 2005) and frontal plane trunk rotations during walking (de Hoon et al. 2003), and the duration and variability of body transfers such as during sit-to-stand (Najafi et al. 2002), have all shown to be sensitive in distinguishing older fallers from non-fallers, or frail from fit elderly. Using wearable sensors, it is possible to monitor such parameters and other parameters, such as instabilities during missteps or tripping, over long duration. However, the predictive validity of these and similar measures still needs to be demonstrated in larger cohorts. Ideally, a monitoring approach would allow to evaluate whether a person is at an increased risk for falling before a fall occurs. Thus, a timely initiation of preventive measures could avoid future falls and injuries. Such preventive measures could encompass exercise-based interventions to optimize balance (i.e. 'capacity') and daily physical activity (i.e. 'performance'), counseling strategies, home-adaptations, or compensating interventions (for example the use of assistive devices such as a cane or a walker, or wearing hip protectors).

Monitoring of Mobility and Fall Incidents in High-Risk Groups

The epidemiology of falls is threatening. Approximately 30% of persons older than 65 years fall each year, and after the age of 75 fall rates are even higher (e.g. O'Loughlin et al. 1993). In Germany more than 5 millions falls occur each year, with a substantial part of these falls leading to hospital admissions. It has been estimated that the fall-related costs in European countries, Australia and the USA are between 0.85% and 1.5% of the total health care expenditures (Heinrich et al. 2009). Given the huge impact of falls, strategies that effectively reduce the number of falls or the consequences of falls are highly relevant. Thus, the development of reliable monitoring approaches which monitor parameters, which indicate fall-risk (cf. the previous sub-section), physical activity patterns and the occurrence of falls is one of the most urgent needs in health care services to older people. Given its relevance, it is no surprise that in the last two decades an increasing effort is made to develop reliable fall detection methods. At present, a number of different approaches, either based on ambient technology (i.e. smart homes) or body worn sensors (e.g. N'I Scanaill et al. 2006), have been reported (see also in earlier section). However, it is astonishing, how little real-life falls data are available and it must be stressed that currently there are no sensor-based fall detection systems available that have been tested in large scale trials. Therefore, the development of adequate sensors and fall-detection algorithms, and their real-life validation in different older populations continues to be an enormous challenge.

The development of automatic fall-alarms needs to encompass an analysis of the fall and its impact as well as the post-fall phase. Sensor-based signals during the falling and impact phase are needed to identify a fall. Depending on sensor type and location, information on body acceleration, jerk, impact height, fall direction, protective mechanisms and body position while hitting the ground can be derived from the data. These can be used to develop algorithms to detect a fall. Figure 1 presents an example of accelerations measured at the lower trunk before, during and after a real-life fall. In this specific example the circumstances of the fall and the nature of the fall itself were well-documented. It should be noted that, given the variety of falls and their pre-conditions, the categorization and recording of different fall types is highly relevant for the development of sensitive fall detection methods in different populations. The movement pattern in the time period following the impact phase reflects the consequences of the fall. Consequently, their interpretation is crucial for the decision whether or not to initiate an automated alarm response. The post-fall situation might be life threatening (e.g. syncope or epilepsy), very serious (fracture), or without serious consequences. From a user perspective it is crucial that a major event is recognized immediately (e.g. calling an emergency) and that a minor event does not result in an overreaction of the social environment.

THE USER PERSPECTIVE

In respect to monitoring solutions over longer durations, questions about the users' acceptance become more and more relevant next to aspects of effectiveness and (social) significance. The successful application of technologies in this field is strongly influenced by factors that relate to the fit between the demands of the technology and the specific capabilities of the user, the obtrusiveness of the monitoring method, and not least by intrinsic

Figure 1. An example of acceleration signals in vertical (x-axis), medio-lateral (y-axis) and sagittal (z-axis) direction during a real-life fall with impact at t = 30 sec

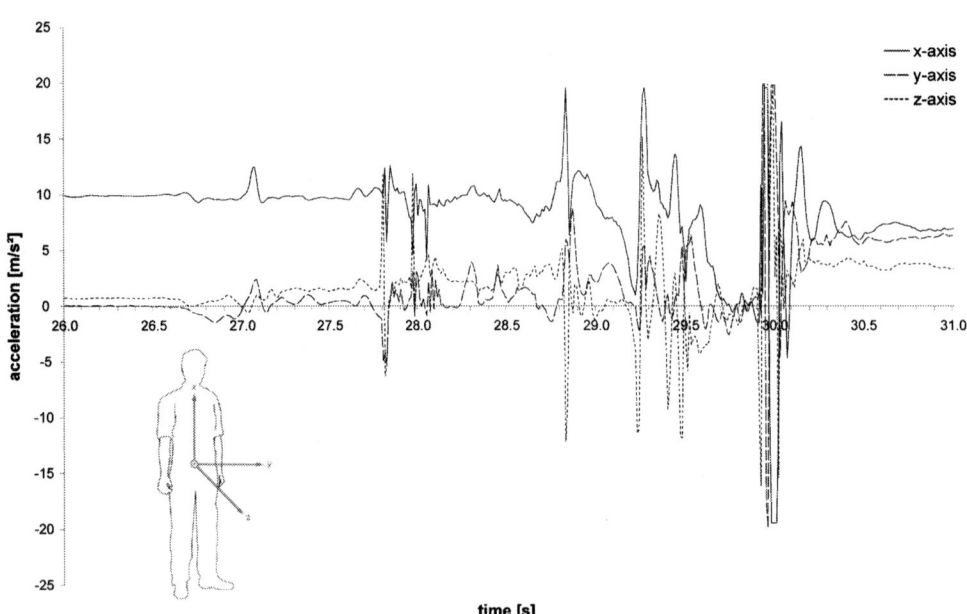

and extrinsic motivational factors. Furthermore non-acceptance and non-usage can be regarded partly as a consequence of the failure of designs and operational procedures to respond to the wishes and feelings (of this very heterogeneous group) of older people (Fisk 1998). This seems to be a very important issue because even very simple and already widely used systems like wearable alarm-buttons seem to be poorly used for their intended purpose: the case of emergency.

In a recent study it was shown that alarm-buttons were not used in most cases where a fall was followed by long period of lying on the floor (Fleming & Brayne 2008). It was shown that 94% of the person who were living in institutional settings, 78% in the community, and 59% in sheltered accommodations did not use their call alarm to summon help after they felt alone and were unable to get up without help. 97% of the person lying on the floor for over one hour did not use their alarm to summon help. "Barriers to using alarms arose at several crucial stages: not seeing any advantage

in having such a system, not developing the habit of wearing the pendant even if the system was installed, and, in the event of a fall, not activating the alarm – either as a conscious decision or as a failed attempt" (Fleming & Brayne 2008). One reason probably could be found in the fact that 35% of the participants were severely cognitive impaired. Another aspect of these results may show the danger in the overemphasis of clinical objectives within service frameworks for tele-care in people's own homes. Technologies in the home may be viewed as more intrusive (and, therefore, less acceptable) than in other, more institutional contexts (Fisk 1997).

For a successful extension of (commercial) monitoring technology and its integration into tele-health systems a better understanding of acceptance and non-acceptance for specific target groups is indispensable. The following briefly outlines three theoretical constructs, which address important key aspects relevant to this question.

Figure 2. Matching system demands to user capabilities (see text for further explanation)

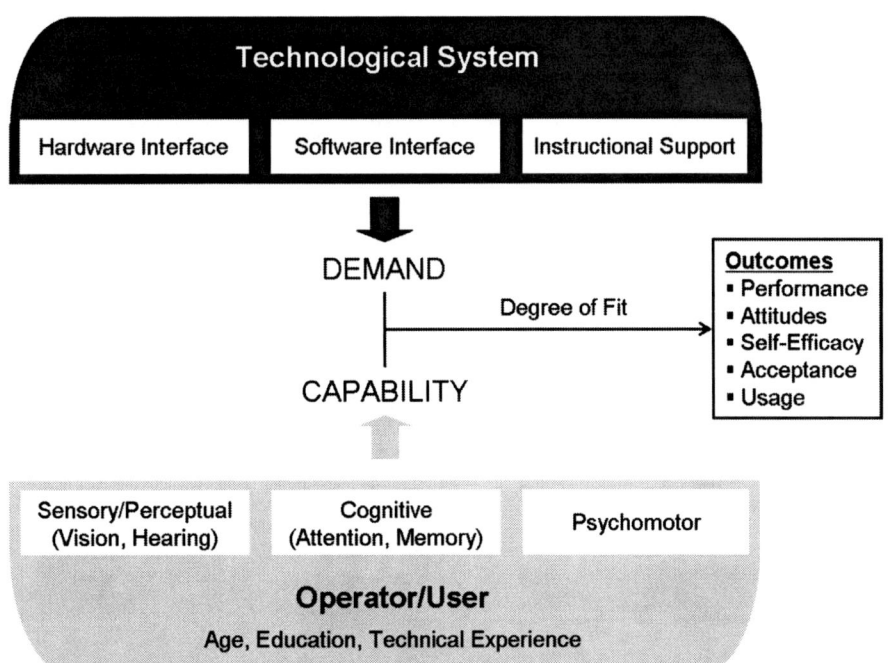

The Human Factors Approach

The human factors approach refers to "the role of humans in complex systems, the design of equipment and facilities for human use, and the development of environments for comfort and safety" (Salvendy 1997). The aim of this approach is to match the demands of a system to the capabilities of the user; as illustrated in Figure 2, described by Rogers & Fisk 2003 and originally adopted by the Center for Research on Aging and Technology Enhancement (Czaja et al. 2001). "The system imposes certain demands on the user as a function of the characteristics of the hardware, software, and instructional support that is provided for it. The operator of the system has certain sensory/perceptual, cognitive, and psychomotor capabilities. The degree of fit between the demands of the system and the capabilities of the user will determine performance of the system as well as attitudes, acceptance, usage of the system, and self-efficacy beliefs about one's own capabilities to use that system" (Rogers & Fisk 2003).

To develop good fitting technologies, various approaches like exact analysis of the necessary tasks when using the technology, observation of users, manipulation of the different designs, and the development of proper training and instructional support are recommended by the authors.

The Obtrusiveness Concept

The obtrusiveness concept in tele-health was defined by (Hensel et al. 2006a) "as a summary evaluation by the user based on characteristics or effects associated with the technology that are perceived as undesirable and physically and/or psychologically prominent". This concept (see Figure 3; Hensel et al 2006a) was constructed inductively by 22 categories found in the literature. It adds some further and more specific aspects compared to the more general "Human factors approach". In a secondary analysis within two studies based on focus groups and interviews with residential care residents 16 of the postulated 22 subcategories could be confirmed (*= con-

Figure 3. The obtrusiveness concept (see text for further explanation)

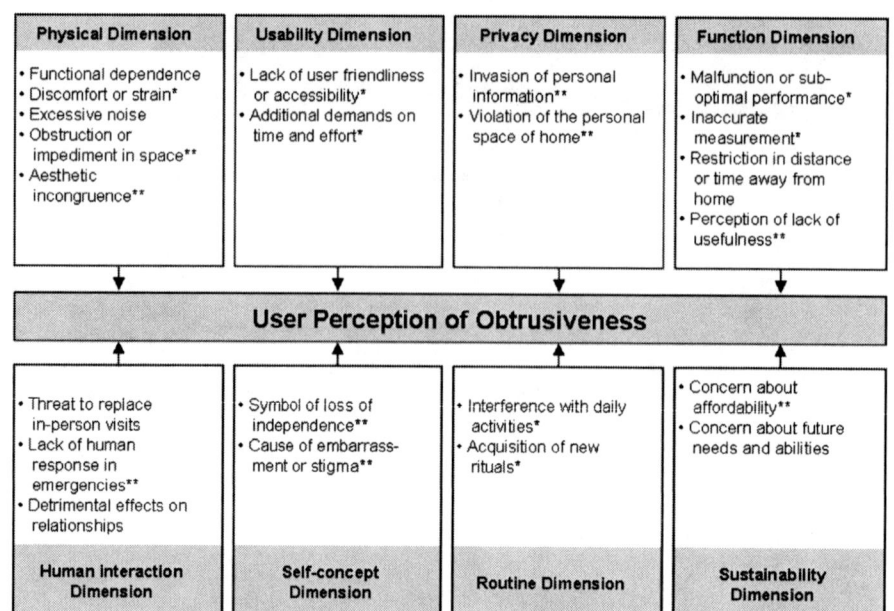

firmed in 1 study, **= in both studies; Courtney, Demiris, & Hensel 2007). Restrictively, it has to be mentioned that only two of the 29 participants of the two studies were using information-based technologies at the time of the interview.

The Expectations-Confirmation Theory

From a consumer behavior perspective the expectations-confirmation theory (ECT) adds a further aspect to user satisfaction with including initial expectations of a specific product or service prior to purchase or delivery. This theoretical construct posits that the expectations lead, after a period of initial experience, to post-purchase satisfaction. The primary reason that we experience disappointment or delight is because our expectations have not been met (negative disconfirmation) or they have been superseded (positive disconfirmation) and we have noticed and responded to the discrepancy (Figure 4; Oliver 1980; Spreng et al. 1996).

Integration of User Perspectives in the Development of Monitoring Approaches

When summarizing the previous three concepts, *user satisfaction* with wearable activity monitoring systems should be seen in the context of a good fit between the demands of the device and the capabilities of the user, and furthermore the meeting or exceeding of the user's expectations in regard of a favorite balance between the perceived benefit and obtrusive aspects. Considering aspects of user satisfaction is becoming more recognized as an important criterion for the development and application of long term and unsupervised monitoring approaches. However, there still seems to be a lack of pertinent data. In a recent systematic review of studies using wearable systems for mobility monitoring in older people (de Bruin et al. 2008), it was noted that only few studies had actually applied monitoring methods over long durations, and that the number of studies that addressed feasibility and user acceptance aspects was even smaller. The identified feasibility and

Figure 4. The expectations-confirmation theory (see text for further explanation)

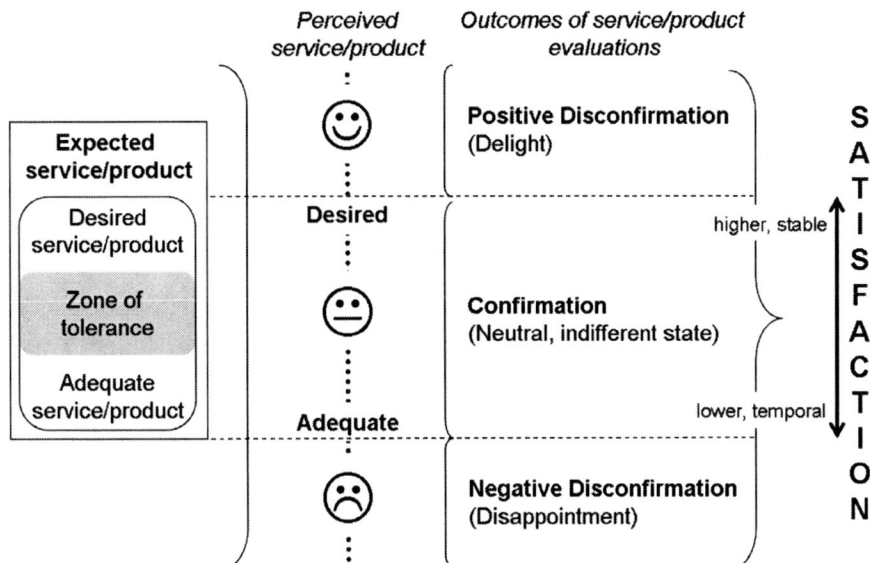

adherence aspects mainly related to the reliability of various devices in unsupervised measurement settings and the acceptance of devices by the populations under study. The user acceptance seemed to vary with sensor location and attachment method. Our own experience in recent or ongoing studies indicates a reasonable user acceptance of single-sensor monitoring techniques. The adherence was above 90% for short periods (24-48 hours) of monitoring with a sensor on the trunk. However, with repeated and extended measurements the acceptability decreased to 50-60%, and in patients with severe cognitive impairment, or during hot periods, adherence can be considerably lower.

These experiences indicate that there is a need for sensor miniaturization and/or the integration of small sensors in clothing. Ultimately, monitoring systems need to be evaluated over longer periods and by taking into account different aspects of user perspectives. To our knowledge, there currently is no comprehensive assessment tool available that evaluates user satisfaction with monitoring technologies. Therefore, we have started to develop a questionnaire with six dimensions and 30 items in total. The five-point level Likert scaled items are

phrased with regard to sensor based applications and comprise the following six dimensions: (perceived) benefit, usability, self-concept, privacy & loss of control, quality of life, wearing comfort. The questionnaire is currently under validation in a number of ongoing studies. Further information is available under www.aktiv-in-jedem-alter.de.

CONCLUSION

Demographic changes confront most industrialized countries with the challenge of an ageing population together with a decreasing work force. Innovative solutions are needed to maintain the quality of our health care systems. Monitoring based health-care services can potentially play a role in decreasing the workload of health care professionals. For example by increasing the effectiveness of existing work routines, or by supporting effective preventive strategies that avoid the extensive use of regular health care services. Given the huge challenges in the next decades, the latter preventive medicine approach deserves increased attention.

The present contribution has shown that basic technical solutions for wearable systems for monitoring mobility are available, and that relevant clinical applications can be identified for different older populations. However, from the preceding sections, it will be clear that there still is a gap to bridge before mobility monitoring approaches can become an accepted part of regular health-care services. Without claiming to be complete, we think at least the following issues need to be resolved to facilitate the successful application of wearable systems for mobility monitoring as part of healthcare services.

First of all, the present evidence-base for the clinical relevance of existing clinical assessment tools for mobility related activities is insufficient, and, at this time, this shortcoming is also true for the new sensor-based assessment tools. Although several studies suggest a high potential for relevant applications in older people, the new sensor-based approaches for mobility assessment and monitoring still need to be applied in appropriately designed clinical studies to unequivocally demonstrate their clinical validity for specific purposes. Evidence-based clinical applications of new monitoring techniques should rely on epidemiological studies with non-selected cohorts as well as in well-defined patient groups. The additional benefit of monitoring should be documented in controlled trials.

Secondly, there is little doubt that ongoing and future research in the next years will only further increase the abundance of different sensor-based assessment approaches. This will lead to further improvements and innovations, but it will also increase the need for standardization of instruments and procedures for data-acquisition and data-analysis. In addition, it can be expected that there will be a need to define standards for the clinical validation procedures, in order to be able to compare different approaches. At present, such considerations have hardly received attention.

Third, the application of monitoring based health-care services requires the development of monitoring approaches which are acceptable to its potential users. Thus, it is essential to assess and incorporate user perspectives in the development process. It should be noted that these user perspectives must not only comprise the patient perspective, but also the perspectives of health care professionals who are involved in using the system. Both types of users will need to be convinced of the potential benefits of the monitoring techniques. It is likely that the willingness to accept will not only depend on an existing evidence-base for the clinical relevance, but also on the practicability of the systems in the home environment and in the clinical environment.

REFERENCES

Allum, J. H. J., & Carpenter, M. G. (2005). A speedy solution for balance and gait analysis: angular velocity measured at the centre of body mass. *Current Opinion in Neurology, 18*, 15–21. doi:10.1097/00019052-200502000-00005

American College of Sports Medicine, Chodzko-Zajko, W.J., Proctor, D.N., Fiatarone Singh, M.A., Minson, C.T., Nigg, C.R., Salem, G.J. & Skinner, J.S. (2009). American College of Sports Medicine position stand. Exercise and physical activity for older adults. *Medicine and Science in Sports and Exercise, 41*(7), 1510–1530.

Aminian, K., & Najafi, B. (2004). Capturing human motion using body-fixed sensors: outdoor measurement and clinical applications. *Computer Animation and Virtual Worlds, 15*(2), 79–94. doi:10.1002/cav.2

Aminian, K., Najafi, B., Bula, C., Leyvraz, P. F., & Robert, P. (2002). Spatio-temporal Parameters of Gait Measured by an Ambulatory System Using Miniature Gyroscopes. *Journal of Biomechanics, 35*(5), 689–699. doi:10.1016/S0021-9290(02)00008-8

Aminian, K., Robert, Ph., Buchser, E., Rutschmann, B., Hayoz, D., & Depairon, M. (1999). Physical activity monitoring based on accelerometry: validation and comparison with video observation. *Medical & Biological Engineering & Computing, 37,* 304–308. doi:10.1007/BF02513304

Bonato, P. (2005). Advances in wearable technology and applications in physical medicine and rehabilitation. *Journal of Neuroengineering and Rehabilitation, 2,* 1–4. doi:10.1186/1743-0003-2-2

Bourke, A. K., O'Brien, J. V., & Lyons, G. M. (2007). Evaluation of a threshold-based tri-axial accelerometer fall detection algorithm. *Gait & Posture, 26,* 194–199. doi:10.1016/j.gaitpost.2006.09.012

Bourke, A. K., van de Ven, P. W. J., Chaya, A. E., Olaighin, G. M., & Nelson, J. (2008). Testing of a long-term fall detection system incorporated into a custom vest for the elderly. Proceedings of 30th Annual *International Conference of the IEEE Engineering in Medicine and Biology Society* (pp. 2844-2847).

Bussmann, J. B. J., Veltink, P. H., Koelma, F., van Lummel, R. C., & Stam, H. J. (1995). Ambulatory monitoring of mobility-related activities: the initial phase of the development of an activity monitor. *European Journal of Physical Medicine and Rehabilitation, 5*(1), 2–7.

Courtney, K. L., Demiris, G., & Hensel, B. K. (2007). Obtrusiveness of information-based assistive technologies as perceived by older adults in residential care facilities: a secondary analysis. *Journal of Medical Internet, 32*(3), 241–249.

Czaja, S. J., Sharit, J., Charness, N., Fisk, A. D., & Rogers, W. A. (2001). The Center for Research and Education on Aging and Technology Enhancement (CREATE): A program to enhance technology for older adults. *Gerontechnology (Valkenswaard), 1,* 50–59. doi:10.4017/gt.2001.01.01.005.00

de Bruin, E. D., Hartmann, A., Uebelhart, D., Murer, K., & Zijlstra, W. (2008). Wearable systems for monitoring mobility related activities in older people. *Clinical Rehabilitation, 22,* 878–895. doi:10.1177/0269215508090675

de Hoon, E. W., Allum, J. H., Carpenter, M. G., Salis, C., Bloem, B. R., Conzelmann, M., & Bischoff, H. A. (2003). Quantitative assessment of the stops walking while talking test in the elderly. *Archives of Physical Medicine and Rehabilitation, 84*(6), 838–842. doi:10.1016/S0003-9993(02)04951-1

Dejnabadi, H., Jolles, B. M., & Aminian, K. (2005). A new approach to accurate measurement of uni-axial joint angles based on a combination of accelerometers and gyroscopes. *IEEE Transactions on Bio-Medical Engineering, 52*(8), 1478–1484. doi:10.1109/TBME.2005.851475

Dejnabadi, H., Jolles, B. M., Casanova, E., Fua, P., & Aminian, K. (2006). Estimation and Visualization of Sagittal Kinematics of Lower Limbs Orientation using Body-Fixed Sensors. *IEEE Transactions on Bio-Medical Engineering, 53,* 1385–1393. doi:10.1109/TBME.2006.873678

Dijkstra, B., Kamsma, Y. P. T., & Zijlstra, W. (2010). Detection of gait and postures using a miniaturized tri-axial accelerometer-based system: accuracy in community-dwelling older adults. *Age and Ageing, 39*(2), 259–262. doi:10.1093/ageing/afp249

Dijkstra, B., Zijlstra, W., Scherder, E., & Kamsma, Y. (2008). Detection of gait episodes and number of steps in older adults and patients with Parkinson's disease: accuracy of a pedometer and an accelerometry based method. *Age and Ageing, 37*(4), 436–441. doi:10.1093/ageing/afn097

Fahn, S. (2010). Parkinson's disease: 10 years of progress, 1997-2007. *Movement Disorders, 25*(Suppl 1), 2–14. doi:10.1002/mds.22796

Fisk, M. J. (1997). Telecare equipment in the home. Issues of intrusiveness and control. *Journal of Telemedicine and Telecare, 3*(Suppl. 1), 30–32. doi:10.1258/1357633971930274

Fisk, M. J. (1998). Telecare at home: factors influencing technology choices and user acceptance. *Journal of Telemedicine and Telecare, 4,* 80–83. doi:10.1258/1357633981931993

Fleming, J., & Brayne, C. (2008). Inability to get up after falling, subsequent time on floor, and summoning help: prospective cohort study in people over 90. *British Medical Journal, 337,* a2227. doi:10.1136/bmj.a2227

Garcia-Aymerich, J., Lange, P., Benet, M., Schnohr, P., & Anto, J. M. (2006). Regular physical activity reduces hospital admission and mortality in chronic obstructive pulmonary disease: a population based cohort study. *Thorax, 61,* 772–778. doi:10.1136/thx.2006.060145

Gates, S., Smith, L. A., Fisher, J. D., & Lamb, S. E. (2008). Systematic review of accuracy of screening instruments for predicting fall risk among independently living older adults. *Journal of Rehabilitation Research and Development, 45,* 1105–1116. doi:10.1682/JRRD.2008.04.0057

Giannakouris, K. (2008). *Eurostat - Statistics in focus.* Population and social conditions. 72/2008: Luxemburg.

Haskell, W. L., Lee, I. M., Pate, R. R., Powell, K. E., Blair, S. N., & Franklin, B. A. (2007). Physical activity and public health: updated recommendation for adults from the American College of Sports Medicine and the American Heart Association. *Medicine and Science in Sports and Exercise, 39,* 1423–1434. doi:10.1249/mss.0b013e3180616b27

Hauer, K., Lamb, S. E., Jorstad, E. C., Todd, C., & Becker, C. (2006). PROFANE-Group. Systematic review of definitions and methods of measuring falls in randomised controlled fall prevention trials. *Age and Ageing, 35,* 5–10. doi:10.1093/ageing/afi218

Hausdorff, J. M., Ashkenazy, Y., Peng, C. K., Ivanov, P. C., Stanley, H. E., & Goldberger, A. L. (2001). When human walking becomes random walking: fractal analysis and modeling of gait rhythm fluctuations. *Physica A, 302*(1-4), 138–147. doi:10.1016/S0378-4371(01)00460-5

Hausdorff, J. M., Edelberg, H. K., Mitchell, S. L., Goldberger, A. L., & Wei, J. Y. (1997). Increased gait unsteadiness in community-dwelling elderly fallers. *Archives of Physical Medicine and Rehabilitation, 78,* 278–283. doi:10.1016/S0003-9993(97)90034-4

Hausdorff, J. M., Ladin, Z., & Wei, J. Y. (1995). Footswitch system for measurement of the temporal parameters of gait. *Biometrical Journal. Biometrische Zeitschrift, 28*(3), 347–351.

Heinrich, S., Rapp, K., Rissmann, U., Becker, C., & König, H. H. (2009). Cost of falls in old age: a systematic review. [Epub ahead of print]. *Osteoporosis International,* (Nov): 19.

Helbostad, J. L., & Moe-Nilssen, R. (2003). The effect of gait speed on lateral balance control during walking in healthy elderly. *Gait & Posture, 18*(2), 27–36. doi:10.1016/S0966-6362(02)00197-2

Hensel, B. K., Demiris, G., & Courtney, K. L. (2006). Defining obtrusiveness in home telehealth technologies: a conceptual framework. *Journal of the American Medical Informatics Association, 13,* 428–431. doi:10.1197/jamia.M2026

Hermens, H. J., & Vollenbroek-Hutten, M. M. (2008). Towards remote monitoring and remotely supervised training. *Journal of Electromyography and Kinesiology, 18*(6), 908–919. doi:10.1016/j.jelekin.2008.10.004

Hillman, C.H., & Erickson, K.I., Kramer, & A.F. (2008). Be smart, exercise your heart: exercise effects on brain and cognition. *Nature Reviews. Neuroscience, 9*(1), 58–65. doi:10.1038/nrn2298

Hoehn, M. M., & Yahr, M. D. (2001). Parkinsonism: onset, progression, and mortality. 1967. *Neurology, 57*(10Suppl 3), S11–S26.

Huxham, F. E., Goldie, P. A., & Patla, A. E. (2001). Theoretical considerations in balance assessment. *The Australian Journal of Physiotherapy, 47*, 89–100.

International Classification of Functioning. Disability and Health (ICF). (n.d.). *World Health Organisation, Geneva.* Retrieved from www.who.int/classification/icf.

Kangas, M., Konttila, A., Lindgren, P., Winblad, I., & Jämsä, T. (2008). Comparison of low-complexity fall detection algorithms for body attached accelerometers. *Gait & Posture, 28*(2), 285–291. doi:10.1016/j.gaitpost.2008.01.003

Karantonis, D. M., Narayanan, M. R., Mathie, M., Lovell, N. H., & Celler, B. G. (2006). Implementation of a real-time human movement classifier using a triaxial accelerometer for ambulatory monitoring. *IEEE Transactions on Information Technology in Biomedicine, 10*(1), 156–167. doi:10.1109/TITB.2005.856864

Kramer, A. F., Erickson, K. I., & Colcombe, S. J. (2006). Exercise, cognition, and the aging brain. *Journal of Applied Physiology, 101*(4), 1237–1242. doi:10.1152/japplphysiol.00500.2006

Lamb, S. E., McCabe, C., Becker, C., Fried, L. P., & Guralnik, J. M. (2008). The optimal sequence and selection of screening test items to predict fall risk in older disabled women: the Women's Health and Aging Study. *The Journals of Gerontology. Series A, Biological Sciences and Medical Sciences, 63*(10), 1082–1088.

Lindeman, U., Claus, H., Stuber, M., Augat, P., Muche, R., Nikolaus, T., & Becker, C. (2003). Measuring power during the sit-to-stand transfer. *European Journal of Applied Physiology, 89*, 466–470. doi:10.1007/s00421-003-0837-z

Lindemann, U., Hock, A., Stuber, M., Keck, W., & Becker, C. (2005). Evaluation of a fall detector based on accelerometers: a pilot study. *Medical & Biological Engineering & Computing, 43*(2), 548–551. doi:10.1007/BF02351026

Luinge, H. J., & Veltink, P. H. (2005). Measuring orientation of human body segments using miniature gyroscopes and accelerometers. *Medical & Biological Engineering & Computing, 43*(2), 273–282. doi:10.1007/BF02345966

Mathie, M. J., Coster, A. C., Lovell, N. H., & Celler, B. G. (2004). Accelerometry: providing an integrated, practical method for long-term, ambulatory monitoring of human movement. *Physiological Measurement, 25*(2), R1–R20. doi:10.1088/0967-3334/25/2/R01

Mayagoitia, R. E., Lötters, J. C., Veltink, P. H., & Hermens, H. (2002). Standing balance evaluation using a triaxial accelerometer. *Gait & Posture, 16*(1), 55–59. doi:10.1016/S0966-6362(01)00199-0

Moe-Nilssen, R., & Helbostad, J. L. (2002). Trunk accelerometry as a measure of balance control during quiet standing. *Gait & Posture, 16*(1), 60–68. doi:10.1016/S0966-6362(01)00200-4

Morlock, M., Schneider, E., Bluhm, A., Vollmer, M., Bergmann, G., Müller, V., & Honl, M. (2001). Duration and frequency of every day activities in total hip patients. *Journal of Biomechanics, 34*, 873–881. doi:10.1016/S0021-9290(01)00035-5

N'I Scanaill, C., Carew, S., Barralon, P., Noury, N., Lyons, D. & Lyons, G.M. (2006). A Review of Approaches to Mobility Telemonitoring of the Elderly in Their Living Environment. *Annals of Biomedical Engineering, 34*, 547–563. doi:10.1007/s10439-005-9068-2

Najafi, B., Aminian, K., Loew, F., Blanc, Y., & Robert, P. (2002). Measurement of stand-sit and sit-stand transitions using a miniature gyroscope and its application in fall risk evaluation in the elderly. *IEEE Transactions on Bio-Medical Engineering*, *49*(8), 843–851. doi:10.1109/TBME.2002.800763

Najafi, B., Aminian, K., Paraschiv-Ionescu, A., Loew, F., Bula, C., & Robert, Ph. (2003). Ambulatory system for human motion analysis using a kinematic sensor: monitoring of daily physical activity in elderly. *IEEE Transactions on Bio-Medical Engineering*, *50*(6), 711–723. doi:10.1109/TBME.2003.812189

Najafi, B., Büla, C., Piot-Ziegler, C., Demierre, M., & Aminian, K. (2003). Relationship between fear of falling and spatio-temporal parameters of gait in elderly persons. *From Basic Motor Control to Functional Recovery III*, Chapter II: From Posture to Gait, 152-158. Ecole Polytechnique Fédérale Lausanne: MCC2003 Book.

Nelson, M. E., Rejeski, W. J., Blair, S. N., Duncan, P. W., Judge, J. O., & King, A. C. (2007). Physical activity and public health in older adults: recommendation from the American College of Sports Medicine and the American Heart Association. *Medicine and Science in Sports and Exercise*, *39*(8), 1435–1445. doi:10.1249/mss.0b013e3180616aa2

Nicolai, S., Benzinger, P., Skelton, D. A., Aminian, K., Becker, C., & Lindemann, U. (2010). Day-to-day variability of physical activity of older adults living in the community. *Journal of Aging and Physical Activity*, *18*(1), 75–86.

Noury, N., Fleury, A., Rumeau, P., Bourke, A. K., Laighin, G. O., Rialle, V., & Lundy, J. E. (2007) Fall detection principles and methods. *Conference Proceedings - IEEE Engineering in Medicine and Biology*, 1663-1666.

O'Loughlin, J. L., Robitaille, Y., Boivin, J. F., & Suissa, S. (1993). Incidence of and risk factors for falls and injurious falls among the community-dwelling elderly. *American Journal of Epidemiology*, *137*(3), 342–354.

Oliver, R. (1980). A cognitive model of the antecedents and consequences of satisfaction decisions. *JMR, Journal of Marketing Research*, *17*, 460–469. doi:10.2307/3150499

Pitta, F., Troosters, T., Probst, V. S., Langer, D., Decramer, M., & Gosselink, R. (2008). Are patients with COPD more active after pulmonary rehabilitation? *Chest*, *134*(2), 273–280. doi:10.1378/chest.07-2655

Pitta, F., Troosters, T., Spruit, M. A., Probst, V. S., Decramer, M., & Gosselink, R. (2005). Characteristics of physical activities in daily life in chronic obstructive pulmonary disease. *American Journal of Respiratory and Critical Care Medicine*, *171*(9), 972–977. doi:10.1164/rccm.200407-855OC

Ploutz-Snyder, L. L., Manini, T., Ploutz-Snyder, R. J., & Wolf, D. A. (2002). Functionally relevant thresholds of quadriceps femoris strength. *Journal of Gerontology: Medical Sciences*, *57A*, M144–M152.

Roetenberg, D., Luinge, H. J., Baten, C. T., & Veltink, P. H. (2005). Compensation of magnetic disturbances improves inertial and magnetic sensing of human body segment orientation. *IEEE Transactions on Neural Systems and Rehabilitation Engineering*, *13*(3), 395–405. doi:10.1109/TNSRE.2005.847353

Rogers, W. A., & Fisk, A. D. (2003). Technology Design, Usability, and Aging: Human Factors Techniques and considerations. In Charness, N., & Schaie, K. W. (Eds.), *Impact of technology on successful aging* (pp. 1–14). New York: Springer.

Sabatini, A. M., Martelloni, C., Scapellato, S., & Cavallo, F. (2005). Assessment of Walking Features From Foot Inertial Sensing. *IEEE Transactions on Bio-Medical Engineering, 52*(3), 486–494. doi:10.1109/TBME.2004.840727

Salvendy, G. (1997). *Handbook of human factors and ergonomics*. New York: Wiley.

Schenkman, M., Hughes, M., Samsa, G., & Studenski, S. (1996). The relative importance of strength and balance in chair rise by functionally impaired older individuals. *Journal of the American Geriatrics Society, 44*(12), 1441–1446.

Skelton, D. A., & Todd, C. (2004). *What are the main risk factors for falls amongst older people and what are the most effective interventions to prevent these falls? How should interventions to prevent falls be implemented? Health Evidence Network*. Denmark: World Health Organisation.

Spreng, R. A., MacKenzie, S. B., & Olshavsky, R. W. (1996). A reexamination of the determinants of consumer satisfaction. *Journal of Marketing, 60*, 15–32. doi:10.2307/1251839

Terrier, P., & Schutz, Y. (2005). How useful is satellite positioning system (GPS) to track gait parameters? A review. *Journal of Neuroengineering and Rehabilitation, 2*, 2–28. doi:10.1186/1743-0003-2-28

U.S. Department of Health and Human Services. (1996). *Physical activity and health: a report of the Surgeon General* (pp. 146–148). Atlanta, GA: U.S. Department of Health and Human Services, Centers for Disease Control and Prevention, National Center for Chronic Disease Prevention and Health Promotion.

van den Akker-Scheek, I., Stevens, M., Bulstra, S. K., Groothoff, J. W., van Horn, J. R., & Zijlstra, W. (2007). Recovery of gait after short-stay total hip arthroplasty. *Archives of Physical Medicine and Rehabilitation, 88*(3), 361–367. doi:10.1016/j.apmr.2006.11.026

van den Akker-Scheek, I., Zijlstra, W., Groothoff, J. W., Bulstra, S. K., & Stevens, M. (2008). Physical functioning before and after total hip arthroplasty: perception and performance. *Physical Therapy, 88*(6), 712–719. doi:10.2522/ptj.20060301

Van Duin, C. (2009). *Bevolkingsprognose 2008–2050:* naar 17,5 miljoen inwoners. Centraal Bureau voor de Statistiek 2009. http://www.cbs.nl/NR/rdonlyres/D49C0D9A-7540-42E9-948D-794EDD3E8443/0/2010bevolkingsprognose20092060art.pdf

Veltink, P. H., Bussmann, H. B. J., de Vries, W., Martens, W. L. J., & van Lummel, R. C. (1996). Detection of static and dynamic activities using uniaxial accelerometers. *IEEE Transactions on Neural Systems and Rehabilitation Engineering, 4*(4), 375–385.

Warburton, D. E., Gledhill, N., & Quinney, A. (2001). The effects of changes in musculoskeletal fitness on health. *Canadian Journal of Applied Physiology, 26*, 161–216.

Warburton, D. E., Gledhill, N., & Quinney, A. (2001). Musculoskeletal fitness and health. *Canadian Journal of Applied Physiology, 26*, 217–237.

Warburton, D. E., Nicol, C. W., & Bredin, S. S. D. (2006). Health benefits of physical activity: the evidence. *Canadian Medical Association Journal, 174*, 801–809. doi:10.1503/cmaj.051351

Winter, D. A. (1995). Human balance and posture control during standing and walking. *Gait & Posture, 3*, 193–214. doi:10.1016/0966-6362(96)82849-9

Zecevic, A. A., Salmoni, A. W., Speechley, M., & Vandervoort, A. A. (2006). Defining a fall and reasons for falling: Comparisons among the views of seniors, health care providers, and the research literature. *The Gerontologist, 46*, 367–376.

Zhang, T., Wang, J., Liu, P., & Hou, J. (2006). Fall Detection by Embedding an Accelerometer in Cellphone and Using KFD Algorithm. *International Journal of Computer Science and Network Security, 6*(10), 277–284.

Zijlstra, W. (2004). Assessment of spatio-temporal parameters during unconstrained walking. *European Journal of Applied Physiology, 92*, 39–44. doi:10.1007/s00421-004-1041-5

Zijlstra, W., & Aminian, K. (2007). Mobility assessment in older people, new possibilities and challenges. *European Journal of Ageing, 4*, 3–12. doi:10.1007/s10433-007-0041-9

Zijlstra, W., & Bisseling, R. (2004). Estimation of Hip Abduction Moment based on Body Fixed Sensors. *Clinical Biomechanics (Bristol, Avon), 19*(8), 819–827. doi:10.1016/j.clinbiomech.2004.05.005

Zijlstra, W., Bisseling, R. W., Schlumbohm, S., & Baldus, H. (2010). A body-fixed-sensor based analysis of power during sit-to-stand movements. *Gait & Posture, 31*(2), 272–278. doi:10.1016/j.gaitpost.2009.11.003

Zijlstra, W., & Hof, A. L. (1997). Displacement of the pelvis during human walking: experimental data and model predictions. *Gait & Posture, 6*, 249–262. doi:10.1016/S0966-6362(97)00021-0

Zijlstra, W., & Hof, A. L. (2003). Assessment of spatio-temporal Gait Parameters from Trunk Accelerations during Human Walking. *Gait & Posture, 18*(2), 1–10. doi:10.1016/S0966-6362(02)00190-X

ADDITIONAL READING

American College of Sports Medicine, Chodzko-Zajko, W.J., Proctor, D.N., Fiatarone Singh, M.A., Minson, C.T., Nigg, C.R., Salem, G.J. & Skinner, J.S. (2009). American College of Sports Medicine position stand. Exercise and physical activity for older adults. *Medicine and Science in Sports and Exercise, 41*(7), 1510–1530.

Aminian, K., & Najafi, B. (2004). Capturing human motion using body-fixed sensors: outdoor measurement and clinical applications. *Computer Animation and Virtual Worlds, 15*(2), 79–94. doi:10.1002/cav.2

Bonato, P. (2005). Advances in wearable technology and applications in physical medicine and rehabilitation. *Journal of Neuroengineering and Rehabilitation, 2*, 1–4. doi:10.1186/1743-0003-2-2

de Bruin, E. D., Hartmann, A., Uebelhart, D., Murer, K., & Zijlstra, W. (2008). Wearable systems for monitoring mobility related activities in older people. *Clinical Rehabilitation, 22*, 878–895. doi:10.1177/0269215508090675

Hausdorff, J. M. (2005). Gait variability: methods, modeling and meaning. *Journal of Neuroengineering and Rehabilitation, 2*, 19. doi:10.1186/1743-0003-2-19

Hermens, H. J., & Vollenbroek-Hutten, M. M. (2008). Towards remote monitoring and remotely supervised training. *Journal of Electromyography and Kinesiology, 18*(6), 908–919. doi:10.1016/j.jelekin.2008.10.004

International Classification of Functioning. Disability and Health (ICF).(n.d.). *World Health Organisation*, Geneva (www.who.int/classification/icf).

Luinge, H. J. (2002). *Inertial sensing of human movement*. PhD thesis. The Netherlands: Twente University Press.

Mathie, M. J., Coster, A. C., Lovell, N. H., & Celler, B. G. (2004). Accelerometry: providing an integrated, practical method for long-term, ambulatory monitoring of human movement. *Physiological Measurement, 25*(2), R1–R20. doi:10.1088/0967-3334/25/2/R01

N'I Scanaill, C., Carew, S., Barralon, P., Noury, N., Lyons, D. & Lyons, G.M. (2006). A Review of Approaches to Mobility Telemonitoring of the Elderly in Their Living Environment. *Annals of Biomedical Engineering, 34*, 547–563. doi:10.1007/s10439-005-9068-2

Noury, N., Fleury, A., Rumeau, P., Bourke, A. K., Laighin, G. O., Rialle, V., & Lundy, J. E. (2007) Fall detection principles and methods. *Conference Proceedings - IEEE Engineering in Medicine and Biology*, 1663-1666.

Roetenberg, D. (2006*). Inertial and magnetic sensing of human motion*. PhD thesis. The Netherlands: University of Twente.

Skelton, D. A., & Todd, C. (2004). *What are the main risk factors for falls amongst older people and what are the most effective interventions to prevent these falls? How should interventions to prevent falls be implemented? Health Evidence Network*. Denmark: World Health Organisation.

Terrier, P., & Schutz, Y. (2005). How useful is satellite positioning system (GPS) to track gait parameters? A review. *Journal of Neuroengineering and Rehabilitation, 2*, 2–28. doi:10.1186/1743-0003-2-28

Winter, D. A. (2009). *Biomechanics and Motor Control of Human Movement* (4th ed.). New York: John Wiley & Sons. doi:10.1002/9780470549148

Zijlstra, W., & Aminian, K. (2007). Mobility assessment in older people, new possibilities and challenges. *European Journal of Ageing, 4*, 3–12. doi:10.1007/s10433-007-0041-9

KEY TERMS AND DEFINITIONS

Movement: Movement is a change of position, or a rotation, of an object or (parts of) the body.

Physical Activity: Physical activity is any body movement produced by skeletal muscles that results in energy expenditure.

Mobility (as used in this contribution): Mobility relates to voluntary movements that involve a change of overall body position, for example rising from a chair, or walking. A person with a mobility impairment may have difficulty with walking, standing, lifting, climbing stairs, carrying, or balancing.

Motion Sensor: An instrument that senses and measures movement.

Assessment (as used in this contribution): The systematic collection of information about an individual's motor and/or cognitive functioning.

Monitoring (as used in this contribution): Repeated assessments of aspects of an individual's motor and/or cognitive functioning.

Fall: An unexpected event in which a person comes to rest on the ground, floor, or a lower level.

Fall Detection: An automated recognition of the occurance of a fall, for example based on video data or based on motion sensors.

Chapter 12

Med–on–@ix:
Real–Time Tele–Consultation in Emergency Medical Services – Promising or Unnecessary?

In-Sik Na
University Hospital Aachen, Germany

Stefan Beckers
University Hospital Aachen, Germany,

Max Skorning
University Hospital Aachen, Germany

Harold Fischermann
University Hospital Aachen, Germany

Arnd T. May
University Hospital Aachen, Germany

Nadja Frenzel
University Hospital Aachen, Germany

Marie-Thérèse Schneiders
RWTH Aachen University, Germany

Tadeusz Brodziak
P3 Communications GmbH, Germany

Michael Protogerakis
RWTH Aachen University, Germany

Rolf Rossaint
University Hospital Aachen, Germany

ABSTRACT

The aim of the project Med-on-@ix is to increase the quality of care for emergency patients by the operationalisation of rescue processes. The currently available technologies will be integrated into a new emergency telemedical service system. The aim is to capture all the necessary information comprising electrocardiogram, vital signs, clinical findings, images and necessary personal data of a patient at the emergency scene and transmit this data in real time to a centre of competence. This would enable a "virtual presence" on site of an Emergency Medical Services physician (EMS-physician, the German Notarzt). Thus, we can raise the quality of EMS in total and counter the growing problem of EMS-physician shortage by exploiting the existing medical resources. In addition, this system offers EMS-physicians and paramedics consultation from a centre of competence. Thereby referring to evidence-based medicine and ensuring the earliest possible information of the hospital.

DOI: 10.4018/978-1-60960-469-1.ch012

INTRODUCTION

At present, emergency calls are condensed to certain keywords, such as *respiratory distress*, and dispatched to both paramedics as well as the EMS-physician. Typically, the ambulance staffed with paramedics is the first on scene and the EMS-physician arrives a few minutes later. In rural areas the arrival period can exceed 30 minutes as there are more ambulance bases than EMS-physician bases. The distances from the bases to the scene are much shorter for ambulances than for the EMS-physician. As a consequence drug free interval vary significantly, depending on whether the emergency is taking place in an urban or rural area. Additionally, the lack of EMS-physicians in times of general shortage of physicians impedes the 24 hours occupation of EMS-physician bases in rural areas (Deutscher Bundestag, 2006) (Behrendt & Schmiedel, 2004).

The Med-on-@ix-project aims at the broad implementation of a telemedical system in EMS enabling support up to a real-time teleconsultation. The basis of the system is a centre of competence with an experienced emergency medical physician (further called *Telenotarzt* in accordance to the German equivalent for EMS-physician, the *Notarzt*). Advanced mobile data transmission enables the real time transmission of all vital parameters of a patient and a video live stream from the ambulance and the scene to the competence centre, where the information is visualized on large screens.

He uses specially designed software, including maps, and he has a documentation software as well as databases. The competence centre is responsible for the contact and data transfer to the hospital and the consultation with other institutions (for example family physician, cardiology, poisoning centre, and so forth). Thus, the rescuers on scene can focus on their main task, which is the manual patient care. German paramedics are restricted in their clinical actions due to legal limitations, for example drug therapy at the emergency scene.

Therefore, the advantage of this system is, that measures reserved normally only for physicians could be begun on the order of the Telenotarzt until the EMS physician arrives on site. Thus, the treatment free interval may be shortened. In cases where the EMS-physician is not present in the foreseeable future, the Telenotarzt could even replace the EMS physician in part. In most cases it is mainly the expertise and decision-making of the physician that is needed, rather than the practical skills (Gries, Helm & Martin, 2003).

The main aim of this research is to improve the quality of medical care and patient safety while speeding up the whole process. Since 2004, this project has been created by the emergency medicine section at the Department of Anaesthesiology, University Hospital of Aachen. In 2006, the merger of the existing consortium of industry and research was completed. The project Med-on-@ix is funded by the Federal Ministry of Economics and Technology funding programme *SimoBIT* (secure use of mobile information technology to increase value creation in small business and government)

The main partners in this consortium listed below:

1. Department of Anaesthesiology at the University Hospital Aachen EMS-physicians are recruited from the Department of Anaesthesiology The department operates a simulation centre (AIXTRA) with a "Full-Scale Simulator" to practice various real emergency situations.

2. Department of Information Management in Mechanical Engineering of the RWTH Aachen University, Germany, (ZLW/IMA) This department focuses on system integration, customer-driven technology development and design of human-technology interfaces. Within the Med-on-@ix project, the ZLW / IMA is responsible for the implementation of scenarios, the design of human-technology interfaces, as well as

the conduct of simulation studies and their evaluation.

3. Philips Healthcare, Hamburg Philips develops and manufactures products for patient monitoring systems for the global market. In the Med-on-@ix project, Philips is involved with the Cardiac & Monitoring Section in Boeblingen and the marketing section in Hamburg.

4. P3 communications GmbH, Aachen (Telecommunications) P3 communications includes the telecommunication activities since 1999 of the P3 SOLUTIONS GmbH Consulting Company for Management & Organisation. P3 is now a Europe-wide company which has specialized in the measurement, analysis and optimisation of mobile networks and services. In our project, P3 is responsible for transmission techniques and hardware devices as well as software development.

BACKGROUND

The trade-off between the best possible care and controllable costs is compounded by other problems in EMS. One of these problems is the Working Hours Act, which took effect in 2007, and is now being implemented for physicians. The act limits the working hours of physicians to twelve hours a day. Hereby, a greater number of EMS-physicians is needed in times of general shortage of physicians (Rieser, 2005). The consequences of the lack of EMS-physicians, especially in rural areas, are a deterioration of quality management and deficiencies in medical care. Additionally, the number of EMS-physician stations will be reduced, and the time of arrival of the emergency patient will be extended (Bundesärztekammer, 2004). However, arrival times have already become prolonged, as shown by a direct comparison of data from the survey periods of 2000/2001 and of 2004/2005, which is the most recent data available. In 95%

of the emergency missions, service arrived within 16.3 minutes (previously 15.9 minutes). An EMS-physician arrived in 95% of cases, at the latest, after 22.3 minutes (Deutscher Bundestag, 2006). In the years 1994/1995, the mean arrival time was 18.6 minutes, in 1998/1999, it was 20.2 minutes and in 2000/2001 it increased to 21.9 minutes (Behrendt & Schmiedel, 2003). These numbers demonstrate the successive deterioration of arrival time. This leads to serious consequences, such as a prolonged drug-free interval and an overall delayed emergency medical care by the physician, especially in rural areas.

In this context, a comparison with other European Rescue Systems in other countries (for example the UK and the Netherlands) is remarkable. In most other European countries the out-of-hospital emergency medical care is exclusively maintained by well qualified paramedics and without physicians, which has not led to poorer results overall.

However, there is evidence that a physician-led EMS is advantageous for invasive measures, such as respiratory protection (Jemmet, Kendal, Fourre & Burton, 2003) (Jones, Murphy & Dickson, 2004) (Katz & Falk, 2001) (Silvestri, Ralls & Krauss, 2005) (Timmermann, Russo, Eich & 2007).

The health sector is one of the most important economic factors in Germany with expenditures of 224.94 billion Euros every year. Of this, 2.39 billion Euros are needed just for the short period of EMS care, which is more than 1%. In particular, the costs for EMS have increased by leaps and bounds in recent years (Statistisches Bundesamt, 2006). The EMS also faces other major challenges. The total quantity of emergency cases has increased from year to year. In Germany, 10.2 millions of rescue missions have been carried out per year according to the most recent survey data, and 4.7 millions of these have been categorised as emergency missions (Deutscher Bundestag, 2006). In parallel with the total number of ambulance calls, the number of emergency cases with involvement of EMS-physicians has also increased. In 1985, the proportion of EMS cases involving EMS-physicians was 33%. In Germany, in 2000, it was already 50%, which corresponded to 1.7 million emergency missions involving physicians (Gries et al., 2003).

More recent nationwide data on the incidence of emergency medical interventions are not available, but a further increase is most likely. This increase also means that there are increases in failed emergency missions, which account for 8.9% of all emergency missions involving physicians (Gesundheitsberichterstattung des Bundes, 2007). This would also entail an increase in emergency missions not requiring EMS-physicians.

Moreover, only a small proportion of emergency medical interventions actually require the manual skills of an EMS-physician on scene. For most provided care, only the expertise and decision-making authority of an EMS-physician is required. EMS-physicians are for example needed for intubation, resuscitation, anaesthesia induction and so forth. Gries et al. (2003) reported that the sum of incidences of individual medical procedures that required an experienced EMS-physician on site was only 14.3% of all assignments. The actual proportion would still be much lower if one considers that many of these measures were performed on the same patients. Messelken, Martin & Milewski (1998) state that the EMS-physicians themselves retrospectively assess that in only 51.5% of their missions, the patient is in a life-threatening (36.4%) or acute life-threatening (15.1%) situation. In at most 4.0% of these missions, resuscitation measures must be taken, but successful resuscitation as the primary goal represents only 1.7% of emergency missions (Messelken, Martin & Milewski, 1998).

Nationally, an emergency operation takes an average of 50.1 minutes to claim (Behrendt & Schmiedel, 2004), and during this time, the EMS-physician is attached to the patient and is not available for other missions. This is despite the fact that the EMS-physician's actual therapeutic activity is often limited to a few minutes (for ex-

ample during the subsequent transportation to the hospital), and in many cases, his primary liability is only to manage the situation. The duration of the emergency mission is correlated primarily to the transportation time to the nearest suitable hospital and thus is longer in rural areas.

MAIN FOCUSES OF THE CHAPTER

The project Med-on-@ix consists of a multidisciplinary team of researchers that all have a distinctive perspective on telemedicine. Therefore, the project has a medical, technical, socio-technical as well as ethical focus. These different perspectives will be elaborated in the following chapter.

Issues, Controversies, Problems

Medical Focus

The Department of Anaesthesiology at the University Hospital Aachen is responsible for all medical aspects of the project Med-on-@ix and elaborates on all clinical issues that arise due to telemedicine in the German EMS.

In international emergency medicine systems, telemedicine applications have been examined for many years and have partly been established. The telemedicine systems for prehospital emergency medicine have their seeds in the United States, where teleconsultation between the physician in the hospital and the paramedics on scene via radio has become standard. In this way, the quality of primary care can be improved and assessed more exactly. In addition, in-hospital procedures could be optimized through better and faster transfer of information (Augustine, 2001) (Erder, Davidson & Cheney, 1989) (Wuerz, Swope, Holliman & Vazquez, 1995). For example, the transfer of a 12-lead electrocardiogram (ECG) to the receiving cardiology department has also become a standard in some German EMS, and it has been shown in international studies to lead to a significant

Figure 1. The Process of an emergency mission with Med-on-@ix

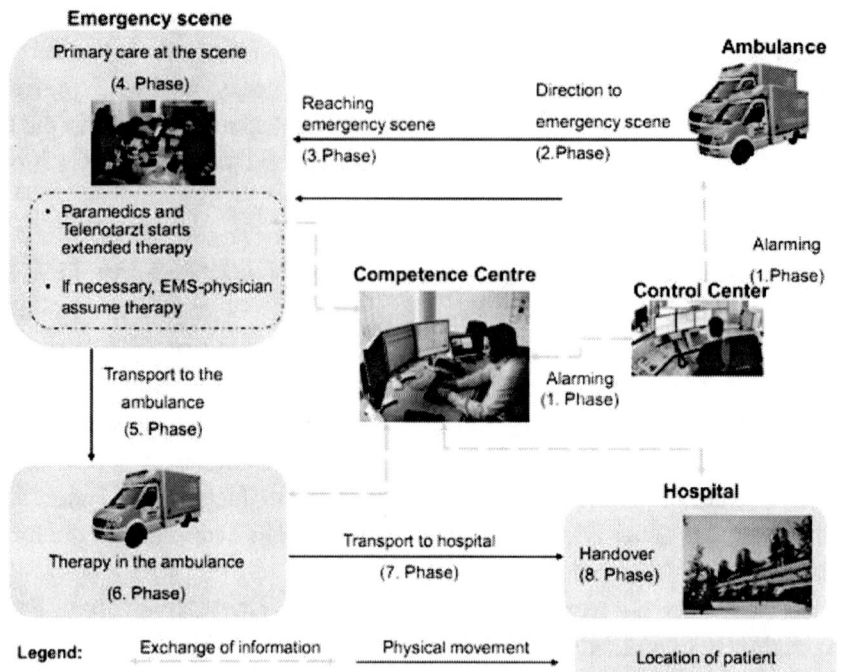

reduction in ischaemia time during ST-elevation myocardial infarction. *Contact-to-balloon time* and *door-to-balloon time* could be reduced through target-oriented confinement of the patient in a centre with cardiac catheterisation and prior information of the hospital staff (Adams, Campbell & Adams, 2006) (Dhruva, Abdelhadi & Anis, 2007) (Sejersten, Sillesen & Hansen, 2008).

But such innovative procedures are carried out mainly by using second-generation mobile phones, without any additional encryption mechanisms and without suitability for larger amounts of data and an accelerated transmission.

The approach of the project Med-on-@ix is the broad implementation of a telemedicine system in the EMS. All mission- and patient-related data, such as ECGs, pulse oximetry, blood pressure, various vital signs, auscultation information, and video live-streams of the rescue unit, can be exchanged in real time between the working on-site rescue personnel and the physician at the centre

of competence. The on-site rescue personnel may consists of paramedics and EMS-physician.

These competence centres are staffed with highly qualified specialists who determine further treatment on site and during transportation based on the information at the scene and the relevant guidelines. These competence centres will also have extensive opportunities to contact other health care providers in order to obtain comprehensive organizational and patient-related information. The competence centre will transmit all relevant information to the designated hospital in advance of the patient arrival. Therefore, the patient benefits from a timely adequate therapy.

Figure 1 shows how an emergency mission would proceed with and without the Med-on-@ ix system.

Normally, there is no EMS physician on the ambulance in the EMS in the city of Aachen. The physician has his own car and meets the ambulance on the scene in a rendezvous system, so he is much more flexible. In our third year, the trial run, we placed an EMS physician on the ambulance, as a backup system.

1. Phase: Incoming emergency call into the control centre, the dispatcher alarms the ambulance and the EMS physician. Depending on the location of the scene, the ambulances start from different bases, while the EMS physician car is placed on the main fire fighter base. With Med-on-@ix: Dispatcher also alarms the Telenotarzt

2. Phase: Ambulance and EMS physician car are on the direction to the scene. With Med-on-@ix: Telenotarzt in the Competence centre gets in contact with the paramedics and the EMS physician who is on the ambulance. There is no separate EMS-physician car on direction to the scene in our trial run.

3. Phase: Ambulance reach the scene, the EMS physician arrives a few minutes later, depending on the location of the scene. With Med-on-@ix: Paramedics and the EMS physician arrive at the scene. Please notice that normally there is no physician on the ambulance. In our research trial, we placed the physician as a backup system for the paramedics on the ambulance.

4. Phase: Paramedics will ask for past medical history and the actual disorders, get the blood pressure and other vital parameters, like ECG and so forth. If extended therapy is necessary they have to wait for the EMS physician for further therapy which are reserved only for physicians (for example application of special medicaments) In this phase or in one of the following phases the paramedics or the physician must inform the hospital, give them the information about the disorders, vital signs or other problems, maybe ask for a free place on the intensive care unit. During this time the paramedic or the physician is not focused to the patient. With Med-on-@ix: Paramedics starts also with asking for past medical history, the actual disorders but starts parallel with the extended therapy, ordered and supported by the Telenotarzt in the Competence Centre. If he has all important information about the patient, he could inform the hospital and organize everything. If the manual skill of the physician is needed, the backup physician could help. (In the future, the system is professional implemented in the EMS, the EMS physician must be reordered in this case, if he was not alarmed parallel to the ambulance)

5. Phase: Transport to the ambulance. While the team is carrying the patient to the ambulance it might not be so much focused on the patient. With Med-on-@ix: During the transport to the ambulance, the Telenotarzt could control the vital signs of the patient, while the team is concentrated on the transport.

6. Phase: The therapy will go on in the ambulance. In the case that the condition of the patient gets worse, he is not available for a new emergency case, because his expertise and decisions is probably needed. With Med-on-@ix: The Telenotarzt in the Competence Centre could support the paramedics with his expertise and decisions and the EMS physician would be free for a new emergency.

7, 8. Phase: Transport to the hospital and handover. If the patient`s condition deteriorated, the paramedic or the physician is occupied with the therapy, to stabilize the patient, but maybe cannot inform the hospital early enough about the new situation. The consequence could be, that the procedure in hospital could take much longer, because they were not well prepared. With Med-on-@ix: There is a constant exchange of information between hospital and paramedics or EMS physician by the Telenotarzt, so the hospital is up to date about the situation of the patient and the therapy, therefore the hospital could better prepare their workflow.

The strategy was to implement the concept above within three years. In the first year, we identified the requirements for a comprehensive telemedicine system and defined the specifications. In close cooperation with our industrial partners, operational systems have been re-evaluated and assessed on how well the system is available and how it can be combined with up-to-date technical equipment. The project started with a technical pre-release (*mock-up*), which showed the transfer functionality in a simulator environment, but lacked the required mobility and security in its entirety. The second year of the project was mainly used for studies on the Emergency and Anaesthesia Simulator Centre, AIXTRA of the University Hospital Aachen. Here, the application of the system was prospectively tested by paramedics and EMS-physicians. In September 2008, the first simulator study, SIMI I, was carried out successfully. In this study, 29 teams, each consisting of one EMS-physician and two paramedics, were confronted with two different emergency scenarios (ST-elevation myocardial infarction and brain trauma), for which there are primary care guidelines. We randomised the Telenotarzt support for each scenario. The teams' treatments of the patients were assessed with video-based evaluations in terms of the differences in adhering to emergency treatment guidelines, conformity and the time requirement, with and without the Telenotarzt. The second simulator study, SIMI II, which was conducted in May 2009, examined to what extent drug therapy by paramedics with telemedicine guidance and control can be performed safely. The quality of the diagnosis and treatment recommendations of the Telenotarzt was compared with those of an EMS-physician treating the patient on scene. In the third project year, the trial run was carried out in the EMS of the City of Aachen, for which an ambulance of the City of Aachen Fire Department has been fully equipped with telemedical devices. Figure 2 shows how the patient data (for example vital parameters, 12 lead-ECG, videos) are transmit-

ted from the emergency scene to the competence centre and to the hospital. It also shows the communication pathways.

This makes the system Med-on-@ix ready for application and testing in real operations in the evaluation phase. Medical assignments in this phase take place only in the presence and supervision of an experienced EMS-physician, so that maximum safety for the patient and legal certainty for the paramedics is guaranteed. Legal aspects have been a key issue in this context. Extensive legal advice was obtained from Professor Christian Katzenmeier, who is specialist in medical law and director of the *Institute of Legal Medicine* at the *University of Cologne*, and Professor Karsten Fehn, who is specialist in medical law, criminal law and professor at the *Cologne University of Applied Sciences*. They discussed the issues of privacy and patient data protection as well as the liabilities including criminal liabilities in case of damage. Legal problems can also result from the interaction of the Telenotarzt working at the competence centre with the staff working on scene. Questions arose on how the authority and responsibility should be allocated between the EMS-physician on the scene and the Telenotarzt in the competence centre. Another scenario had to be considered in which paramedics had to be delegated by the Telenotarzt in the physical absence of a physician on site, for example in the administration of certain intravenously applied medications. In summary, the Telenotarzt is responsible for medical decisions and instruction to the paramedics, unless an EMS-physician is on site. The on-site EMS-physician has the final responsibility for making decisions.

Technical Focus

In this section, the requirements for the telematic support system will be outlined. These requirements have led to a technical system summarised separated into the hardware and software system architecture. Ancillary to an appropriate system

Figure 2. Data transmission in Med-on-@ix

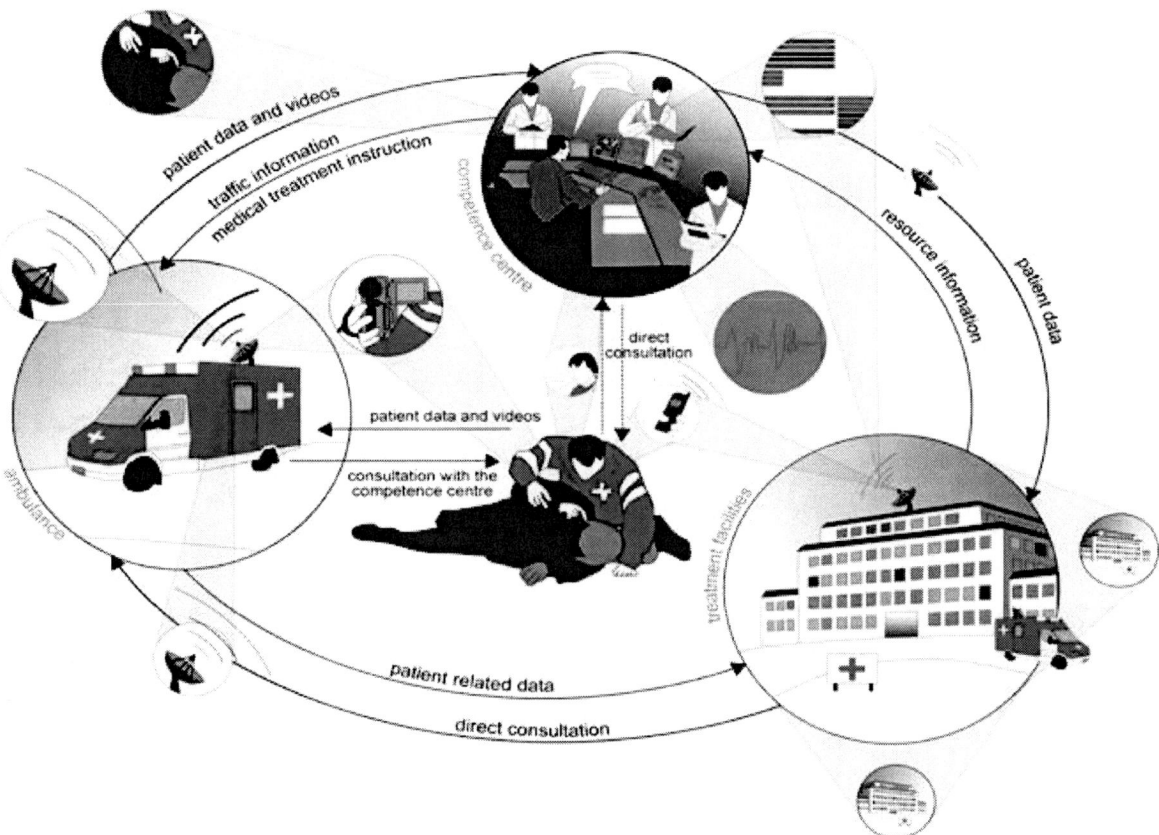

architecture a methodology to reduce technical risk in the development and the realisation is needed (Müller, Protogerakis & Henning, 2009)

Requirements. The condensed functional and non-functional requirements concerning the system design, which were based on discussions from two expert workshops with physicians and paramedic staff, are presented below.

Functional Requirements. Table 1 shows the necessary signals to be transmitted from the emergency site that would serve as the basis for decisions by the physician at the centre of competence for classification of cases into continuous live or intermittent transmission and for classification of cases into high or low priority for transmission. No need could be identified by the experts for a more dynamic prioritisation or control of these priorities by the centre of competence.

All vital parameters shown in Table 1 are measured under optimal circumstances by one single monitor/defibrillator device. Because we were limited by technical factors, we had to work with a single monitor and extra defibrillator. The device supports the real-time export of all signals except the 12-lead ECG. An electronic stethoscope allows the live wireless transmission of auscultation. The ambulance is equipped with at least one fixed remote control camera to allow the transmission of live video stream and high quality pictures. A portable camera provides a video live stream and high-resolution steady pictures from the place of emergency. Up to three wireless headsets are used for voice communication at the place of emergency. The microphones of the on-site staff can be activated by a central control device on site. The quality of the headsets is of diagnostic

Table 1. Signals to be transferred from site and their priorities

Signal	Continuous / Intermittent Transmission	Priority
12-Lead-ECG	Intermittent (5-30 min)	1A
Voice Communication	Continuous	1B
Rhythm ECG	Continuous	2
Non-Invasive Blood Pressure	Intermittent (1-5 min)	3
Pulse Oximetry	Intermittent Continuous	4 10
Kapnometry	Intermittent Continuous	5 8
Defibrillator	Intermittent	6
Invasive Blood Pressure	Intermittent Continuous	7 9
Central Venous Pressure	Continuous	11
High Resolution Pictures	Intermittent	12
~30 sec Video Sequences	Intermittent	13
Video	Continuous	14
Stethoscope	Intermittent	15

quality for auscultation. As an important step towards better quality control, the system features the documentation of the medical and mission data by software on site and by the software at the competence centre (Bergrath, 2006). The documented data from the place of emergency is displayed in real-time at the centre of competence. The documentation software receives and displays textual commands from the centre of competence, for example for the application of drugs. The documentation software allows an automatic data import of patient data from the medical devices. Pictures taken with a camera device are embedded in the documentation. Commercial mobile radio networks are well established and available at reasonable prices in most countries. If they are used redundantly, they can also be utilised for critical safety applications to take advantage of

the huge capabilities in data transfer, which contrasts with the *Professional Mobile Radio Standards*, such as the *Terrestrial Trunked Radio* (TETRA). *Global System for Mobile Communications* (GSM) and TETRA can be used for voice communication where their high availability can be utilized. All transmitted data from the place of emergency is archived for later evaluation and quality management. The latter access to anonymised archive data is restricted with the use of an appropriate authentication system.

Non-functional Requirements. To be easily adapted to the heavily varying local conditions for EMS, the system architecture must be configurable in a modular way. This applies especially to medical devices and to mobile communication technologies. The main issues concerning safety, security and reliability that have to be ensured in the system design are

1. the safety from interception of patient related data,
2. the prevention of unauthorised access to the system and
3. the data privacy of staff and patient related data.

Thus, all wireless communication must be secured by signing and encrypting of the data. A mobile device, such as a Tablet PC, is used as the central control unit and for the documentation software on site. The audio transmission of auscultation from the stethoscope is of diagnostic quality. Therefore, the stethoscope allows for wireless transmission e.g., via Bluetooth with the *Advanced Audio Distribution Profile* (A2DP) standard. The video cameras feature a resolution of at least 640x480 pixels and a frame rate of at least fifteen frames per second. A change of the frame rate must be possible during online operation. For energy and weight efficiency reasons, a fixed camera in the ambulance vehicle features a hardware compression of the video stream. A portable camera is either mounted on a small telescope tripod that is fixed onto one of the other units or be a head mounted model.

Bluetooth 2.0 is used for the connection between the communication unit and the headsets. The headsets features the *Headset-Profil* (HSP*)* and *Handsfree-Profil* (HFP) as well as the A2DP profile to allow for listening to the stethoscope signal. The system provides a middleware solution to ensure its extensibility and adaptability. It re-establishes lost connections due to problems on the underlying communication channels. It supports the abstraction of hardware vendor specific interfaces, such as the real-time interface of the ECG/defibrillator unit, by means of adapters between the vendor specific device driver and a middleware interface. In the case of insufficient bandwidth, it must feature the prioritisation of the data according to Table 1. The system must ensure the synchronicity of signals in configurable groups.

The communication unit offers a dedicated *Internet Protocol* (IP) based packet tunnel and a separate voice service to the middleware. It supports the use of the *Professional Mobile Radio* services (PMR), such as TETRA and a *Circuit Switched GSM* mode for voice communication. Common mobile network technologies, such as *General Packet Radio Service* (GPRS) with *Enhanced Data Rates for GSM Evolution* (EDGE), and *Universal Mobile Telecommunications System* (UMTS) with *High Speed Packet Access* (HSPA), support through a generic interface for the IP-based communication. The unit offers one tunnel through the parallel channels of different providers. It uplinks bandwidth information to the middleware.

Hardware Network Architecture. The distribution of hardware components and the physical network architecture is shown in Figure 2. The components on site are connected to the communication unit according to the requirements described above. The communication unit is an embedded computer that hosts the middleware, the networking logics and the hardware network interfaces. It connects to the ambulance vehicle

via an 802.11 network or directly to the *Public Switched Telephone Network* (PSTN) and the Internet through GSM/TETRA and GPRS/UMTS. Multiple GPRS/UMTS data connections to different providers ensure higher mobile network coverage and/or higher bandwidth. Bundling the different connections is a task to be realised in the network layer of the system's software. The communication unit in the ambulance connects to the mobile networks in the same way. The connection between the On-Site Communication Unit and the Ambulance Vehicle Communication Unit is for redundancy only. Additional peripheral devices such as a printer are connected to the *Ambulance Vehicles Communication Unit* by *Ethernet*. On the centre of competence's side, the servers are connected to the PSTN via ISDN and to the Internet. The Clients in the centre of competence connect to the Servers through a local network.

Software Layer Architecture. As for most communication systems, a layered architecture was also chosen for the software architecture of the telematic support system. The software architecture of the telematic support system is divided into the Application Layer, the Session Layer and the Network Layer as shown in Figure 3.

The Application Layer encapsulates the medical devices and other sensors as well as the clients and servers in the centre of competence. The interfaces between the session layer and the application layer is clearly described. That makes it easy to exchange single components of the application layer to meet the different demands of different emergency medical services. When using components with proprietary interfaces adapters can be implemented to adapt them to the defined interface.

The Session Layer consists of the Middleware and is responsible for the session management and the conditioning of all outgoing data. The session management holds the state of the actual connection. That makes it possible to use stateless applications as components on the application layer. For example an ECG sender application on

Figure 3. Hardware distribution and network architecture overview

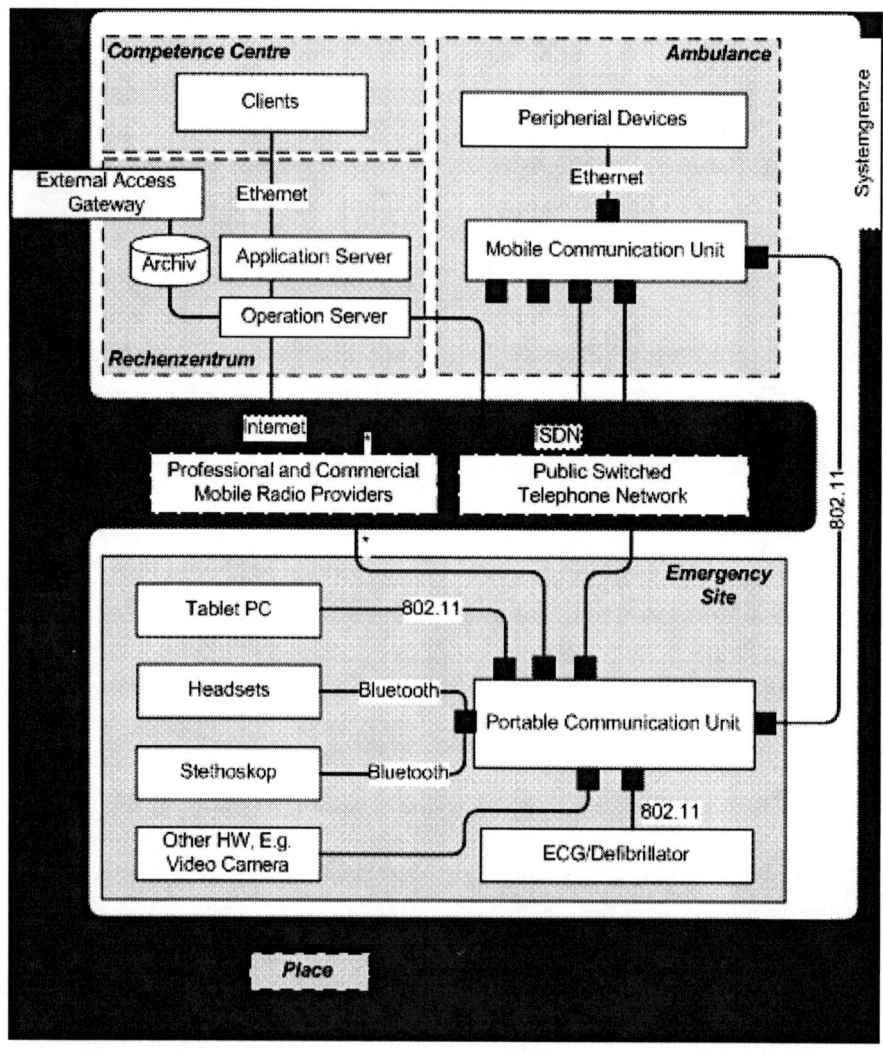

Figure 4. Overview of the different logistical layers in the system

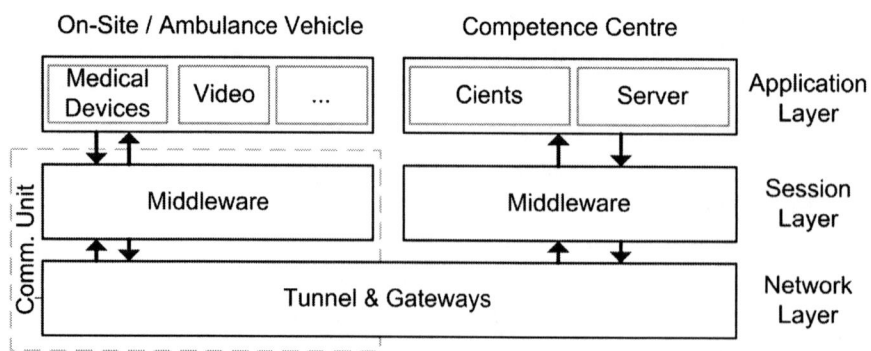

the application layer sends data to a not specified receiver. The middleware decides about the routing of this data to the appropriate receiver. That approach supports loser couplings of applications into the architecture. The conditioning of the outgoing data by the session layer is mainly the prioritization of the signals to be transferred according to Table 1 and the adaptive compression of streams like video, according to the actual available bandwidth resulting from the network coverage.

In the Network Layer multiple encrypted VPN Tunnels in the Network Layer are established over multiple concurrent physical links and bonded to one virtual tunnel interface. While techniques for vertical handovers like Mobile IP and the Session Initiation Protocol (SIP) in mobile networks have been well established over the last few years (Good & Ventura, 2006), the parallel use of multiple links to increase bandwidth is still a challenge (Li & Brassil, 2006). The resulting networking properties of the bonded tunnel are determined by the fact that the order of arriving packets on the receiver side is non-deterministic due to the different behaviours of the underlying communication channels. That makes it useless to have protocols like *User Datagram Protocol* (UDP) that lack robustness against the reordering of packets. The Transmission Control Protocol (TCP) is much more robust against packet reordering. Bohacek, Hespanha, Lee, Lim and Obraczka (2006) described a new TCP with high resistance against packet reordering. The Real-Time Transport Protocol (RTP) extends UDP with a reordering robustness and is well suited for real-time streaming applications (Iren, Amer & Conrad, 1999) (Schulzrinne, Casner, Frederick & Jacobson, 2006).

Streaming Services. To achieve the integration of services with real-time and synchronicity requirements, the *Streaming Part* must balance different directives for the streaming services. It must ensure the synchronicity of different signals in "synchronisation groups" such as the different

ECG leads. In the case of an insufficient total available bandwidth, it should prevent the "stuttering" of the signal output on the receiver side (continuity). The minimal length of continuous data is determined by the minimal length needed for diagnostic purposes. The Middleware should not present data that is too old to the receiver side (timeliness). Only the most recent parts of a minimum useful length must be transmitted from the sender's side. Therefore, in order to achieve a trade-off between both continuity and timeliness, streams have been broken down into smallest segments that are still medically interpretable. To achieve this, the *Streaming Part* design contains two buffers and a *resampler* or *recoder* in between. A controller calculates the parameters to achieve the described balance for the buffer and resampling/recoding parameters. There is one *Packer* for each synchronisation group of streaming signals. It fetches data from outgoing buffers of all signal paths in one synchronisation group and multiplexes them.

Socio-Technical Focus

Socio-technical aspects are relevant in a telemedical context. The Department of Information Management in Mechanical Engineering of the RWTH Aachen University has elaborated on the implementation of scenarios, the design of human-technology interfaces, the conduct of simulation studies and their evaluation.

Evaluation of User Acceptance within Med-on-@ix.

To ensure a user oriented development of the telematic support system, the researchers relied on an iterative development process characterized by a consequent dialogue between developers and users of the system. To illustrate the user integration some of the evaluation results gathered so far within the project are described within the following lines. Until now findings derived from simulation studies realised within Med-on-@ix can provide an indication on the acceptance of the system by the different involved user groups and constituted an important basis for a user-centred technical development.

The user acceptance is one decisive factor to guarantee a successful development and implementation of the telematic support system. Various theories of user acceptance had been developed, describing user satisfaction as one major key to success in the development of new technologies. Davis (1993) describes acceptance in line with the *technology acceptance model* (TAM), correlating perceived usefulness, perceived ease of use, attitude towards use and actual system use. Generally, user acceptance reflects whether a technology fits the requirements of the user as well as the characteristics of the task. The process-oriented approach of Kollmann (1998) focuses on acceptance developed within three phases, distinguishing the attitude, the acting and the long-term user acceptance. Regarding the arrangement of a user-centred development strategy, this theoretical approach offers the possibility to evaluate acceptance at different stages within the research project. Usability aspects and user acceptance were therefore reflected in the technical development in keeping with the holistic research strategy of Med-on-@ix (Skorning et al., 2009). Besides various technical and medical requirements, economical, judicial and safety-related specifications were analysed to set up the broad trial operation in Aachen. At different stages of development of the telematic support system, simulation studies were conducted at the *Interdisciplinary Medical Simulation Centre* (AIXSIM) of the University Hospital Aachen, Germany. In September 2008 and in June 2009, the simulation studies were carried out to validate the identified requirements by involving EMS workers as well as a full-scale patient simulator. EMS Teams and EMS-physicians had the opportunity to test the telematic support system in different simulated rescue scenarios. The researchers focused on the effect of using a telematic support system in

EMS missions on the quality of medical care. Following the scenarios performed by EMS Teams, different social research methods were applied to examine the factors of acceptance and utilisation issues amongst EMS. The results from both studies were partly published within the Proceeding of the International Conference on Successes & Failures in Telehealth 2009, which took place in Brisbane, Australia.

A questionnaire with both open-ended and closed-ended questions were designed and used to gather feedback from the different stakeholders – EMS-physicians, paramedics and the Telenotarzt. The questions referred to the general attitude towards the application of telemedicine in EMS, the evaluation of the scenarios with and without the support of the telematic system, the support by the remote EMS-physician and especially the impact of the telemedical assistance on communication- or work-related processes, the perception of the role of the team members as well as the perceived quality of care and guideline conformity of the treatment processes. The respondents specified their level of agreement on a six-point Likert scale. The semi-structured interviews were carried out by using an issue-focused interview guide. Gathering data by moderated group discussions offered the interviewer the possibility to react individually to the issues that the respondents wanted to focus on. Following the methods described by Mayring (2000), the transcript video-documented interviews underwent a rule-guided qualitative content analysis. The approach is advantageous because it combines the methodological strengths of quantitative content analysis and the concept of qualitative procedure. The textual data was coded into thematic categories representing the different aspects of interpretation in terms of the underlying textual material.

In the first study, 87 subjects from 29 EMS-teams (one EMS-physician and two paramedics) took part in the interview, whereas 48 test persons (16 EMS-physicians and 32 paramedics) took part in the second run in 2009. In both studies, the test subjects were divided into half, with one half assigned to the control group without the telematic support system to allow a comparison of the quality of treatment with and without the application of telematics. The first simulation study addressed the support of an EMS-physician, who was informed about the scenarios. The second simulation study tackled the support of an EMS Team consisting of two paramedics by a trained EMS-physician in the competence centre who was uninformed about the course of the scenarios. Another decisive difference between both studies was the number and type of the simulated scenarios: in the first run, only two standardised scenarios (ST-elevation myocardial infarction and severe traumatic brain injury) were performed, while in the second study, five different scenarios (a diving accident, a renal colic, a second-degree burn, an intoxication and a hypoglycaemia) were performed by actors as patient simulators, and they offered a wide scope of scenarios for testing (Schneiders, Protogerakis & Isenhardt, 2009). The first survey showed a positive attitude of the respondents towards the use of a telematic support system in the emergency care. For 83% of the EMS-physicians and almost 93% of the questioned paramedics, the implementation of an always available EMS-physician in a competence centre was viewed as a great support in their everyday work. The interviewees especially approved of the support by the telematic system in case of doubt or rare conditions as well as for inexperienced physicians. Critics were concerned about the encroachment on usual operational procedures by the telematic support system. In particular, experienced EMS-Teams had difficulties handling the interventions from the EMS-physician in the competence centre and complained about the fact of not knowing the physician and hence having some problems of communication within the team. It was significant that the unusual working situation had a crucial impact on the information exchange between the medical services as well as with the patient.

The feedback and results from questionnaires and interviews were integrated into further development of the system itself and the organisational implementation into the EMS. For example, the project aims to provide the needed confidence towards the EMS-physician in the competence centre by the rotation of physicians working on site and the physicians working in the competence centre. The teamwork on site provides the required routine and trust towards the involved co-workers. All subjects called for continued training with the system to get used to the new working situation. To guarantee efficient teamwork, some crucial rules, concerning the timing and modalities of communication, were defined and disseminated in line with necessary training courses for the user groups. Those defined rules underwent an in-depth analysis within the second simulation study in 2009 and had a positive impact on user acceptance. Although the critical voices constituted 83% in the first study, only 45% of the test subjects criticised the communication during the scenarios in the second run (Schneiders et al., 2009). The acceptance of the telematic support systems was 91.6% in the second study, highlighting all the positive aspects of the system on the diagnostic confidence and the operational procedures on site – like the preparation of hospitalisation or the management of additional or specialised rescue units. Most of the interviewed persons estimated that the use of such a system would reduce the pressure of work on site. A significant positive development of the teamwork and the communication between the participants was observed over the course of the five scenarios. The interviewees confirmed a training effect and underscored the needed routine in working with the telematic support system (Schneiders et al., 2009). The intensified exchange between researchers, developers and potential users of the described studies offered a wide range of feedback and points of criticisms from the user groups. The consideration of the documentation requirements during the development process was crucial to improve the system and strengthen the acceptance of the telematic support system by the EMS teams. A high involvement of the user had a positive impact on earning their trust in the research activities and the developed system. To achieve user-centred development and an acceptable result, the project has to take into account the requirements and suggestions for improvement. A user- and market-focused design of new technologies for the healthcare sector can be achieved by using an iterative and cooperative user-centred developing strategy, which incorporates acceptability factors, criticisms and statements of distrust on the part of test users to overcome possible market barriers in an early stage of development.

Ethical Focus

Telemedicine and especially the Telenotarzt enable a higher standard of care with a shorter time for treatment from paramedic care for patients. The principle of care and beneficence for the patient is enhanced by a trained EMS-physician who supports the EMS-physician at the emergency scene via telemedicine equipment. The teamwork between the EMS-physician at the emergency scene and the Telenotarzt has to be trained in order to achieve optimal medical competence for the patient. In a traditional patient-doctor relationship, it is preferable that the physician sees the patient in a face-to-face consultation. In contrast to the on-scene EMS-physician, the Telenotarzt's impression of the situation of the patient is limited to the information he gets via telemedicine. The Telenotarzt only gets in contact with other professionals such as the EMS-physician or trained paramedics. The direct communication of the patient and the Telenotarzt is not a focus of the project.

Even if an EMS-physician is not present, the patient would presumably seek telemedicine consultation because even the limited communication of the patient with an off-scene EMS-physician is preferable to the situation where only paramedics are involved. The organizing principle of emergency medical service in Germany is still to send an EMS-physician to the emergency scene to support the paramedics. In cases where the EMS-physician is expected to arrive at the emergency scene after the paramedics due to traffic or distance, then the telemedicine system reduces the time that a physician is not involved to a minimum. The principle of beneficence of Beauchamp and Childress (2009) requires agents to provide benefits to others. In the absence of a clearly formulated and known wish of the patient, the paramedics and the EMS-physician are in charge to provide the best possible medical treatment. Therefore, it is a moral obligation to involve an EMS-physician via telemedicine to shorten the time without involvement of a physician. It is a moral duty to reduce the time of treatment if the telemedicine system is available because the alternative would be a longer period of time of not being treated by a physician. The telemedicine system in Aachen comes into effect if a person is in danger, and therefore, the best possible medical treatment is in the interest of the patient. The patient can expect the best possible treatment, and it is a strong ethical imperative that physicians act for the benefit of their patients. The involvement of the telemedicine system in emergency medical service in Germany is a moral obligation if the system is available, and no other form of involvement of an EMS-physician is possible. The involvement of an EMS-physician via telemedicine is demanded by the patient because a competent patient interacts with the physician in a special way. The principle of informed consent requests a communication of the patient with the physician. For the interpretation and acknowledgment of an Advance Directive, it is necessary to have the qualification of a physician. In such a situation, an EMS-physician via telemedicine can make treatment decisions that paramedics are not allowed to make. For the situation where there is an absence of an emergency physician on the scene, the involvement of an EMS-physician via telemedicine secures the respect for autonomy of the patient. The principle of justice is a focus of the telemedicine system for emergency treatment in Aachen, and the telemedicine system values efficiency in allocating the on-duty personnel. On the other hand, the possibility of involving an emergency physician via telemedicine reduces the risk of accidents on the way to the patient. Not all patients need the treatment of an EMS-physician, and the physician at the hospital can take care of the patient when there is no life-threatening situation. Paramedics can be directed via telemedicine support by an emergency physician, the use of this needed competence is fair, equitable and appropriate for the patient, and more patients can benefit from the higher availability of EMS-physician competence. The activation of the EMS-physicians by the coordinating fire department strictly follows medical principles and depends on the need of the patient and is not determined by other factors, such as insurance status or neighbourhood of the patient. It would be unethical to send paramedics only, if it is clear by the information provided in the emergency call that the help of an EMS-physician is needed. Another situation would be when all on-duty EMS-physician are busy in treating patients, and the support of an EMS-physician via telemedicine for a colleague is stopped when a paramedic orders support of an EMS-physician via telemedicine. The quality of the treatment of a patient by an EMS-physician, if substituted with an EMS-physician via telemedicine, might slightly decline, but the quality of treatment for the patient with only paramedics at the scene will considerable improve. The principle of justice demands the support of an EMS-physician via telemedicine for patients who need a physician.

FUTURE RESEARCH DIRECTIONS

The Med-on-@ix systems may be used in other medical applications as well as in non-medical areas. Due to the open interfaces and the individual components of the system, Med-on-@ix could

be further broadened or supplemented and thus could be adjusted to individual needs. The use of the specific system components for less complex applications is also possible. In particular, the application of the secure transmission technology, which was developed in the framework of the Med-on-@ ix project, could be of use for many other industries. Wherever rapid expert consultation in an emergency is necessary, the patient sensor and the transmission technology of Med-on-@ix can be used. For example:

1. Emergency care provided through the general practitioner by the Resident Doctors` Association
2. Emergency care provided in commercial airliner or on cruise ships
3. Emergency care in remote areas, e.g., on expeditions
4. Emergency care in difficult terrain, such as in a mountain rescue

Additionally, the concept of Med-on-@ix could be transferred to other sectors of health care, such as developing interfaces to home monitoring, digital health recordings or nursing homes. To implement the technology in clinical practice, one goal must be further miniaturisation and weight reduction of mobile technologies for data transmission, which may also allow the launching of these technologies to the commercial market.

Another interesting aspect is the extension of the evaluation phase and the involvement of more ambulances equipped with telematic techniques from the Med-on-@ix project, for evaluating not only the situation in an urban environment but also in rural regions. It would be of particular interest to assess long distance teleconsultations to see if it is possible to compensate for the lack of EMS-physicians and to assess what kinds of technical problems may arise compared to an urban environment. Another conceivable area of application for the Med-on-@ix technology would be during a major crisis with mass numbers of injured people, in which there might be a shortage of EMS-physicians, especially at the beginning of such as crisis. Here, the Telenotarzt could perform mainly organizational tasks, such as alerting hospitals and asking for free intensive care unit capacities, even in hospitals at a larger radius from the incident. Easy implementation, continuous updating of all relevant medical guidelines, usability and teaching concepts in combination with telematic techniques remain major important themes, especially in the EMS sector, where the shortage of well qualified EMS-physicians is challenged by the steadily increasing number of missions. Therefore, a continuing discourse is needed in society about the quality of care. Also, a continuing dialog between governmental policies, health authorities and medical industries is mandatory to allow the economisation of the health system as well as the optimisation of the quality of care within the EMS.

Projects such as the EU projects "MyHeart" (MyHeart, n.d.) "6WINIT" (Rall et al., 2004), and "MobiHealth" (MobiHealth, 2010), which consist of several individual projects on telemedicine (van Halteren et al. 2004), or the "Tele-trauma system" project (Chu & Ganz, 2004) show how much potential can be found in the area of telemedicine and how challenging it is to explore the opportunities and the complexity of the interactions between men and machines.

CONCLUSION

There is a need for new strategies to face the current and future problems in the German Emergency Medical Services. The lack of quality management and the increasing costs in the presence of a shortage of EMS-physicians are typical challenges, resulting in an increasingly inadequate medical care. In addition, the information and communication technology used in the German EMS is out of date. The physician-powered EMS has to be modernized to increase the quality and

to show measurable evidence of its effectiveness. Otherwise, its future existence is at serious risk. Therefore, the project Med-on-@ix was created by the Department of Anesthesiology at the University Hospital Aachen, Germany.

After the three-year project period, we expect that there will be a safe functioning telemedicine system that is available for use in the German EMS.

A comprehensive telemedicine system needs to solve the above mentioned problems through the optimisation of the emergency process in the German physician-led EMS.

This system offers EMS-physicians and paramedics an additional consultation by a specialized centre of competence, thus assuring medical therapy that is compliant with evidence-based guidelines. Several prospective studies have been conducted to analyse this system in comparison to the conventional EMS.

The efficiency and quality of emergency care can only be improved by taking the telemedicine approach for the entire process of emergency care from receiving a distress call to care for the patient.

Therefore, the Med-on-@ix project includes in its action plan, a modeling system that connects technical challenges with organizational and human aspects. First, all partners of the consortium, including the emergency physicians, lawyers and engineers, helped to define all the requirements for a telemedical emergency assistance system. These various requirements included security, speed and reliability of data transmission, but also the ergonomics of the controls.

Telematic assistance in the safety of EMS can be achieved with the already established Professional Mobile Radio in combination with commercial mobile network technologies. The parallel use of multiple physical links adds reliability and can be secured by using VPN mechanisms. A middleware architecture based on this technology is restricted in the choice of usable transport protocols. It must offer different channels for message-oriented communication and streaming-oriented communication with real-time and synchronicity requirements. In the future, the architecture will be extended to fulfill the needs for the interoperability with other centers of competence and for the interconnection with hospital information systems. Med-on-ix @ ensures integration of all relevant actors in the EMS, including the emergency physicians, paramedics, control room staff and patients.

We are now in the third year of the project and testing the system in real time in real operations. The results of the evaluation phase will be presented in the future.

REFERENCES

Adams, G. L., Campbell, P. T., & Adams, J. M. (2006). Effectiveness of prehospital wireless transmission of to a cardiologist via handheld device for patients with acute myocardial infarction. *The American Journal of Cardiology, 98*, 1160–1164. doi:10.1016/j.amjcard.2006.05.042

Augustine, J. J. (2001). Medical direction and EMS. *Emergency Medical Services, 30*, 65–69.

Beauchamp, T. L., & Childress, J. F. (2009). *Principles of Biomedical Ethics*. New York: Oxford University Press.

Behrendt, H., & Schmiedel, R. (2003). *Ausgewählte Ergebnisse der Leistungsanalyse 2000/2001*. In K. Mendel. Handbuch des Rettungswesens. Witten, Germany: Mendel Verlag.

Behrendt, II. & Schmiedel, R. (2004). Die aktuellen Leistungen des Rettungsdienstes in der Bundesrepublik Deutschland im zeitlichen Vergleich (Teil II). *Notfall- & Rettungsmedizin*. 7, 59-70.

Bergrath, S. (2006). *Retrospektive Analyse der Datenqualität eines kommerziellen Datenbanksystems für den Notarztdienst und der Dokumentationscompliance des Notarztdienstes der Stadt Aachen. Universitätsklinikum der RWTH Aachen: Ph. D. Dissertationen.*

Bohacek, S., Hespanha, J. P., Lee, J., Lim, C., & Obraczka, K. (2006). A new tcp for persistent packet reordering. *IEEE/ACM Transactions on Networking, 14*(2), 369–382. doi:10.1109/TNET.2006.873366

Bundesärztekammer (2004). Tätigkeitsbericht der Bundesärztekammer: Entschließungen zum Tagesordnungspunkt VI. *Deutsches Ärzteblatt, 101* (22), A1584, B1313, C1266.

Chu, Y., & Ganz, A. (2004). A mobile teletrauma system using 3G networks. *IEEE Transactions on Information Technology in Biomedicine, 8*(4), 456–462. doi:10.1109/TITB.2004.837893

Davis, F. D. (1993). User acceptance of information technology: System characteristics, user perceptions and behavioural impacts. *International Journal of Man-Machine Studies, 38*, 475–487. doi:10.1006/imms.1993.1022

Deutscher Bundestag. (2006). *Unfallverhütungsbericht Straßenverkehr 2004/2005*. Retrieved from www.dip.bundestag.de

Dhruva, V. N., Abdelhadi, S. I., & Anis, A. (2007). ST-Segment analysis using wireless technology in acute myocardial infarction (STAT-MI) trial. *Journal of the American College of Cardiology, 50*, 509–513. doi:10.1016/j.jacc.2007.04.049

Erder, M. H., Davidson, S. J., & Cheney, R. A. (1989). Online medical command in theory and praxis. *Annals of Emergency Medicine, 18*, 261–268. doi:10.1016/S0196-0644(89)80411-1

Gesundheitsberichterstattung des Bundes. (2007). *Ad-hoc-Tabellen*. Retrieved 06.03.2007 from www.gbe-bund.de

Good, R., & Ventura, N. (2006). *A multilayered hybrid architecture to support vertical handover between ieee802.11 and umts*. In IWCMC '06: Proceedings of the 2006 international conference on Wireless communications and mobile computing(pp.257-262). New York: ACM.

Gries, A., Helm, M., & Martin, E. (2003). Zukunft der präklinischen Notfallmedizin in Deutschland. *Der Anaesthesist, 52*, 718–724. doi:10.1007/s00101-003-0548-1

Iren, S., Amer, P. D., & Conrad, P. T. (1999). The transport layer: tutorial and survey. *ACM Computing Surveys, 31*(4), 360–404. doi:10.1145/344588.344609

Jemmet, M. E., Kendal, K. M., Fourre, M. W., & Burton, J. H. (2003). Unrecognized misplacement of endotracheal tubes in a mixed urban to rural emergency medical services setting. *Academic Emergency Medicine, 10*, 961–965. doi:10.1111/j.1553-2712.2003.tb00652.x

Jones, J. H., Murphy, M. P., & Dickson, R. L. (2004). Emergency physician-verified out-of-hospital intubation: miss rates by paramedics. *Academic Emergency Medicine, 11*, 707–709.

Katz, S. H., & Falk, J. L. (2001). Misplaced endotracheal tubes by paramedics in an urban emergency medical services system. *Annals of Emergency Medicine, 37*, 32–37. doi:10.1067/mem.2001.112098

Kollmann, T. (1998). *Akzeptanz innovativer Nutzungsgüter und -systeme.* Wiesbaden, Germany: Gabler.

Li, J., & Brassil, J. (2006). *On the performance of traffic equalizers on heterogeneous communication links.* QShine, Proceedings of the 3rd international conference on Quality of service in heterogeneous wired/wireless networks. New York: ACM.

Mayring, P. (2000). *Qualitative Content Analysis.* Forum Qualitative Sozialforschung / Forum: Qualitative Social Research. Retrieved 2000 from http://nbnresolving. de/urn:nbn:de:0114-fqs0002204

Messelken, M., Martin, J., Milewski, P. (1998). Ergebnisqualität in der Notfallmedizin. *Notfall-& Rettungsmedizin.* 1, 143-149.

MobiHealth. (2010). *MobiHealth – shaping the future of Healthcare.* Retrieved 29.03.10 from http://www.mobihealth.org/

Müller, M., Protogerakis, M., & Henning, K. (2009). *A methodology to reduce technical risk in the development of telematic rescue assistance systems.* Proceedings of the second international conference on computer and electrical engineering. Dubai: UAE.

MyHeart. (n.d.). *Forschungsprojekt im 6. EU-Rahmenprogramm.* Retrieved 30.11.2009 from www.hitech-projects.com/euprojects/myheart/

Rall, M., Reddersen, S., Schädle, B., Zieger, J., Christ, P., Scheerer, J., & Liang, Y. (2004). *Das Schutz-Engel- System - Telemedizinische Unterstützung in Echtzeit.* In A. Jäckel, Telemedizinführer Deutschland (pp. 51–64). Witte, Germany: Mendel Verlag.

Rieser, S. (2005). Arbeitsbedingungen schrecken viele ab. *Deutsches Arzteblatt, 102*, C629.

Schneiders, M., Protogerakis, M., & Isenhardt, I. (2009). *User acceptance as a key to success for the implementation of a Telematic Support System in German Emergency Medical Services.* Proceedings of The International Conference on Successes & Failures in Telehealth 2009: SFT-09 Australia. 2009.

Schulzrinne, H., Casner, S., Frederick, R., & Jacobson, V. (2003). *RTP: A Transport Protocol for Real-Time Applications RFC 3550 (Standard).* Retrieved 30.11.2009 from http://www.ietf.org/rfc/rfc3550.txt

Sejersten, M., Sillesen, M., & Hansen, P. R. (2008). Effect on treatment delay of prehospital teletransmission of 12-lead electrocardiogram to a cardiologist for immediate triage and direct referral of patients with ST-segment elevation acute myocardial infarction to primary percutaneous coronary intervention. *The American Journal of Cardiology, 101*, 941–946.

Silvestri, S., Ralls, G. A., & Krauss, B. (2005). The effectiveness of out-of hospital use of continuous endtidal carbon dioxide monitoring on the rate of unrecognized misplaced intubation within a regional emergency medical services system. *Annals of Emergency Medicine, 45*, 497–503. doi:10.1016/j.annemergmed.2004.09.014

Skorning, M., Bergrath, S., Rörtgen, D., Brokmann, J., Beckers, S., & Protogerakis, M. (2009). E-Health in der Notfallmedizin – das Forschungsprojekt Med-on-@ix. *Der Anaesthesist, 58*, 285–292. doi:10.1007/s00101-008-1502-z

Statistisches Bundesamt. (2006). *Gesundheit – Ausgaben, Krankheitskosten und Personal 2004.* Retrieved 16.08.2006 from www.destatis.de

Timmermann, A., Russo, S. G., & Eich, C. (2007). The out-of-hospital esophageal and endobronchial intubations performed by emergency physicians. *Anesthesia and Analgesia, 104*, 619–623. doi:10.1213/01.ane.0000253523.80050.e9

van Halteren, A., Bults, R., Wac, K., Dokovsky, N., Koprinkov, G., & Widya, I. (2004). Wireless body area networks for healthcare: the MobiHealth project. *Studies in Health Technology and Informatics, 108*, 181–193.

Wuerz, R. C., Swope, G. E., Holliman, C. J., & Vazquez-de Miguel, G. (1995). Online medical direction: a prospective study. *Prehospital and Disaster Medicine, 10*, 174–177.

ADDITIONAL READING

Arntz, H. R., & Somasundaram, R. (2008). Internistische Notfallmedizin. *Intensivmedizin, 45*, 212–216..doi:10.1007/s00390-008-0879-x

Gries, A., Zink, W., Bernhard, M., Messelken, M., & Schlechtriemen, T. (2005). Einsatzrealität im Notarztdienst. *Notfall und Rettungsmedizin, 8*, 391–398..doi:10.1007/s10049-005-0756-0

Heidenreich, G., & Blobel, B. (2009). IT-Standards für telemedizinische Anwendungen - Der Weg zum effizienten Datenaustausch in der Medizin. *Bundesgesundheitsblatt, Gesundheitsforschung, Gesundheitsschutz, 52*, 316–323. doi:10.1007/s00103-009-0788-6

Norgall, T. (2009). Fit und selbstständig im Alter durch Technik - Von der Vision zur Wirklichkeit? *Bundesgesundheitsblatt, Gesundheitsforschung, Gesundheitsschutz, 52*, 297–305. doi:10.1007/s00103-009-0789-5

Perlitz, U. (2010) *Telemedizin verbessert Patientenversorgung.* Deutsche Bank Research. Retrieved 31.01.2010 from www.dbresearch.de

Protogerakis, M., Gramatke, A., & Henning, K. (2009a). A Software Architecture for a Telematic Rescue Assistance Systerm. InIFMBE Proceedings Vol. 25, WC2009. Hrsg. v. Dössel, O.; Schlegel, W., 1–4. www.springerlink.com

Röhrig, R., & Rüth, R. (2009). Intelligente Telemedizin in der Intensivstation-Patientennaher Einsatz von Medizintechnik und IT in der Intensivmedizin. *Bundesgesundheitsblatt, Gesundheitsforschung, Gesundheitsschutz, 52*, 279–286.

Schmidt, S., & Grimm, A. (2009). Versorgungsforschung zur telemedizinische Anwendung. *Bundesgesundheitsblatt, Gesundheitsforschung, Gesundheitsschutz, 52*, 270–278. doi:10.1007/s00103-009-0794-8

Thomas, E. J., Lucke, J. F., & Wueste, L. (2009). Association of Telemedicine for Remote Monitoring of Intensive Care Patients With Mortality, Complications, and Length of Stay. *Journal of the American Medical Association, 302*(24), 2671–2678. doi:10.1001/jama.2009.1902

KEY TERMS AND DEFINITIONS

Telenotarzt: An experienced Emergency Medical Services (EMS) physician who is situated at the competence centre and support the paramedics and the EMS physician on scene in medical and organizational questions.

Telemedicine: Support in medical therapy and diagnosis by advanced mobile data transmission between the medical personal on scene and a highly expert physician who is not on site.

Competence Centre: The competence centre is responsible for the contact and data transfer to the hospital, the consultation with other institutions (for example family physician, cardiology, poisoning centre, and so forth) and is staffed with the Telenotarzt.

Teleconsultation: Consultation between the Telenotarzt and paramedics or EMS physician at the emergency scene.

Emergency Medical System (EMS): German Emergency Medical System is physician based

Live Vital Data Transmission: Real time transmission of all vital parameters of a patient and a video live stream from the ambulance and the scene to the Telenotarzt in the competence centre.

Quality Management: The Telenotarzt can initiate a shorter drug free interval if the paramedics are the first on scene and can also support a better guideline compliant therapy.

Chapter 13
The Smart Condo Project:
Services for Independent Living

Nicholas M. Boers
University of Alberta, Canada

Robert Lederer
University of Alberta, Canada

David Chodos
University of Alberta, Canada

Lili Liu
University of Alberta, Canada

Pawel Gburzynski
University of Alberta, Canada

Ioanis Nikolaidis
University of Alberta, Canada

Lisa Guirguis
University of Alberta, Canada

Cheryl Sadowski
University of Alberta, Canada

Jianzhao Huang
University of Alberta, Canada

Eleni Stroulia
University of Alberta, Canada

ABSTRACT

Most would agree that older adults want affordable, high-quality healthcare that enables them to live independently longer and in their own homes. To this end, ambient assisted living environments have been developed that are able to non-intrusively monitor the health of people at-home and to provide them with improved care. The authors have designed an environment, the Smart Condo, to support seniors and rehabilitating patients. They have embedded a wireless sensor network into a model living space, which incorporates universal design principles. Information from the sensor network is archived in a server, which supports a range of views via APIs. One such view is a virtual world, which is realistic and intuitive, while remaining non-intrusive. This chapter examines computing technologies for smart healthcare-related environments and the needs of elderly patients. It discusses the Smart Condo architecture, reviews key research challenges, and presents the lessons learned through the project.

DOI: 10.4018/978-1-60960-469-1.ch013

INTRODUCTION AND MOTIVATION

As baby boomers grow older and life expectancies increase, we need advances in health service-delivery models that address an increasing number of chronic conditions in ways that are appropriate for an increasingly informed older population. The healthcare and social implications of aging populations, and the need to enable them to live independently at home longer, is a priority for governments, industry, and researchers to address. Motivated by this need, an increasing number of industrial products and research prototypes today envision *ambient assisted living environments* that are able to non-intrusively monitor the health of people at-home and to guide and support more specialized, timely, and cost-effective care to them. The substantial and increasing wave of new research in this area is a testament to the social importance of the problem and the technical challenges involved. The technical challenges span a range of disciplines.

1. What types of monitoring technologies can be deployed for assisted living purposes? Today, we have a wide variety of technologies at our disposal, ranging from passive and active RFIDs[1], to sensors that can be embedded in the environment or to the patients' clothing and bodies, to wireless devices that are (or can be) integrated with home devices to communicate data on their status and readings.

2. How can data from the various technologies above be fused to infer clinically relevant information about patients? How can the inferred information be communicated to patients and their caregivers (health professionals and family members) in order to be effectively acted upon? And what healthcare disciplines might benefit from information thus obtained?

3. What types of physical, psychological, and cognitive assistance can be possible through digital technologies? Individual patients may suffer from a variety of ailments, such as limited mobility, diabetes with its variety of implications to stability and food concerns, and forgetfulness.

4. How should care-delivery activities be effectively orchestrated between the patients themselves and their caregivers? Depending on their condition, abilities, and their social environment, patients may be more or less able to manage their own conditions. How can the monitoring infrastructure flexibly support them, while also recognizing exceptional situations and triggering alarms to responsible health professionals?

Hand-in-hand with the above technical challenges (and the functional requirements they imply for an assisted-living infrastructure) come a variety of social requirements. These are distinct yet equally important as the technical requirements, and their fulfillment is a prerequisite for the eventual adoption of any such infrastructure.

1. First is the issue of ethical concerns around privacy, ownership of the collected data, patient access to it, and fair use. Patients, although they may appreciate the increased sense of safety that comes with the monitoring infrastructure, are leery of having their every move monitored. The question then becomes the identification of an acceptable trade-off between data collection and safety.

2. Second is the issue of adaptability. Patients come with different needs, and as their conditions progress, their needs change. This evolution of patient needs implies the need for an extendible assistive infrastructure that can evolve as necessary.

3. Third is the issue of training healthcare professionals. New technologies are only as effective as the people who are using them are knowledgeable; thus, an education program is needed for training health-sciences

professionals to effectively use the at-home health monitoring and care technologies to access rich information about the patient's health status, so that they can better serve these patients.

Our team has been involved in the Smart Condo project[2] for approximately a year and a half. Our objective is to design an environment, including the physical and the computing infrastructures, to support seniors and patients living at home in the community or in congregate housing. Although these individuals are, by and large, able to live independently, they are still susceptible to harmful incidents related to complex physical and cognitive impairments. Thus, we are developing a model Smart Condo, designed according to universal design principles (Center for Universal Design, 1997), within which we have embedded a wireless sensor network. Information from the sensor network is archived in a server, which supports a range of REST APIs through which the information is visualized as a range of views. Among the most useful views is a virtual world (currently, Second Life), in which a model of the Smart Condo has been built. This view into the patient's activity is realistic and intuitive, while at the same time non-intrusive, since personal-appearance details are not actually monitored or recorded. A reengineered SL client accesses information regarding the patient's activities, as inferred by the sensor data stream through the server's REST APIs, and uses it to control an avatar mirroring the patient's activity in the real world.

Our intent is to make the live stream of the person's activity available to their caregivers and potentially healthcare professionals, who can recognize potentially subtle harmful events and communicate with the condo occupant through this low-bandwidth videoconferencing tool. Event detection is, of course, not delegated simply to caregivers "watching" the virtual-world feed: we are developing stream-mining methods for recognizing pre-specified patterns of sensor readings indicative of potential problems in order to alert caregivers and cause them to intervene. Finally, analytics methods inspect the archive of recorded sensor readings in order to extract patterns and to recognize trends associated with clinically significant symptoms. In addition to enabling better care for independent individuals, this infrastructure can advance the state of health-care knowledge and delivery practices through the systematic collection and analysis of evidence. A recording of the virtual-world activity, "annotated" with the readings of the various sensors, can also serve as an aspect of the patient's health record, providing detailed and contextual information on the patient's history. It can be replayed at an accelerated rate, to allow quick viewing of large spans of time for diagnostic purposes. Recordings of "pedagogically interesting" activity segments can also be used for simulation training of health-sciences students. We believe that this integration of sensor networks with virtual worlds represents a "sweet spot" in the spectrum of at-home health monitoring and care delivery.

The rest of this chapter is organized as follows. We first review the broad background of this work. We examine the computing technologies that have been developed in the service of smart environments, with a special focus on environments designed for healthcare related purposes. We also review, at a rather high level of abstraction, the needs of elderly people living independently at home or in long-term care facilities. Next, we discuss the overall architecture of our Smart Condo. We then review what we perceive as key research challenges in this area. Finally, we conclude with a summary of the lessons we have learned in the context of this project.

UBIQUITOUS COMPUTING TO SUPPORT OLDER ADULTS

In this paper, our use of the term *Smart Home* means a home that has both a set of sensors to observe the environment and a set of devices/ actuators to improve the inhabitant's experience at home. Our use of the term home may refer to one in the community or one in an assisted living or congregate living situation. A Smart Home can provide a variety of services from simple task automations, such as room temperature control, to more complex analyses, such as inference of the occupants' activities. Smart-home technologies are being deployed in a variety of application domains, including real-estate security monitoring, home energy consumption reduction, cognitive and memory aiding to people with special needs, and remote patient monitoring by healthcare professionals. Our Smart Condo work is motivated by the last type of applications, and thus, in the remainder of this section, we review (a) the potential applications of these technologies for supporting elderly people to live independently in their homes and (b) the technological advances in implementing smart homes.

Smart Homes in Service of an Aging Population

In healthcare, the concepts of *continuing care*, *assisted living*, and *aging in place* are recent when compared to the substantial amount of work that has been carried out under the heading of *long-term care* (LTC) in specialized facilities. To some extent, it is this large body of research in LTC that has motivated the idea of using technology to support people to continue living independently, in their own homes, as they age. For example, healthcare researchers found that the quality of life for LTC residents was enhanced if their physical and social environment were more homelike, with minimal institutional features (Morgan and Stewart, 1997; Morgan and Stewart, 1998; Zingmark, Sandman, and Norberg, 2002). More specifically, non-institutional environments were found to enhance mealtime experience. Gruber-Baldini et al. (2005) examined food and fluid intake of 407 residents in 45 assisted living facilities and discovered that,

in addition to appropriate lighting and reduced noise levels (McDaniel, Hunt, Hackes, and Pope, 2001), staff monitoring of residents, dining in a public area, and non-institutional environmental features were associated with higher food and fluid intake. Furthermore, engagement in meaningful activities has been associated with less depression and better cognitive and physical function (Dobbs et al., 2005). Programming engaging activities in LTC facilities is challenging since it has to be balanced with personal choice and opportunities for appropriate levels of involvement. On the other hand, one can imagine that living in one's own home environment would enhance the degree of one's engagement in typical activities.

Having established as a desirable objective supporting people to stay and age in their homes as long as possible, there is a need to identify simple technological supports that could be used to address problematic behaviors observed in LTC facilities such as sundowning[3] (Nowak and Davis, 2007) and wandering[4] (Beattie, Song, and LaGore, 2005), to monitor activity engagement, to help ensure safety, and to provide therapeutic interventions. More specifically, these technologies could potentially (a) minimize the visible barriers that typical community homes place to independent living, while still ensuring an appropriate level of safety; (b) augment the normal care available to the elderly in their physical/ social environments; and (c) expand the range of ways for family members and healthcare professionals to appropriately and respectfully monitor the movements of the individual for the purpose of providing help at the right moment. The first dimension of improvement is the subject of *universal design* research. The term universal design recognizes the importance of how things look and encompasses a set of principles that can lead to designs that delight and are accessible to users with a variety of abilities and disabilities. The latter two dimensions of improvement can be accomplished with sensor technologies. Sensors can be used to unobtrusively monitor people, recognize when they may need assistance from family members and care providers, and involve the necessary helpers in a timely manner. Alternatively, sensors and actuators can be used to control the environment and effectively assist people in their regular activities. For example, automatic lighting can simplify night-time activities and minimize fall risk. Technology can also help notify staff, who can offer care and support or provide automatic reminders for routine or *event-triggered* activities (e.g., electronic notification of individual medication needs and recording of documentation).

Another service of potentially high value to the increasing population of seniors – they account for almost 14% of the Canadian population (Statistics Canada, 2006) – is effective medication management. There is increasing medication use with age, with those aged 80 years and older receiving the greatest number of prescriptions. In Canada, 76.3% of senior households used any medications in the preceding 2 days, and there was an association between multiple medication use and ill health (Ramage-Morin, 2009). Seniors also account for half of visits to physician specialists (US Department of Health, 2009). Older adults also have an increased disease burden. Many seniors have at least three chronic medication conditions, and these seniors consume a disproportionate amount of healthcare resources (Boyd et al., 2005). Disease states often present atypically in older adults, and geriatric syndromes are common (Tinetti and Fried, 2004).

Cassel (2009) has identified six characteristics of optimal quality of care for older adults with frailty, including reducing the risk of medications in older adults, communications, and managing healthcare across the healthcare system. Due to the significant use of medications by seniors and the associated risks, monitoring is an extremely important issue. In fact, pharmacists are usually the first healthcare professional to have regular contact with people as they are approaching their "elderly" years, even before they have health concerns serious enough to require regular con-

tact with other specialists. In addition to being accessible, pharmacist care has been shown to enhance medication management and the health of patients (Beney, Bero, and Bond, 2000; Roughead, Semple, and Vitry, 2005). The role of the pharmacists in North America has been expanding. The profession has moved its mandate from a provider of medication to a care provider who accepts responsibility for medication-related outcomes. Their role in providing patient care can be considered in the context of the medication management process (Bajcar, Kennie, and Einarson, 2005), which includes identifying the need for therapy, prescribing, dispensing, packaging, administration, and monitoring. There is a strong societal need for pharmacists to provide increased medication monitoring to reduce the patient burden of inappropriate medication use and identify unmet needs for therapy. Financial and healthcare system structures are emerging to support pharmacist's provision of care beyond dispensing. Smart technologies will allow them to monitor patients' use of medications and health outcomes.

Information and communication technology has been identified and accepted nationally as one of five key areas required to help pharmacists reach their vision of optimal drug therapy outcomes for Canadians through patient-centered care (Task Force on a Blueprint for Pharmacy, 2008). The challenge is to connect pharmacists and patients in an ongoing and systematic way. One means to connect them is via electronic medication monitoring systems that have been integrated into caps on vials, e.g., the Medication Event Monitoring Systems (MEMS), or into calendar packaging, e.g., a blister package (Santschi, Wuerzner, Schneider, Bugnon, and Burnier, 2007). These devices collect data regarding the day and time that the medication is accessed and communicate it to an external site. This technology has been used frequently in trials related to medication adherence. Unfortunately, they do not measure the medication administration or consumption, are quite large in contrast to contemporary medication packaging, remain expensive, and are not designed to be childproof. Due to these deficiencies, electronic medication monitoring has been predominantly used for research purposes and has failed to be integrated into clinical practice.

Establishing acceptance of technology-based health monitoring systems through pharmacy care is, we believe, an important step in introducing and widely disseminating this technology. We are interested in drug dispensation and usage monitoring as a clinically relevant application in the assisted-living area. At this time, we have not yet incorporated such technology into our project. However, since we have recognized its importance early, we have been aiming to explore the relevant technologies and incorporate them to some extent in the Smart Condo. We are now piloting a new project that will attempt to identify the types of patients who can benefit the most from technological support for medication reminders and intake monitoring.

There is evidence that monitoring, information, and feedback does increase adherence to medication regimens (Haynes, Ackloo, Sahota, McDonald, and Yao, 2008). While there is support for monitoring, it is important to ensure that such technology is integrated with software and systems used in clinical practice. Community pharmacies, for example, use one of many different software programs for dispensing and patient information. A monitoring system must be integrated seamlessly into the client's living environment and must also interface productively with the healthcare professionals who are providing care.

Smart-Home Technologies

There has been substantial research and development of smart-home technologies. Among the earliest projects in this area is most likely Georgia Tech's *Aware Home,* which is "devoted to the multidisciplinary exploration of emerging technologies and services based in the home" (Kientz,

Patel, Jones, et al., 2008, p. 3675) and seeks to provide services to aging residents that enhance their quality of life and support aging-in-place. Rather than developing a general smart-home software platform, the project has been an umbrella under which a variety of distinct research activities have been carried out, most focusing on developing effective human-computer interfaces through which to support people with cognitive and memory impairments. For example, Fetch assists visually impaired people to locate misplaced objects (Kientz, Patel, Tyebkhan, et al., 2006) and Cook's Collage assists seniors in following recipes (Tran, Calcaterra, and Mynatt, 2005).

The Ambient Assisted Living Environment (AAL Environment) (Kleinberger, Becker, Ras, Holzinger, and Müller, 2007; Ras, Becker, and Koch, 2007), developed by the Fraunhofer Institute for Experimental Software Engineering in Germany, is an apartment-like environment for developing, integrating, and analyzing ambient intelligence technologies. A number of health-related research projects use this space as a realistic testing environment for new technology. Another project, the WASP architecture (Atallah, Lo, Yang, and Siegemund, 2008), is not motivated by specific healthcare concerns but focuses on the design of a software infrastructure for effectively integrating a population of wireless sensors to recognize events in a living environment and provide aural feedback. The system requires that the occupant wear an active radio-frequency identification (RFID) tag to help localization tasks and uses acceleration sensors to detect doors opening and closing.

The Sensorized Elderly Care Home (Hori, Nishida, Aizawa, Murakami, and Mizoguchi, 2004) is a system installed in a nursing home in Tokyo. This work is motivated by the desire to alleviate the routine workload of nursing personnel through automation. More specifically, a sensor-based system is used for localizing patients in a nursing home (LTC scenario), monitoring their status, and raising alarms as necessary so that

Figure 1. *The software architecture used in the MavHome project*

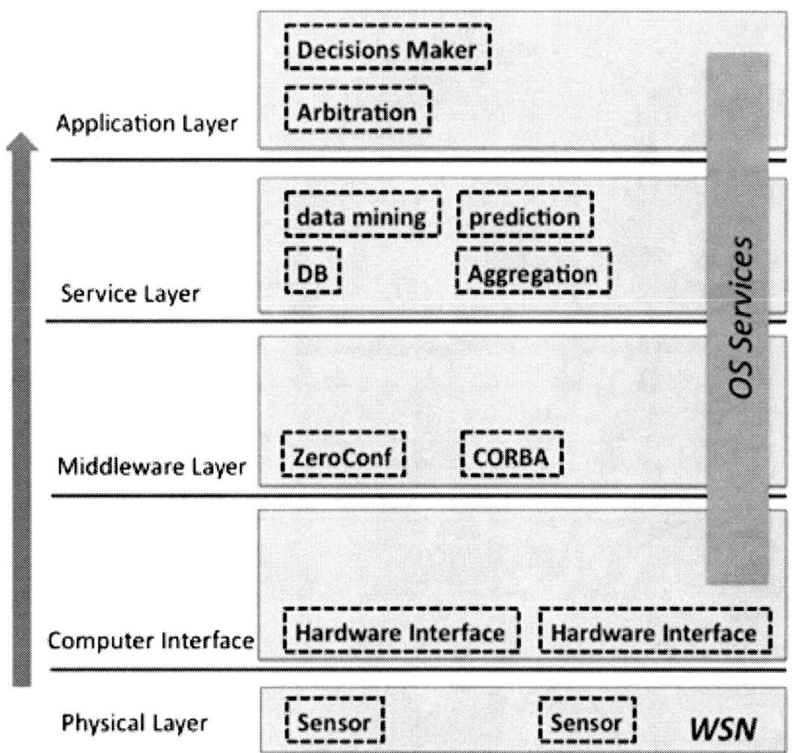

nurses do not have to do routine rounds. The system assumes a relatively limited level of activity on the part of the patients. It relies on "Ultra Badge" transmitters, placed on wheelchairs, and receivers, placed in several locations in the nursing home, to monitor wheelchair movement. Furthermore, a specially designed placement of transmitters and receivers on the ceiling monitors the patient's head position while on the bed to predict when the patient may leave the bed (Hori, Nishida, and Murakami, 2006).

The MavHome and Gator Tech House projects focused on the development of a general extendible software architecture for smart homes that monitor and actively help their occupants, essentially sharing the same goal as our Smart Condo project. The MavHome project (Cook, 2006) uses a variety of sensors (light, temperature, humidity, motion, and door/seat status sensors) to monitor the state of the environment and analyzes the collected data

to (a) identify lifestyle trends through sequential pattern mining, (b) provide reminders to the home occupants through prediction of future activities, and (c) detect anomalies in the current data when the actual sensed events are considered unlikely according to the system's predictions. MavHome's power-line control automates all lights and appliances, as well as HVAC, fans, and mini-blinds.

MavHome uses a layered software architecture, as shown in Figure 1. Perception of light, humidity, temperature, smoke, gas, motion, and switch settings is performed through a sensor network developed in-house. Sensors monitor the environment in the physical layer, and this information is available through the interface layer for components in higher layers, such as the database, the data-mining component, the prediction module, and the decision-making units. Each device in the physical layer registers itself using ZeroConf[5] (Zero Configuration) and

Figure 2. The software architecture used by the Gator Tech House project

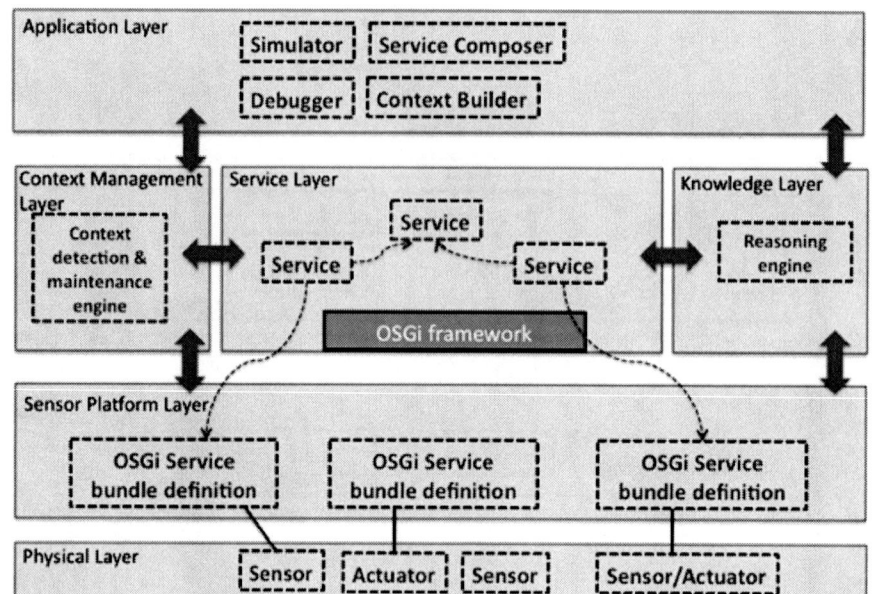

CORBA[6] handles the communication in higher layers. Environment perception is a bottom-up flow; actions follow a top-down trajectory, where each action is invoked by the application layer, is subsequently recorded by the service layer, and finally is enacted by devices in the physical layer. For example, MavHome can perceive the room temperature and respond to that by sending an action to related actuators for automated temperature control.

The Gator Tech Smart House at the University of Florida (Helal et al., 2005) is yet another high-tech house that embeds a variety of sensors to assist with the behavioral monitoring (and alteration) of elderly occupants or patients suffering from diabetes and obesity. Its envisioned software architecture is shown in Figure 2. The space incorporates technology into many aspects of the home. For example, their Smart Front Door allows keyless entry using radio frequency identification (RFID) and incorporates a microphone, camera, text LCD display, and speaker in order for the occupant to communicate with visitors. Their Smart (Micro)Wave also uses RFID to detect the

type of food to cook, and a screen displays a video instructing how to open the item. The sensor-platform layer adopts the OSGi (Open Services Gateway Initiative) framework to maintain the service definitions of the underlying devices and make them available to application developers. A sensor is registered when it is powered on by sending its "service bundle definition" to OSGi. The application developers can write new services or use available services in this layer for their applications. The knowledge layer is envisioned to contain an ontology of the available services and a reasoning engine that identifies valid composite service requests (i.e., composite services that can be performed). The context-management layer enables application developers to build new context for new services in their application. Finally, the application layer includes a graphical development environment for creating contexts or activating services, a simulator, and a debugger.

Yet another system is the one deployed in Tiger Place (Skubic, Alexander, Popescu, Rantz, and Keller, 2009), which is among the longer and more mature projects in the area, having been deployed in 17 apartments for between 2 and 3 years. The system sensors (motion, bed pressure, and stove on-off) communicate with the X10 protocol with a PC that collects the information from a home and pushes it in regular intervals to a central database that makes it available through a web application to care providers. The system architecture's design appears to be primarily motivated by the technologies adopted, but the project is especially interesting because it involves a substantial team of researchers across disciplines who have conducted very interesting case studies with their installation. The Tiger Place team interviewed elderly volunteers about their acceptance of being monitored by video cameras and found that, although they disliked in principle the idea of cameras, they liked the less fuzzified silhouettes when they reviewed their own videos. This finding sheds an interesting light on the acceptability of video monitoring, which appears to be a primary objective of this project. Another interesting contribution of this project is the fact that it has empirically demonstrated the social value of such monitoring installations, as both the elderly participating in the program and their family members agreed that they had an increased peace of mind with the system than without. The researchers also raised the very important question of the clinical value of such installations being conditional upon the ability to correlate the sensor data stream with clinical observations by the healthcare providers.

Of the above projects, MavHome and Tiger Place focused more on the data analyses and the information extraction that it could support, where the more recent Gator Tech Smart House – similar to our Smart Condo – attempts to consider the software-architecture issues in a more systematic manner. Indeed, as the available sensor types increase and development kits, such as the Arduino (2010) and the Sun SPOTs (Oracle, 2010) for example, make programming with sensors more accessible, the question of a flexible architecture

that can integrate new sensor types communicating through different protocols with a common data repository becomes increasingly important. There is increasing attention being given to this question, with much of the work appearing under the heading of "Ambient Intelligence". The term refers to environments that integrate a variety of sensors through which to perceive the presence and activities of people so that they can transparently respond to them in a way that supports these activities by controlling the environment – i.e., lighting, sound, temperature – and the appliances included in it. Mukherjee, Aarts, and Doyle (2009) recently reviewed the research objectives of the field as context awareness, ubiquitous access, and natural interaction. There has been substantial work in this area, much more than what we can review in this paper. An interesting recent example of this field is Amelie (Metaxas, Markopoulos, and Aarts, 2009) a service-oriented framework designed to support the implementation of awareness systems based on a recombinant-computing paradigm. In this paradigm, devices implement a limited set of *recombinant interfaces* that enable them to interact with one another dynamically. In Amelie, these interfaces enable the dynamic specification of the information each entity exposes to others (nimbus) and the information each entity acquires from other (focus) entities in a given situation. Another approach focusing more on a standardized implementation – as opposed to a theoretical specification framework – is the Shaspa framework (2009) that aims at simplifying the development of smart environments by enabling users to visualize, monitor, and manage their environments. At the same time, interactive interfaces provide immediate feedback to users. Shaspa "provides a smart interface to the most widely used industry-standard protocols for assembling real-world data from different input streams to manage physical spaces", thus fundamentally simplifying the interfacing of the physical layer with the higher analysis and decision-making modules.

THE SMART CONDO AT THE UNIVERSITY OF ALBERTA

The Health Sciences Education and Research Commons (HSERC) at the University of Alberta promotes and facilitates inter-professional education and research. It supports the *Smart Condo* project that brings together researchers from occupational therapy, industrial design, pharmacy, and computing science to integrate universal-design concepts with sensor technologies to address the needs of older adults living in their community[7]. While we await the completion of the actual Smart Condo, we designed a mock Smart Condo located in a single large room (of approximately 850 square feet) in a building on the University of Alberta campus for the purpose of student learning and research. The project was originally inspired by the independent-living suite at the Glenrose Rehabilitation Hospital in Edmonton, where patients can stay for up to three days to help ensure that they are ready for discharge home. During this stay, they are supposed to live independently, i.e., take care of themselves as if they were at home. Healthcare personnel are supposed to unobtrusively monitor them and only become involved when needed. Thus, the primary research objective in the development of our Smart Condo has been to establish that, through sensors only, we can record a precise picture of the condo's occupant, which can be unobtrusive and equally useful as if the healthcare personnel were actually monitoring the occupant through video cameras.

Teams of Industrial Design and Occupational Therapy (OT) students converted this area into a six-room condominium. Inside each room, they created prototypes for appliances, furniture, and other fixtures. Inside this space, we have deployed our wireless sensor network (WSN), which currently consists of nineteen nodes. These nodes contain four types of sensors, including (a) two types of motion sensors, (b) tactile pressure sensors, (c) reed switches, and (d) accelerometers.

In terms of motion sensors, we have deployed six passive-infrared motion sensors for spot detection (Panasonic AMN43121) and seven passive-infrared motion sensors for wide-area detection (Panasonic AMN44121). Spaced throughout the condominium, the thirteen motion sensors cover the unit adequately to correctly locate the condo's occupant. Pressure sensors (FlexiForce A201, 1 pound) have been embedded in several chairs. They enable us to detect when someone sits on these chairs. We attached reed switches to the front door and the door of the microwave to determine whether they are open. Finally, we attached an accelerometer to the front door to detect knocking. Figure 3 diagrammatically depicts the software architecture of our Smart Condo infrastructure. The collection of the nodes we discussed above constitutes the WSN component, shown as a small "cloud" at the bottom of the figure.

The WSN communicates wirelessly with one (or more) sink(s). Through a wireless module peripheral, the sink receives packets generated in the WSN and passes them to the Operations Support System (OSS) on a server for parsing and acknowledgement generation. Acknowledgements then flow back to the sink where the attached wireless module transmits them to the WSN. The OSS component also generates a raw data stream of parsed sensor observations. It feeds these into a simple stream-processing component, which examines the data stream within a predefined time window and identifies sequences that conform to any of a set of predefined rules of interest. Finally, it archives the raw data stream, as well the instances of rules that have been matched by it to the Smart Condo repository, the SensorDB.

To support a variety of client applications a set of REST (representational state transfer) APIs (application programming interfaces) have been implemented to provide data of interest in a standardized XML schema to potential consumer applications.

Currently, two clients use these APIs: Second Life for 3D visualizations and SensorGIS for 2D

Figure 3. The Smart Condo's software architecture

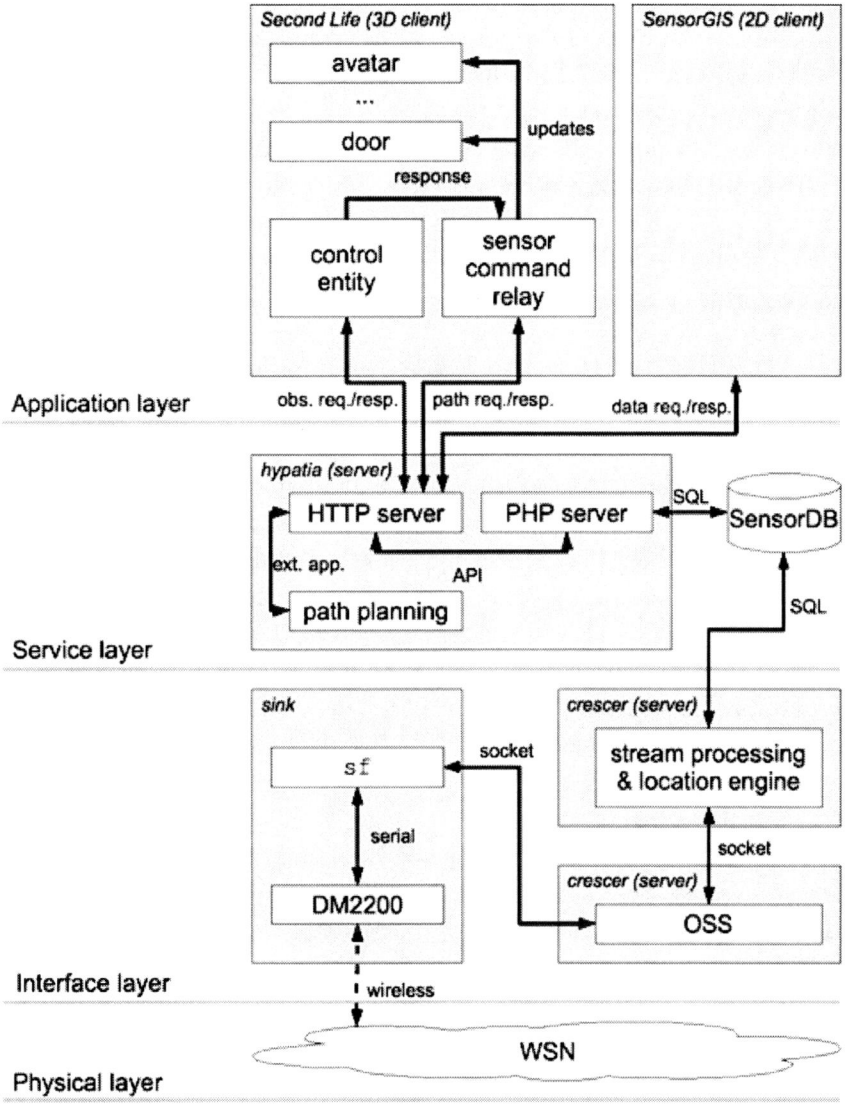

visualizations. Second Life (SL) uses the information to change the state of the virtual world (e.g., location of the avatar and state of other objects) to reflect the sensed reality. SensorGIS uses the same APIs to reflect the information as points on a map and to generate a variety of tables and graphs, illustrating the history of the WSN readings over a time window and their statistics.

In the next four subsections, we discuss in more detail each of the four layers of the Smart Condo architecture.

Wireless Sensor Network (WSN)

As we have already mentioned, our first objective in the Smart Condo has been to unobtrusively, yet in a precise and timely fashion, recognize the occupant's location and activities. To this end, we have deployed several passive-infrared motion sensors throughout the environment. To augment these observations, we have deployed tactile pressure sensors on chairs to detect sitting and a bed occupancy sensor to detect presence on the bed. Moreover, by observing changes in the state of furniture and appliances we can further recognize the occupant's activities in the environment, e.g., whether he or she is opening or closing appliance doors, for example. Thus, we have deployed magnetic reed switches on both the entrance and microwave doors.

The sensors are connected to wireless nodes, currently the DM2200 module from RF Monolithics[8]. Each WSN node consists of (a) a microcontroller, (b) a radio transceiver, and (c) an energy source. The microcontroller enables the node to interface with sensors and executes a simple "observe sensor value, sleep, and wake up" application. The radio transceiver enables the node to communicate the observed data wirelessly with other nodes. Typically, wireless modules use simple microcontrollers and transceivers. They tend to have very limited processing and storage ability (e.g., the MSP430F148 microcontroller: 8 MHz, 48 KB flash memory, and 2 KB RAM). They also tend to communicate data at slow data rates (e.g., the TR8100 transceiver: 9600 bps). These characteristics stem from both the application requirements and a desire to keep both costs and energy consumption low. Each of our nodes runs the PicOS operating system (Akhmetshina, Gburzynski, and Vizeacoumar, 2003). The development tools associated with PicOS are reviewed in the section titled The Development Toolkit.

In a wireless network, there are two primary techniques for moving data from a sender to a receiver: single-hop and multi-hop communication. In the former case, the two nodes must be within each other's radio-transceiver range, in which case the sender transmits the data directly to the receiver. When the receiver is outside of the sender's transmission range, the sender relies on intermediate nodes to forward its data toward

the receiver through multiple hops. The Smart Condo space is small enough that all nodes can communicate directly, in a single hop, with the sink node.

The Network-Service Interface Layer

The sink node is a node of the same type as described above with the exception that it is connected to an interface board, which is connected as a peripheral to a more capable host through a USB interface. It is actually this combination of wireless module, interface board, and host that we call a sink. These sink nodes bridge the WSN with a typically wired (Ethernet) backbone network. When observations arrive wirelessly from the sensor network to the sink, the wireless node encapsulates them in the TinyOS serial message format (Levis et al., 2005) and transmits them to the attached host through a socket. The Operations Support System (OSS), implemented in Perl, connects to this socket and sees all packets received at the sink. It parses the packets, generates acknowledgments for the WSN nodes in the WSN, and makes the data stream available to any other application that might need to process it, thus allowing the same WSN to be shared among multiple applications.

We see several benefits to this sink-to-OSS forwarding approach. First, it offloads all data processing on more capable servers. The sink node, even though more powerful than a WSN node, is still assumed to have limited resources of its own. Second, through its particular acknowledgement strategy, it enforces end-to-end reliability between each individual sensor node and the OSS. This is important for handling failures at any intermediate step and for removing stored sensed data at the sensor nodes only after it is absolutely certain that the data have been delivered to the application. Third, the approach simplifies maintenance. As we add new types of sensors, we only need to update the software on a central server rather than each individual sink node.

Figure 4. The SensorDB ER diagram

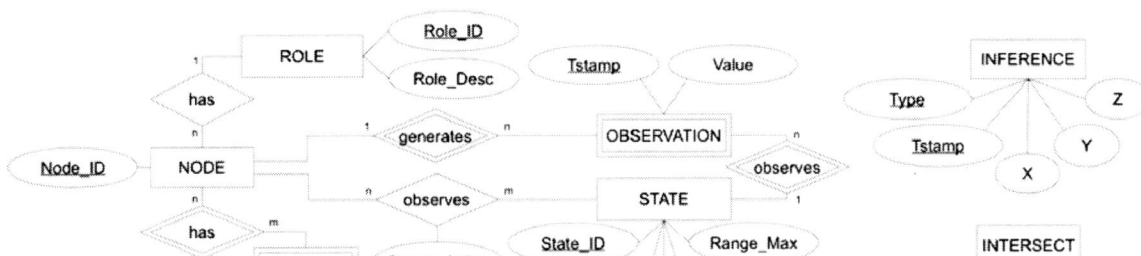

The OSS generated data stream is in the form of tuples, consisting of (a) time-stamp, (b) network ID, (c) node ID, (d) sensor ID, (e) sensor type, and (f) event type. The *time-stamp* indicates when the event occurred. The *network ID* allows several independent WSN deployments to report to a single OSS, and the *node ID* identifies a single node within each network. The *sensor ID* and *sensor type* together distinguish a specific peripheral connected to a wireless module. Finally, *event type* describes the observation made by an attached sensor.

In our application, the OSS is connected to the stream-processing engine that is responsible for saving all received observations in the Smart Condo repository, SensorDB, and inferring higher-order information by recognizing simple patterns on the data stream within a short time window. The basic intuition here is that, in some cases, co-occurring readings of individual sensors are caused by a single complex phenomenon in the world. Therefore, the hypothesis is that one can define the patterns of sensor readings that correspond to such phenomena of interest and then recognize instances of these patterns in the data stream as evidence of the occurrence of this phenomenon. In the Smart Condo, we use the stream-mining component to infer the occupant's location. Specifically, passive-infrared motion sensors have a view that ranges from around 38°

(for the spot variety) to 116° (for the wide-angle variety) to a distance of either five or ten meters, respectively. The sensor's binary output simply indicates whether it detected movement within this field of view. As viewable regions overlap, patterns of independent sensor readings correspond to the recognition of the occupant in a location within their area overlap. Therefore, the smaller the area, the more precise is the inferred location.

Note that, at this point, we assume only a single occupant with the condo. Given multiple occupants, radio-frequency identification (RFID) could help distinguish between them (Kanai, Nakada, Hanbat, and Kunifuji, 2008).

The Service Layer: SensorDB and the REST APIs

The SensorDB serves as the long-term repository of (a) the collected sensor data, (b) the information derived from it through the stream-mining component, and (c) the data extracted by a standard data-mining component. It contains five primary tables (see Figure 4).

1. NODE, with attribute Node_ID, records the sensor node IDs deployed in the network.
2. LOCATION, with attributes for the longitude, latitude, altitude, and a time-stamp, identifies the physical location of each node.

We include a time-stamp field to support mobile nodes.

3. STATE lists all the possible states/phenomena that a node may observe.

4. OBSERVATION contains the actual state measurements. Each observation must come from a node and measure one of the observed states.

5. ROLE lists the possible functions a node may assume in the network (e.g., sensor or sink). At any given moment, each node is associated with one of these roles.

Two additional tables, INTERSECT and INFERENCES, support the stream processing. We use an intersection analysis tool to convert possibly overlapping passive-infrared sensor polygons to non-overlapping regions; INTERSECT stores the results from this analysis. The localization procedure uses data from this table to compute the occupant's location and stores the results in the table INFERENCES.

The data hosted in SensorDB is made available to client applications in a service-oriented manner through a set of REST APIs (Fielding and Taylor, 2002). Service orientation is a new, increasingly adopted software-engineering paradigm, which advocates the design and development of complex software systems through the composition of (independently designed and developed) *services*. These services, although implemented in a variety of platforms and programming languages, are interoperable through open XML-based specifications of their interfaces. Today, under the term *service interface*, two distinct types of specifications are understood: (a) operation-based APIs specified in WSDL and accessed at run-time through SOAP and (b) data-centric APIs specified in terms of the XML schemas of the data communicated and accessed at run-time through HTTP. The latter type is simpler to implement, typically requires less parsing at run time, and, more importantly, makes no commitment to a standardized set of operations to be performed on the repository data,

which is the case with WSDL APIs. These are the primary reasons why we chose this style for the Smart Condo architecture.

The decision to use REST was also validated by the fact that it accommodates the restrictions imposed by the Second Life programming environment, which we subsequently adopted as a 3D world in which to reflect the condo's state and the occupant's activities.

This environment limits communication with external web-based applications to a URL-based request and the receipt of the response as a string of text, which can then be parsed by the limited text-processing functions. Fortunately, these limited capabilities are sufficient for a REST-based system, and thus the SL client is able to communicate effectively with the intermediary program.

Second Life: The 3D Mirror of the Smart Condo

As we mentioned in the beginning of this section, SensorGIS (Huang, Boers, Stroulia, Gburzynski, and Nikolaidis, 2010) is one of the applications accessing the Smart Condo APIs to visualize the sensor data on a map and through graphs. We will not discuss this application in detail here. In this chapter, we will focus on the Second Life-based application (Boers et al., 2009) that reflects the state of the condo and the occupant's activities.

The Second Life-based application is composed of (a) a conversion utility that can turn a 2D blueprint of a home into a 3D model, (b) an automated character module that is responsible for moving the occupant's avatar through the locations at which the occupant has been detected by the stream miner, (c) a path-planning algorithm to extrapolate the occupant's avatar path around obstacles between these locations, and (d) a control system to coordinate these components.

We discuss the first component in the next section titled The Development Toolkit. Once the virtual space has been created, the occupant's avatar can be placed in an initial position within that space and given instructions on where it should move. The actual movement of the occupant's avatar is controlled by a Second Life script. This module essentially serves as the controller of the SL avatar of the occupant, instead of an actual user of the SL client, by interpreting a sequence of geographic (latitude/longitude) co-ordinates and associated time-stamps, accessed through the service-layer APIs, into instructions for movement and actions (sitting on a chair, opening/closing doors, lying on a bed). These data are then converted in both space and time: the spatial co-ordinates are translated to the virtual-world co-ordinates, and their associated time-stamps are translated to match the replay speed chosen by the user. Thus, the control system creates a list of local destination co-ordinates along with the appropriate delay between each destination. Before these co-ordinates are used to move the occupant's avatar, however, they are converted to a set of intermediate points using the path-planning algorithm. This component, a C implementation of a potential-fields algorithm (Greytak, 2005), ensures that the character does not walk through any obstacles on its way to a destination.

Our use of Second Life as a means of visualizing the activities of the Smart Condo occupant is motivated by several reasons. First it enables an intuitive comparison of the correctness of the system inferences against the video recording of the space. Video recording provides a very precise record of the occupant's life but it raises many challenges, both technical with respect to storage requirements and information extraction, as well as social, around privacy. The Second Life visualization is generated through the sensor data-stream analysis and need not be stored as it can be regenerated upon demand. At the same time, it provides an intuitive interface for health professionals and family members alike, who can be aware of the occupant's activities as opposed to simply being alerted to exceptional problematic events. Even if health professionals and family members want to only be alerted upon such events,

the Second-Life visualization – regenerated upon demand – can potentially provide more context about the person's activities before the event of interest. Finally, we envision Second Life will be useful, not simply as a visualization environment, but also as a bidirectional communication platform between the Smart-Condo occupant and his/her health providers and family members. We would like to encourage the occupant's friends to visit with him/her in the Second Life Smart Condo as well as enable the occupant to visit other places and potentially develop a parasocial life in the virtual world. By no means, would we want to encourage further alienation of he elderly by "locking" them in the virtual world, as opposed to encouraging them to participate in real-world activities. However, in some cases (mobility issues, lack of family members in the vicinity, long winters), this environment can provide a rich alternative and augmentation medium of the occupant's social life.

The Development Toolkit

In this section, we discuss the utilities that we have developed to support the deployment of the Smart Condo. The first tools relate to the wireless sensor network and the later tools relate to the virtual world and visualization.

To develop our software, we relied extensively on the emulation environment named SIDE (Gburzynski, 1995; Dobosiewicz and Gburzynski, 1997; Gburzynski and Nikolaidis, 2006) and its API for PicOS named VUE[2] (Boers, Gburzynski, Nikolaidis, and Olesinski, 2010). These tools allowed us to build our application for either the actual hardware or the emulated environment simply by running the appropriate compiler. With only a little extra effort, we then built our Operations Support System (OSS) to work seamlessly with both the real and emulated system. This integrated combination allowed us to test the WSN node software, the OSS, and the stream processing components before actually

Figure 5. The Smart Condo rendered in SL

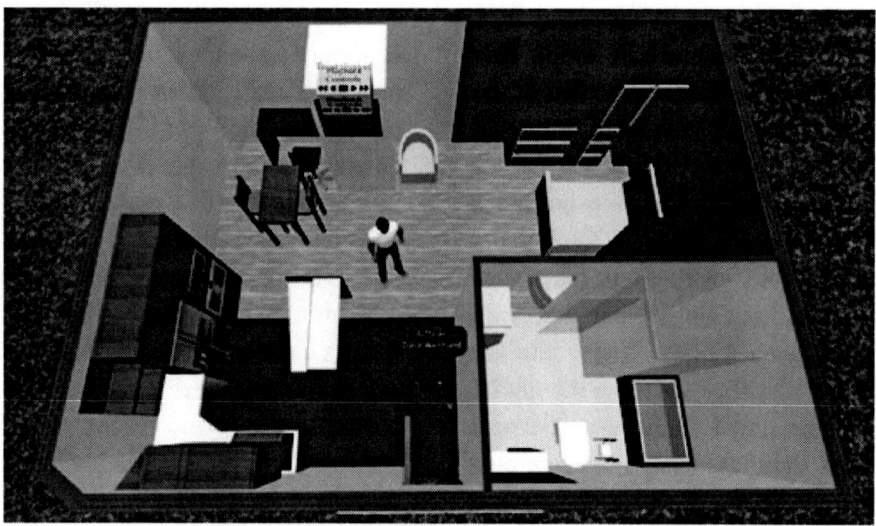

deploying any hardware. It allowed us to debug our code with ease.

In terms of the virtual world, the first tool supports the development of the 3D model of the particular space in which the infrastructure is deployed. The user can trace the location of the walls and indicate the location of furniture using a web-based blueprint creation tool. The tool stores these locations in a database. Once this input process is complete, a program written within SL reads the information from the database and creates walls and furniture in the specified locations. Finally, color and textures can be added, through built-in SL tools, to improve the appearance of the virtual condo. At the same time, the wall and furniture locations are used to create a grid-based obstacle map, which guides the path-planning algorithm. Figure 5 shows a top-down view of the Smart Condo, created in Second Life. Figure 6 shows a close-up of both an occupant's avatar and an observer.

Another development tool is designed to help with the deployment of the various sensors in the space. As we already mentioned, the occupant's location is inferred by recognizing patterns of related sensor readings in the data stream. Though each sensor detects environmental changes independently and has its own detection zone, different zones might overlap. A single movement of the patient may trigger multiple readings from different sensors, which, when detected, indicate that the patient is somewhere within the intersection of the detection zones. It is therefore essential to place sensors in such a way that we maximize the coverage of the space while taking advantage of any overlap. To determine sensor placement, an analysis tool was developed. The analysis tool imports the floor plan of the Smart Condo and, through a user interface, receives possible locations for the available sensors. Based on the sensor specifications, it then visualizes their coverage and overlap on the floor plan. The user can adjust the sensor layout easily and re-compute the visual coverage when that layout changes. After the user comes up with a satisfactory layout, he or she can save it for further adjustment and/or use the tool to export the respective table entries into the database for localization lookup. This way, the analysis tool can save the network developer much effort in identifying the intersections.

Figure 6. The occupant's avatar, wearing a white shirt, in the SL condo with an observer

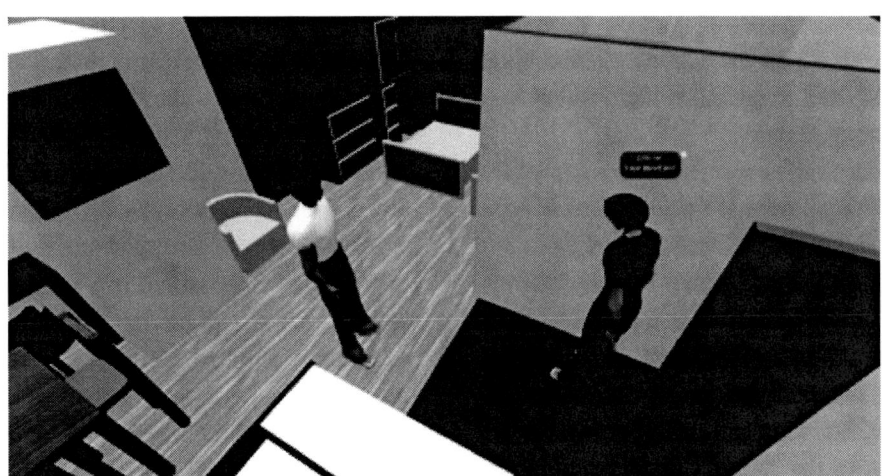

Experience with the Smart Condo

After placing sensors within the unit, we worked with our colleagues in occupational therapy (OT) to evaluate our work. A test subject followed a number of scripts within the unit while the OTs evaluated the virtual representation. The Smart Condo contains a number of video cameras (which were installed in the room for a different project), which we used to verify inferences about the location of the occupant. Our OT colleagues matched the script with their observations of both the video feed and the virtual representation. The scripts included such actions as moving from room to room, sitting on chairs, and opening and closing doors. The initial reaction of our colleagues was positive: they were very satisfied with the fidelity of the virtual representation with respect to the real world and felt that this would be a useful tool for monitoring patients undergoing rehabilitation.

RESEARCH CHALLENGES

In our short experience setting up the condo with our colleagues in Occupational Therapy, Pharmacy, and Industrial Design, one challenge we had to meet was our differences in "language"

and methodological assumptions. As Computing-Science researchers, we were primarily concerned with the technical capabilities of the infrastructure, its potential for extendibility and scalability, and its technical constraints. Our colleagues were very much guided by the needs of the personas for whom they were designing the space and had to ensure that all functions developed made sense to (and were usable by) these personas. As a team, we are continuously adjusting to each other and the experience has been interesting and rewarding. Having acknowledged this social/methodological challenge, in this section, we discuss the technical research challenges we see for the next stages of the project, as we move to develop an extendible, easily deployable system.

WSNs for Smart Indoor Environments

The task of integrating new types of sensors to wireless nodes still requires specialized programming skills, not necessarily taught as part of most computing-science degree programs. To simplify this process, a development-support toolkit is required, including tools to support (a) the development of new sensor drivers and core applications and (b) the deployment of the heterogeneous sensors within an interior space to maximize the coverage of the space (thus improving the degree to which the occupant's activities are recognized) and to optimize the number and type of necessary sensors.

The integration of new sensor types in a WSN requires the development of a standard set of core software services at the WSN node level, i.e., data packetization, duty-cycle (sleep vs. processing) of the sensor node, selection of a (variant of an existing) communication protocol, and message routing. This software has to be optimized for code-footprint, data-loss, and energy-consumption minimization. In the Smart Condo installation, for example, we had to fine-tune the node sleep-processing cycle in order to make sure that the delay between the activity in the real world and its reflection in the virtual world was less than 20 seconds. The long-term objective of our WSN research is to develop a service-oriented model for sensor applications, and a corresponding IDE[9] for model-driven engineering (Schmidt, 2006) of such applications.

Beyond the development of software for new sensors, this envisioned IDE should also support the design, development, testing, and simulation of the overall sensor-network application; as long as the types of sensors used in the network are known, domain experts (e.g., residential property managers) should be able to deploy their applications (e.g., temperature sensing and HVAC controlling) and know in advance, possibly though model checking and/or simulation, its properties (e.g., the temperature will not be above 20°C for more than 3 minutes). An essential step in this process is the placement of the sensors themselves, which is currently an empirical, experience-based activity. The automation of the placement of heterogeneous sensors in order to meet the monitoring and control requirements of the application is an important challenge that has to be met if these systems are to be widely adopted.

Finally, in addition to the IDE for WSN application development, another essential activity for effective health management and care delivery is the reengineering of existing health-monitoring devices in order for them to serve as "sensors" in our sensor networks. Patients are increasingly using commercially available off-the-shelf devices to monitor and manage their health, e.g., blood glucose meters, blood pressure monitors, etc. Information arising from the use of these devices (possibly stored in a proprietary format) can be essential to having a complete picture of the patient's current status and history. This is of special interest to pharmacists who can use this information when interacting with patients to renew medications.

SOA Systems for Monitoring, Analysis, and Control

The core objective in developing the software architecture of the Smart Condo system has been to support the flexible integration of various data streams, whether from sensor networks or from home-care devices potentially, and to accommodate multiple types of data analyses and user views and the flexible integration of new analyses and views.

We have considered both the REST and WS* SOA styles for our system and we decided to adopt the REST style, since the implied data-centric application model is simpler to conceptualize and enables more flexible integration of future modules, as it does not assume any agreement on standard operations. REST APIs are also very appropriate for communication between the Rich Internet Clients, through which the archived information may be communicated to its different classes of users (i.e., patients, their families, healthcare professionals, educators, and students). To date, our work has focused mostly on a variety of views for effectively communicating the sensed information through standard graphs and plots, a 2D GIS view, a 3D virtual-world visualization, and a wiki through which patients and healthcare professionals can record their observations on the recorded information.

Clearly, as can be seen by reviewing the "smart homes" listed previously, the primary functionalities of interest are (a) mining the collected data to extract higher-order information and (b) using the inferred information to control the environment or somehow support the resident. Several types of data-mining services are potentially useful. In a short time scale (seconds), data streams can be examined to recognize patterns on the basis of which to raise alarms, such as for example, recognizing falls based on accelerometers either worn on the person or embedded in the floor (Rajendran, Corcoran, Kinosian, and Alwan, 2008; Alwan et al., 2006). In a longer time scale (days), data can be mined to recognize patterns in the residents' behavior. These patterns can be associated with specific control actions or interactions with the residents. For example, recognizing the completion of the resident's nightly routine, the system may switch off all lights and remind the resident of his nightly medicine. Recognizing near misses from well-established routines, such as for example sleeping unusually late, may also trigger alarms to family members and health professionals. Finally, special purpose mining algorithms are necessary for analyzing patterns of physiological variables recorded by wearable and embedded sensors, such as for example, gait analysis based on sensors embedded in footwear and sleep-pattern analysis based on bed sensors. In addition to these services, research is required to address the following issues.

Further support is necessary for users interested in accessing and visualizing information. Instead of having a pre-designed set of views to the information, high-level domain-specific languages are necessary to enable domain experts to query the collected data for information of interest. For example, a health professional may be interested in knowing the longest segment of continuous standing or walking activity by the patient and he should be able to specify this query, have the system translate it into an efficient SQL query, and visualize the results in an appropriate view.

Finally, in order to better support the interpretation of the collected data, it is essential to enable the appropriate stakeholders to annotate information of interest with their observations. We envision that the information sensed by the Smart Condo, aggregated and abstracted through data mining and further redacted by the resident patient and his healthcare providers, will be part of his electronic health record. To enable this vision, the system users, both patient and healthcare professionals, should be able to review the collected information and annotate it with their (self) observations and interpretations. We are experimenting with an access-controlled wiki for that purpose.

Virtual Worlds for Simulation and Training

One of the most innovative aspects of the Smart Condo infrastructure, we believe, is the use of a virtual-world platform (Second Life, more specifically) for visualizing the activities of the condo tenant through an avatar. We believe that this type of view into the patient's everyday life can fundamentally enhance the interaction between patients and their healthcare providers and family members. This view is more intuitive than information visualization and enables realistic communication between the patients and their pharmacists, nurses, doctors, and family who can "visit" the patients in their own (virtual) home. This increased realism can potentially improve the social life of patients who may have difficulties getting out of their homes, without compromising their privacy to the degree video-based monitoring systems do. As the technologies mature, we expect health professionals to visit patients in a virtual world and interact with them in a context that should be more engaging, and with a higher-degree of social presence. Furthermore, recordings of clinically relevant resident behaviors are available to be reviewed by healthcare teams for education purposes.

Clearly, there are a variety of concerns to be addressed by further research on the potential benefits that these platforms may bring and the potential issues they may bring forward. There are still technical problems involved in reflecting the physical environment in the virtual world in a way that is precise. Collada (https://collada.org) is an emerging standard, supported by several virtual worlds, although not Second Life, for digital-asset exchange within the interactive 3D industry. In parallel with the development of these aware environments, there is a need to also develop corresponding virtual-world-based instructional programs for health science students, so that they can effectively use the system to improve patient care and potentially decrease its costs. Finally, the psychological and social effect of enabling virtual socialization needs to be studied. Although, it has been shown that virtual worlds enable a sense of communication among people, it is not clear how this can benefit patient support and healthcare team communication and not lead to even more isolation for patients who are not as motivated to visit their healthcare team as often.

CONCLUSION

In this chapter, we discussed our work in the Smart Condo project. Our interdisciplinary team includes researchers from Occupational Therapy, Industrial Design, Pharmacy, and Computing Science. Together, we have developed a model condo, designed according to universal design principles, within which we have embedded a wireless network with a variety of sensors. The raw observations recorded by the sensor network, as well as the information inferred based on this raw data, are archived in a server, which supports a range of REST APIs. Using these APIs, the information is visualized in a 2D GIS and a 3D virtual world.

Our Smart Condo is one of a new breed of smart-home applications, all of which envision the (semi)automated monitoring and control of buildings, in order to improve interior climate control, reduce energy consumption, and support residents with physical and cognitive disabilities to live independently longer. There are three specific innovations in our work that distinguish it from the other research in the area. First, we are experimenting with a variety of sensor types, and we are looking into integrating commodity home-care device sensors in our networks. Second, we have developed an integrated software architecture with a component for collecting and archiving sensor-network data which is unaffected by changes in the sensor network topology, a stream-data mining component for synthesizing raw sensor network data into higher-order information, and a set of APIs through which the information can be provided to different clients for different types of visualization. Finally, we are using a virtual world, i.e., SL, as a highly realistic visualization of the condo and the activities of its occupant. This visualization is intuitive and easy to use for all healthcare professionals, who do not need to interpret graphs to infer information about the patient. Moreover it can also serve as a communication channel between the patient and the caregivers. At the same time, the system is minimally intrusive, since the patient is not required to wear any special-purpose devices and their appearance is not monitored or recorded – people, in general, do not like to be monitored by cameras and are generally resistant to wearing a "tag" with an RFID.

This work is in its initial stages, but based on our preliminary evaluation, our virtual-world visualization shows promising results. We have established that our approach is effective and capable of driving such visualizations.

ACKNOWLEDGMENT

The authors are grateful to the support of NSERC (the Natural Sciences and Engineering Research Council), iCORE (the Informatics Circle Of Research Excellence), the Alberta Ministry of Advanced Education and Technology, and IBM. We also wish to thank the anonymous reviewers who, with their thoughtful comments, helped us improve this chapter.

REFERENCES

Akhmetshina, E., Gburzynski, P., & Vizeacoumar, F. (2003). PicOS: A tiny operating system for extremely small embedded platforms. In *ESA '03: Proceedings of the International Conference on Embedded Systems and Applications* (pp. 116-122). Las Vegas, NV:CSREA Press.

Alwan, M., Rajendran, P. J., Kell, S., Mack, D., Dalal, S., Wolfe, M., & Felder, R. (2006). A smart and passive floor-vibration based fall detector for elderly. In *ICTTA '06: Proceedings of the International Conference on Information and Communication Technologies* (pp. 1003-1007).

Arduino. (2010). *Arduino website.* Retrieved January 5, 2010, from http://www.arduino.cc/

Atallah, L., Lo, B., Yang, G. Z., & Siegemund, F. (2008). Wirelessly accessible sensor populations (WASP) for elderly care monitoring. In *PervasiveHealth '08: Proceedings of the Second International Conference on Pervasive Computing Technologies for Healthcare* (pp. 2-7).

Bajcar, J. M., Kennie, N., & Einarson, T. R. (2005). Collaborative medication management in a team-based primary care practice: An explanatory conceptual framework. *Research in Social & Administrative Pharmacy, 1*(3), 408–429. doi:10.1016/j.sapharm.2005.06.003

Beattie, E. R. A., Song, J. A., & LaGore, S. (2005). A comparison of wandering behaviour in nursing homes and assisted living facilities. *Research and Theory for Nursing Practice. International Journal (Toronto, Ont.), 19*(2), 181–192.

Beney, J., Bero, L. A., & Bond, C. M. (2000). Expanding the roles of outpatient pharmacists: Effects on health services utilisation, costs, and patient outcomes. *Cochrane Database of Systematic Reviews, 2*, CD000336. doi:. doi:10.1002/14651858.CD000336

Boers, N. M., Chodos, D., Huang, J., Gburzynski, P., Nikolaidis, I., & Stroulia, E. (2009). The Smart Condo: Visualizing independent living environments in a virtual world. In *PervasiveHealth '09: Proceedings of the Third International Conference on Pervasive Computing Technologies for Healthcare*, 1-8.

Boers, N. M., Gburzynski, P., Nikolaidis, I., & Olesinski, W. (2010). Developing wireless sensor network applications in a virtual environment. *Telecommunication Systems, 45*, 165–176. doi:10.1007/s11235-009-9246-x

Boyd, C. M., Darer, J., Boult, C., Fried, L. P., Boult, L., & Wu, A. W. (2005). Clinical practice guidelines and quality of care for older patients with multiple comorbid diseases. *Journal of the American Medical Association, 293*, 716–724. doi:10.1001/jama.294.6.716

Cassel, C. K. (2009). Policy for an aging society. Review of systems. *Journal of the American Medical Association, 302*, 2701–2702. doi:10.1001/jama.2009.1901

Cook, D. J. (2006). Health monitoring and assistance to support aging in place. *Journal of Universal Computer Science, 12*(1), 15–29.

Dobbs, D., Munn, J., Zimmerman, S., Boustani, M., Williams, C. S., & Sloane, P. D. (2005). Characteristics associated with lower activity involvement in long-term care residents with dementia. *The Gerontologist, 12*(1), 81–86.

Dobosiewicz, W., & Gburzynski, P. (1997). Protocol design in SMURPH. In *State of the Art in Performance Modeling and Simulation* (pp. 255-274).

Fielding, R. T., & Taylor, R. N. (2002). Principled design of the modern Web architecture. *ACM Transactions on Internet Technology, 2*(2), 115–150. doi:10.1145/514183.514185

Gburzynski, P. (1995). *Protocol design for local and metropolitan area networks*. Upper Saddle River, NJ: Prentice Hall PTR.

Gburzynski, P., & Nikolaidis, I. (2006). Wireless network simulation extensions in SIDE/ SMURPH. In *Proceedings of the 38th Winter Simulation Conference* (pp. 2225-2233).

Greytak, M. (2005). *Numerical potential field path planning tutorial*. Retrieved January 4, 2010, from http://ocw.mit.edu/NR/rdonlyres/Aeronautics-and-Astronautics/16-410Fall-2005/E6469924-5AE3-41C0-AA36-145D20739B7E/0/greytak.pdf

Gruber-Baldini, A. L., Zimmerman, S., Boustani, M., Watson, L. C., Williams, C. S., & Reed, P. S. (2005). Characteristics associated with depression in long-term care residents with dementia. *The Gerontologist, 45*(1), 50–55.

Haynes, R. B., Ackloo, E., Sahota, N., McDonald, H. P., & Yao, X. (2008). Interventions for enhancing medication adherence. *Cochrane Database of Systematic Reviews, 2*, CD000011. doi:. doi:10.1002/14651858.CD000011.pub3

Helal, S., Mann, W. C., El-Zabadani, H., King, J., Kaddoura, Y., & Jansen, E. (2005). The Gator Tech Smart House: A programmable pervasive space. *IEEE Computer, 38*(3), 50–60.

Hori, T. Nishida, Y. Aizawa, H. Murakami, S., & Mizoguchi, H. (2004). Sensor network for supporting elderly care home. In *Proceedings of IEEE Sensors: Vol. 2* (pp. 575-578).

Hori, T., Nishida, Y., & Murakami, S. (2006). Pervasive sensor system for evidence-based nursing care support. In *ICRA '06: Proceedings of the IEEE International Conference on Robotics and Automation* (pp. 1680-1685).

Huang, J., Boers, N. M., Stroulia, E., Gburzynski, P., & Nikolaidis, I. (2010). SensorGIS: An integrated architecture for information systems based on sensor networks. In *WEBIST '10: Proceedings of the 6th International Conference on Web Information Systems and Technologies*.

Kanai, H., Nakada, T., Hanbat, Y., & Kunifuji, S. (2008). A support system for context awareness in a group home using sound cues. In *PervasiveHealth '08: Second International Conference on Pervasive Computing Technologies for Healthcare* (pp. 264-267).

Kientz, J. A., Patel, S. N., Jones, B., Price, E., Mynatt, E. D., & Abowd, G. D. (2008). The Georgia Tech Aware Home. In *CHI '08: Extended Abstracts on Human Factors in Computing Systems* (pp. 3675-3680).

Kientz, J. A., Patel, S. N., Tyebkhan, A. Z., Gane, B., Wiley, J., & Abowd, G. D. (2006). Where's my stuff?: Design and evaluation of a mobile system for locating lost items for the visually impaired. In *ASSETS '06: Proceedings of the 8th International ACM SIGACCESS Conference on Computers and Accessibility* (pp. 103-110).

Kleinberger, T., Becker, M., Ras, E., Holzinger, A., & Müller, P. (2007). Ambient intelligence in assisted living: Enable elderly people to handle future interfaces. In *Lecture Notes in Computer Science: Vol. 4555/2007. Universal Access in Human-Computer Interaction. Ambient Interaction* (pp. 103-112). Germany: Springer Verlag.

Levis, P., Madden, S., Polastre, J., Szewczyk, R., Whitehouse, K., Woo, A., & Gay, D. Hill, J., Welsh, M., Brewer, E., & Culler D. (2005). TinyOS: An operating system for sensor networks. In *Ambient Intelligence* (pp. 115-148). The Netherlands: Springer Verlag.

McDaniel, J. H., Hunt, A., Hackes, B., & Pope, J. F. (2001). Impact of dining room environment on nutritional intake of Alzheimer's residents: A case study. *American Journal of Alzheimer's Disease and Other Dementias, 16*(5), 297–302. doi:10.1177/153331750101600508

Metaxas, M. Markopoulos. P., Aarts, E. H. L. (2009). Amelie: A Recombinant Computing Framework for Ambient Awareness. In *Ambient Intelligence 2009* (pp. 88-100).

Morgan, D. G., & Stewart, N. M. (1997). The importance of the social environment in dementia care. *Western Journal of Nursing Research, 19*(6), 740–761. doi:10.1177/019394599701900604

Morgan, D. G., & Stewart, N. M. (1998). Multiple occupancy versus private rooms on dementia care units. *Environment and Behavior, 30*(4), 487–503. doi:10.1177/001391659803000404

Mukherjee, S., Aarts, E. H. L., & Doyle, T. (2009). Special issue on Ambient Intelligence. *Information Systems Frontiers, 11*(1), 1–5. doi:10.1007/s10796-008-9146-8

Nowak, L. A., & Davis, J. E. (2007). A qualitative examination of the phenomenon of sundowning. *Journal of Nursing Scholarship, 39*(3), 256–258. doi:10.1111/j.1547-5069.2007.00177.x

Oracle Corporation. (2010). *Sun SPOTS*. Retrieved on January 5, 2010 from http://planets.sun.com/SunSPOT/

Rajendran, P., Corcoran, A., Kinosian, B., & Alwan, M. (2008). Falls, fall prevention, and fall detection technologies. In R. J. Pignolo, M. A. Forciea, & J. C. Johnson (Series Eds.) & R. Felder & M. Alwan (Vol. Eds.), *Aging medicine: Eldercare technology for clinical practitioners* (pp. 187-202). Totowa, NJ: Humana Press.

Ramage-Morin, P. L. (2009). Medication use among senior Canadians. *Health Reports, 20*(1), 1–8.

Ras, E., Becker, M., & Koch, J. (2007). Engineering tele-health solutions in the ambient assisted living lab. In *AINAW '07: 21st International Conference on Advanced Information Networking and Applications Workshops: Vol 2* (pp. 804-809).

Roughead, E. E., Semple, S. J., & Vitry, A. I. (2005). Pharmaceutical care services: A systematic review of published studies, 1990 to 2003, examining effectiveness in improving patient outcomes. *International Journal of Pharmacy Practice, 13*, 53–70. doi:10.1211/0022357055551

Santschi, V., Wuerzner, G., Schneider, M., Bugnon, O., & Burnier, M. (2007). Clinical evaluation of IDAS II, a new electronic device enabling drug adherence monitoring. *European Journal of Clinical Pharmacology, 63*(12), 1179–1184. doi:10.1007/s00228-007-0364-7

Schmidt, D. C. (2006). Guest editor's introduction: Model-driven engineering. *Computer, 39*(2), 25–31. doi:10.1109/MC.2006.58

Shaspa Smart Home Kit. (2009). Retrieved from http://www.shaspa.com

Skubic, M., Alexander, G., Popescu, M., Rantz, M., & Keller, J. (2009). A Smart Home Application to Eldercare: Current Status and Lessons Learned. *Technology and Health Care, 17*(3), 183–201.

Statistics Canada. (2006). *2006 Census: Portrait of the Canadian Population in 2006, by Age and Sex: National portrait*. Retrieved on January 6, 2010, from http://www12.statcan.ca/census-recensement/2006/as-sa/97-551/p3-eng.cfm

Task Force on a Blueprint for Pharmacy. (2008). *Blueprint for pharmacy: the vision for pharmacy*. Ottawa, ON: Canadian Pharmacists Association.

The Center for Universal Design. (1997). *The principles of universal design, version 2.0*. Raleigh, NC: North Carolina State University.

Tinetti, M. E., & Fried, T. (2004). The end of the disease era. *The American Journal of Medicine, 116*(3), 179–185. doi:10.1016/j.am-jmed.2003.09.031

Tran, Q., Calcaterra, G., & Mynatt, E. (2005). Cook's collage: Deja vu display for a home kitchen. In *HOIT '05: Proceedings of Home-Oriented Informatics and Telematics* (pp. 15-32).

US Department of Health and Human Services. (2010). *Exhibit 2.11 estimated percentage of physician's time spent providing care to patients, by age of patient.* Retrieved on January 6, 2010, from http://bhpr.hrsa.gov/healthworkforce/reports/changedemo/images/2.11.htm

Zingmark, K., Sandman, P. O., & Norberg, A. (2002). Promoting a good life among people with Alzheimer's disease. *Journal of Advanced Nursing, 38*(1), 50–58. doi:10.1046/j.1365-2648.2002.02145.x

ADDITIONAL READING

Abowd, G. D., Atkeson, C. G., Bobick, A. F., Essa, I. A., MacIntyre, B., Mynatt, E. D., & Starner, T. E. (2000). Living laboratories: the future computing environments group at the Georgia Institute of Technology. In *CHI '00 extended abstracts on Human factors in computing systems* (pp. 215-216).

Brumitt, B., Meyers, B., Krumm, J., Kern, A., & Shafer, S. A. (2000). EasyLiving: Technologies for Intelligent Environments. In *Proceedings of the 2nd international symposium on Handheld and Ubiquitous Computing* (pp.12-29).

Canadian Healthcare Association. (2009). *New directions for facility-based long-term care.* Ottawa: Canadian Healthcare Association.

Carswell, W., McCullagh, P. J., Augusto, J. C., Martin, S., Mulvenna, M. D., & Zheng, H. (2009). A review of the role of assistive technology for people with dementia in the hours of darkness. *Technology and Health Care, 17*, 281–304.

Chan, M., Estève, D., Escriba, C., & Campo, E. (2008). A review of smart homes-Present state and future challenges. *Computer Methods and Programs in Biomedicine, 91*(1), 55–81. doi:10.1016/j.cmpb.2008.02.001

Christensen, D. B., & Farris, K. B. (2006). Pharmaceutical care in community pharmacies: Practice and research in the US. *The Annals of Pharmacotherapy, 40*(7), 1400–1406. doi:10.1345/aph.1G545

Das, S., Cook, D. J., Bhattacharya, A., Heierman, I. E. O., & Lin, T.-Y. (2003). *The role of prediction algorithms in the MavHome smart home architecture.* IEEE Wireless Communications.

Emiliani, P. L., & Stephanidis, C. (2005). Universal access to ambient intelligence environments: Opportunities and challenges for people with disabilities. *IBM Systems Journal, 44*(3), 605–619. doi:10.1147/sj.443.0605

Fuchsberger, V. (2008). Ambient assisted living: elderly people's needs and how to face them. In *SAME '08: Proceeding of the 1st ACM international workshop on Semantic ambient media experiences* (pp. 21-24).

Hanák, D., Szijarto, G., & Takacs, B. (2007). A Mobile Approach to Ambient Assisted Living. In *IADIS Wireless Applications and Computing* (pp. 1-8).

Hayes, G. R., Shehan, E., Iachello, G., Patel, S. N., Grimes, A., Abowd, G. D., & Truong, K. N. Physical, Social, and Experiential Knowledge of Privacy and Security in a Pervasive Computing Environment. In *IEEE Pervasive Computing*, Oct. – Dec. 2007.

Henkler, S., Greenyer, J., Hirsch, M., Schäfer, W., Alhawash, K., Eckardt, T., et al. (2009). Synthesis of timed behavior from scenarios in the Fujaba real-time tool suite. In *ICSE '09: Proceedings of the 31st International Conference on Software Engineering* (pp. 615-618).

Jones, E. J., MacKinnon, N. J., & Tsuyuki, R. T. (2005). Pharmaceutical care in community pharmacies: Practice and research in Canada. *The Annals of Pharmacotherapy, 39*(9), 1527–1533. doi:10.1345/aph.1E456

King, J., Bose, R., Zabadani, H., Yang, H., & Helal, A. (2006). Atlas: A Service-Oriented Sensor Platform. In *Proceedings of the 31st IEEE Conference on Local Computer Networks* (pp.630-638).

Kohler, M., Patel, S. N., Summet, J. W., Stuntebeck, E. P., & Abowd, G. D. (2007). TrackSense: Infrastructure Free Precise Indoor Positioning using Projected Patterns. In *Proceedings of the 5th International Conference on Pervasive Computing*, 334-350.

Lesser, V., Atighetchi, M., Benyo, B., Horling, B., Raja, A., Vincent, R., et al. (1999). The intelligent home testbed. In *Proceedings of the Autonomy Control Software Workshop.*

Lester, J., Choudhury, T., & Borriello, G. (2006). A Practical Approach to Recognizing Physical Activities. In *Proceedings of the 4th International Conference on Pervasive Computing* (pp. 1-16).

Mynatt, E. D., & Rogers, W. A. (2002). Developing technology to support the functional independence of older adults. *Ageing International, 27*(1), 24–41. doi:10.1007/s12126-001-1014-5

Nehmer, J., Karshmer, A., Becker, M., & Lamm, R. (2006). Living Assistance Systems – An Ambient Intelligence Approach. In *Proceedings of the 28th International Conference on Software Engineering* (pp. 43-50).

Perry, M., Dowdall, A., Lines, L., & Hone, K. (2004). Multimodal and ubiquitous computing systems: Supporting independent-living older users. *IEEE Transactions on Information Technology in Biomedicine, 8*(3), 258–270. doi:10.1109/TITB.2004.835533

Spanoudakis, N., Moraitis, P., & Dimopoulos, Y. (2009). Engineering an Agent-based Approach to Ambient Assisted Living. In *Ambient Inelligence '09: Workshop on Interactions Techniques and Metaphors in Assistive Smart Environments* (pp. 268-271).

Tapia, E. M., Intille, S. S., & Larson, K. (2004) Activity recognition in the home using simple and ubiquitous sensors. In *Proceedings of Pervasive Computing* (pp. 158-175).

Weippl, E., Holzinger, A., & Tjoa, A. M. (2006). Security aspects of ubiquitous computing in health care. *Elektrotechnik and Informationstechnik, 123*(4), 156–162. doi:10.1007/s00502-006-0336

Welch, G., & Foxlinv, E. (2002). Motion Tracking: No Silver Bullet, But a Respectable Arsenal. *IEEE Computer Graphics and Applications, 22*(6), 24–38. doi:10.1109/MCG.2002.1046626

Yang, H., King, J., Helal, A., & Jansen, E. (2007). A Context-Driven Programming Model for Pervasive Spaces. *Proceeding of the 5th International Conference on Smart Homes and Health Telematics (ICOST)* (pp. 31-43).

KEY TERMS AND DEFINITIONS

Smart Home: In this paper, our use of the term *Smart Home* means a home that has both a set of sensors to observe the environment and a set of devices/actuators to improve the inhabitant's experience at home.

Wireless Sensor Network: A network that consists of distributed sensors that monitor physical or environmental conditions and are integrated on network nodes that wirelessly communicate these measurements through radio-frequency communication.

Virtual World: A 3D computer-based virtual environment, in which users can socialize, form communities and interact with one another and objects in the world.

Ambient Intelligence: Technologies that integrate a variety of sensors through which to perceive the presence and activities of people so that they can transparently respond to them in a way that supports these activities by controlling the environment.

Assisted Living: Physical and technological support for daily-life activities, for elderly and people with disabilities.

ENDNOTES

[1] Radio Frequency Identification devices

[2] http://ssrg.cs.ualberta.ca/index.php/Smart_Condo

[3] Sundowning is a syndrome of six behaviors: physical aggression, resistiveness, disconcerted verbalizing, night-time sleeplessness, wandering, and daytime sleepiness.

[4] Wandering is associated with complex physical and mental co-morbidities in people, who tend to be socially isolated, have limited attention span, and have impaired verbal communication skills.

[5] ZeroConf is a protocol that provides self-configuration, i.e., without any user involvement, of devices joining a network and enables them to be accessible using IP protocols.

[6] Common Object Request Broker Architecture enables inter operation of programs in different languages regardless of their operating system.

[7] http://www.healthscience.ualberta.ca/nav02.cfm?nav02=87350&nav01=15074

[8] The choice of hardware was completely pragmatic; nothing in our architecture depends on this particular piece of hardware.

[9] Integrated Development Environment

Compilation of References

Aaltonen, S., Nurminen, M., Rejonen, P., & Vuorenheimo, J. (2002, August). *User-driven Implementation of Information Systems*. Paper presents at the 25th Information System Research Seminar in Scandinavia, Bautahol, Denmark.

Acharya, R., Anand, D., Bhat, S., & Niranjan, U. C. (2001). Compact storage of medical images with patient information. *IEEE Transactions on Information Technology in Biomedicine*, *5*, 320–323. doi:10.1109/4233.966107

Ackerman, M. (3 May). *Personnal Interview. Lister Hill National Center for Biomedical Communications of the NLM* .

Adami, A. M., Hayes, T. L., Pavel, M., & Singer, C. M. (2005). Detection and Classification of Movements in Bed using Load Cells: Engineering in Medicine and Biology Society, 2005. IEEE-EMBS 2005. 27th Annual International Conference of the. *Engineering in Medicine and Biology Society, 2005. IEEE-EMBS 2005. 27th Annual International Conference of the* (pp. 589-592).

Adams, G. L., Campbell, P. T., & Adams, J. M. (2006). Effectiveness of prehospital wireless transmission of to a cardiologist via handheld device for patients with acute myocardial infarction. *The American Journal of Cardiology*, *98*, 1160–1164. doi:10.1016/j.amjcard.2006.05.042

Adlam, T. D., & Orpwood, R. D. (2003). Technology, Autonomy and Cognitive Disability. In *Proceedings of The 2nd International Workshop on Ubiquitous Computing for Pervasive Healthcare Applications (UbiHealth '03)*, Seattle, WA.

Agrawal, R., & Srikant, R. (2000). Privacy-preserving data mining. [New York: ACM.]. *SIGMOD Record*, *29*(2), 439–450. doi:10.1145/335191.335438

Agrawal, R., & Johnson, C. (2007). Securing electronic health records without impeding the flow of information. *International Journal of Medical Informatics*, *76*(5-6), 471–479. doi:10.1016/j.ijmedinf.2006.09.015

Akhmetshina, E., Gburzynski, P., & Vizeacoumar, F. (2003). PicOS: A tiny operating system for extremely small embedded platforms. In *ESA '03: Proceedings of the International Conference on Embedded Systems and Applications* (pp. 116-122). Las Vegas, NV: CSREA Press.

Alagöz, F., Wilkowska, W., Roefe, D., & Klack, L. Ziefle, M. & Schmitz-Rode (2010). Technik ohne Herz? Nutzungsmotive und Akzeptanzbarrieren medizintechnischer Systeme aus der Sicht von Kunstherzpatienten. *In Proceedings of the Third Ambient Assisted Living Conference (AAL '10)*, Berlin, Germany: VDE. CD-ROM.

Alavi, M. (1984). An Assessment of the Prototyping Approach to Information Systems Development . *Communications of the ACM*, *27*, 556–563. doi:10.1145/358080.358095

Alberta Health Services. (n.d.). Engaging the Patient in Healthcare: An Overview of Personal Health Record Systems and Implications for Alberta, *White Paper*.

Alexandrou, M. (n.d.). *Joint Application Development (JAD) Methodology*. Retrieved August 16, 2009, from http://searchsoftwarequality.techtarget.com/sDefinition/0,sid92_gci820966,00.ht ml

Algase, D., Moore, D., Vandeweerd, C., & Gavin-Dreschnack, D. J. (2007). Mapping the maze of terms and definitions in dementia-related wandering. *Aging & Mental Health*, *11*(6), 686–698. doi:10.1080/13607860701366434

Algase, D., Moore, D., Gavin-Dreschnack, D., & Vande-Weerd, C. (2007). Wandering Definitions and Terms . In Nelson, A., & Algase, D. L. (Eds.), *Evidence-Based Protocols for Managing Wandering Behaviors*. New York: Springer Publishing Company

Allum, J. H. J., & Carpenter, M. G. (2005). A speedy solution for balance and gait analysis: angular velocity measured at the centre of body mass. *Current Opinion in Neurology*, *18*, 15–21. doi:10.1097/00019052-200502000-00005

Alwan, M., Rajendran, P. J., Kell, S., Mack, D., Dalal, S., Wolfe, M., & Felder, R. (2006). A smart and passive floor-vibration based fall detector for elderly. In *ICTTA '06: Proceedings of the International Conference on Information and Communication Technologies* (pp. 1003-1007).

Alzheimer's Association. (2009). 2009 Alzheimer's disease facts and figures. *Alzheimer's & Dementia, 5*(3), 234–270. doi:10.1016/j.jalz.2009.03.001

American Academy of Pediatrics, American Academy of Family Physicians, American College of Physicians, American Osteopathic Association. (2007). *Joint principles of the patient-centered medical home.* Retrieved January 6, 2010, from http://www.medicalhomeinfo.org/joint 20Statement.pdf.

American College of Sports Medicine, Chodzko-Zajko, W.J., Proctor, D.N., Fiatarone Singh, M.A., Minson, C.T., Nigg, C.R., Salem, G.J. & Skinner, J.S. (2009). American College of Sports Medicine position stand. Exercise and physical activity for older adults. *Medicine and Science in Sports and Exercise, 41*(7), 1510–1530.

Aminian, K., & Najafi, B. (2004). Capturing human motion using body-fixed sensors: outdoor measurement and clinical applications. *Computer Animation and Virtual Worlds, 15*(2), 79–94. doi:10.1002/cav.2

Aminian, K., Najafi, B., Bula, C., Leyvraz, P. F., & Robert, P. (2002). Spatio-temporal Parameters of Gait Measured by an Ambulatory System Using Miniature Gyroscopes. *Journal of Biomechanics, 35*(5), 689–699. doi:10.1016/S0021-9290(02)00008-8

Aminian, K., Robert, Ph., Buchser, E., Rutschmann, B., Hayoz, D., & Depairon, M. (1999). Physical activity monitoring based on accelerometry: validation and comparison with video observation. *Medical & Biological Engineering & Computing, 37,* 304–308. doi:10.1007/BF02513304

Amit, R., & Schoemaker, P. J. H. (1993). Strategic assets and organizational rent. *Strategic Management Journal, 14*(1), 33. doi:10.1002/smj.4250140105

Anderson, J. G., Jay, S. J., Perry, J., & Anderson, M. (1989). Increasing Physician Use of Computerized Hospital Information System. In B. Barber, D. Cao, D. Qin, & G. Wagner (Eds), *Proccedings of the 6ᵗʰ World Conference on Medical Informatics,* North-Holland.

Arduino. (2010). *Arduino website.* Retrieved January 5, 2010, from http://www.arduino.cc/

Armac, I., Panchenko, P., Pettau, M., & Retkowitz, R. (2009). Privacy-Friendly Smart Environments. In K. Al-Begain (Ed.). *Proceedings of the Third International Conference and Exhibition on Next Generation Mobile Applications, Services and Technologies (NGMAST 2009),* Cardiff, U (pp. 425-431). London: IEEE Computer Society, 2009.

Arning, K., & Ziefle, M. (2009). Effects of cognitive and personal factors on PDA menu navigation performance. *Behaviour & Information Technology, 28*(3), 251–268. doi:10.1080/01449290701679395

Arning, K., & Ziefle, M. (2009). Different Perspectives on Technology Acceptance: The Role of Technology Type and Age . In Holzinger, A., & Miesenberger, K. (Eds.), *Human – Computer Interaction for eInclusion. LNCS 5889* (pp. 20–41). Berlin, Heidelberg: Springer.

Assimacopoulos, A., Elsig, R. N., Griesser, V., & Scherrer, J. R. (1988). End User Training for Hospital Information Systems: Catching Up with Technology . In Bakker, A. R., Ball, M. J., Scherrer, J. R., & Willems, J. L. (Eds.), *Towards New Hospital Information Systems.* North-Holland.

ASTM E2147 - 01(2009). *Standard Specification for Audit and Disclosure Logs for Use in Health Information Systems.* Retrieved from http://www.astm.org/Standards/E2147.htm

Atallah, L., Lo, B., Yang, G. Z., & Siegemund, F. (2008). Wirelessly accessible sensor populations (WASP) for elderly care monitoring. In *PervasiveHealth '08: Proceedings of the Second International Conference on Pervasive Computing Technologies for Healthcare* (pp. 2-7).

Augustine, J. J. (2001). Medical direction and EMS. *Emergency Medical Services, 30,* 65–69.

Aziz, O., Lo, B., Pansiot, J., Atallah, L., Yang, G.-Z., & Darzi, A. (2008). From computers to ubiquitous computing by 2010: health care. *Philosophical Transactions of the Royal Society A: Mathematical, Physical and Engineering Sciences, 366*(1881), 3805-3811.

Bajcar, J. M., Kennie, N., & Einarson, T. R. (2005). Collaborative medication management in a team-based primary care practice: An explanatory conceptual framework. *Research in Social & Administrative Pharmacy, 1*(3), 408–429. doi:10.1016/j.sapharm.2005.06.003

Baker, L., Wagner, T., Singer, S., & Bundorf, K. (2003). Use of the Internet and e-mail for health care information: Results from a national survey. *Journal of the American Medical Association, 289,* 2400–2406. doi:10.1001/jama.289.18.2400

Barber, B. (1983). *The Logic and Limits of Trust*. New Brunswick, NJ: Rutgers University Press.

Bardini, T. (n.d.). *What is Actor-Network Theory?* Retrieved March 20, 2010, from http://carbon.ucdenver.edu/~mryder/itc_data/ant_dff.html.

Bardram, J. E. (2005). (JCAF) – A Service Infrastructure and Programming Framework for Context-Aware Applications . In *Pervasive Computing* (pp. 98–115). The Java Context Awareness Framework. doi:10.1007/11428572_7

Barley, S. R. (1986). Technology as an Occasion for Structuring: Evidence from Observations of CT Scanners and the Social Order of Radiology Departments. *Administrative Science Quarterly*, *31*(1), 78. doi:10.2307/2392767

Barley, S. R. (1990). The Alignment Of Technology And Structure Through Roles And. *Administrative Science Quarterly*, *35*(1), 61. doi:10.2307/2393551

Barney, J., & Hansen, M. (1994). Trustworthiness as a source of competitive advantage. *Strategic Management Journal*, *15*, 175–190. doi:10.1002/smj.4250150912

Baroudi, J. J., Olson, M. H., & Ives, B. (1986). *An Empirical Study of the Impact of User Involvement on System Usage and Information Satisfaction*.

Bashshur, R. L., Sanders, J., & Shannon, G. W. (1997). *Telemedicine: Theory and practice*. Springfield: Charles Thomas.

Beaglehole, E. (1932). *A Study in Social Psychology*. New York: Mcmillan.

Beattie, E. R. A., Song, J. A., & LaGore, S. (2005). A comparison of wandering behaviour in nursing homes and assisted living facilities. *Research and Theory for Nursing Practice . International Journal (Toronto, Ont.)*, *19*(2), 181–192.

Beauchamp, T. L., & Childress, J. F. (2009). *Principles of Biomedical Ethics*. New York: Oxford University Press.

Becker, S. (2004). A study of web usability for older adults seeking online health resources. *ACM Transactions on Computer-Human Interaction*, (April): 11, 387–406.

Beggan, J. K. (1992). On the Social Nature of Nonsocial Perception: The Mere Ownership Effect. *Journal of Personality and Social Psychology*, *62*(2), 229. doi:10.1037/0022-3514.62.2.229

Behrendt, H. & Schmiedel, R. (2004). Die aktuellen Leistungen des Rettungsdienstes in der Bundesrepublik Deutschland im zeitlichen Vergleich (Teil II). *Notfall- & Rettungsmedizin*. 7, 59-70.

Behrendt, H., & Schmiedel, R. (2003). *Ausgewählte Ergebnisse der Leistungsanalyse 2000/2001*. In K. Mendel. Handbuch des Rettungswesens. Witten, Germany: Mendel Verlag.

Belanger, F., Hiller, J., & Smith, W. (2002). Trustworthiness in electronic commerce: the role of privacy, security, and site attributes. *The Journal of Strategic Information Systems*, *11*(3&4), 245–270. doi:10.1016/S0963-8687(02)00018-5

Benaloh, J., Chase, M., Horvitz, E., & Lauter, K. (2009). *Patient Controlled Encryption: Ensuring Privacy of Electronic Medical Records*. Retrieved December 20, 2009, from: http://research.microsoft.com/en-us/um/people/horvitz/ccsw_2009_benaloh_chase_horvitz_lauter.pdf.

Beney, J., Bero, L. A., & Bond, C. M. (2000). Expanding the roles of outpatient pharmacists: Effects on health services utilisation, costs, and patient outcomes. *Cochrane Database of Systematic Reviews*, *2*, CD000336. doi:. doi:10.1002/14651858.CD000336

Benhamou, S., & Bovet, P. (1992). Distinguishing between elementary orientation mechanisms by means of path analysis. *Animal Behaviour*, *43*, 371–377. doi:10.1016/S0003-3472(05)80097-1

Berg, M. (1999). Patient care information systems and health care work: a sociotechnical approach. *International Journal of Medical Informatics*, *55*(2), 87–101. doi:10.1016/S1386-5056(99)00011-8

Berg, M. (2001). Implementing Information Systems in Health Care Organizations: Myths and Challenges. *International Journal of Medical Informatics*, *64*(2-3), 143–156. doi:10.1016/S1386-5056(01)00200-3

Berg, M., Langenberg, C., Berg, I., & Kwakkernaat, J. (1998). Considerations for sociotechnical design: experiences with an electronic patient record in a clinical context. *International Journal of Medical Informatics*, *52*(1-3), 243–251. doi:10.1016/S1386-5056(98)00143-9

Berg, M., & Toussaint, P. (2003). The mantra of modelling and the forgotten powers of paper: A sociotechnical view on the development of process-oriented ICT in healthcare. *International Journal of Medical Informatics*, *69*(2-3), 223–234. doi:10.1016/S1386-5056(02)00178-8

Bergrath, S. (2006). *Retrospektive Analyse der Datenqualität eines kommerziellen Datenbanksystems für den Notarztdienst und der Dokumentationscompliance des Notarztdienstes der Stadt Aachen. Universitätsklinikum der RWTH Aachen: Ph. D. Dissertationen*.

Bethencourt, J., Sahai, A., & Waters, B. (2007). Ciphertext-policy attribute-based encryption. In *Proceedings of the 28th IEEE Symposium on Security and Privacy (Oakland)* (pp. 321-334).

Beul, S., Klack, L., Kasugai, K., Möllering, C., Röcker, C., Wilkowska, W., & Ziefle, M. (2010). Between Innovation and Daily Practice in the Development of AAL Systems: Learning from the experience with today's systems. *3rd International ICST Conference on Electronic Healthcare for the 21st century* (ehealth 2010).

Beul, S., Mennicken, S., Ziefle, M., & Jakobs, E.-M. (2010). What Happens After Calling the Ambulance: Information, Communication, and Acceptance Issues in a Telemedical Workflow. In C.A Shoniregun & G.A. Akmayeva (Eds.). In *Proceedings of the International Conference on Information Society* (pp. 111-116). London: Infonomics Society.

Beyer, H., & Holtzblatt, K. (1998). *Contextual Design: Defining Customer-Centered Systems*. San Francisco: Morgan Kaufmann.

Bharadwaj, A., Sambamurthy, V., & Zmud, R. W. (1999). IT Capabilities: Theoretical Perspectives and Operationalization. *Proceedings of the Twentieth International Conference on Informations Systems, Charlotte, NC*.

Bhattacherjee, A. (2002). Individual trust in online firms: Scale development and initial test. *Journal of Management Information Systems, 19*(1), 211–241.

Bilterys, R., & Milord, F. (2008). Preventing nosocomial infections: a topic of concern in developing countries as well. *Perspective Infirmiere, 5*(7), 21–26.

BioHealth: Security and Identity Management Standards in eHealth including Biometrics. Retrieved December 23, 2009, from http://biohealth.helmholtz-muenchen.de/

BIS Berliner Institut für Sozialforschung. DZFA Deutsches Zentrum für Alternsforschung (Ed.) (2002). *Technik im Alltag von Senioren. Arbeitsbericht zur vertiefenden Auswertung der sentha-Repräsentativerhebung*. Heidelberg

Bishop, J. E., O'Reilly, R. L., Daddox, K., & Hutchinson, K. (2002). Client Satisfaction in a faisability Study Comparing face-to-face Interviews with Telepsychiatry. *Journal of Telemedicine and Telecare, 8*(4). doi:10.1258/135763302320272185

Bland, R. (1999). Independence, privacy and risk: two contrasting approaches to residential care for older people. *Ageing and Society, 19*(5), 539–560. doi:10.1017/S0144686X99007497

Blois, K. J. (1999). Trust in business to business relationships: an evaluation of its status. *Journal of Management Studies, 36*(2), 197–215. doi:10.1111/1467-6486.00133

Bodenheimer, T. (2006). Primary care – will it survive? *The New England Journal of Medicine, 355*(9), 861–864. doi:10.1056/NEJMp068155

Boers, N. M., Gburzynski, P., Nikolaidis, I., & Olesinski, W. (2010). Developing wireless sensor network applications in a virtual environment. *Telecommunication Systems, 45*, 165–176. doi:10.1007/s11235-009-9246-x

Boers, N. M., Chodos, D., Huang, J., Gburzynski, P., Nikolaidis, I., & Stroulia, E. (2009). The Smart Condo: Visualizing independent living environments in a virtual world. In *PervasiveHealth '09: Proceedings of the Third International Conference on Pervasive Computing Technologies for Healthcare*, 1-8.

Bohacek, S., Hespanha, J. P., Lee, J., Lim, C., & Obraczka, K. (2006). A new tcp for persistent packet reordering. *IEEE/ACM Transactions on Networking, 14*(2), 369–382. doi:10.1109/TNET.2006.873366

Bonato, P. (2005). Advances in wearable technology and applications in physical medicine and rehabilitation. *Journal of Neuroengineering and Rehabilitation, 2*, 1–4. doi:10.1186/1743-0003-2-2

Bonatti, P., & Samarati, P. (2002). A unified framework for regulating access and information release on the web. [Amsterdam: IOS Press.]. *Journal of Computer Security, 10*(3), 241–271.

Boneh, D., & Franklin, M. K. (2001) Identity-based encryption from the weil pairing. In *J. Kilian, editor, Advances in Cryptology - CRYPTO 2001, 21st Annual International Cryptology Conference* (pp 213–229), vol. 2139 of LNCS. New York: Springer.

Bortz, J., & Döring, N. (1995). *Forschungsmethoden und Evaluation*. Berlin: Springer.

Bos, N., Olson, J., Gergle, D., Olson, G., & Wright, Z. (2002). *Effects of four computer-mediated communications channels on trust development. Proceedings of Human Factors in Computing Systems. CHI2002* (pp. 135–140). ACM.

Bourke, A. K., O'Brien, J. V., & Lyons, G. M. (2007). Evaluation of a threshold-based tri-axial accelerometer fall detection algorithm. *Gait & Posture, 26*, 194–199. doi:10.1016/j.gaitpost.2006.09.012

Bourke, A. K., van de Ven, P. W. J., Chaya, A. E., Olaighin, G. M., & Nelson, J. (2008). Testing of a long-term fall detection system incorporated into a custom vest for the elderly. *Proceedings of 30ᵗʰ Annual International Conference of the IEEE Engineering in Medicine and Biology Society* (pp. 2844-2847).

Boyd, C. M., Darer, J., Boult, C., Fried, L. P., Boult, L., & Wu, A. W. (2005). Clinical practice guidelines and quality of care for older patients with multiple comorbid diseases. *Journal of the American Medical Association, 293,* 716–724. doi:10.1001/jama.294.6.716

BPPC (2006). *IHE, Patient Care Coordination Technical Framework, Supplement 2005-2006, Basic Patient Privacy Consents (BPPC),* Trial Implementation Version, Draft

Brady, J. L. (2005). Telemedicine behind bars: a cost-effective and secure trend. *Biomedical Instrumentation & Technology, 39*(1), 7–8.

Brenkert, G. G. (1998). Trust, morality and international business. *Business Ethics Quarterly, 8*(2), 293–317. doi:10.2307/3857330

Briggs, P., Burford, B., DeAngeli, A., & Lunch, P. (2002). Trust in online advice. [March.]. *Social Science Computer Review, 20,* 321–334.

Brinkmann, M., Floeck, M., & Litz, L. (2008). Concept and Design of an AAL home monitoring system based on a personal computerized assistive unit . In Mühlhäuser, M., Ferscha, A., & Aitenbichler, E. (Eds.), *Constructing Ambient Intelligence: AmI 2007 Workshops* (pp. 218–227). Berlin: Springer. doi:10.1007/978-3-540-85379-4_27

Broadbent, M., & Weill, P. (1997). Management by Maxim: How Business and IT Managers Can Create IT Infrastructures. *Sloan Management Review, 38*(3), 77.

Broadbent, M., Weill, P., Brien, T., & Neo, B.-S. (1996). Firm context and pattern of IT infrastructure capability. *The International Conference on Information Systems.*

Bruegge, B., & Klinker, G. (2005). *DWARF - Distributed Wearable Augmented Reality Framework* (White Paper). Technische Universität München, Chair for Applied Software Engineering.

Bui, F. M., & Hatzinakos, D. (2008). Biometric methods for secure communications in body sensor networks: resource-efficient key management and signal-level data scrambling. *EURASIP Journal of Advance Signal Processesing, 8*(2), 1–16. doi:10.1155/2008/529879

Bundesärztekammer (2004). Tätigkeitsbericht der Bundesärztekammer: Entschließungen zum Tagesordnungspunkt VI. *Deutsches Ärzteblatt, 101* (22), A1584, B1313, C1266.

Buskens, V. (1998). The social structure of trust. *Social Networks, 20*(3), 265–289. doi:10.1016/S0378-8733(98)00005-7

Bussmann, J. B. J., Veltink, P. H., Koelma, F., van Lummel, R. C., & Stam, H. J. (1995). Ambulatory monitoring of mobility-related activities: the initial phase of the development of an activity monitor. *European Journal of Physical Medicine and Rehabilitation, 5*(1), 2–7.

Byun, J. W., Bertino, E., & Li, N. (2005). Purpose based access control of complex data for privacy protection. *In Proceedings of the tenth ACM symposium on Access control models and technologies* (pp. 102-110). New York: ACM.

Cabral, K. P. (2009). How to meet national quality initiatives: best practices. [Epub ahead of print]. *Journal of Thrombosis and Thrombolysis,* (Nov): 12.

Cabrera, A., Cabrera, E., & Barajas, S. (2001). The key role of organizational culture in a multi-system view of technology-driven change. *International Journal of Information Management, 21*(3), 245–261. doi:10.1016/S0268-4012(01)00013-5

Campion, M. A., Medsker, G. J., & Higgs, A. C. (1993). Relations between work group characteristics and effectiveness: Implications for designing effective work groups. *Personnel Psychology, 46*(4), 823. doi:10.1111/j.1744-6570.1993.tb01571.x

Čapkun, S., Hubaux, J., & Buttyán, L. (2003). Mobility helps security in ad hoc networks. In *Proceedings of the 4th ACM international Symposium on Mobile Ad Hoc Networking and Computing* (pp. 46-56). New York: ACM Press.

Caplan, S. (1990). Using focus groups methodology for economic design. *Ergonomics, 33,* 527–533. doi:10.1080/00140139008927160

Carroll, J. M., & Rosson, M. B. (1992). Getting around the task-artifact cycle: How to make claims and design by scenario. *ACM Transactions on Information Systems, 10,* 181–212. doi:10.1145/146802.146834

Cassel, C. K. (2009). Policy for an aging society. Review of systems. *Journal of the American Medical Association, 302,* 2701–2702. doi:10.1001/jama.2009.1901

Chae, B., & Poole, M. S. (2005). The surface of emergence in systems development: agency, institutions, and large-scale information systems. *European Journal of Information Systems, 14*, 19–36. doi:10.1057/palgrave. ejis.3000519

Chae, B. (2002). *Understanding information systems as social institutions: Dynamic institutional theory.* Unpublished doctoral dissertation, Texas A&M University, Texas, USA

Chan, M., Esteve, D., Escriba, C., & Campo, E. (2008). A review of smart homes- present state and future challenges. *Computer Methods and Programs in Biomedicine, 91*(1), 55–81. doi:10.1016/j.cmpb.2008.02.001

Chan, D. (1998). Functional relations among constructs in the same content domain at different levels of analysis: A typology of composition models. *The Journal of Applied Psychology, 83*(2), 234. doi:10.1037/0021-9010.83.2.234

Chao, H. M., Hsu, C. M., & Miaou, S. G. (2002). A data-hiding technique with authentication, integration, and confidentiality for electronic patients records. *IEEE Transactions on Information Technology in Biomedicine, 6*, 46–53. doi:10.1109/4233.992161

Chatterjee, D., Grewal, R., & Sambamurthy, V. (2002). Shaping up for e-commerce: Institutional enablers of the organizational assimilation of web technologies. *Management Information Systems Quarterly, 26*(2), 65. doi:10.2307/4132321

Chatterjee, D., & Segars, A. H. (2001). Transformation of the Enterprise through E-Business: An Overview of Contemporary Practices and Trends. *Report to the Advanced Practices Council of the Society for Information Management,* (July).

Cherukuri, S., Venkatasubramanian, K. K., & Gupta, S. K. S. (2003). BioSec: A biometric based approach for securing communication in wireless networks of biosensors implanted in the human body. In *Proceedings of the 1ˢᵗ Workshop on Wireless Security and Privacy* (pp. 432-439).

Cheskin Research & Studio Archetype/Sapient. (1999). *Ecommerce trust study.* Retrieved May 5, 2007 from http://www.sapient.com/cheskin.

Chevrollier, N., & Golmie, N. (2005). On the Use of Wireless Network Technologies in Healthcare Environments. In *Proceedings of the fifth IEEE Workshop on Applications and Services in Wireless Networks* (pp. 147-152).

Chhanabhai, P., & Holt, A. (2007). Consumers Are Ready to Accept the Transition to Online and Electronic Records if they can be assured of the Security Measures. *MedGenMed, 9*(1), 8-20. Retrieved December 23, 2009, from http://www.ncbi.nlm.nih.gov/pmc/articles/PMC1924980/? tool=pubmed

Chiu, Y. C., Algase, D., Whall, A., Liang, J., Liu, H. C., & Lin, K. N. (2004). Getting lost: Directed attention and executive functions in early Alzheimer's disease patients. *Dementia and Geriatric Cognitive Disorders, 17*(3), 174–180. doi:10.1159/000076353

Chor, B. Z., & Goldreich, O. Kushilevitz, E.(1998). Private Information Retrieval. *Journal of the ACM, 45*(6), 965-982. Retrieved December 20, 2009, from: http://citeseerx.ist.psu.edu/viewdoc/download?doi=10.1.1.126.9441&rep=rep1&type=pdf.

Chu, Y., & Ganz, A. (2004). A mobile teletrauma system using 3G networks. *IEEE Transactions on Information Technology in Biomedicine, 8*(4), 456–462. doi:10.1109/TITB.2004.837893

Codling, E. A., Plank, M. J., & Benhamou, S. (2008). Random walk models in biology. *Journal of the Royal Society, Interface.* .doi:10.1098/rsif.2008.0014

Cohn, J. R., & Goodenough, B. (2002). Health Professionals Attitudes to Videoconferencing in Pediatric Heathcare. *Journal of Telemedicine and Telecare, 8*(5). doi:10.1258/135763302760314243

COM. (2004). Communication from the Commission to the Council, the European Parliament. *the European Economic and Social Committee and the Committee of the Regions: e-Health-making healthcare better for European citizens: an action plan for a European e-Health Area.* Retrived December 23, 2009, from http://eur-lex.europa.eu/LexUriServ/LexUriServ.do?uri=CELEX:52004DC0356:ES:HTML

Commins, J. (2009). *Patient knowledge of their meds woeful, says stud: Health leaders media,* December 10, 2009. Retrieved January 5, 2010, from http://www.healthleadersmedia.com/content/243355/topic/WS_HLM2_QUA/Patient-Knowledge-of-Their-Meds-Woeful-Says-Study.html.

Continua. (2007). Retrieved from http://www.continuaalliance.org/home.

Cook, D. J. (2006). Health monitoring and assistance to support aging in place. *Journal of Universal Computer Science, 12*(1), 15–29.

Cooper, R. B., & Zmud, R. W. (1990). Information Technology Implementation Research: A Technological Diffusion Approach. *Management Science, 36*(2), 123. doi:10.1287/mnsc.36.2.123

Corbitt, B. J., Thanasankit, T., & Yi, H. (2003). Trust and ecommerce: a study of consumer perceptions. *Electronic Commerce Research and Applications, 2*, 203–215. doi:10.1016/S1567-4223(03)00024-3

Corritore, C., Kracher, B., & Wiedenbeck, S. (2003). On-line trust: concepts, evolving themes, a model. *International Journal of Human-Computer Studies, 58*, 737–758. doi:10.1016/S1071-5819(03)00041-7

Courtney, K. L., Demiris, G., & Hensel, B. K. (2007). Obtrusiveness of information-based assistive technologies as perceived by older adults in residential care facilities: a secondary analysis. *Journal of Medical Internet, 32*(3), 241–249.

Cox, I. J., & Miller, M. L. (2002). The first 50 years of electronic watermarking. *EURASIP Journal on Applied Signal Processing, 2*, 126–132. doi:10.1155/S1110865702000525

Cox, I. J., Miller, M. L., & Bloom, J. A. (2000). *Digital Watermarking*. San Francisco: Morgan Kaufmann.

CPC-DAM. (2009). *HL-7 Composite Privacy Consent Directive Topic*. Retrieved from http://www.hl7.org/v3ballot/html/domains/uvmr/uvmr_CompositePrivacyConsentDirective.htm#RCMR_DO000010UV-Privacyconsent-ic.

Craik, F. I. M., & Salthouse, T. A. (1992). *Handbook of Ageing and Cognition*. Hillsdale, NJ: Lawrence Erlbaum Associates.

Crossan, M. M., Lane, H. W., & White, R. E. (1999). An organizational learning framework: From intuition to institution. Academy of Management. *Academy of Management Review, 24*(3), 522. doi:10.2307/259140

Croteau, A.-M., & Vieru, D. (2002). *Telemedicine Adoption by Different Group of Physicians*. Proceedings of the 35th Hawaii International Conference on System Sciences IEEE.

Cvrcek, D. Kumpost, M., Matyas, V., & Danezis, G. (2006). A Study on the Value of Location Privacy. In: *Proceedings of the ACM Workshop on Privacy in the Electronic Society* (pp. 109-118). New York: ACM.

Czaja, S. J., Sharit, J., Charness, N., Fisk, A. D., & Rogers, W. A. (2001). The Center for Research and Education on Aging and Technology Enhancement (CREATE): A program to enhance technology for older adults. *Gerontechnology (Valkenswaard), 1*, 50–59. doi:10.4017/gt.2001.01.01.005.00

Daemen, J., & Rijmen, V. (2002). *The design of Rijndael: AES-the Advanced Encryption Standard*. New York: Springer Verlang.

Daft, R., & Weick, K. E. (1984). Toward a Model of Organizations as Interpretation Systems. *Academy of Management Review, 9*, 284–295. doi:10.2307/258441

Daft, R. L. (1995). *Organization Theory and Design* (5th ed.). Minneapolis: West Publishing Co.

D'Amour, D., Ferrada-Videla, M., San Martin Rodriguez, F., & Beaulieu, M. D. (2005). The conceptual basis for interprofessional collaboration: Core concepts and theoretical frameworks. *Journal of Interprofessional Care, 1*(Supplement), 116–131. doi:10.1080/13561820500082529

D'Amour, D. (Centre Mont-Royal, Montréal, 2006). *Collaboration interprofessionnelle: Bien saisir les enjeux. Colloque: L'Interdisciplinarité, Défi Ou Déni.*

Dasgupta, P. (1988). Trust as a commodity . In Gambetta, D. (Ed.), *Trust: Making and Breaking Cooperative Relations* (pp. 49–72). New York: Basil Blackwell.

Davenport, T. (1995). *Reengineering a business process*. Harvard Business School Case Studies.

Davis, F. (1989). Perceived usefulness, perceived ease of use and user acceptance of information technology. *Management Information Systems Quarterly, 13*(3), 319–340. doi:10.2307/249008

Davis, F., Bagozzi, R., & Warshaw, P. (1989). User acceptance of computer technology: A comparison of two theoretical models. *Management Science, 35*(8), 982–1003. doi:10.1287/mnsc.35.8.982

Davis, R., Buchanan-Oliver, M., & Brodie, R. (1999). Relationship marketing in electronic commerce environments. *Journal of Information Technology, 14*, 319–331. doi:10.1080/026839699344449

Davis, F. D. (1993). User acceptance of information technology: System characteristics, user perceptions and behavioural impacts. *International Journal of Man-Machine Studies, 38*, 475–487. doi:10.1006/imms.1993.1022

Davis, J., Morrell, J., & McFaddin, G. (1999, November). *Workflow-based Lifecycle Modeling: A Paradigm for the Analysis and Architecture of Enterprise-wide-e-Health Applications*. Paper presented at OOPSLA Workshop on Objects, Workflow and the Virtual Enterprise. OOPSLA-99 Conference on Object-Oriented Programming, Systems, Languages and Applications, Denver, Colorado.

Dawson, J. F., Gonzalez-Roma, V., Davis, A., & West, M. A. (2008). Organizational climate and climate strength in UK hospitals. *European Journal of Work and Organizational Psychology, 17*(1), 89. doi:10.1080/13594320601046664

de Bruin, E. D., Hartmann, A., Uebelhart, D., Murer, K., & Zijlstra, W. (2008). Wearable systems for monitoring mobility related activities in older people. *Clinical Rehabilitation, 22*, 878–895. doi:10.1177/0269215508090675

De Carvalho Bastone, A., & Filho, W. J. (2004). Effect of an exercise program on functional performance of institutionalized elderly. *Journal of Rehabilitation Research and Development, 41*(5), 659–668. doi:10.1682/JRRD.2003.01.0014

de Hoon, E. W., Allum, J. H., Carpenter, M. G., Salis, C., Bloem, B. R., Conzelmann, M., & Bischoff, H. A. (2003). Quantitative assessment of the stops walking while talking test in the elderly. *Archives of Physical Medicine and Rehabilitation, 84*(6), 838–842. doi:10.1016/S0003-9993(02)04951-1

de Leon, M. J., Potegal, M., & Gurland, B. (1984). Wandering and parietal signs in senile dementia of Alzheimer's type. *Neuropsychobiology, 11*(3), 155–157. doi:10.1159/000118069

De Moor, G. J. E., & Claerhout, B. (2004). Privacy enhancing techniques in E-Health: an overview. In G. Demiris (Ed.), *Studies in Health Technology and Informatics: Vol. 106. eHealth: Current Status and Future Trends* (pp. 75-82). Netherlands: IOS Press.

Dejnabadi, H., Jolles, B. M., & Aminian, K. (2005). A new approach to accurate measurement of uniaxial joint angles based on a combination of accelerometers and gyroscopes. *IEEE Transactions on Bio-Medical Engineering, 52*(8), 1478–1484. doi:10.1109/TBME.2005.851475

Dejnabadi, H., Jolles, B. M., Casanova, E., Fua, P., & Aminian, K. (2006). Estimation and Visualization of Sagittal Kinematics of Lower Limbs Orientation using Body-Fixed Sensors. *IEEE Transactions on Bio-Medical Engineering, 53*, 1385–1393. doi:10.1109/TBME.2006.873678

Demiris, G., Rantz, M. J., Aud, M. A., Marek, K. D., Tyrer, H. W., & Skubic, M. (2004). Older adults' attitudes towards and perceptions of smart home technologies: A pilot study. *Informatics for Health & Social Care, 29*(2), 87–94. doi:10.1080/14639230410001684387

Deng, J., Han, R., & Mishra, S. (2006). INSENS: Intrusion-tolerant routingn for wireless sensor networks. *Computer Communications, 29*, 216–230. doi:10.1016/j.comcom.2005.05.018

Denning, P., Horning, J., Parnas, D., & Weinstein, L. (2005). Wikipedia risks. *CACM, 48*, 152.

DeSanctis, G., & Poole, M. S. (1994). Capturing the Complexity in Advanced Technology Use: Adaptive Structuration Theory. *Organization Science, 5*(2), 121–147. doi:10.1287/orsc.5.2.121

Deutsch, M. (1958). Trust and suspicion. *Conflict Resolution, 2*(4), 265–279. doi:10.1177/002200275800200401

Deutsch, M. (1962). Cooperation and trust: Some theoretical notes. *Nebraska Symposium on Motivation. Nebraska Symposium on Motivation, 10*, 275–318.

Deutsch, M. (1949). An experimental study of cooperation and competition upon group process. *Human Relations, 2*, 199–231. doi:10.1177/001872674900200301

Deutsch, M. (1973). *The resolution of conflict: Constructive and destructive process*. New Haven, CT: Yale University Press.

Deutscher Bundestag. (2006). *Unfallverhütungsbericht Straßenverkehr 2004/2005*. Retrieved from www.dip.bundestag.de

Dhruva, V. N., Abdelhadi, S. I., & Anis, A. (2007). ST-Segment analysis using wireless technology in acute myocardial infarction (STAT-MI) trial. *Journal of the American College of Cardiology, 50*, 509–513. doi:10.1016/j.jacc.2007.04.049

DHSS. (2001). *Report to Congress on Telemedicine*: Secretary of Health and Human Services.

Dijkstra, B., Kamsma, Y. P. T., & Zijlstra, W. (2010). Detection of gait and postures using a miniaturized tri-axial accelerometer-based system: accuracy in community-dwelling older adults. *Age and Ageing, 39*(2), 259–262. doi:10.1093/ageing/afp249

Dijkstra, B., Zijlstra, W., Scherder, E., & Kamsma, Y. (2008). Detection of gait episodes and number of steps in older adults and patients with Parkinson's disease: accuracy of a pedometer and an accelerometry based method. *Age and Ageing, 37*(4), 436–441. doi:10.1093/ageing/afn097

DiMaggio, P. J., & Powell, W. W. (1983). The Iron Cage Revisited: Institutional Isomorphism and Collective Rationality in Organizational Fields. *American Sociological Review, 48*(2), 147–160. doi:10.2307/2095101

Dirks, K. T., Cummings, L. L., & Pierce, J. L. (1996). Psychological ownership in organizations: Conditions under which individuals promote and resist change . In Woodman, R. W., & Pasmore, A. W. (Eds.), *Research in organizational change and development* (*Vol. 9*, pp. 1–23). Greenwich, CT: JAI Press.

Dix, A., Finlay, J., Abowd, G., & Beale, R. (2003). *Human-Computer Interaction* (3rd ed.). Upper Saddle River, NJ: Prentice Hall.

Dobbs, D., Munn, J., Zimmerman, S., Boustani, M., Williams, C. S., & Sloane, P. D. (2005). Characteristics associated with lower activity involvement in long-term care residents with dementia. *The Gerontologist, 12*(1), 81–86.

Dobosiewicz, W., & Gburzynski, P. (1997). Protocol design in SMURPH. In *State of the Art in Performance Modeling and Simulation* (pp. 255-274).

Doh, M., & Kaspar, R. (2006). Entwicklung und Determinanten der Internetdiffusion bei älteren Menschen . In Hagenah, J., & Meulemann, H. (Eds.), *Sozialer Wandel und Mediennutzung in der Bundesrepublik Deutschland* (pp. 139–156). Münster, Germany: LIT.

Doney, P. & Canon, J. (1997). An examination of the nature of trust in buyer-seller relationships. *Journal of Marketing*, February, 61, 35-51.

Donggang, L., Peng, N., & Wenliang, D. (2005). Group-based key predistribution in wireless sensor networks. In *Proceedings of the 4th ACM Workshop on Wireless Security* (pp. 11-20). New York: ACM Press.

Drazin, R., Glynn, M. A., & Kazanjian, R. K. (1999). Multilevel theorizing about creativity in organizations: A sensemaking perspective. *Academy of Management. Academy of Management Review, 24*(2), 286. doi:10.2307/259083

Duberstein, P., Meldrum, S., Fiscella, K., Shields, C. G., & Epstein, R. M. (2007). Influences on patients' ratings of physicians: Physicians demographics and personality. *Patient Education and Counseling, 65*(2), 270–274. doi:10.1016/j.pec.2006.09.007

Dutertre, B., Cheung, S., & Levy, J. (2004). *Lightweight key management in wireless sensor networks by leveraging initial trust*. Technical Report SRI-SDL-04-02, SRI International.

Effken, J. (2002). Different lenses, improved outcomes: a new approach to the analysis and design of healthcare information systems. *International Journal of Medical Informatics, 65*(1), 59–74. doi:10.1016/S1386-5056(02)00003-5

Einwiller, S. (2003). When reputation engenders trust: An empirical investigation in business-to-consumer electronic commerce. *Electronic Markets*, (March): 13, 196–209.

Erder, M. H., Davidson, S. J., & Cheney, R. A. (1989). Online medical command in theory and praxis. *Annals of Emergency Medicine, 18*, 261–268. doi:10.1016/S0196-0644(89)80411-1

Erickson, E. G. (1963). *Childhood and Society*. New York: W.W. Norton.

EUA (2005). *IHE, "IT Infrastructure Technical Framework Volume 1 (ITI TF-1) Integration Profiles; Revision 2.0 - Final Text*. August 15, 2005

European Commission. (2004). *ISTAG Report on Experience and Application Research- Involving Users in the Development of Ambient Intelligence*. Luxembourg: Office for Official Publications of the European Communities.

Eveland, J. D., & Tornatzky, L. (1990). The Deployment of Technology . In In Tornatzky, L., & Fleischer, M. (Eds.), *The Processes of Technological Innovation*. Lexington: Lexington Books.

Evfimievski, A., Srikant, R., Agrawal, R., & Gehrke, J. (2002). *Privacy preserving mining of association rules*, In Proceedings of the 8th ACM SIGKDDD International Conference on Knowledge Discovery and Data Mining.

Fahn, S. (2010). Parkinson's disease: 10 years of progress, 1997-2007. *Movement Disorders, 25*(Suppl 1), 2–14. doi:10.1002/mds.22796

Falcão-Reis, F., Costa-Pereira, A., & Correia, M. E. (2008). Access and privacy rights using web security standards to increase patient empowerment. In L. Bos, B. Blobel, A. Marsh, & D. Carroll (Eds.), *Studies in Health Technology and Informatics: Vol. 137. Medical and Care Compunetics 5 (pp. 275-285)*. Netherlands: IOS Press.

Feng, J., & Potkonjak, M. (2003). Real-time watermarking techniques for sensor networks. *Proceedings of the Society for Photo-Instrumentation Engineers, 5020*(391), 391–402.

Ferraiolo, D. F., & Kuhn, D. R. (1992). Role Based Access Control. In *Proceedings of the NIST–NSA National (USA) Computer Security Conference* (pp. 554–563).

Ferreira, A., et al. (2006). How to break access control in a controlled manner. *19th IEEE International Symposium on Computer-Based Medical Systems (CBMS 2006)*, IEEE Press, 2006, pp. 847–854.

Fichman, R. G., & Kemerer, C. F. (1997). The assimilation of software process innovations: An organizational learning perspective. *Management Science, 43*(10), 1345. doi:10.1287/mnsc.43.10.1345

Fichman, R. G., & Kemerer, C. F. (1999). The illusory diffusion of innovation: An examination of assimilation gaps. *Information Systems Research, 10*(3), 255. doi:10.1287/isre.10.3.255

Fielding, R. T., & Taylor, R. N. (2002). Principled design of the modern Web architecture. *ACM Transactions on Internet Technology, 2*(2), 115–150. doi:10.1145/514183.514185

Finney, M., & Mitroff, I. I. (1986). Strategic Plans Failures: The organization as its own worst enemy. *The Thinking Organization* (317-335). San Francisco: Jossey-Bass.

Fishbein, M., & Ajzen, I. (1975). *Belief, Attitude, Intention and Behavior: An Introduction to Theory and Research.* Reading, MA: Addison-Wesley Publishing Company.

Fisk, A. D., & Rogers, W. A. (1997). *Handbook of Human Factors and the Older Adult.* San Diego, CA: Academic Press.

Fisk, M. J. (1997). Telecare equipment in the home. Issues of intrusiveness and control. *Journal of Telemedicine and Telecare, 3*(Suppl. 1), 30–32. doi:10.1258/1357633971930274

Fisk, M. J. (1998). Telecare at home: factors influencing technology choices and user acceptance. *Journal of Telemedicine and Telecare, 4*, 80–83. doi:10.1258/1357633981931993

Fleming, J., & Brayne, C. (2008). Inability to get up after falling, subsequent time on floor, and summoning help: prospective cohort study in people over 90. *British Medical Journal, 337*, a2227. doi:10.1136/bmj.a2227

Floeck, M., & Litz, L. (2008). Lange selbstbestimmt leben mit geeigneter Hausautomatisierung und einem persönlichen technischen Assistenten. *Ambient Assisted Living, 1. Deutscher Kongress mit Ausstellung,* 30.1.-1.2.2008. (pp. S. 287 – 290). Berlin.

Floeck, M., & Litz, L. (2009). Inactivity Patterns and Alarm Generation in Senior Citizens' Houses. In *Proceedings of the European Control Conference (ECC) 2009, Budapest,* 26 August 2009.

Fogg, B. & Tseng, H. (1999). The elements of computer credibility. *Proceedings of Human Factors in Computing Systems,* CHI1999, ACM, 80-87.

Fogg, B., Marshall, J., Kameda, T., Solomon, J., Rangnekar, A., Body, J., & Brown, B. (2001). Web credibility research: A method for online experiments and early study results. *Proceedings of Human Factors in Computing Systems,* CHI2001, ACM, 295-296.

Fogg, B., Marshall, J., Laraki, O., Osipovich, A., Varma, C., Fang, N., et al. (2001). What makes web sites credible? A report on a large quantitative study. *Proceedings of the Conference on Human Factors in Computing Systems* CHI 2001, ACM, 3(1), 61-8.

Fogg, B., Osipovich, A., Varma, C., Laraki, O., Fang, N., Paul, J., et al. (2000). Elements that affect web credibility: Early results form a self-reported study. *Proceedings of the 2000 Conference on Designing for User Experiences,* CHI 2000, ACM, 287-288.

Fogg, B., Soohoo, C., Danielson, D. R., Marable, L., Stanford, J., & Tauber, E. R. (2003). How do users evaluate the credibility of web sites? A study with over 2500 participants. *Proceedings of the 2003 Conference on Designing for User Experiences,* ACM, 1-15.

Fontana, R. J., & Gunderson, S. J. (2002). Ultra-wideband precision asset location system: Ultra Wideband Systems and Technologies, 2002. Digest of Papers. 2002 IEEE Conference on. *Ultra Wideband Systems and Technologies, 2002. Digest of Papers. 2002 IEEE Conference on* (pp. 147-150).

Fox, S., & Jones, S. (2009). *The social life of health information: Americans' pursuit of health takes place within a widening network of both online and offline sources.* PEW Report. Retrieved December 15, 2009 from http://www.pewInternet.org/Reports/2009/8-The-Social-Life-of-Health-Information.aspx.

Fozard, J. (2005). Impacts of technology on health and self esteem. *Gerontechnology (Valkenswaard), 4*(2), 63–76. doi:10.4017/gt.2005.04.02.002.00

Fozard, J., & Kearns, W. (2006). Persuasive GERONtechnology: Reaping Technology's Coaching Benefits at Older Age. W. In *Ijsselsteijn, Y. de Kort, C. Midden, B. Eggen, & E. van den HovenPersuasive Technology,3962* (pp. 199–202). Berlin, Heidelberg: Springer-Verlag.

Fozard, J. (2000). How ten years with ageless rats and college sophomores led to a thirty something career in geropsychology . In Birren, J. E., & Schroots, J. H. H. (Eds.), *History of Geropsychology through autobiography* (pp. 91–108). Washington, DC: American Psychological Assn. doi:10.1037/10367-008

Fozard, J. L., & Heikkinen, E. (1997). Maintaining movement ability in old age . In Graafinans, J. A. M., Taipale, V., & Charness, N. E. (Eds.), *Gerontechnology: A sustainable investment in the future* (pp. 48–61). Amsterdam: IOS Press.

Fragopoulos, A., Gialelis, J., & Serpanos, D. (2009). Security Framework for Pervasive Healthcare Architectures Utilizing MPEG-21 IPMP Components. *International Journal of Telemedicine and Applications, 2009*, 1–9. doi:10.1155/2009/461560

Friedman, M. A., Schueth, A., & Bell, D. S. (2009). Interoperable electronic prescribing in the United States: a progress report. *Health Affairs, 28*(2), 393–403. doi:10.1377/hlthaff.28.2.393

Friedman, B., Kahn, P. H., & Howe, D. C. (2000). Trust online. *Communications of the ACM, 43*(12), 34–40. doi:10.1145/355112.355120

Fromkin, H. L., & Streufert, S. (1976). Laboratory experimentation . In Dunnette, B. (Ed.), *Handbook of Industrial and Organizational Psychology* (pp. 415–465). Chicago: Rand McNally College Publishing Company.

Fruhling, A., & Lee, S. M. (2006). The Influence of User Interface Usability on Rural Consumers' Trust of e-Health Services. *International Journal of Electronic Healthcare, 2*(4), 305–321.

Gallivan, M. J. (2001). Organizational adoption and assimilation of complex technological innovations: Development and application of a new framework. *The Data Base for Advances in Information Systems, 32*(3), 51.

Ganesen, S. (1994). Determinants of long-term orientation in buyer-seller relationship. *Journal of Marketing, 58*, 1–19. doi:10.2307/1252265

Garcia-Aymerich, J., Lange, P., Benet, M., Schnohr, P., & Anto, J. M. (2006). Regular physical activity reduces hospital admission and mortality in chronic obstructive pulmonary disease: a population based cohort study. *Thorax, 61*, 772–778. doi:10.1136/thx.2006.060145

Garfinkel, H. (1963). A conception of, and experiments with, 'Trust' as a condition of stable concerted actions . In Harvey, O. J. (Ed.), *Motivation and Social Interaction: Cognitive Determinants* (pp. 187–238). New York: Ronald Press.

Gates, S., Smith, L. A., Fisher, J. D., & Lamb, S. E. (2008). Systematic review of accuracy of screening instruments for predicting fall risk among independently living older adults. *Journal of Rehabilitation Research and Development, 45*, 1105–1116. doi:10.1682/JRRD.2008.04.0057

Gattuso, S. (1996). The meaning of home for older women in rural Australia. *Australian Journal on Ageing, 4*(15), 172–176. doi:10.1111/j.1741-6612.1996.tb00024.x

Gaul, S., & Ziefle, M. (2009). Smart Home Technologies: Insights into Generation-Specific Acceptance Motives . In Holzinger, A. (Eds.), *Human – Computer Interaction for eInclusion. LNCS 5889* (pp. 312–332). Berlin, Heidelberg: Springer.

Gburzynski, P. (1995). *Protocol design for local and metropolitan area networks*. Upper Saddle River, NJ: Prentice Hall PTR.

Gburzynski, P., & Nikolaidis, I. (2006). Wireless network simulation extensions in SIDE/SMURPH. In *Proceedings of the 38th Winter Simulation Conference* (pp. 2225-2233).

Gefen, D. (2000). Ecommerce: The role of familiarity and trust. *Omega, 28*(6), 725–737. doi:10.1016/S0305-0483(00)00021-9

Gefen, D., Karahanna, E., & Straub, D. (2003a). Inexperience and experience with online stores: The importance of TAM and trust. *IEEE Transactions on Engineering Management, 50*(3), 307–321. doi:10.1109/TEM.2003.817277

Gefen, D., Karahanna, E., & Straub, D. (2003b). Trust and TAM in online shopping: an integrated model. *Management Information Systems Quarterly, 27*(1), 51–90.

Gefen, D. & Straub, D. (2003). Managing user trust in B2C e-services. *e-Service Journal*, 7-24.

Geldmacher, D. S. (2004). Donepezil (Aricept) for treatment of Alzheimer's disease and other dementing conditions. *Expert Review of Neurotherapeutics, 4*(1), 5–16. doi:10.1586/14737175.4.1.5

Gentry, C., & Silverberg, A. (2002). Hierarchical ID-based cryptography. In *Asiacrypt 2002* (LNCS, vol. 2501, pp. 149-155).Berlin: Springer Berlin / Heidelberg.

Gesundheitsberichterstattung des Bundes. (2007). *Ad-hoc-Tabellen*. Retrieved 06.03.2007 from www.gbe-bund.de

Giani, A., Roosta, T., & Sastry, S. (2008). Integrity checker for wireless sensor networks in health care applications. In *Proceedings of the 2nd International Conference on Pervasive Computing Technologies for Healthcare* (pp. 135-138).

Giannakouris, K. (2008). *Eurostat - Statistics in focus*. Population and social conditions. 72/2008: Luxemburg.

Giddens, A. (1990). *The Consequences of Modernity*. Cambridge, U.K.: Polity Press.

Giddens, A. (2005). *La Constitution de la Société: éléments de la théorie de la structuration (traduit de l'anglais par Michel Audet)*. Paris: Quadridge PUF (1ère édition).

Giffen, K. (1967). The contribution of studies of source credibility to a theory of inter-personal trust in the communications process. [February.]. *Psychological Bulletin*, *68*, 104–120. doi:10.1037/h0024833

Gineste, Y. Pellissier & Humanitude, J. (2007). *Comprendre la vieillesse, prendre soin des Hommes vieux*. Paris: Armand Colin.

Goffman, I. (1974). *Frame Analysis*. New York: Harper & Row.

Goldman, A. E., & McDonald, S. S. (1987). *The Group Depth Interview: Principles and Practice*. Upper Saddle River, NJ: Prentice Hall.

Goldreich, O., Micali, S., & Wigderson, A. (1987). How to play ANY mental game. In *Proceedings of the nineteenth annual ACM conference on Theory of computing* (pp. 218-229), New York: ACM Press.

Good, D. (1988). Individuals, interpersonal relations, and trust . In Gambetta, D. (Ed.), *Trust: Making and Breaking Cooperative Relations* (pp. 32–47). New York: Basil Blackwell.

Good, R., & Ventura, N. (2006). *A multilayered hybrid architecture to support vertical handover between ieee802.11 and umts*. In IWCMC '06: Proceedings of the 2006 international conference on Wireless communications and mobile computing(pp.257-262). New York: ACM.

Goodwin, B. J., Bender, D. J., Contreras, T. A., Fahrig, L., & Wegner, J. F. (1999). Testing for habitat detection distances using orientation data. *Oikos*, *84*(1), 160–163. doi:10.2307/3546877

Gosain, S. (2004). Enterprise Information Systems as Objects and Carriers of Institutional Forces: The New Iron Cage. *Journal of the Association for Information Systems*, *5*(4), 151–182.

Graeber, S. (1997). *The Impact of Workflow Management Systems on the Design of Hospital Information Systems*. Paper presented at the American Medical Informatics Association (AMIA) Annual Fall Symposium, Vol. 856.

Graham, G. S., & Denning, P. J. (1972). *Protection: principles and practice*. In Proceedings of AFIPS (pp. 417-429). Montvale, NJ, USA.

Grauel, J., & Spellerberg, A. (2007). Akzeptanz neuer Wohntechniken für ein selbständiges Leben im Alter – Erklärung anhand sozialstruktureller Merkmale, Technikkompetenz und Technikeinstellungen. *Zeitschrift fur Sozialreform*, *53*(2), 191–215.

Grauel, J., & Spellerberg, A. (2008). Wohnen mit Zukunft - Soziologische Begleitforschung zu Assisted Living-Projekten. In E. Maier & P. Roux (Ed.), *Seniorengerechte Schnittstellen zur Technik: Zusammenfassung der Beiträge zum Usability Day VI, 16. Mai 2008* (pp. 36-43). Lengerich: Pabst Science Publishers.

Grauel, J., Spellerberg, A., Leschke, B., & Schelisch, L. (2008). Acceptance of Assisted Living Solutions. In R. Anderl, B. Arich-Gerz & R. Schmiede (Ed.), *Technologies of Globalization. Intenational Conference*. October 2008 (pp. 328-343). Darmstadt.

Grayson, J. P. (1997). Technology and home adaptations. Landspery S, & Hyde J (Eds), *Staying put: Adapting the places instead of the people* (pp. 55-74). Amityville, NY: Baywood.

Grazioli, S., & Jarvenpaa, S. L. (2000). Perils of Internet fraud: An empirical investigation of deception and trust with experienced Internet consumers. *IEEE Transactions on Systems, Man, and Cybernetics*, *30*(4), 395–410. doi:10.1109/3468.852434

Greenbaum, T. L. (1988). *The Practical Handbook and Guide to Focus Group Research*. Lexington, MA: D.C. Heath & Co.

Gregory, K. L. (1983). Native-View Paradigms: Multiple ultures and culture conflicts in organization. *Administrative Science Quarterly*, *28*(3), 359–376. doi:10.2307/2392247

Grémy, F., & Bonnin, M. (1995). Evaluation of Automatic Health Informations Systems. What and How? E. In Van Gennip, et J. Talmon (Eds.), *Assessment and Evaluation of Information Technologies in Medicine*. Amsterdam: IOS Press.

Greytak, M. (2005). *Numerical potential field path planning tutorial*. Retrieved January 4, 2010, from http://ocw.mit.edu/NR/rdonlyres/Aeronautics-and-Astronautics/16-410Fall-2005/E6469924-5AE3-41C0-AA36-145D20739B7E/0/greytak.pdf

Gries, A., Helm, M., & Martin, E. (2003). Zukunft der präklinischen Notfallmedizin in Deutschland. *Der Anaesthesist*, *52*, 718–724. doi:10.1007/s00101-003-0548-1

Grigsby, J., Schlenker, R., Kaehny, M. M., Shaughnessy, P. W., & Sandberg, E. J. (1995). Analytic framework for evaluation of telemedicine. *Telemedicine Journal, 1*(1), 31–39.

Großschadl, J. (2006). TinySA: A security architecture for wireless sensor networks. In *Proceedings of the 2nd International Conference on Emerging Networking Experiments and Technologies*.

Gruber-Baldini, A. L., Zimmerman, S., Boustani, M., Watson, L. C., Williams, C. S., & Reed, P. S. (2005). Characteristics associated with depression in long-term care residents with dementia. *The Gerontologist, 45*(1), 50–55.

Gulliksen, J., Goransson, B., Boivie, I., Blomkvist, S., Persson, J., & Cajander, A. (2003). Key Principles for User-centred Systems Design. *Behaviour & Information Technology, 22*(6), 397–410. doi:10.1080/0144929031 0001624329

Gummerus, J., & Liljander, V. (2004). Customer loyalty to content-based Web sites: The case of an online health-care service. *Journal of Services Marketing, 18*(2/3), 175–186. doi:10.1108/08876040410536486

Hackman, J. R., & Oldham, G. R. (1975). Development of the Job Diagnostic Survey. *The Journal of Applied Psychology, 60*(2), 159–170. doi:10.1037/h0076546

Hadim, S., & Mohamed, N. (2006). Middleware Challenges and Approaches for Wireless Sensor Networks. *IEEE Distributed Systems Online, 7*.

Halamka, J., Juels, A., Stubblefield, A., & Westhues, J. (2006). The Security Implications of VeriChip Cloning. *Journal of the American Medical Informatics Association, 13*(6), 601–607. doi:10.1197/jamia.M2143

Hall, G., & Loucks, S. (1977). A developmentla Model for Determining Wether the Treatment is Actually Implemented. *American Educational Research Journal, 14*(3), 263–276.

Halperin, D., Heydt-Benjamin, T. S., Fu, K., Kohno, T., & Maisel, W. H. (2008). Security and Privacy for Implantable Medical Devices. *IEEE Pervasive Computing / IEEE Computer Society [and] IEEE Communications Society, 7*(1), 30–39. doi:10.1109/MPRV.2008.16

Halperin, D., Heydt-Benjamin, T. S., Ransford, B., Clark, S. S., Defend, B., Morgan, W., et al. (2008). Pacemakers and Implantable Cardiac Defibrillators: Software Radio Attacks and Zero-Power Defenses. In *Proceedings of IEEE Symposium on Security and Privacy* (pp. 129-142).

Hamill, M., Young, V., Boger, J., & Mihailidis, A. (2009). Development of an automated speech recognition interface for Personal Emergency Response Systems. *Journal of Neuroengineering and Rehabilitation, 6*, 26. doi:10.1186/1743-0003-6-26

Harre, R., & Madden, E. H. (1975). *Causal Powers: A Theory of Natural Necessity*. Oxford: Blackwell.

Harris, L. C., & Goode, M. M. H. (2004). The four levels of loyalty and the pivotal role of trust: A study of online service dynamics. *Journal of Retailing, 80*, 139–158. doi:10.1016/j.jretai.2004.04.002

Hartwick, J., & Barki, H. (1994). Explaining the Role of User Participation in Information System Use. *Management Science, 40*, 440–465. doi:10.1287/mnsc.40.4.440

Harvey, N., Zhou, Z., Keller, J. M., Rantz, M., & He, Z. (2009). Automated estimation of elder activity levels from anonymized video data. *Conference Proceedings; ... Annual International Conference of the IEEE Engineering in Medicine and Biology Society. IEEE Engineering in Medicine and Biology Society. Conference, 1*, 7236–7239.

Haskell, W. L., Lee, I. M., Pate, R. R., Powell, K. E., Blair, S. N., & Franklin, B. A. (2007). Physical activity and public health: updated recommendation for adults from the American College of Sports Medicine and the American Heart Association. *Medicine and Science in Sports and Exercise, 39*, 1423–1434. doi:10.1249/mss.0b013e3180616b27

Hauber, J., Regenbrecht, H., Billinghurst, M., & Cockburn, A. (2006). Spatiality in videoconferencing: tradeoffs between efficiency and social presence. In CSCW '06: *Proceedings of the 20th anniversary conference on computer supported cooperative work* (pp. 413–422). New York: ACM.

Hauer, K., Lamb, S. E., Jorstad, E. C., Todd, C., & Becker, C. (2006). PROFANE-Group. Systematic review of definitions and methods of measuring falls in randomised controlled fall prevention trials. *Age and Ageing, 35*, 5–10. doi:10.1093/ageing/afi218

Hausdorff, J., Rios, D., & Edelberg, H. (2001). Gait variability and fall risk in community-living older adults: A 1-year prospective study. *Archives of Physical Medicine and Rehabilitation, 82*(8), 1050–1056. doi:10.1053/apmr.2001.24893

Hausdorff, J. M., Ashkenazy, Y., Peng, C. K., Ivanov, P. C., Stanley, H. E., & Goldberger, A. L. (2001). When human walking becomes random walking: fractal analysis and modeling of gait rhythm fluctuations. *Physica A, 302*(1-4), 138–147. doi:10.1016/S0378-4371(01)00460-5

Hausdorff, J. M., Edelberg, H. K., Mitchell, S. L., Goldberger, A. L., & Wei, J. Y. (1997). Increased gait unsteadiness in community-dwelling elderly fallers. *Archives of Physical Medicine and Rehabilitation, 78*, 278–283. doi:10.1016/S0003-9993(97)90034-4

Hausdorff, J. M., Ladin, Z., & Wei, J. Y. (1995). Footswitch system for measurement of the temporal parameters of gait. *Biometrical Journal. Biometrische Zeitschrift, 28*(3), 347–351.

Haynes, R. B., Ackloo, E., Sahota, N., McDonald, H. P., & Yao, X. (2008). Interventions for enhancing medication adherence. *Cochrane Database of Systematic Reviews, 2*, CD000011. doi:.doi:10.1002/14651858.CD000011.pub3

Heinrich, S., Rapp, K., Rissmann, U., Becker, C., & König, H. H. (2009). Cost of falls in old age: a systematic review. [Epub ahead of print]. *Osteoporosis International*, (Nov): 19.

Helal, S., Mann, W. C., El-Zabadani, H., King, J., Kaddoura, Y., & Jansen, E. (2005). The Gator Tech Smart House: A programmable pervasive space. *IEEE Computer, 38*(3), 50–60.

Helbostad, J. L., & Moe-Nilssen, R. (2003). The effect of gait speed on lateral balance control during walking in healthy elderly. *Gait & Posture, 18*(2), 27–36. doi:10.1016/S0966-6362(02)00197-2

Henderson, V. W., Mack, W., & Williams, B. W. (1989). Spatial disorientation in Alzheimer's disease. *Archives of Neurology, 46*(4), 391–394.

Hensel, B. K., Demiris, G., & Courtney, K. L. (2006). Defining obtrusiveness in home telehealth technologies: a conceptual framework. *Journal of the American Medical Informatics Association, 13*, 428–431. doi:10.1197/jamia.M2026

Hermens, H. J., & Vollenbroek-Hutten, M. M. (2008). Towards remote monitoring and remotely supervised training. *Journal of Electromyography and Kinesiology, 18*(6), 908–919. doi:10.1016/j.jelekin.2008.10.004

Hickey, J. (2010). Caring for the Patient with Cerebrovascular Disorders . In Osborn, K., Wraa, C., & Watson, A. (Eds.), *Medical Surgical Nursing*. Boston: Pearson.

Hillman, C.H., & Erickson, K.I., Kramer, & A.F. (2008). Be smart, exercise your heart: exercise effects on brain and cognition. *Nature Reviews. Neuroscience, 9*(1), 58–65. doi:10.1038/nrn2298

HIMSS. (2003). *EHR Definition, Attributes and Essential Requirements*. Retrieved from: http://www.himss.org/content/files/EHRAttributes.pdf.

Hirschheim, R. A. (1985). User Experience with and Assessment of Participative Systems Design. *Management Information Systems Quarterly, 9*(3), 295–304. doi:10.2307/249230

Hitt, G., & Adam, J. (2009, December 25). Senate passes sweeping health-care bill. *Wall Street Journal*. Retrieved January 5, 2010, from http://online.wsj.com/article/SB126165317923104141.html.

HL-7. (2007). Retrieved from http://www.hl7.org.

Hoehn, M. M., & Yahr, M. D. (2001). Parkinsonism: onset, progression, and mortality. 1967. *Neurology, 57*(10Suppl 3), S11–S26.

Hong, T. (2006). The influence of structural ad message features on web site credibility. [January.]. *Journal of the American Society for Information Science and Technology, 57*, 114–127. doi:10.1002/asi.20258

Hori, T. Nishida, Y. Aizawa, H. Murakami, S., & Mizoguchi, H. (2004). Sensor network for supporting elderly care home. In *Proceedings of IEEE Sensors: Vol. 2* (pp. 575-578).

Hori, T., Nishida, Y., & Murakami, S. (2006). Pervasive sensor system for evidence-based nursing care support. In *ICRA '06: Proceedings of the IEEE International Conference on Robotics and Automation* (pp. 1680-1685).

Houghton, D., Hurtig, H., & Brandabur, M. (2008). *Parkinson's Disease: Medications*. Miami, Florida: Parkinson's Disease Foundation.

Hu, Y.-C., Perrig, A., & Johnson, D. B. (2002). Ariadne: a secure on-demand routing protocol for ad hoc networks. *Wireless Networks, 11*(1-2), 21–38. doi:10.1007/s11276-004-4744-y

Hu, P., & Chau, P. (1999). Physician acceptance of telemedicine technology: an empirical investigation. *Topics in Health Information Management, 19*(4), 20–35.

Hu, P. J., Chau, P. Y. K., & Sheng, O. L. (2000). Investigation of factors affecting healthcare organization's adoption of telemedicine technology. *Proceedings of the 33rd Hawaii International Conference on System Sciences*.

Hu, P. J.-H., Wei, C.-P., & Cheng, T.-H. (2002). Investigating Telemedicine Developments in Taiwan: Implications for Telemedicine Program. *Proceedings of the 35th Hawaii International Conference on System Sciences*.

Hu, Y.-C., Johnson, D. B., & Perrig, A. (2002). SEAD: secure efficient distance vector routing for mobile wireless ad hoc networks. In *Proceedings of the 4th IEEE Workshop on Mobile Computing Systems and Applications* (pp. 3–13).

Huang, J., Boers, N. M., Stroulia, E., Gburzynski, P., & Nikolaidis, I. (2010). SensorGIS: An integrated architecture for information systems based on sensor networks. In *WEBIST '10: Proceedings of the 6th International Conference on Web Information Systems and Technologies*.

Hurley, B. F., Hanson, E. D., & Sheaff, A. K. (in press). Strength Training as a Countermeasure to Age Related Disease. *Sports Medicine (Auckland, N.Z.)*.

Huxham, F. E., Goldie, P. A., & Patla, A. E. (2001). Theoretical considerations in balance assessment. *The Australian Journal of Physiotherapy*, *47*, 89–100.

Ibraimi, L., Asim, M., & Petkovic, M. (2009). *Secure Management of Personal Health Records by Applying Attribute-Based Encryption*. Centre for Telematics and Information Technology, University of Twente.

Ibraimi, L., Petkovic, M., Nikova, S., Hartel, P., & Jonker, W. (2009). Mediated Ciphertext-Policy Attribute-Based Encryption and Its Application. In *Information Security Applications: 10th International Workshop-WISA* (pp. 309-323), Springer-Verlag.

Ibraimi, L., Tang, Q., & Hartel, P. Jonker. W. (2009). Efficient and provable secure ciphertext-policy attribute-based encryption schemes. In *Proceedings of Information Security Practice and Experience* (pp. 1-12), vol. 5451 of *LNCS*, Springer.

IHE. (2005). *IHE IT Infrastructure, Technical Framework, Volume 3 – Document Content Profiles*. Retrieved December 20, 2009, from: http://www.ihe.net/Technical_Framework/upload/IHE_ITI_TF-Supplement_Digital_Signature-TI_2005-08-15.pdf.

Ihgb, Ramakers, Visser, P. J., Aalten, P., Boesten, J. H. M., Metsemakers, J. F. M., Jolles, J. et al. (2007). Symptoms of Preclinical Dementia in General Practice up to Five Years Before Dementia Diagnosis. *Dementia and Geriatric Cognitive Disorders*, *24*(4), 300–306. doi:10.1159/000107594

Illich, I. (1973). *Tools for conviviality*. New York: Harper and Row.

Impicciatore, P., Pandolfini, C., Casella, N., & Bonzti, M. (1997). Reliability of health information for the public on the World Wide Web: Systematic survey of advice on managing fever in children at home. *British Medical Journal*, *314*, 1875–1881.

InfoWay. (2007). Retrieved from http://www.infoway-inforoute.ca.

Institute of Medicine. Workshop Proceedings. *Health literacy, eHealth, and communication: Putting the consumer first*. (March 24, 2009). Retrieved January 6, 2010, from http://www.iom.edu/Reports/2009/Health-Literacy-eHealth-and-Communication-utting-the-Consumer-First-Workshop-Summary.aspx.

International Classification of Functioning. Disability and Health (ICF). (n.d.). *World Health Organisation, Geneva*. Retrieved from www.who.int/classification/icf.

International Organization for Standardization. ISO/*FDIS 9241-110. Ergonomics of human-system interaction -- Part 110: Dialogue principles*. International Organization for Standardization. ISO/*FDIS 9241-210. Ergonomics of human-system interaction -- Part 210: Human-centred design for interactive systems*. Retrieved December 28, 2009, from http://www.iso.org/iso/catalogue_detail.htm?csnumber=52075.

Iren, S., Amer, P. D., & Conrad, P. T. (1999). The transport layer: tutorial and survey. *ACM Computing Surveys*, *31*(4), 360–404. doi:10.1145/344588.344609

Isaacs, S. (1933). *Social Development in Young Children*. London: Routledge and Kegan Paul.

ISO 21298 (2007). *ISO/TC 215/WG 4, ISO TS 21298 Health Informatics - Functional and structural roles*.

ISO 22600 (2007). *ISO/TC 215/WG 4, ISO/IS 22600 Privilege management and access control*.

Iwarsson, S. (2003). Assessing the fit between older people and their physical home environments: An occupational therapy research perspective. In Wahl WE, Scheidt RJ, & Windley PG (Eds), *Annual Review of Gerontology and Geriatrics. Focus on aging in context: socio-physical environments* (Vol. 23pp. 85-109). New York: Springer.

Jajodia, S., & Sandhu, R. (1991). Toward a multilevel secure relational data model. *In Proceedings of the ACM SIGMOD Conference on Management of Data* (pp. 50-59). Denver, CO, USA.

Jarvenpaa, S., Tractinsky, N., & Vitale, M. (2000). Consumer trust in Internet store. *Information Technology Management*, *1*(1-2), 45–71. doi:10.1023/A:1019104520776

Jarvenpaa, S. L., Tractinsky, N., & Saarinen, L. (1999). Consumer trust in an Internet store: A cross-cultural validation. *Journal of Computer-Mediated Communication 5*(2). Retrieved on March 3, 2010 at http://www.ascusc.org/jcmc/vol5/issue2.

Jeffcott, M. (2001, September) *Technology Alone Will Never Work: Understanding How Organisational Issues Contribute to User Neglect and Information Systems Failure in Healthcare*. Paper presented at the IT in Healthcare: Sociotechnical Approaches International Conference, Rotterdam, The Netherlands.

Jemmet, M. E., Kendal, K. M., Fourre, M. W., & Burton, J. H. (2003). Unrecognized misplacement of endotracheal tubes in a mixed urban to rural emergency medical services setting. *Academic Emergency Medicine, 10*, 961–965. doi:10.1111/j.1553-2712.2003.tb00652.x

Jenkins, C., Corritore, C., & Wiedenbeck, S. (2003). Patterns of information seeking on the web: A qualitative study of domain expertise and web expertise. *Information Technology & Society, 1*(3), 64–89.

Jensen, J., Nyberg, L., Gustafson, Y., & Lundin-Olsson, L. (2003). Fall and injury prevention in residential care--effects in residents with higher and lower levels of cognition. *Journal of the American Geriatrics Society, 51*(5), 627–635. doi:10.1034/j.1600-0579.2003.00206.x

Johnson, K., & Wiedenbeck, S. (2009). Enhancing perceived credibility of citizen journalism web sites. *Journalism & Mass Communication Quarterly, 86*(2), 332–348.

Johnson, D. K., Storandt, M., Morris, J. C., & Galvin, J. E. (2009). Longitudinal Study of the Transition From Healthy Aging to Alzheimer Disease. *Archives of Neurology, 66*(10), 1254–1259. doi:10.1001/archneurol.2009.158

Johnson-George, C., & Swap, W. (1982). Measurement of specific interpersonal trust: Construction and validation of a scale to assess trust in a specific other. *Journal of Personality and Social Psychology, 43*(6), 1306–1317. doi:10.1037/0022-3514.43.6.1306

Jones, M. C., & Beatty, R. C. (1998). Towards the development of measures of perceived benefits and compatibility of EDI: a comparative assessment of competing first order factor models. *European Journal of Information Systems, 7*(3), 210–220. doi:10.1057/palgrave.ejis.3000299

Jones, J. H., Murphy, M. P., & Dickson, R. L. (2004). Emergency physician-verified out-of-hospital intubation: miss rates by paramedics. *Academic Emergency Medicine, 11*, 707–709.

Joshi, A., Finin, T., Kagal, L., Parker, J., & Patwardhan, A. (2008) Security policies and trust in ubiquitous computing. *Philosophical Transactions of the Royal Society A: Mathematical, Physical and Engineering Sciences, 366*(1881), 3769-3780.

Kahn, W. A. (1990). Psychological Conditions of Personal Engagement and Disengagement at Work. *Academy of Management Journal, 33*(4), 692. doi:10.2307/256287

Kanai, H., Nakada, T., Hanbat, Y., & Kunifuji, S. (2008). A support system for context awareness in a group home using sound cues. In *PervasiveHealth '08: Second International Conference on Pervasive Computing Technologies for Healthcare* (pp. 264-267).

Kangas, M., Konttila, A., Lindgren, P., Winblad, I., & Jämsä, T. (2008). Comparison of low-complexity fall detection algorithms for body attached accelerometers. *Gait & Posture, 28*(2), 285–291. doi:10.1016/j.gaitpost.2008.01.003

Kao, A., Gree, D., Zaslavsky, A., Koplan, J., & Cleary, P. (1998). The relationship between method of physician payment and patient trust. *Journal of the American Medical Association, 280*, 1708–1715. doi:10.1001/jama.280.19.1708

Karantonis, D. M., Narayanan, M. R., Mathie, M., Lovell, N. H., & Celler, B. G. (2006). Implementation of a real-time human movement classifier using a triaxial accelerometer for ambulatory monitoring. *IEEE Transactions on Information Technology in Biomedicine, 10*(1), 156–167. doi:10.1109/TITB.2005.856864

Karl, H., & Willing, A. (2005). *Protocols and Architectures for Wireless Sensor Networks*. West Sussex, England: John Willy & Sons. doi:10.1002/0470095121

Karlof, C., & Wagner, D. (2003). Secure routing in wireless sensor networks: attacks and countermeasures. *Ad Hoc Networking, 1*(2-3), 293–315. doi:10.1016/S1570-8705(03)00008-8

Karlof, C., Sastry, N., & Wagner, D. (2004). TinySec: A link layer security architecture for wireless sensor networks. In *Proceedings of the 2nd ACM Conference on Embedded Networked Sensor Systems* (162–175).

Kasugai, K., Ziefle, M., Röcker, C., & Russell, P. (2010). Creating spatio-temporal contiguities between real and virtual rooms in an assistive living environment . In Bonner, J., Smyth, M., O'Neill, S., & Mival, O. (Eds.), *Proceedings of create 10* (pp. 62–67). Loughborough, UK: Institute of Ergonomics & Human Factors.

Katsikas, S., Lopez, J., & Pernul, G. (2008). The challenge for security and privacy services in distributed health settings. In B. Blobel, P. Pharow, & M. Nerlich (Eds.), *Studies in Health Technology and Informatics: Vol. 134. eHealth: Combining Health Telematics, Telemedicine, Biomedical Engineering and Bioinformatics to the Edge-Global Experts Summit Textbook* (pp. 113-125). Netherlands: IOS Press.

Katz, S. H., & Falk, J. L. (2001). Misplaced endotracheal tubes by paramedics in an urban emergency medical services system. *Annals of Emergency Medicine, 37*, 32–37. doi:10.1067/mem.2001.112098

Katzenbeisser, S., & Petkovic, M. (2008). *Privacy-preserving recommendation systems for consumer healthcare services ARES 2008* (pp. 889–895). Washington, DC: IEEE Computer Society Press.

Kayworth, T. R., Chatterjee, D., & Sambamurthy, V. (2001). Theoretical justification for IT infrastructure investments. *Information Resources Management Journal, 14*(3), 5.

Kearns, W., Algase, D., Moore, D., & Ahmed, S. (2008). Ultra wideband radio: A novel method for measuring wandering in persons with dementia. *Gerontechnology (Valkenswaard), 7*(1), 48–57. doi:10.4017/gt.2008.07.01.005.00

Kearns, W., & Fozard, J. L. (2009). Evaluation of Wandering by Residents in an Assisted Living Facility (ALF) using Ultra Wideband Radio RTLS. *The Journal of Nutrition, Health & Aging, 13*, S54.

Kearns, W., & Moore, D. (2008). RFID: A tool for measuring wandering in persons with dementia. A. Mihailidis, J. Boger, H. Kautz, & L. Normie (Eds.), *Technology and Aging: Selected Papers from the 2007 International Conference on Technology and Aging* (Vol. 21pp. 154-164). Amsterdam: IOS Press.

Kee, H., & Knox, R. (1970). Conceptual and methodological considerations in the study of trust and suspicion. *Conflict Resolution, 14*(3), 357–366. doi:10.1177/002200277001400307

Keen, P., & McDonald, M. (2000). *The eProcess Edge: Creating Customer Value and Business Wealth in Internet Era*. Berkeley, CA: McGraw Hill.

Kenny, R. (2005). Mobility and Falls . In Johnson, M., Bengston, V., Coleman, P., & Kirkwood, T. (Eds.), *The Cambridge Handbook of Age and Ageing* (pp. 131–134). Cambridge, UK: Cambridge University Press. doi:10.1017/CBO9780511610714.012

Kettelhut, M. C. (1993). JAD Methodology and Group Dynamics. *Information Systems Management, 10*, 46–53. doi:10.1080/10580539308906912

Kientz, J. A., Patel, S. N., Jones, B., Price, E., Mynatt, E. D., & Abowd, G. D. (2008). The Georgia Tech Aware Home. In *CHI '08: Extended Abstracts on Human Factors in Computing Systems* (pp. 3675-3680).

Kientz, J. A., Patel, S. N., Tyebkhan, A. Z., Gane, B., Wiley, J., & Abowd, G. D. (2006). Where's my stuff?: Design and evaluation of a mobile system for locating lost items for the visually impaired. In *ASSETS '06: Proceedings of the 8th International ACM SIGACCESS Conference on Computers and Accessibility* (pp. 103-110).

Kim, D. J., & Ferrin, D. L. (2009). Trust and satisfaction, two stepping stones for successful ecommerce relationships: A longitudinal exploration. *Information Systems Research, 20*(2), 237–257. doi:10.1287/isre.1080.0188

Kim, H., Xu, Y., & Koh, J. (2004). A comparison of online trust building factors between potential customers and repeat customers. *Journal of the Association for Information Systems*, (October): 5, 392–420.

Kim, J., & Moon, J. Y. (1998). Designing towards emotional usability in customer interfaces-trustworthiness of cyber-banking system interfaces. *Interacting with Computers, 10*(1), 1–29. doi:10.1016/S0953-5438(97)00037-4

Kim, S., & Stoel, L. (2004). Apparel retailers: Website quality dimensions and satisfaction . *Journal of Retailing and Consumer Services, 11*(2), 109–117. doi:10.1016/S0969-6989(03)00010-9

Kim, D. J., Song, Y., Braynov, S. B., & Rao, H. R. (2001). A B-to-C trust model for on-line exchange. *Proceedings for the Seventh Americas Conference on Information Systems*, 784-787.

Kim, Y. (2004). *Pedagogical agents as learning companions: the effects of agent affect and gender on student learning, interest, self-efficacy, and agent persona*. PhD thesis, Tallahassee, USA.

King, W. R., & Lee, T. H. (1991, January). *The Effects of User Participation on System Success: Toward a Contingency Theory of User Satisfaction*. Paper presented at the 12th International Conference on Information Systems, New York, USA.

Kisely, S. (2002). Treatments for chronic fatigue syndrome and the Internet: a systematic survey of what your patients are reading. *The Australian and New Zealand Journal of Psychiatry, 36*, 240–245. doi:10.1046/j.1440-1614.2002.01017.x

Klack, L., Kasugai, K., Schmitz-Rode, T., Röcker, C., Ziefle, M., Möllering, C., et al. (2010). A Personal Assistance System for Older Users with Chronic Heart Diseases. In: *Proceedings of the Third Ambient Assisted Living Conference (AAL'10)*. Berlin, Germany: VDE (CD-ROM).

Klack, L., Möllering, C., Ziefle, M., & Schmitz-Rode, T. (2010). Future Care Floor: A sensitive floor for movement monitoring and fall detection in home environments, *1st International ICST Conference on Wireless Mobile Communication and Healthcare* - MobiHealth 2010.

Klecun-Dabrowska, E., & Cornford, T. (2002). *The Organizing Vision of Telehealth*. Gdansk, Poland: ECIS.

Klein, H. K., & Myers, M. D. (1999). A set of principles for conducting and evaluating interpretive field studies in information systems. *Management Information Systems Quarterly, 23*(1), 67–93. doi:10.2307/249410

Klein, K. J., Dansereau, F., & Hall, R. J. (1994). Levels issues in theory development, data collection, and analysis. *Academy of Management. Academy of Management Review, 19*(2), 195. doi:10.2307/258703

Kleinberger, T., Becker, M., Ras, E., Holzinger, A., & Müller, P. (2007). Ambient intelligence in assisted living: Enable elderly people to handle future interfaces. In *Lecture Notes in Computer Science: Vol. 4555/2007. Universal Access in Human-Computer Interaction. Ambient Interaction* (pp. 103-112). Germany: Springer Verlag.

Kling, R., & Iacono, C. (1989). The Institutional Character of Computerized Information System. *Office Technology & People, 1*(1), 24–43.

Kling, R. (1987). Defining the Boundaries of Computing Accross Complex Organizations . In Bolland, R., & Hirscheim, R. A. (Eds.), *Critical Issues in Information Systems Research*. London: John Wiley.

Kling, R., & Dutton, W. H. (1982). The computer package, dynamic complexity. In J. N. Danziger, D. W. H., R. Kling,& K. L. Kraemer (eds) *Computers and Politics: High Technolgy in American Local Governments*. (p.22-50). New York: Columbia University Press.

Kling, R., & Scacchi, W. (1982). The Web of Computing: Computer technology as Social Organization. *Advances in Computers*, (21), 1-90.

Koda, T., & Maes, P. (1996). Agents with faces: The effects of personification of agents. *5th IEEE International Workshop on Robot and Human Communication*, Tsukuba, Japan.

Koehn, D. (2003). The nature of and conditions for online trust. *Journal of Business Ethics, 43*, 3–19. doi:10.1023/A:1022950813386

Kohl, J., & Neuman, C. (1993). *RFC 1510: The Kerberos network authentication service (v5)*. Citeseer.

Kollmann, T. (1998). *Akzeptanz innovativer Nutzungsgüter und -systeme*. Wiesbaden, Germany: Gabler.

Konstantas, D., Jones, V., & Herzog, R. (2002) Mobi-Health-Innovative 2.5/3G mobile services and applications for health care. In *Proceedings of the IST Mobile and Wireless Telecommunications Summit*.

Korupp, S., & Szydlik, M. (2005). Causes and Trends of the Digital Divide. *European Sociological Review, 4*, 409–422. doi:10.1093/esr/jci030

Kostova, T. (1998). Quality of inter-unit relationships in MNEs as a source of competitive advantage. M. Hitt, J. Ricart, & R. Nixon (Eds.), *New Managerial Mindsets: Organizational transformation and strategy implementation*. Chichester, UK: Wiley.

Kotonya, G., & Sommerville, I. (1998). *Requirements Engineering - Processes and Techniques*. Chichester, UK: John Wiley & Sons Inc.

Koufi, V., & Vassilacopoulos, G. (2008). *HDGPortal: A Grid Portal Application for Pervasive Access to Process-Based Healthcare Systems*. Paper presented at the 2nd International Conference in Pervasive Computing Technologies in Healthcare (PervasiveHealth'08), Tampere, Finland.

Kozlowski, S. W. J., & Hults, B. M. (1987). An Exploration of Climates for Technical Updating and Performance. *Personnel Psychology, 40*, 539–563. doi:10.1111/j.1744-6570.1987.tb00614.x

Kozlowski, S. W. J., & Klein, J. K. (2000). A Multilevel Approach to Theory and Research in Organizations: Contextual, Temporal, and Emergent Process. In J. K. Klein, & S. W. J. Kozlowski (eds.), *Multilevel Theory, Research, and Methods in Organizations* (3-90). San Francisco: Jossey-Bass.

Kramer, A. F., Erickson, K. I., & Colcombe, S. J. (2006). Exercise, cognition, and the aging brain. *Journal of Applied Physiology, 101*(4), 1237–1242. doi:10.1152/japplphysiol.00500.2006

Krontiris, I., & Dimitriou, T. (2006). Authenticated in-network programming for wireless sensor networks. In *Proceedings of the 5th International Conference on AD-HOC Networks & Wireless* (pp. 390-403).

Krontiris, I., Dimitriou, T., & Giannetsos, T. (2008). LIDeA: A distributed lightweight intrusion detection architecture for sensor networks. In *Proceeding of the fourth International Conference on Security and Privacy for Communication*.

Krotish, D., Mitchell, P., Hirth, V., & Shin, Y. J. (2010). The use of time-frequency analysis using electromyography and foot pressure distribution for the determination of gait disorders. *Proceedings of the 3rd International Congress on Gait & Mental Functions: The Interplay Between Walking, Behavior and Cognition.* Geneva: Kenes.

Kubitschke, L., & Meyer, I. (2007). WING - Watching IST Innovation and Knowledge. *Impact Analysis in the Domain of eInclusion – Final Report.* Bonn, Brussels.

Kubzansky, P. E., & Druskat, V. U. (1993). Psychological sense of ownership in the workplace: Conceptualisation and measurement. *Paper Presented at the Annual Meeting of the American Psychological Association, Toronto, Canada.*

Kueng, P. (1998). *Impact of Workflow Systems on People, Task, and Structure: a Post-implementation Evaluation.* In A. Brown, D. Remenyi (Eds), *Proceedings of the Fifth European Conference on the Evaluation of Information Technology* (pp. 67-75) Reading University, UK.

Künzi, J., Koster, P., & Petkovic, M. (2009). Emergency Access to Protected Health Records . In Adlassnig, K.-P. (Eds.), *Medical Informatics in a United and Healthy Europe, MIE 2009* (pp. 705–709). IOS Press.

Kwon, T. H. (1987). *A Study of the Influence of Communication Network on MIS Institutionalization.* Unpublished doctoral dissertation, The University of North Carolina at Chapel Hill, United States -- North Carolina.

Lamb, S. E., McCabe, C., Becker, C., Fried, L. P., & Guralnik, J. M. (2008). The optimal sequence and selection of screening test items to predict fall risk in older disabled women: the Women's Health and Aging Study. *The Journals of Gerontology. Series A, Biological Sciences and Medical Sciences, 63*(10), 1082–1088.

Lamm, R., & Lamm, E. (2008). *Aging and Technology. Dagstuhl Seminar on Assisted Living Systems.* LZI.

Land, F. F., & Hirschheim, R. A. (1983). Participative Systems Design: Rationale, Tools, and Techniques. *Journal of Applied Systems Analysis, 10,* 327–338.

Larzelere, R. E., & Huston, T. L. (1980). The dyadic trust scale: Toward understanding interpersonal trust in close relationships. *Journal of Marriage and the Family,* (Aug): 595–604. doi:10.2307/351903

Latour, B. (1992). The sociology of a few mundane artifacts. B. In Bijker, and J. Law (eds.), *Shaping Technology/ Building Society Studies in Sociotechnological Change* (135-150). Cambridge, MA: MIT Press.

Lau, G. T., & Sook, H. L. (1999). Consumers' trust in a brand and the link to brand loyalty. *Journal of Market Focused Management, 4,* 341–370. doi:10.1023/A:1009886520142

Lauer, G. (2009). *Health Record Banks Gaining Traction in Regional Projects.* Retrieved December 15, 2009, from http://www.ihealthbeat.org/features/2009/health-record-banks-gaining-traction-in-regional-projects.aspx

Lauriol, J. (1998). Les représentations sociales dans la décision. In H.Laroche, et J-P. Nioche (dir.), *Repenser la stratégie.* France: Vuibert.

Lee, J., & Moray, N. (1992). Trust, control strategies and allocation of function in human-machine systems. *Ergonomics, 35*(10), 1243–1270. doi:10.1080/00140139208967392

Lee, M. K. O., & Turban, E. (2001). A trust model for consumer Internet shopping. *International Journal of Electronic Commerce, 6*(1), 75–91.

Lee, J., Kim, J. & Moon, J. (2000). What makes Internet users visit cyber stores again? Key design factors for customer loyalty. *Proceedings of Human Factors in Computing Systems,* CHI2000, ACM, 305-312.

Leonard-Barton, D. (1988). Implementation as mutual adaptation of technology and organization. *Research Policy, 17*(5), 251–267. doi:10.1016/0048-7333(88)90006-6

Leonhardt, S. (2005). Personal Healthcare Devices. In S. Mekherjee et al. (Eds.), *Malware: Hardware Technology Drivers of AI* (pp. 349-370). Dordrecht, NL: Springer.

Levis, P., Madden, S., Polastre, J., Szewczyk, R., Whitehouse, K., Woo, A., & Gay, D. Hill, J., Welsh, M., Brewer, E., & Culler D. (2005). TinyOS: An operating system for sensor networks. In *Ambient Intelligence* (pp. 115-148). The Netherlands: Springer Verlag.

Lewicki, R. J., & Bunker, B. (1996). Developing and maintaining trust in work relationships . In Kramer, R., & Tyler, T. (Eds.), *Trust in Organizations: Frontiers of Theory and Research* (pp. 114–139). Newbury Park, CA: Sage.

Lewicki, R. J., & Bunker, B. B. (1995). Trust in relationships: A model of development and decline. In B.B. Bunker & J.Z. Rubin (Eds.), *Conflict, Cooperation, and Justice: Essays Inspired by the Work of Morton Deutsch* (pp. 133-173). San Fransisco: Jossey-Bass.

Lewin, K. (1947). Frontiers in Group Dynamics: Concept, Method and Reality in Social Science; Social Equilibra and Social Change. *Human Relations, 1*(5).

Lewis, D., & Weigert, A. (1985). Trust as a social reality. *Social Forces, 63*(4), 967–985. doi:10.2307/2578601

Li, J., & Brassil, J. (2006). *On the performance of traffic equalizers on heterogeneous communication links.* QShine, Proceedings of the 3rd international conference on Quality of service in heterogeneous wired/wireless networks. New York: ACM.

Lindeman, U., Claus, H., Stuber, M., Augat, P., Muche, R., Nikolaus, T., & Becker, C. (2003). Measuring power during the sit-to-stand transfer. *European Journal of Applied Physiology, 89,* 466–470. doi:10.1007/s00421-003-0837-z

Lindemann, U., Hock, A., Stuber, M., Keck, W., & Becker, C. (2005). Evaluation of a fall detector based on accelerometers: a pilot study. *Medical & Biological Engineering & Computing, 43*(2), 548–551. doi:10.1007/BF02351026

Liu, A., & Ning, P. (2008). TinyECC: A configurable library for elliptic curve cryptography in wireless sensor networks. In . *Proceedings of the International Conference on Information Processing in Sensor Networks, 1,* 245–256.

Lorincz, K., Malan, D. J., & Fulford-Jones, T. R. F., Nawoj. A., Clavel, A., Shnayder, V., Mainland, G., Welsh, M., & Moulton, S. (2004). Sensor networks for emergency response: challenges and opportunities. *IEEE Pervasive Computing / IEEE Computer Society [and] IEEE Communications Society, 3,* 16–23. doi:10.1109/MPRV.2004.18

Lovis, C. (2006). Comprehensive management of the access to the electronic patient record: Towards trans-institutional networks. *International Journal of Medical Informatics, 176*(5-6), 466–470.

Luhmann, N. (1979). *Trust and Power.* Chichester, UK: Wiley.

Luinge, H. J., & Veltink, P. H. (2005). Measuring orientation of human body segments using miniature gyroscopes and accelerometers. *Medical & Biological Engineering & Computing, 43*(2), 273–282. doi:10.1007/BF02345966

Luis, C. A., & Brown, L. M. (2007). Neuropsychological correlates of wanderers . In Nelson, A. L., & Algase, D. L. (Eds.), *Evidence-based protocols for managing wandering behaviors* (pp. 65–74). New York: Springer.

Luo, W., & Najdawi, M. (2004). Trust-building measures: A review of consumer health portals. *Communications of the ACM, 47,* 108–113. doi:10.1145/962081.962089

Lupu, E., Dulay, N., Sloman, M., Sventek, J., Heeps, S., & Strowes, S. (2007). AMUSE: autonomic management of ubiquitous e-Health systems. *Concurrency and Computation, 20*(3), 277–295. doi:10.1002/cpe.1194

Machanavajjhala, A., Kifer, D., Gehrke, J., & Venkitasubramaniam, M. (2007). l-diversity: Privacy beyond k-anonymity. In *ACM Transactions on Knowledge Discovery from Data (TKDD), 1,* (3), New York: ACM.

Macy, M. W., & Skvoretz, J. (1998). The evolution of trust and cooperation between strangers: A computational model. *American Sociological Review, 63*(10), 638–660. doi:10.2307/2657332

Malamateniou, F., & Vassilacopoulos, G. (2002). Developing a Virtual Patient Record as a Web-based Workflow System. In G. Surján, R. Engelbrecht & P. McNair (Eds), *Medical Informatics Europe: Vol. 90. Studies in Health Technology and Informatics 2002* (pp. 298-304). Amsterdam: IOS Press.

Malasri, K., & Wang, L. (2007). Addressing security in medical sensor networks. In *Proceedings of the 1st ACM SIGMOBILE International Workshop on Systems and networking support for healthcare and assisted living environments* (pp. 7-12). New York: ACM Press.

Mandell, S. F. (1987). Resistance to Computerization. *Journal of Medical Systems, 11*(4), 311–318. doi:10.1007/BF00994015

Manzo, M., Roosta, T., & Sastry, S. (2005). Time synchronization attacks in sensor networks. In *Proceedings of the 3rd ACM Workshop on Security of Ad Hoc and Sensor Networks* (pp. 107-116). New York: ACM Press.

Marcus, M. L. (1983). Power, politics, and MIS implementation. *Communications of the ACM, 26,* 430–444. doi:10.1145/358141.358148

Markle. (2003). *The personal health working group. Markle foundation. Connecting for health: a public-private collaborative, final report.* Retrieved December 20, 2009, from: http://www.connectingforhealth.org/resources/wg_eis_final_report_0704.pdf.

Marohn, D. (2006) Biometrics in Healthcare. *Biometric Technology Today, 14*(9), 9-11. New York: Elsevier.

Marschollek, M., & Demirbilek, E. (2006). Providing longitudinal health care information with the new German Health Card—a pilot system to track patient pathways. [New York: Elsevier]. *Journal of Computer Methods and Programs in Biomedicine, 81,* 266–271. doi:10.1016/j.cmpb.2006.01.001

Marshall. P. (2007). *Personal Health Records - An Overview.* Retrieved December 20, 2009, from: http://www.ncvhs.hhs.gov/050106p1.pdf.

Marti, R., Delgado, J., & Perramon, X. (2004). Network and Application Security in Mobile e-Health Applications. In L. Bos, B. Blobel, A. Marsh, & D. Carroll (Eds.), *Lecture Notes in Computer Science: Vol. 3090. Information Networking (pp. 995-1004)*. Berlin/Heidelberg: Spriger-Verlag.

Martinsons, M. (1995). Radical Process Innovation Using Information Technology: The Theory, the Practice and the Future of Reengineering. *International Journal of Information Management, 15*(4), 253–269. doi:10.1016/0268-4012(95)00023-Z

Maslow, A. (1954). *Motivation and Personality*. New York: Harper.

Mather, A. S., Rodriguez, C., Guthrie, M. F., McHarg, A. M., Reid, I. C., & McMurdo, M. E. T. (2002). Effects of exercise on depressive symptoms in older adults with poorly responsive depressive disorder. *The British Journal of Psychiatry, 180*, 411–415. doi:10.1192/bjp.180.5.411

Mathews, A. W. (2009, October 27). Compare and contrast. *Wall Street Journal*, R4.

Mathie, M. J., Coster, A. C., Lovell, N. H., & Celler, B. G. (2004). Accelerometry: providing an integrated, practical method for long-term, ambulatory monitoring of human movement. *Physiological Measurement, 25*(2), R1–R20. doi:10.1088/0967-3334/25/2/R01

Mayagoitia, R. E., Lötters, J. C., Veltink, P. H., & Hermens, H. (2002). Standing balance evaluation using a triaxial accelerometer. *Gait & Posture, 16*(1), 55–59. doi:10.1016/S0966-6362(01)00199-0

Mayer, R. C., Davis, J. H., & Schoorman, F. D. (1995). An integrative model of organizational trust. *Academy of Management Review, 20*(3), 709–734. doi:10.2307/258792

Mayhew, D. J. (1999). *The usability engineering lifecycle*. San Francisco: Morgan Kaufmann.

Mayring, P. (2000). *Qualitative Content Analysis*. Forum Qualitative Sozialforschung / Forum: Qualitative Social Research. Retrieved 2000 from http://nbnresolving. de/urn:nbn:de:0114-fqs0002204

McCulloch, C. E., & Cain, M. L. (1989). Analyzing discrete movement data as a correlated random walk. *Ecology, 70*, 383–388. doi:10.2307/1937543

McDaniel, J. H., Hunt, A., Hackes, B., & Pope, J. F. (2001). Impact of dining room environment on nutritional intake of Alzheimer's residents: A case study. *American Journal of Alzheimer's Disease and Other Dementias, 16*(5), 297–302. doi:10.1177/153331750101600508

McKee, J. J., Evans, N. E., & Owens, F. J. (1996). Digital Transmission of 12-Lead Electrocadiograms and Duplex Speech in the Telephone Bandwith. *Journal of Telemedicine and Telecare, 2*(1). doi:10.1258/1357633961929150

McKnight, D., & Chervaney, N. (2001). Trust and distrust definitions: One bit at a time . In Falcone, R., Singh, M., & Tan, Y. (Eds.), *Trust in Cyber-societies* (pp. 27–54). Berlin: Springer-Verlag. doi:10.1007/3-540-45547-7_3

McKnight, D. H., & Chervany, N. L. (2000). What is trust? A conceptual analysis and an interdisciplinary model. In Chung, M. H. (Ed.), *Proceedings of the Americas Conference on Information Systems,* August, 2000, (pp. 827-833). Long Beach, California.

McKnight, D. H., & Kacmar, C. J. (2007). Factors and effect of information credibility. *Proceedings of the ninth international conference on Electronic commerce,* ICEC2007, ACM, 423-432.

McKnight, D., Choudhury, V., & Kacmar, C. (2000). Trust in ecommerce vendors: A two-stage model. *Proceedings of the Twenty First International Conference on Information Systems,* 532-536.

Mechanic, D. (2004). In my chosen doctor I trust. *British Medical Journal, 329*(7480), 1418–1419. doi:10.1136/bmj.329.7480.1418

Melenhorst, A.-S., Rogers, W., & Bouwhuis, D. (2006). Older Adults' Motivated Choice for Technological Innovation. *Psychology and Aging, 21*(1), 190–195. doi:10.1037/0882-7974.21.1.190

Messelken, M., Martin, J., Milewski, P. (1998). Ergebnisqualität in der Notfallmedizin. *Notfall-& Rettungsmedizin*. 1, 143-149.

Metaxas, M. Markopoulos. P., Aarts, E. H. L. (2009). Amelie: A Recombinant Computing Framework for Ambient Awareness. In *Ambient Intelligence 2009* (pp. 88-100).

Meyer, A. D., & Goes, J. B. (1988). Organizational Assimilation of Innovations: A Multilevel Contextual Analysis. *Academy of Management Journal, 31*(4). doi:10.2307/256344

Meyer, S., & Schulze, E. (2008). *Smart Home für ältere Menschen. Handbuch für die Praxis*. Berlin: Berliner Institut für Sozialforschung GmbH.

Meyerson, D., Weick, K. E., & Kramer, R. M. (1996). Swift trust and temporary groups . In Kramer, R. M., & Tyler, T. R. (Eds.), *Trust in Organizations: Frontiers of Theory and Research* (pp. 166–195). Thousand Oaks, CA: Sage Publications.

Mihailidis, A., Cockburn, A., Longley, C., & Boger, J. (2008). The acceptability of home monitoring technology among community-dwelling older adults and baby boomers. *Assistive Technology*, 20(1), 1–12. doi:10.108 0/10400435.2008.10131927

Mikkelsen, A., & Gronhaug, K. (1999). Measuring Organizational Learning Climate. *Review of Public Personnel Administration*, 19(4), 31. doi:10.1177/0734371X9901900404

Milne, G. R., & Boza, M.-E. (1999). Trust and concern in consumers' perceptions of marketing information management practices. *Journal of Interactive Marketing*, 13(1), 5–24. doi:10.1002/(SICI)1520-6653(199924)13:1<5::AID-DIR2>3.0.CO;2-9

Mintzberg, H. (1981). Organiser l'entreprise: Prêt-à-porter ou sur mesure? *Harvard, L'Expansion,* (été), 9-23.

Mishra, A., Nadkarni, K., & Patcha, A. (2004). Intrusion detection in wireless ad hoc networks. *IEEE Wireless Communications*, 11, 48–60. doi:10.1109/MWC.2004.1269717

Misztal, B. A. (1996). *Trust in Modern Societies: The Search for the Bases of Social Order*. New York: Polity Press.

Mitchell, B. R., Mitchell, J. G., & Disney, A. P. (1996). User adoption Issues in Renal Telemedicine. *Journal of Telemedicine and Telecare*, 2(2). doi:10.1258/1357633961929835

Mitchell, T. R., & Silver, W. S. (1990). Individual and Group Goals When Workers Are Interdependent. *The Journal of Applied Psychology*, 75(2), 185. doi:10.1037/0021-9010.75.2.185

MobiHealth. (2010). *MobiHealth – shaping the future of Healthcare*. Retrieved 29.03.10 from http://www.mobihealth.org/

Moe-Nilssen, R., & Helbostad, J. L. (2002). Trunk accelerometry as a measure of balance control during quiet standing. *Gait & Posture*, 16(1), 60–68. doi:10.1016/S0966-6362(01)00200-4

Mohan, J. (2004). Health attitudes, health cognitions, and health behaviors among Internet health information seekers: Population-based survey, *Journal of Medical Internet Research*, vol. 6. Retrieved January 14, 2009 from http://www.jmir.org/.

Mollenkopf, H., Marcellini, F., Ruoppila, I., & Tacken, M. (2004). *Ageing and Outdoor Mobility. A European Study*. Amsterdam: IOS Press.

Mollenkopf, H., & Kaspar, R. (2004). Technisierte Umwelten als Handlungs- und Erlebensraeume aelterer Menschen . In Backes, G., Clemens, W., & Kuenemund, H. (Eds.), *Lebensformen und Lebensführung im Alter* (pp. 193–221). Wiesbaden: Verlag für Sozialwissenschaften.

Mollenkopf, H., Oswald, F., & Wahl, H.-W. (2007). Neue Personen-Umwelt-Konstellationen im Alter: Befunde und Perspektiven zu Wohnen, außerhäuslicher Mobilität und Technik . In Wahl, H.-W., & Mollenkopf, H. (Eds.), *Alternsforschung am Beginn des 21. Jahrhunderts: Alterns- und Lebenslaufkonzeptionen im deutschsprachigen Raum* (pp. 361–380). Berlin: AKA Verlag.

Moore, J. (2000). Placing home in context. *Journal of Environmental Psychology*, 20, 207–217. doi:10.1006/jevp.2000.0178

Morgan, R. M., & Hunt, S. D. (1994). The commitment-trust theory of relationship marketing. *Journal of Marketing*, 58, 20–38. doi:10.2307/1252308

Morgan, D. G., & Stewart, N. M. (1997). The importance of the social environment in dementia care. *Western Journal of Nursing Research*, 19(6), 740–761. doi:10.1177/019394599701900604

Morgan, D. G., & Stewart, N. M. (1998). Multiple occupancy versus private rooms on dementia care units. *Environment and Behavior*, 30(4), 487–503. doi:10.1177/001391659803000404

Morgeson, F. P., & Hofmann, D. A. (1999). The structure and function of collective constructs: Implications for multilevel research and theory development. *Academy of Management. Academy of Management Review*, 24(2), 249. doi:10.2307/259081

Morlock, M., Schneider, E., Bluhm, A., Vollmer, M., Bergmann, G., Müller, V., & Honl, M. (2001). Duration and frequency of every day activities in total hip patients. *Journal of Biomechanics*, 34, 873–881. doi:10.1016/S0021-9290(01)00035-5

Muir, B. M., & Moray, N. (1996). Trust in automation: Part II, Experimental studies of trust and human intervention in a process control simulation. *Ergonomics*, 39(3), 429–460. doi:10.1080/00140139608964474

Mukherjee, S., Aarts, E. H. L., & Doyle, T. (2009). Special issue on Ambient Intelligence. *Information Systems Frontiers*, 11(1), 1–5. doi:10.1007/s10796-008-9146-8

Müller, M., Protogerakis, M., & Henning, K. (2009). *A methodology to reduce technical risk in the development of telematic rescue assistance systems.* Proceedings of the second international conference on computer and electrical engineering. Dubai: UAE.

Mumford, E. (1981). *Participative Systems Design: Structure and Method: Systems, Objectives, Solutions.* North-Holland.

Mumford, E. (1983). *Designing Participatively.* Manchester, UK: Manchester Business School.

Mumford, E. (2000). A Socio-Technical Approach to Systems Design. *Requirements Engineering, 5*(2), 125–133. doi:10.1007/PL00010345

Mura, T., Dartigues, J. F., & Berr, C. (2009). How many dementia cases in France and Europe? Alternative projections and scenarios 2010-2050. *European Journal of Neurology.*

Murray, D., Hannan, P. J., Jacobs, D. R., McGoven, P. J., Schmid, L., Baker, W. L., & Gray, C. (1994). Assessing Intervention Effects in the Minnesota Heart Health Program. *American Journal of Epidemiology, 139,* 91–103.

MyHeart. (2003). Retrieved from http://www.hitech-projects.com/euprojects/myheart/.

MyHeart. (n.d.). *Forschungsprojekt im 6. EU-Rahmenprogramm.* Retrieved 30.11.2009 from www.hitech-projects. com/euprojects/myheart/

N'I Scanaill, C., Carew, S., Barralon, P., Noury, N., Lyons, D. & Lyons, G.M. (2006). A Review of Approaches to Mobility Telemonitoring of the Elderly in Their Living Environment. *Annals of Biomedical Engineering, 34,* 547–563. doi:10.1007/s10439-005-9068-2

Najafi, B., Aminian, K., Loew, F., Blanc, Y., & Robert, P. (2002). Measurement of stand-sit and sit-stand transitions using a miniature gyroscope and its application in fall risk evaluation in the elderly. *IEEE Transactions on Bio-Medical Engineering, 49*(8), 843–851. doi:10.1109/TBME.2002.800763

Najafi, B., Aminian, K., Paraschiv-Ionescu, A., Loew, F., Bula, C., & Robert, Ph. (2003). Ambulatory system for human motion analysis using a kinematic sensor: monitoring of daily physical activity in elderly. *IEEE Transactions on Bio-Medical Engineering, 50*(6), 711–723. doi:10.1109/TBME.2003.812189

Najafi, B., Büla, C., Piot-Ziegler, C., Demierre, M., & Aminian, K. (2003). Relationship between fear of falling and spatio-temporal parameters of gait in elderly persons. *From Basic Motor Control to Functional Recovery III,* Chapter II: From Posture to Gait, 152-158. Ecole Polytechnique Fédérale Lausanne: MCC2003 Book.

Nams, V. O. (2005). Using animal movement paths to measure response to spatial scale. *Oecologia, 143,* 179–188. doi:10.1007/s00442-004-1804-z

Nams, V. (1997-2001). *Fractal computer program, version 3.16.* Web site: URL http://www.nsac.ns.ca/envsci/staff/vnams/Fractal.htm

Nardi, B. A., & O'Day, V. L. (1999). *Information Ecologies: Using Technologies with Heart.* Cambridge, MA: MIT Press.

Nass, C., Fogg, B. J., & Moon, Y. (1996). Can computers be teammates? *International Journal of Human-Computer Studies, 45,* 669–678. doi:10.1006/ijhc.1996.0073

Nathan, R., Getz, W. M., Revilla, E., Holyoak, M., Kadmon, R., & Saltz, D. (2008). A movement ecology paradigm for unifying organismal movement research. *Proceedings of the National Academy of Sciences of the United States of America, 105*(49), 19052–19059. doi:10.1073/pnas.0800375105

National Archives and Records Administration. *President Truman's proposed health program.* November 19, 1945. Retrieved January 5, 2010, from http://www.trumanlibrary.org/publicpapers/index.php?pid=483&st=&st1.

Naveen, S., & David, W. (2004). Security considerations for IEEE 802.15.4 networks. In *Proceedings of the ACM Workshop on Wireless Security* (pp. 32-42). New York: ACM Press.

Nelson, M. E., Rejeski, W. J., Blair, S. N., Duncan, P. W., Judge, J. O., & King, A. C. (2007). Physical activity and public health in older adults: recommendation from the American College of Sports Medicine and the American Heart Association. *Medicine and Science in Sports and Exercise, 39*(8), 1435–1445. doi:10.1249/mss.0b013e3180616aa2

Neves, P., Stachyra, M., & Rodrigues, J. (2008). Application of Wireless Sensor Networks to Healthcare Promotion. *Journal of Communications Software and Systems, 4*(3), 181–190.

Ng, H. S., Sim, M. L., & Tan, C. M. (2006). Security issues of wireless sensor networks in healthcare applications. *BT Technology Journal, 24*(2), 138–144. doi:10.1007/s10550-006-0051-8

Ng, J. W. P., Lo, B. P. L., Wells, O., Sloman, M., Toumazou, C., Peters, N., et al. (2004). *Ubiquitous Monitoring Environment for Wearable and Implantable Sensors (UbiMon)*. Paper presented at UbiComp, Nottingham.

Nguyen, D. & Canny, J. (2007). MultiView: Improving trust in group video conferencing through spatial faithfulness. *Proceedings of Human Factors in Computing Systems*, CHI 2007, ACM, 1465-1474.

Ni Scanaill, C., Carew, S., Barralon, P., Noury, N., Lyons, D., & Lyons, G. M. (2006). A review of approaches to mobility telemonitoring of the elderly in their living environment. *Annals of Biomedical Engineering, 34*(4), 547–563. doi:10.1007/s10439-005-9068-2

Nicogossian, A. E., Pober, D. F., & Roy, S. A. (2001). Evolution of telemedicine in the space program and earth applications. *Telemedicine Journal and e-Health, 7*(1), 1–15. doi:10.1089/153056201300093813

Nicolai, S., Benzinger, P., Skelton, D. A., Aminian, K., Becker, C., & Lindemann, U. (2010). Day-to-day variability of physical activity of older adults living in the community. *Journal of Aging and Physical Activity, 18*(1), 75–86.

NICTIZ. (2007). Retrieved from http://www.nictiz.nl.

Nielsen, J., Molich, R., Snyder, C., & Farrell, S. (2000) E-commerce user experience: trust. Fremont, CA, USA, Nielsen Norman Group, http://www.nngroup.com/reports/ecommerce, accessed 3/2001.

Nielson, J. (1993). *Usability Engineering*. New York: Academic Press.

Noe, B., et al. (2009). Home Centric ICT Services for the Ageing Society. In *Ambient Assisted Living 2*, German AAL-Congress, Conference Proceeding, Berlin, Germany, January 27-28, 2009.

Nordal, E. J., Moseng, D., Kvammen, B., & Lochen, M. (2001). A Comparative Study of Teleconsultation versus Face-to-Face Consultations. *Journal of Telemedicine and Telecare, 7*(5). doi:10.1258/1357633011936507

Noury, N., Fleury, A., Rumeau, P., Bourke, A. K., Laighin, G. O., Rialle, V., & Lundy, J. E. (2007) Fall detection principles and methods. *Conference Proceedings - IEEE Engineering in Medicine and Biology*, 1663-1666.

Nowak, L. A., & Davis, J. E. (2007). A qualitative examination of the phenomenon of sundowning. *Journal of Nursing Scholarship, 39*(3), 256–258. doi:10.1111/j.1547-5069.2007.00177.x

O'Donnell, P. J., Scobie, G., & Baxter, I. (1991). The use of focus groups as an evaluation technique in HCI. In Diaper, D. & Hammond, N. (Eds.). *People and Computers VI*, 211-224. Cambridge, UK: Cambridge University Press.

ODRL. (2009), *Open Digital Rights Language*. Retrieved from http://odrl.net/

Oliver, R. (1980). A cognitive model of the antecedents and consequences of satisfaction decisions. *JMR, Journal of Marketing Research, 17*, 460–469. doi:10.2307/3150499

O'Loughlin, J. L., Robitaille, Y., Boivin, J. F., & Suissa, S. (1993). Incidence of and risk factors for falls and injurious falls among the community-dwelling elderly. *American Journal of Epidemiology, 137*(3), 342–354.

Oracle Corporation. (2010). *Sun SPOTS*. Retrieved on January 5, 2010 from http://planets.sun.com/SunSPOT/

Orlikowski, W., & Baroudi, J. (1991). Studying information technology in organizations: Research approaches and assumptions. *Information Systems Research, 2*(1), 1–28. doi:10.1287/isre.2.1.1

Orlikowski, W. J. (1993). Learning from notes: Organizational issues in groupware implementation. *The Information Society, 9*(3), 237. doi:10.1080/01972243.1993.9960143

Orlikowski, W. J., & Gash, D. C. (1994). Technological frames: making sense of information technology in organizations. *ACM Transactions on Information Systems, 12*(2), 174–207. doi:10.1145/196734.196745

Orlikowski, W. J., & Iacono, C. S. (2001). Research commentary: Desperately seeking "IT" in IT research - A call to theorizing the IT artifact. *Information Systems Research, 12*(2), 121. doi:10.1287/isre.12.2.121.9700

Ortiz, M. P. C. A., Oyarzun, D., Yanguas, J. J., Buiza, C., González, M. F., & Etxeberria, I. (2007). Elderly Users in Ambient Intelligence: Does an Avatar Improve the Interaction? *Proceedings of 9th ERCIM Workshop 'User Interfaces For All'*, pp. 99-114.

Osborn, K., Wraa, C., & Watson, A. (2010). *Medical Surgical Nursing*. Boston: Pearson.

Oswald, F., Wahl, H. W., Schilling, O., Nygren, C., Fange, A., & Sixsmith, A. (2007). Relationships between housing and healthy aging in very old age. *The Gerontologist, 47*(1), 96–107.

Pak, R. (2001). A Further Examination of the Influence of Spatial Abilities on Computer Task Performance in Younger and Older Adults. In *Proceedings of the Human Factors and Ergonomics Society 48th Annual Meeting* (pp. 1551 – 1555). Santa Monica, CA: The Human Factors and Ergonomic Society.

Paré, G., & Sicotte, C. (2004). Les technologies de l'information et la transformation de l'offre de soins. *Cahier Du GReSI,* (04-04).

Passini, R., Rainville, C., Marchand, N., & Joanette, Y. (1995). Wayfinding in dementia of the Alzheimer type: planning abilities. *Journal of Clinical and Experimental Neuropsychology*, *17*(6), 820–832. doi:10.1080/01688639508402431

Pavel, M., Hayes, T. L., Adami, A., Jimison, H., & Kaye, J. (2006). Unobtrusive assessment of mobility. *Conference Proceedings; ... Annual International Conference of the IEEE Engineering in Medicine and Biology Society. IEEE Engineering in Medicine and Biology Society. Conference*, *1*, 6277–6280. doi:10.1109/IEMBS.2006.260301

Pavel, M., Hayes, T., Tsay, I., Erdogmus, D., Paul, A., Larimer, N., et al. (2007). *Continuous assessment of gait velocity in Parkinson's disease from unobtrusive measurements: CNE '07*. 3rd International IEEE/EMBS Conference on Neural Engineering, 2007. 5/2/2007-5/5/2007 Hawaii, USA 700-703.

Pavlou, P. (2001). Integrating trust in electronic commerce with the technology acceptance model: Model development and validations. *Proceedings of the Seventh Americas Conference on Information Systems, Association of Information Systems*, 816-822.

Payette, M. (2001). Interdisciplinarité: Clarification des concepts. *Interaction*, *5*(1).

Pearce, J. L., & Gregersen, H. B. (1991). Task Interdependence and Extrarole Behavior: A Test of the Mediating Effects of Felt Responsibility. *The Journal of Applied Psychology*, *76*(6), 838. doi:10.1037/0021-9010.76.6.838

Pearson, S. D., Schneider, E. C., Kleinman, K. P., Coltin, K. L. & Singer, J. A. (2008). The impact of pay-for-performance on health care quality in Massachusetts, 2001-2003. *Health Affairs*.

Peimann, J. C. (1998). Modeling Hospital Information Systems with Petri Nets. *Methods of Information in Medicine*, *27*, 17–22.

Penders, J., van de Molengraft, J., Brown, L., Grundlehner, B., Gyselinckx, B., & van Hoof, C. (2009). Potential and challenges of body area networks for personal health. In *Proceedings of the Annual International Conference of the IEEE Engineering in Medicine and Biology Society* (pp. 6569-6572). IEEE Engineering in Medicine and Biology Society. Washington, DC: IEEE Press.

Penninx, B., van Tilburg, T., Kriegsman, D., Boeke, A., Deeg, D., & van Eijk, J. (1999). Social network, social support, and loneliness in older persons with different chronic diseases. *Journal of Aging and Health*, *11*(2), 151–168. doi:10.1177/089826439901100202

Penninx, B. W., Messier, S. P., Rejeski, W. J., Williamson, J. D., DiBari, M., & Cavazzini, C. (2001). Physical exercise and the prevention of disability in activities of daily living in older persons with osteoarthritis. *Archives of Internal Medicine*, *161*(19), 2309–2316. doi:10.1001/archinte.161.19.2309

Perrig, A., Szewczyk, R., Tygar, J., Wen, V., & Culler, D. E. (2002). SPINS: security protocols for sensor networks. *Wireless Networks*, *8*, 521–534. doi:10.1023/A:1016598314198

Petković, M., Katzenbeisser, S., & Kursawe, K. (2007). *Rights Management Technologies: A Good Choice for Securing Electronic Health Records?* International Conference on Information Security Solutions Europe (ISSE), Warsaw, Poland

Pew Internet Research. (2002). Vital decisions: How Internet users decide what information to trust when they or their loved ones are sick. Retrieved November 22, 2008 from http://www.pewInternet.org.

Pickering, A. (1995). *The Mangle of Practice*. Chicago: The University of Chicago Press.

Picolo, D., Smolle, D., Argenziano, G., Wolf, I. H., Braun, R., & Cerroni, L. (2000). Teledermoscopy: Results of a Multicentre Study on 43 Pigmented Skin Lesions. *Journal of Telemedicine and Telecare*, *6*(3). doi:10.1258/1357633001935202

Pierce, J. L., Kostova, T., & Dirks, K. T. (2001). Toward a theory of psychological ownership in organizations. *Academy of Management. Academy of Management Review*, *26*(2), 298. doi:10.2307/259124

Pierce, J. L., Rubenfeld, S. A., & Morgan, S. (1991). Employee Ownership: A Conceptual Model of Process and Effects. *Academy of Management. Academy of Management Review*, *16*(1), 121. doi:10.2307/258609

Pilemalm, S., Lindell, P., Hallberg, N., & Eriksson, H. (2007). Integrating the Rational Unified Process and participatory design for development of socio-technical systems: a user participative approach. *Design Studies*, *28*, 263–288. doi:10.1016/j.destud.2007.02.009

Pinch, T., & Bijker, W. (1987). The social connstruction of facts and artifacts. W. In Bijker, T. Hughes and T. Pinch (eds.), *The Social Construction of Technological Systems* (159-187). Cambridge, MA: MIT Press.

Pitta, F., Troosters, T., Probst, V. S., Langer, D., Decramer, M., & Gosselink, R. (2008). Are patients with COPD more active after pulmonary rehabilitation? *Chest*, *134*(2), 273–280. doi:10.1378/chest.07-2655

Pitta, F., Troosters, T., Spruit, M. A., Probst, V. S., Decramer, M., & Gosselink, R. (2005). Characteristics of physical activities in daily life in chronic obstructive pulmonary disease. *American Journal of Respiratory and Critical Care Medicine*, *171*(9), 972–977. doi:10.1164/rccm.200407-855OC

Ploutz-Snyder, L. L., Manini, T., Ploutz-Snyder, R. J., & Wolf, D. A. (2002). Functionally relevant thresholds of quadriceps femoris strength. *Journal of Gerontology: Medical Sciences*, *57A*, M144–M152.

Poole, M. S., & DeSanctis, G. (1990). Understanding the Use of Group Decision Support Systems: The Theory of Adaptive Structuration. In Fulk and Steinfield (eds), *Organizations and Communication Technology*. (173-193). Newbury Park, CA: Sage Publications.

Porac, J. F., Thomas, H., & Baden-Fuller, C. (1989). Competitive groups as cognitive communities: The case of Scottish knitwear manufacturers. *Journal of Management Studies*, *26*(4), 397–416. doi:10.1111/j.1467-6486.1989.tb00736.x

Pratt, M. G., & Dutton, J. E. (2000). Owning up or opting out: The roles of identity and emotions in issue of ownership. In N. Ashkanasy, C. Hartel, & W. Zerbe (eds.), *Emotions in the workplace: Research, theory, and practice* (103-129). New York: Quorum.

Prendinger, H., Ma, C., Yingzi, J., Nakasone, A., & Ishizuka, M. (2005). Understanding the effect of life-like interface agents through users' eye movements. *Proceedings of the 7th international conference on Multimodal interfaces* (pp. 108-115), New York: ACM Press.

Purvis, R. L., Sambamurthy, V., & Zmud, R. (2001). The assimilation of knowledge platforms in organizations: An empirical investigation. *Organization Science*, *12*(2), 117. doi:10.1287/orsc.12.2.117.10115

Putnam, R. D. (1995). Bowling alone: America's declining social capital. *Journal of Democracy*, *6*(1), 3–10. doi:10.1353/jod.1995.0002

Quang, P. T., & Chartier-Kastler, C. (1991). *Merise in Practice* (Avison, D. E., Trans.). Basingstoke: Macmillan.

Raghavendra, C. S., Sivalingam, K. M., & Znati, T. (Eds.). (2004). *Wireless Sensor Networks*. Berlin, Heidelberg: Spriger-Verlag. doi:10.1007/b117506

Rajendran, P., Corcoran, A., Kinosian, B., & Alwan, M. (2008). Falls, fall prevention, and fall detection technologies. In R. J. Pignolo, M. A. Forciea, & J. C. Johnson (Series Eds.) & R. Felder & M. Alwan (Vol. Eds.), *Aging medicine: Eldercare technology for clinical practitioners* (pp. 187-202). Totowa, NJ: Humana Press.

Rall, M., Reddersen, S., Schädle, B., Zieger, J., Christ, P., Scheerer, J., & Liang, Y. (2004). *Das Schutz-Engel-System - Telemedizinische Unterstützung in Echtzeit. In A. Jäckel, Telemedizinführer Deutschland* (pp. 51–64). Witte, Germany: Mendel Verlag.

Ramage-Morin, P. L. (2009). Medication use among senior Canadians. *Health Reports*, *20*(1), 1–8.

Ras, E., Becker, M., & Koch, J. (2007). Engineering tele-health solutions in the ambient assisted living lab. In *AINAW '07: 21st International Conference on Advanced Information Networking and Applications Workshops*: Vol 2 (pp. 804-809).

Ratajczak, S. (2005). *Electronic Health Record Infostructure (EHRi) Privacy and Security Conceptual Architecture, v1.1* (p. 171). Canada Health Infoway Inc.

Ratnasingam, P., & Pavlov, P. (2003). Technology trust in Internet-based interorganizational electronic commerce. *Journal of Electronic Commerce in Organizations*, *1*(1), 17–41.

Reeves, B., & Nass, C. (1996). *The Media Equation: How People Treat Computers, Television, and New Media Like Real People and Places*. California: CSLI Publications and Cambridge: Cambridge University Press.

Reichert, M., & Dadam, P. (1998, September). *Towards Process-oriented Hospital Information Systems: Some Insights into Requirements, Technical Challenges and Possible Solutions*. Paper presented at 43 Jahrestagung der GMDS (GMDS'98) (pp. 175-180), Bremmen, Germany.

Ribbink, D., van Riel, A., Liljander, V., & Streukens, S. (2004). Comfort your online customer: Quality, trust and loyalty on the Internet. *Managing Service Quality*, *16*(6), 446–456. doi:10.1108/09604520410569784

Rieback, M., Crispo, B., & Tanenbaum, A. (2005). RFID Guardian: A Battery-Powered Mobile Device for RFID Privacy Management. In C. Boyd, J. M. G. Nieto (Eds.), Lecture Notes in Computer Science: *Vol. 3574. Information Security and Privacy* (pp. 184-194). Berlin/Heidelberg: Spriger-Verlag.

Riegelsberger, J., & Sasse, M. (2001) Trust builders and trustbusters: the role of trust cues in interfaces to e-commerce applications, in *Towards the E-Society: Proceedings of the First IFIP Conference on E-Commerce, E-Society, and E-Government*,17-30.London: Kluwer.

Riegersberger, J., Sasse, M., & McCarthy, J. (2003). Shiny happy people building trust? Photos on e-commrece websites and consumer trust. *Proceedings of Human Factors in Computing Systems*, CHI2003, ACM, 1465-1474.

Riegersberger, J., Sasse, M., & McCarthy, J. (2005). Rich media: Poor judgments? A study of media effects on users' trust in expertise. *Proceedings of the British HCI Conference*, British Computer Society, 267-284.

Rieser, S. (2005). Arbeitsbedingungen schrecken viele ab. *Deutsches Arzteblatt, 102*, C629.

Rippen, H. (1999). Criteria for assessing the quality of health information on the Internet. *Health Summit Working Group,* Retrieved November 24, 2009 from http://hitiweb.mitretek.org/docs/policy.html.

Ritti, R., & Silver, J. (1986). Early Processes of Institutionalization: The Dramaturgy of Exchange in Interorganizational Relations. *Administrative Science Quarterly, 31*, 25–42. doi:10.2307/2392764

Riva, G. (2003). Ambient intelligence in health care. *Cyberpsychology & Behavior, 6*(3), 295–300. doi:10.1089/109493103322011597

Rivest, R. L., Shamir, A., & Adleman, L. (1978). A method for obtaining digital signatures and public-key cryptosystems. [ACM]. *Communications of the ACM, 21*(2), 120–126. doi:10.1145/359340.359342

Rivest, R. L. (2006). The RC5 encryption algorithm. In B. Preneel (Eds.), *Lecuture Notes in Computer Science: Vol. 1008. Fast software encryption* (pp. 86-96). Berlin/Heidelberg: Springer-Verlag.

Robeznieks, A. (2005). In no big hurry. Physicians still slow to adopt EMR systems: survey. *Modern Healthcare, 35*(38), 17.

Robinson, D. F., Savage, Gr. T.,& Campbell, K. S. (2003). Organizational Learning, Diffusion of Innovation, and International Collaboration in Telemedicine. *Health Care Management Review, 28*(1), 68.

Röcker, C., & Feith, A. Revisiting Privacy in Smart Spaces: Social and Architectural Aspects of Privacy in Technology-Enhanced Environments. *Proceedings of the International Symposium on Computing, Communication and Control* (2009) 201-205.

Röcker, C., Wilkowska, W., Ziefle, M., Kasugai, K., Klack, L., Möllering, C., & Beul, S. (2010). Towards Adaptive Interfaces for Supporting Elderly Users in Technology-Enhanced Home Environments. In *Proceedings of the 18th Biennial Conference of the International Communications Society: Culture, Communication and the Cutting Edge of Technology*. Tokyo, Japan. CD-ROM.

Rodgers, L., & Freundlich, F. (1998). *Employee Ownership Report.* Oakland, CA: National Center for Employee Ownership.

Roetenberg, D., Luinge, H. J., Baten, C. T., & Veltink, P. H. (2005). Compensation of magnetic disturbances improves inertial and magnetic sensing of human body segment orientation. *IEEE Transactions on Neural Systems and Rehabilitation Engineering, 13*(3), 395–405. doi:10.1109/TNSRE.2005.847353

Rogers, W. A., & Fisk, A. D. (2003). Technology Design, Usability, and Aging: Human Factors Techniques and considerations . In Charness, N., & Schaie, K. W. (Eds.), *Impact of technology on successful aging* (pp. 1–14). New York: Springer.

Rogers, W. A., Meyer, B., Walker, N., & Fisk, A. D. (1998). Functional Limitations to Daily Living Tasks in the Aged: A focus Group Analysis. *Human Factors. The Journal of the human factors and ergonomics society, 40 (1)*, 111-125.

Rosemberg, N. (1994). *Exploring the Black Box: Technology, Economics and History.* Cambridge, UK: Cambridge University Press. doi:10.1017/CBO9780511582554

Rosson, M. B., & Carroll, J. M. (2002). *Usability Engineering. Scenario-Based Development of Human-Computer Interaction.* San Francisco: Morgan Kaufmann Publishers.

Roter, D. L., & Hall, J. A. (1989). Studies of Doctor-Patient Interaction. *Annual Review of Public Health, 10*, 163–180. doi:10.1146/annurev.pu.10.050189.001115

Roth, E., & Laurent-Bopp, D. (2004). Challenges of treating dyslipidemia in patients with the metabolic syndrome. *American Journal for Nurse Practitioners, 8*(4), 58–66.

Rotter, J. (1967). A new scale for the measurement of interpersonal trust. *Journal of Personality, 35*, 651–665. doi:10.1111/j.1467-6494.1967.tb01454.x

Rotter, J. (1971). Generalized expectancies for interpersonal trust. *The American Psychologist, 26*, 443–452. doi:10.1037/h0031464

Rotter, J. (1980). Interpersonal trust, trustworthiness, and gullibility. *The American Psychologist, 35*(1), 1–7. doi:10.1037/0003-066X.35.1.1

Roughead, E. E., Semple, S. J., & Vitry, A. I. (2005). Pharmaceutical care services: A systematic review of published studies, 1990 to 2003, examining effectiveness in improving patient outcomes. *International Journal of Pharmacy Practice, 13*, 53–70. doi:10.1211/0022357055551

Rousseau, D. M. (1985). Issues of Level in Organizational Research: Multi-Level and Cross-Level Perspectives . In Cummings, L. L., & Staw, B. M. (Eds.), *Research in Organizational Behavior (Vol. 7)*. Greenwich, CT: JAI Press.

Routasalo, P., Airaksinen, M., Mäntyranta, T., & Pitkälä, K. (2009). Supporting a patient's self-management. *Duodecim, 125*(21), 2351–2359.

Rowe, M., Lane, S., & Phipps, C. (2007). CareWatch: A home monitoring system for use in homes of persons with cognitive impairment. *Topics in Geriatric Rehabilitation, 23*(1), 3.

Rubenstein, L. Z. (2006). Falls in older people: epidemiology, risk factors and strategies for prevention. *Age and Ageing, 35*(Suppl 2), ii37–ii41. doi:10.1093/ageing/afl084

Ruis de Sherbrooke. (2007). La téléassistance en soins de plaies, orientée vers une amélioration continue de la qualité des soins. *Manuel D'Organisation De Projet*, 1-63.

Ruuskanen, J. M., & Ruoppila, I. (1995). Physical activity and psychological well-being among people aged 65 to 84 years. *Age and Ageing, 24*(4), 292–296. doi:10.1093/ageing/24.4.292

Ryan, J. P., McGowan, J., McCaffrey, N., Ryan, G. T., Zandi, T., & Brannigan, G. G. (1995). Graphomotor perseveration and wandering in Alzheimer's disease. *Journal of Geriatric Psychiatry and Neurology, 8*(4), 209–212.

Sabatini, A. M., Martelloni, C., Scapellato, S., & Cavallo, F. (2005). Assessment of Walking Features From Foot Inertial Sensing. *IEEE Transactions on Bio-Medical Engineering, 52*(3), 486–494. doi:10.1109/TBME.2004.840727

Saga, V., & Zmud, R. (1994). The nature and determinants of information technology acceptance, routinization and infusion. In Levine. L. (ed.), *Diffusion, Transfer, and Implementation of Information Technology* (67-68). Noth-Holland, Amsterdam.

Salam, A., Rao, H., & Pegels, C. (2001). Consumer-perceived risk in ecommerce transactions . *Communications of the ACM*, (December): 46, 325–331.

Salvendy, G. (1997). *Handbook of human factors and ergonomics*. New York: Wiley.

Samarati, P., & Sweeney, L. (1998). Protecting privacy when disclosing information: k-anonymity and its enforcement through generalization and suppression. *In Proceedings of the IEEE Symposium on Research in Security and Privacy* (pp. 384-393), Citeseer.

Sambamurthy, V., & Zmud, R. W. (2000). Research commentary: The organizing logic for an enterprise's IT activities in the digital era - A prognosis of practice and a call for research. *Information Systems Research, 11*(2), 105. doi:10.1287/isre.11.2.105.11780

SAML. (2005). *Security Assertion Markup Language. Version 2.0*. OASIS Security Service TC. Retrieved from http://www.oasis-open.org/specs/index.php#saml2.0.

Sample, A. P., Yeager, D. J., Powledge, P. S., & Smith, J. R. (2007). Design of a passively-powered, programmable platform for UHF RFID systems. In *Proceedings of IEEE International Conference on RFID* (pp. 149-156).

Sanford, J. A., Pynoos, J., Tejral, A., & Browne, A. (2001). Development of a Comprehensive Assessment for Delivery of Home Modifications. *Physical & Occupational Therapy in Geriatrics, 20*(2), 43–55.

Santschi, V., Wuerzner, G., Schneider, M., Bugnon, O., & Burnier, M. (2007). Clinical evaluation of IDAS II, a new electronic device enabling drug adherence monitoring. *European Journal of Clinical Pharmacology, 63*(12), 1179–1184. doi:10.1007/s00228-007-0364-7

Sarfaty, M. (n.d.). American Public Health Association. *The Rise of the patient centered medical home: What is it? What does it mean?* Retrieved January 6, 2010, from http://www.apha.org/membergroups/newsletters/sectionnewsletters/medical/winter09/pcmh.htm.

Savastano, M., Hovsto, A., Pharow, P., & Blobel, B. (2008). Security, Safety, and Related Technology-The Triangle of eHealth Service Provision. In S. K. Andersen, G. O. Klein, S. Schulz, J. Aarts, & M. C. Mazzoleni (Eds.), *Studies in Health Technology and Informatics: Vol. 136. eHealth Beyond the Horizon-Get IT There* (pp. 709-714). Netherlands: IOS Press.

Schein, E. (1985). *Organizational Culture and Leadership*. San Francisco: Jossey-Bass.

Schenkman, M., Hughes, M., Samsa, G., & Studenski, S. (1996). The relative importance of strength and balance in chair rise by functionally impaired older individuals. *Journal of the American Geriatrics Society*, *44*(12), 1441–1446.

Schmidt, D. C. (2006). Guest editor's introduction: Model-driven engineering. *Computer*, *39*(2), 25–31. doi:10.1109/MC.2006.58

Schneider, B. (1990). The Climate for Service: An application of the climate construct . In *Social and Behavioral Science Series., Organizational Climate and Culture*. San Francisco: Jossey-Bass.

Schneider, B., & Reichers, A. E. (1983). On the Etiology of Climates. *Personnel Psychology*, *36*(1), 19–39. doi:10.1111/j.1744-6570.1983.tb00500.x

Schneiders, M., Protogerakis, M., & Isenhardt, I. (2009). *User acceptance as a key to success for the implementation of a Telematic Support System in German Emergency Medical Services*. Proceedings of The International Conference on Successes & Failures in Telehealth 2009: SFT-09 Australia. 2009.

Schulzrinne, H., Casner, S., Frederick, R., & Jacobson, V. (2003). *RTP: A Transport Protocol for Real-Time Applications RFC 3550 (Standard)*. Retrieved 30.11.2009 from http://www.ietf.org/rfc/rfc3550.txt

Schumm, W., Bugaighis, M., Buckler, D., Green, D., & Scanton, E. (1985). Construct validity of the dyadic trust scale. *Psychological Reports*, *56*, 1001–1002.

Scott, W. R. (2001). *Institutions and Organizations* (2nd ed.). Thousand Oaks, CA: Sage Publications.

Secker, J., Hill, R., Villeneau, L., & Parkman, S. (2003). Promoting independence: but promoting what and how. *Ageing and Society*, *23*(3), 375–391. doi:10.1017/S0144686X03001193

Sejersten, M., Sillesen, M., & Hansen, P. R. (2008). Effect on treatment delay of prehospital teletransmission of 12-lead electrocardiogram to a cardiologist for immediate triage and direct referral of patients with ST-segment elevation acute myocardial infarction to primary percutaneous coronary intervention. *The American Journal of Cardiology*, *101*, 941–946.

Semmes, C. (1991). Developing trust: Patient-practitioner encounters in natural health care. *Journal of Contemporary Ethnography*, *19*, 450–470. doi:10.1177/089124191019004004

Shamir, A. (1985). Identity-based cryptosystems and signature schemes. In *Proceedings of CRYPTO on Advances in Cryptology* (pp. 47-53).

Shapiro, D. L., Sheppard, B. H., & Cheraskin, L. (1992). Business on a handshake. *Negotiation Journal*, *8*(4), 365–377. doi:10.1111/j.1571-9979.1992.tb00679.x

SharpHealthcare. (2009). *Enabling strong authentication with biometrics*. Retrieved from http://www.sourcesecurity.com/markets/healthcare/application/co-854-ga.64.html

Shaspa Smart Home Kit. (2009). Retrieved from http://www.shaspa.com

Shea, G. P., & Guzzo, R. A. (1987). Groups as human resources. G.R. Ferris and K.M. Rowland (eds.), *Research in personnel and human resources management* (Vol. 5) (323-356). Greenwich, CT: JAI Press.

Sheppard, N. P., Safavi-Naini, R., & Jafari, M. (2009). A Digital Rights Management Model for Healthcare. *Policies for Distributed Systems and Networks, IEEE International Workshop on*, pp. 106-109, 2009 IEEE International Symposium on Policies for Distributed Systems and Networks

Shreeve, S. (2007). http://scottshreeve.blogspot.com. Retrieved on December 31, 2009.

Sillence, E., Briggs, P., Harris, P., & Fishwick, L. (2007). Health websites that people can trust – the case of hypertension. *Interacting with Computers*, *19*(1), 32–42. doi:10.1016/j.intcom.2006.07.009

Sillence, E., Briggs, P., Fishwick, L., & Harris, P. (2004). Trust and mistrust of online health sites. *Proceedings of the Conference on Human Factors in Computing Systems* CHI 2004.New York: ACM Press.

Silvestri, S., Ralls, G. A., & Krauss, B. (2005). The effectiveness of out-of hospital use of continuous endtidal carbon dioxide monitoring on the rate of unrecognized misplaced intubation within a regional emergency medical services system. *Annals of Emergency Medicine*, *45*, 497–503. doi:10.1016/j.annemergmed.2004.09.014

Simon, E., & Madsen, P. Adams, C., (2001). *An Introduction to XML Digital Signatures*. Retrieved from http://www.xml.com/pub/a/2001/08/08/xmldsig.html.

Simons, D., Egami, T., & Perry, J. (2006). Remote Patient Monitoring Solutions . In Spekowius, G., & Wendler, T. (Eds.), *Advances in Health care Technology* (pp. 505–516). The Netherlands: Springer. doi:10.1007/1-4020-4384-8_30

Singh, M. A. F. (2002). Exercise Come of Age: Rationale and Recommendations for a Geriatric Exercise Prescription. *Journal of Gerontology: Medical Sciences*, *57*(5), 262–282.

Singh, V. K., Pirsiavash, H., Rishabh, I., & Jain, R. (2008). Towards environment-to-environment (e2e) multimedia communication systems. *In Same '08: Proceeding of the 1st ACM international workshop on semantic ambient media experiences* (pp. 31–40). New York: ACM.

Sisko, A., Truffer, C., Smith, S., Keehan, S., Cylus, J., et al. (2009). OECD health data 2008: statistics and indicators for 30 countries. Organisation for economic co-operation and development; Health spending projections through 2018: Recession effects add uncertainty to the outlook. *Health Affairs*.

Sixsmith, A. J. (2000). An evaluation of an intelligent home monitoring system. *Journal of Telemedicine and Telecare*, *6*(2), 63–72. doi:10.1258/1357633001935059

Sixsmith, A. (2008). *Ambient technologies: developing user-driven approaches to research and development.* Paper presented at the Gerontological Society of America 61st Annual Scientific Meeting, Gaylord National Resort and Convention Center . *MD Medical Newsmagazine*, (November): 21–25.

Sixsmith, A. (1986). Independence and home in later life. In Phillipson, C., Bernard, M. & Strang, P. (Eds.), *Dependency and interdependency in old age- theoretical perspectives and policy alternatives* (pp. 338- 347). London, Croom Helm in association with The British Society of Gerontology.

Skelton, D. A., & McLaughlin, A. W. (1996). Training Functional Ability in Old Age. *Physiotherapy*, *82*(3), 159–167. doi:10.1016/S0031-9406(05)66916-7

Skelton, D. A., & Todd, C. (2004). *What are the main risk factors for falls amongst older people and what are the most effective interventions to prevent these falls? How should interventions to prevent falls be implemented? Health Evidence Network*. Denmark: World Health Organisation.

Skorning, M., Bergrath, S., Rörtgen, D., Brokmann, J., Beckers, S., & Protogerakis, M. (2009). E-Health in der Notfallmedizin – das Forschungsprojekt Med-on-@ix. *Der Anaesthesist*, *58*, 285–292. doi:10.1007/s00101-008-1502-z

Skubic, M., Alexander, G., Popescu, M., Rantz, M., & Keller, J. (2009). A Smart Home Application to Eldercare: Current Status and Lessons Learned. *Technology and Health Care*, *17*(3), 183–201.

Snijders, C., & Keren, G. (1999). Determinants of trust. In Budescu, D.V., Erev, I., Zwick, R. (Eds.) *Games and Human Behavior: Essays in Honor of Amnon Rapoport*(355-383). Mahwah, NJ: Lawrence Erlbaum.

Snyder, L., Rupprecht, P., Pyrek, J., Brekhus, S., & Moss, T. (1978). Wandering. *The Gerontologist*, *18*(3), 272.

Solomon, R., & Flores, F. (2001). *Building Trust in Business, Politics, Relationships, and Life*. New York: Oxford University Press.

Spine (2009). *NHS Connecting for Health*. Retrieved from http://www.connectingforhealth.nhs.uk/systemsandservices/spine

Spirduso, W. W. (1995). *Balance, Posture and Locomotion. In W. W. Spirduso Physical Dimensions of Aging*. Champaign, Illinois: Human Kinetics.

Spreng, R. A., MacKenzie, S. B., & Olshavsky, R. W. (1996). A reexamination of the determinants of consumer satisfaction. *Journal of Marketing*, *60*, 15–32. doi:10.2307/1251839

Staccini, P., Joubert, M., Quaranta, J., Fieschi, D., & Fieschi, M. (2001). Modelling health care processes for eliciting user requirements: a way to link a quality paradigm and clinical information system design. *International Journal of Medical Informatics*, *64*(2-3), 129–142. doi:10.1016/S1386-5056(01)00203-9

Stanford, J., Tauber, E., Fogg, H., & Marable, L. (2003). Experts vs. online consumers: A comparative credibility study of health and finance Web sites. *Consumer Web Watch Research Report*, Retrieved May 20, 2007 from http://www.consumerwebwatch.org/dynamic/web-credibility-reports-experts-vs-online-abstract.cfm.

Statistics Canada. (2006). *2006 Census: Portrait of the Canadian Population in 2006, by Age and Sex: National portrait*.Retrieved on January 6, 2010, from http://www12.statcan.ca/census-recensement/2006/as-sa/97-551/p3-eng.cfm

Statistisches Bundesamt. (2006). *Gesundheit – Ausgaben, Krankheitskosten und Personal 2004*. Retrieved 16.08.2006 from www.destatis.de

Steinbrück, U., Schaumburg, H., Duda, S., & Krüger, T. (2002) A picture says more than a thousand words – photographs as trust builders in e-commerce websites, in *Proceedings of Conference on Human Factors in Computing Systems CHI 2002, Extended Abstracts*, 748-749. New York: ACM Press

Stingl, C., & Slamanig, D. (2008). Privacy-enhancing methods for e-health applications: how to prevent statistical analyses and attacks. *International Journal of Business Intelligence and Data Mining, 3*(3), 236–254. doi:10.1504/IJBIDM.2008.022135

Stohr, E., & Zhao, L. (2001). Workflow Automation: Overview and Research Issues. *Information Systems Frontiers, 3*(3), 281–296. doi:10.1023/A:1011457324641

Stojmenovic, I., & Olariu, S. (2005). Data-centric protocols for Wireless Sensor Networks . In Stojmenovic, I. (Ed.), *Handbook of Sensor Networks* (pp. 417–456). Sussex, England: John Willy & Sons. doi:10.1002/047174414X.ch13

Strauss, A. (1978). A Social World Perspective. *Studies in Symbolic Interaction, 4*, 171–190.

Succi, M. J., & Walter, Z. D. (1999). Theory of user acceptance of information technologies: An examination of health care professionals. *32nd Hawaii International Conference on System Sciences* IEEE Computer Society.

Suzuki, T, Murase, S, Tanaka, T. & Okazawa, T. (2007). New *approach for the early detection of dementia by recording in-house activities, 13*(1), 41-44.

Swanson, B. E., & Ramiller, N. C. (1997). The Organizing Vision in Information Systems Innovation. *Organization Science, 8*(5), 458. doi:10.1287/orsc.8.5.458

Sweeney, L. (2002). k-anonymity: A model for protecting privacy. *International Journal of Uncertainty Fuzziness and Knowledge Based Systems, 10*(5), 557–570. doi:10.1142/S0218488502001648

Szczechowiak, P., Oliveira, L. B., Scott, M., Collier, M., & Dahab, R. (2008). NanoECC: Testing the limits of elliptic curve cryptography in sensor networks. In R. Verdone (Ed.), *Lecture Notes in Computer Science: Vol. 4913. Wireless Sensor Networks* (pp. 305-320). Berlin/Heidelberg: Spriger-Verlag.

Tan, C. C., Wang, H., Zhong, S., & Li, Q. (2009). IBE-lite: A lightweight identity based cryptography for body sensor networks. *IEEE Transactions on Information Technology in Biomedicine, 13*(6), 926–932. doi:10.1109/TITB.2009.2033055

Tan, C. C., Wang, H., Zhong, S., & Li, Q. (2008). Body sensor network security: an identity-based cryptography approach. In *Proceedings of the first ACM conference on Wireless network security* (pp. 148-153). New York: ACM Press.

Tang, P. C., Ash, J. S., Bates, D. W., Overhage, J. M., & Sands, D. Z. (2006). Personal health records: definitions, benefits, and strategies for overcoming barriers to adoption. [JAMIA]. *Journal of the American Medical Informatics Association, 13*(2), 121–126. doi:10.1197/jamia.M2025

Tanner, D. (2003). Older people and access to care. *British Journal of Social Work, 33*(4), 499–515. doi:10.1093/bjsw/33.4.499

Task Force on a Blueprint for Pharmacy. (2008). *Blueprint for pharmacy: the vision for pharmacy.* Ottawa, ON: Canadian Pharmacists Association.

Tattersall, G. (2002). *Supporting Iterative Development Through Requirements Management.* Retrieved March 3 2010 from: http://www.ibm.com/developerworks/rational/library/2830.html.

Terrier, P., & Schutz, Y. (2005). How useful is satellite positioning system (GPS) to track gait parameters? A review. *Journal of Neuroengineering and Rehabilitation, 2*, 2–28. doi:10.1186/1743-0003-2-28

Terry, M. (2009). Twittering healthcare: social media and medicine. *Telemedicine Journal and e-Health, 15*(6), 507–510. doi:10.1089/tmj.2009.9955

The Center for Universal Design. (1997). *The principles of universal design, version 2.0.* Raleigh, NC: North Carolina State University.

The Lewin Group. (2000). *Assessment of Approaches to Evaluating Telemedicine. Final report prepared for the Office of the Assistant Secretary for Planning and Evaluation, of.* Department of Health and Human Services.

Thom, D., & Campbell, B. (1997). Patient-physician trust: an exploratory study. *The Journal of Family Practice, 44*, 169–177.

Thompson, J. W., Bost, J., Ahmed, F., Ingalls, C. E., & Sennett, C. (1998). The NCQA's quality compass: Evaluating managed care in the United States. A brief look at the NCQA's comparison of health plan performance. *Health Affairs, 17*(1).

Thompson, J. D. (1967). *Organizations in action.* New York: McGraw-Hill.

Thorne, S., & Robinson, C. (1998). Reciprocal trust in health care relationships. *Journal of Advanced Nursing, 13*, 782–789. doi:10.1111/j.1365-2648.1988.tb00570.x

Timmermann, A., Russo, S. G., & Eich, C. (2007). The out-of-hospital esophageal and endobronchial intubations performed by emergency physicians. *Anesthesia and Analgesia, 104*, 619–623. doi:10.1213/01.ane.0000253523.80050.e9

Tinetti, M. E., & Fried, T. (2004). The end of the disease era. *The American Journal of Medicine, 116*(3), 179–185. doi:10.1016/j.amjmed.2003.09.031

TinyOS project. (2004). Berkeley University.(n.d.). Retrived December 23, 2009, from http://webs.cs.berkeley.edu/tos/

Tornatzky, L., & Klein, K. J. (1982). Innovation Characteristics and Innovation-Implementation: A Meta-Analysis of Findings. *IEEE Transactions on Engineering Management, 29*(1), 28–45.

Tracey, J. B., Tannenbaum, S. I., & Kavanagh, M. J. (1995). Applying Trained Skills on the Job: The Importance of the Work Environment. *The Journal of Applied Psychology, 80*(2), 239–252. doi:10.1037/0021-9010.80.2.239

Tran, Q., Calcaterra, G., & Mynatt, E. (2005). Cook's collage: Deja vu display for a home kitchen. In *HOIT '05: Proceedings of Home-Oriented Informatics and Telematics* (pp. 15-32).

Tsai, H.-H., Cheng, J.-S., & Yu, P.-T. (2003). Audio Watermarking Based on HAS and Neural Networks in DCT domain. *EURASIP Journal on Applied Signal Processing, (3)*: 252–263. doi:10.1155/S1110865703208027

Tyre, M. J., & Orlikowski, W. J. (1994). Windows of opportunity: Temporal patterns of technological adaptation in organizations. *Organization Science, 5*(1), 98. doi:10.1287/orsc.5.1.98

U.S. Department of Health and Human Services. (1996). *Physical activity and health: a report of the Surgeon General* (pp. 146–148). Atlanta, GA: U.S. Department of Health and Human Services, Centers for Disease Control and Prevention, National Center for Chronic Disease Prevention and Health Promotion.

Uhsadel, L., Poschmann, A., & Paar, C. (2007). Enabling Full-Size Public-Key Algorithms on 8-bit Sensor Nodes. In F. Stajano, C. Meadows, S. Capkun, & T. Moore (Eds.), *Lecture Notes in Computer science: Vol. 4572. Security and Privacy in Wireless Sensor Networks* (pp. 73-86). Berlin/Heidelberg: Spriger-Verlag.

Urban, G., Sultan, F., & Qualls, W. (1998). Trust-based marketing on the Internet. *MIT Sloan School of Management Working Paper* #4035-98.

US Centers for Disease Control. (2003). Public Health and Aging: Trends in Aging-United States and Worldwide. *Morbidity and Mortality Weekly Report, 52*(6), 101–106.

US Department of Health and Human Services. (2010). *Exhibit 2.11 estimated percentage of physician's time spent providing care to patients, by age of patient.* Retrieved on January 6, 2010, from http://bhpr.hrsa.gov/healthworkforce/reports/changedemo/images/2.11.htm

Vallée, M., Ramparany, F., & Vercouter, L. (2005). A Multi-Agent System for Dynamic Service Composition in Ambient Intelligence Environments. In: *Advances in Pervasive Computing, Adjunct Proceedings of the Third International Conference on Pervasive Computing* (Pervasive'05), May 8-11, 2005, Munich, Germany.

Van De Ven, A. H., Delbecq, A. L., & Koenig, R. J. (1976). Determinants of coordination modes within organizations. *American Sociological Review, 41*, 322–338. doi:10.2307/2094477

van den Akker-Scheek, I., Stevens, M., Bulstra, S. K., Groothoff, J. W., van Horn, J. R., & Zijlstra, W. (2007). Recovery of gait after short-stay total hip arthroplasty. *Archives of Physical Medicine and Rehabilitation, 88*(3), 361–367. doi:10.1016/j.apmr.2006.11.026

van den Akker-Scheek, I., Zijlstra, W., Groothoff, J. W., Bulstra, S. K., & Stevens, M. (2008). Physical functioning before and after total hip arthroplasty: perception and performance. *Physical Therapy, 88*(6), 712–719. doi:10.2522/ptj.20060301

Van der Vegt, G., Emans, B., & Van de Vliert, E. (1998). Motivating Effects of Task and Outcome Interdependence in Work Teams. *Group & Organization Management, 23*(2), 124. doi:10.1177/1059601198232003

Van Deursen, T., Koster, P., & Petkovic, M. (2008). Hedaquin: A reputation-based health data quality indicator. In *Electronic Notes in Theoretical Computer Science* (pp. 159-167). Elsevier.

Van Duin, C. (2009). *Bevolkingsprognose 2008–2050: naar 17,5 miljoen inwoners.* Centraal Bureau voor de Statistiek 2009. http://www.cbs.nl/NR/rdonlyres/D49C0D9A-7540-42E9-948D-794EDD3E8443/0/2010bevolkingsprognose20092060art.pdf

Van Dyne, L., & Pierce, J. L. (2004). Psychological ownership and feelings of possession: three field studies predicting employee attitudes and organizational citizenship behavior. *Journal of Organizational Behavior, 25*(4), 439. doi:10.1002/job.249

van Halteren, A., Bults, R., Wac, K., Dokovsky, N., Koprinkov, G., & Widya, I. (2004). Wireless body area networks for healthcare: the MobiHealth project. *Studies in Health Technology and Informatics, 108*, 181–193.

Van Maanen, J., & Schein, E. (1979). Toward a theory of organizational socialization. *Research in Organizational Behavior, 1*, 209–264.

Varadharajan, V. A. (1991). Petri Nat Model for System Design and Refinement. *Journal of Systems and Software, 15*, 239–250. doi:10.1016/0164-1212(91)90040-D

Vassilacopoulos, G., & Paraskevopoulou, E. (1997). A Process Model Basis for Evolving Hospital Information Systems. *Journal of Medical Systems, 21*(3), 141–153. doi:10.1023/A:1022808222057

Veltink, P. H., Bussmann, H. B. J., de Vries, W., Martens, W. L. J., & van Lummel, R. C. (1996). Detection of static and dynamic activities using uniaxial accelerometers. *IEEE Transactions on Neural Systems and Rehabilitation Engineering, 4*(4), 375–385.

Venkatasubramanian, K., & Gupta, S. K. S. (2007). Security for Pervasive Healthcare. In Y. Xiao (Eds.), *Security in Distributed, Grid, Mobile, and Pervasive Computing* (pp. 443-464). Berlin: Auerbach Publications, CRC Press.

Venkatesh, V., & Davis, F. D. (2000). A theoretical extension of the Technology Acceptance Model: Four longitudinal field studies. *Management Science, 46*(2), 186–204. doi:10.1287/mnsc.46.2.186.11926

Verghese, J., Holtzer, R., Lipton, R. B., & Wang, C. (2009). Quantitative Gait Markers and Incident Fall Risk in Older Adults. *The Journals of Gerontology. Series A, Biological Sciences and Medical Sciences, 64A*(8), 896–901. doi:10.1093/gerona/glp033

Verghese, J., Lipton, R., Hall, C., Kuslansky, G., Katz, M., & Buschke, H. (2002). Abnormality of Gait as a Predictor of Non-Alzheimer's Dementia. *The New England Journal of Medicine, 347*(22), 1761–1768. doi:10.1056/NEJMoa020441

Viens, N. (2006). L'interdisciplinarité dans un CHU: Vers une approche contingente de soins. *Institut D'Adminatation Publique Du Québec* .

Vogel, S., Hulsbusch, M., Hennig, T., Blazek, V., & Leonhardt, S. (2009). In-Ear Vital Signs Monitoring Using a Novel Microoptic Reflective Sensor. *IEEE Transactions on Information Technology in Biomedicine, 13*(6), 882–889. doi:10.1109/TITB.2009.2033268

Volkema, R. J., Farquhar, K., & Bergmann, T. J. (1996). Third-party sensemaking in interpersonal conflicts at work: A theoretical framework. *Human Relations, 49*(11), 1437. doi:10.1177/001872679604901104

Vouyioukas, D., Kambourakis, G., Maglogiannis, I., Rouskas, A., Kolias, C., & Gritzalis, S. (2008). Enabling the provision of secure web based m-health services utilizing XML based security models. *Journal Security and Communication Networks, 1*(5), 375–388. doi:10.1002/sec.46

Vredenburg, K., Isensee, S., & Righi, C. (2002). *User-centred design.* Upper Saddle River, NJ: Prentice Hall.

Wageman, R. (1995). Interdependence and Group Effectiveness. *Administrative Science Quarterly, 40*(1), 145. doi:10.2307/2393703

Walsham, G., & Waema, T. (1994). Information systems strategy and implementation: A case study of a building society. *ACM Transactions on Information Systems, 12*(2), 150–173. doi:10.1145/196734.196744

Walter, T., & Herrmann, T. (1998). The Relevance of showcases for the participative improvement of business processes and workflow management. In R. Chatfiled, S. Kuhn & M. Muller (Eds), *Proceedings of the participatory design conference* (pp. 117-127). Seattle, WA, USA.

Walther, J., Pingree, S., Hawkins, R., & Buller, D. (2005). Attributes of interactive online health information systems. *Journal of Medical Internet Research,* March, 7, Retrieved December 4, 2008 from http://www.jmir.org.

Wang, S., Skubic, M., & Zhu, Y. (2009). Activity density map dis-similarity comparison for eldercare monitoring. *Conference Proceedings; ... Annual International Conference of the IEEE Engineering in Medicine and Biology Society. IEEE Engineering in Medicine and Biology Society. Conference, 1*, 7232–7235.

Warburton, D. E., Gledhill, N., & Quinney, A. (2001). The effects of changes in musculoskeletal fitness on health. *Canadian Journal of Applied Physiology, 26*, 161–216.

Warburton, D. E., Gledhill, N., & Quinney, A. (2001). Musculoskeletal fitness and health. *Canadian Journal of Applied Physiology, 26*, 217–237.

Warburton, D. E., Nicol, C. W., & Bredin, S. S. D. (2006). Health benefits of physical activity: the evidence. *Canadian Medical Association Journal, 174*, 801–809. doi:10.1503/cmaj.051351

Warren, S., & Craft, R. L. (1999). Designing Smart Health Care Technology into the Home of the Future. *Engineering in Medicine and Biology, 2*, 677–681.

Warren, S., Lebak, J., Yao, J., Creekmore, J., Milenkovic, A., & Jovanov, E. (2005) Interoperability and security in wireless body area network infrastructures. In *Proceedings of the 27th Annual International Conference of the IEEE Engineering in Medicine and Biology Society* (pp. 3837–3840).

Waterman, J., Curtis, D., Goraczko, M., Shih, E., Sarin, P., & Pino, E. (2005). (Scalable Medical AlertResponse Technology). In *Proceeding of Washington DC, American Medical Informatics Association* (pp. 1182–1183). Demonstration of SMART.

Wathen, C., & Burkell, J. (2002). Believe it or not: Factors influencing credibility on the web. *Journal of the American Society for Information Science and Technology, 53*, 134–144. doi:10.1002/asi.10016

WeightWatchers. (2007). Retrieved from http://www.weightwatchers.com.

Weill, P., Subramani, M., & Broadbent, M. (2002). Building IT infrastructure for strategic agility. *MIT Sloan Management Review, 44*(1), 57.

Weiner, M., Callahan, C., Tierney, W., Overhage, M., Mamlin, B., Dexter, P., & McDonald, C. (2003). Using Information Technology To Improve the Health Care of Older Adults. *Annals of Internal Medicine, 139*, 430–436.

Weinstein, R. (2005). RFID: a technical overview and its application to the enterprise. *IT Professional*.

Wenger, G. C., Davies, R., Shahtahmasebi, S., & Scott, A. (1996). Social isolation and loneliness in old age: Review and model refinement. *Ageing and Society, 16*(03), 333–358. doi:10.1017/S0144686X00003457

Wenliang, D., Jing, D., Yunghsiang, S. H., Pramod, K. V., Jonathan, K., & Aram, K. (2005). A pairwise key predistribution scheme for wireless sensor networks. *ACM Transactions on Information and System Security, 8*, 228–258. doi:10.1145/1065545.1065548

Werbler, C., & Harris, C. (2009). *Consumers pay little or no attention to drug company's advertised risk disclosures*. Retrieved on December 21, 2009 from http://www.orcguideline.com/about_us_news.aspx.

Wiljer, D., Urowitz, S., Apatu, E., DeLenardo, C., Eysenbach, G., & Harth, T. (2008). Patient accessible electronic health records: exploring recommendations for successful implementation strategies. *Journal of Medical Internet Research, 10*(4). doi:10.2196/jmir.1061

Wilkowska, W., & Ziefle, M. (2009). Which Factors Form Older Adults' Acceptance of Mobile Information and Communication Technologies? In Holzinger, A., & Miesenberger, K. (Eds.), *Human – Computer Interaction for eInclusion. LNCS 5889* (pp. 81–101). Berlin: Springer.

Wilson, B. (1984). *Systems: Concepts, Methodologies and Applications*. New York: Wiley.

Winter, D. A. (1995). Human balance and posture control during standing and walking. *Gait & Posture, 3*, 193–214. doi:10.1016/0966-6362(96)82849-9

Wirtz, S., Jakobs, E.-M., & Beul, S. (2010) Passenger Information Systems in Media Networks – Patterns, Preferences, Prototypes. *In Proceedings of the International Professional Communication Conference 2010 – Communication in a self-service society (IPCC 2010)*, Twente, Netherlands.

Wittenberg, R., Comas-Herrera, A., King, D., Malley, J., Pickard, L., & Darton, R. (2006). Future Demand for Long-Term Care, 2002 to 2041: Projections of Demand for Long-Term Care for Older People in England (PDF). *PSSRU Discussion Paper 2330*. London: London School of Economics.

Wixon, D., & Wilson, C. (1997). The Usability Engineering Framework for Product Design and Evaluation . In Helander, M., Landauer, T. K., & Prabhu, P. (Eds.), *Handbook of Human-Computer Interaction*. Englewood Cliffs, N.J.: Elsevier Science.

Wolf, P., Schmidt, A., & Klein, M. (2008). SOPRANO - An Extensible, Open AAL Platform for Elderly People Based on Semantical Contracts. Paper presented at the *3rd Workshop on Artificial Intelligence Techniques for Ambient Intelligence (AITAmI'08)*, 18th European Conference on Artificial Intelligence (ECAI 08), Patras, Greece.

Wong, J. L., Feng, J., Kirovski, D., & Potkonjak, M. (2006). Security in Sensor Networks: Watermarking Techniques . In Raghavendra, C. S., Sivalingam, K. M., & Znati, T. (Eds.), *Wireless Sensor Networks* (pp. 305–323). Berlin, Heidelberg: Spriger-Verlag.

Wong, A. W., McDonagh, D., Omeni, O., Nunn, C., Hernandez-Silveira, M., & Burdett, A. J. (2009). Sensium: an ultra-low-power wireless body sensor network platform: design & application challenges. In *Proceedings of the Annual International Conference of the IEEE Engineering in Medicine and Biology Society* (pp.6576-6579). IEEE Engineering in Medicine and Biology Society. IEEE Press.

Wood, A. D., & Stankovic, J. A. (2002). Denial of service in sensor networks. *IEEE Computer, 35*(10), 54–62.

Wood, A., Virone, G., Doan, T., Cao, Q., Selavo, L., Wu, Y., et al. (2006). *ALARM-NET: Wireless sensor networks for assisted-living and residential monitoring.* Technical Report CS-2006-1, Department of Computer Science, University of Virginia. Retrieved December 23, 2009 from http://www.cs.virginia.edu/wsn/medical/about/publications

Woolham, J., & Frisby, B. (2002). Building a Local Infrastructure that Supports the Use of Assistive Technology in the Care of People with Dementia. *Research Policy and Planning, 20*(1), 11–24.

Wright, P., McCarthy, J., & Meekison, L. (2005). Making sense of experience . In Blythe, M., Overbeeke, K., Monk, A., & Wright, P. (Eds.), *Funology: from usability to enjoyment* (pp. 43–53). Norwell, MA: Kluwer Academic Publishers.

Wu, D., Kong, W., Yang, B., & Niu, X. (2008). A fast SVD based video watermarking algorithm compatible with MPEG2. *Standard Soft Computing-A Fusion of Foundations . Methodologies and Applications, 13*(4), 375–382.

Wuerz, R. C., Swope, G. E., Holliman, C. J., & Vazquez-de Miguel, G. (1995). Online medical direction: a prospective study. *Prehospital and Disaster Medicine, 10,* 174–177.

Wyld, D. (2006). RFID 101: the next big thing for management. *Management Research News, 29*(4), 154–173. doi:10.1108/01409170610665022

XACML. (2007). *OASIS eXtensible Access Control Markup Language (XACML) TC.* http://www.oasis-open.org/committees/download.php/2406/oasis-xacml-1.0.pdf.

XrML. (2009). *Extensible Rights Markup Language.* Retrieved from http://www.xrml.org/

XSPA. (2008). *OASIS Cross-Enterprise Security and Privacy Authorization (XSPA) TC.* http://www.oasis-open.org/committees/tc_home.php?wg_abbrev=xspa.

XUA. (2005). *IHE, Cross-Enterprise User Authentication (XUA) Integration Profile; Rev 1.1.* Public Comment II Version.

Yasnoff, W. A. (2008). *Electronic Records are Key to Health-care Reform, BusinessWeek.*

Yoon, C., & Kim, S. (2009). Developing the causal model of online store success. *Journal of Organizational Computing and Electronic Commerce, 19*(4), 265. doi:10.1080/10919390903262644

Yu, T., Winslett, M., & Seamons, K. E. (2000). Prunes: An Efficient and complete strategy for automated trust negotiation over internet. *In Proceedings of the 7th ACM Conference on Computer and Communications Security* (pp. 210-219). New York: ACM.

Zajonc, R. B. (1980). Feeling and thinking: Preferences need no inferences. *The American Psychologist, 35*(2), 151–175. doi:10.1037/0003-066X.35.2.151

Zand, D. E. (1972). *Trust and managerial problem solving.* Administrative Science.

Zecevic, A. A., Salmoni, A. W., Speechley, M., & Vandervoort, A. A. (2006). Defining a fall and reasons for falling: Comparisons among the views of seniors, health care providers, and the research literature. *The Gerontologist, 46,* 367–376.

Zhang, Y., Huang, Y.-A., & Lee, W. (2003). Intrusion detection techniques for mobile wireless networks. *Wireless Networks, 9,* 545–556. doi:10.1023/A:1024600519144

Zhang, T., Wang, J., Liu, P., & Hou, J. (2006). Fall Detection by Embedding an Accelerometer in Cellphone and Using KFD Algorithm. *International Journal of Computer Science and Network Security, 6*(10), 277–284.

Zhang, Y., & Lee, W. (2000). Intrusion detection in wireless ad-hoc networks. In *Proceedings of the 6th Annual ACM International Conference on Mobile Computing and Networking* (pp. 275-283).

Zhao, F., & Guibas, L. (2004). *Wireless Sensor Networks: an information processing approach.* San Francisco: Morgan Kaufmann, Elsevier.

Zhou, X. Q., Huang, H. K., & Lou, S. L. (2001). Authenticity and integrity of digital mammography images. *IEEE Transactions on Medical Imaging, 20,* 784–791. doi:10.1109/42.938246

Ziefle, M., & Bay, S. (2006). How to Overcome Disorientation in Mobile Phone Menu. A Comparison of Two Different Navigation Aids. *Human-Computer Interaction, 21*(4), 393–432. doi:10.1207/s15327051hci2104_2

Ziefle, M. (2010). Modeling Mobile Devices for the Elderly. *Proceedings of the 3rd International Conference on Applied Human Factors and Ergonomics* (AHFE'10): Miami, Florida.

Ziefle, M., Röcker, C., Kasugai, K., Klack, L., Jakobs, E.-M., Schmitz-Rode, T., et al. (2009). eHealth – Enhancing Mobility with Aging. In M. Tscheligi, B. de Ruyter, J. Soldatos, A. Meschtscherjakov, C. Buiza, W. Reitberger, N. Streitz, T. Mirlacher (Eds.), *Roots for the Future of Ambient Intelligence, Adjunct Proceedings of the Third European Conference on Ambient Intelligence* (AmI'09 (pp.25-28). Salzburg, Austria.

Zijlstra, W. (2004). Assessment of spatio-temporal parameters during unconstrained walking. *European Journal of Applied Physiology, 92*, 39–44. doi:10.1007/s00421-004-1041-5

Zijlstra, W., & Aminian, K. (2007). Mobility assessment in older people, new possibilities and challenges. *European Journal of Ageing, 4*, 3–12. doi:10.1007/s10433-007-0041-9

Zijlstra, W., & Bisseling, R. (2004). Estimation of Hip Abduction Moment based on Body Fixed Sensors. *Clinical Biomechanics (Bristol, Avon), 19*(8), 819–827. doi:10.1016/j.clinbiomech.2004.05.005

Zijlstra, W., Bisseling, R. W., Schlumbohm, S., & Baldus, H. (2010). A body-fixed-sensor based analysis of power during sit-to-stand movements. *Gait & Posture, 31*(2), 272–278. doi:10.1016/j.gaitpost.2009.11.003

Zijlstra, W., & Hof, A. L. (1997). Displacement of the pelvis during human walking: experimental data and model predictions. *Gait & Posture, 6*, 249–262. doi:10.1016/S0966-6362(97)00021-0

Zijlstra, W., & Hof, A. L. (2003). Assessment of spatio-temporal Gait Parameters from Trunk Accelerations during Human Walking. *Gait & Posture, 18*(2), 1–10. doi:10.1016/S0966-6362(02)00190-X

Zimmer, Z., & Chappell, N. (1999). Receptivity to New Technology among Older Adults. *Disability and Rehabilitation, 21*(5/6), 222–230.

Zingmark, K., Sandman, P. O., & Norberg, A. (2002). Promoting a good life among people with Alzheimer's disease. *Journal of Advanced Nursing, 38*(1), 50–58. doi:10.1046/j.1365-2648.2002.02145.x

Zmud, W. R., & Apple, L. E. (1992). Measuring Technology Incorporation/Infusion. *Journal of Product Innovation Management*, (9): 148–155. doi:10.1016/0737-6782(92)90006-X

Zucker, L. (1977). The Role of Institutionalization in Cultural Persistence. *American Sociological Review, 42*(5), 726–743. doi:10.2307/2094862

Zwar, N. A. (2010). Health care reform in the United States: An opportunity for primary care? *The Medical Journal of Australia, 192*(1), 8.

About the Contributors

Martina Ziefle, Ph.D., is Professor for Communication Science at RWTH Aachen University, Germany and head of a research group at the Human Technology Centre (HumTec). HumTec is funded by the Excellence Initiative of the German federal and state governments and aims at fostering high level interdisciplinary research between the humanities/social sciences and the engineering/natural sciences. Prof. Ziefle's research addresses human factors in different technology types and using contexts, taking demands of user diversity into account. Her methodological competence regards the experimental and empirical evaluation of human computer interaction. A special research focus is directed to the usability and acceptance of mobile devices, which are increasingly used in novel contexts. Her main research concern is to shape technology innovation in ways that technology development is truly balanced with the human factor. In addition to teaching and directing research on campus, Prof. Ziefle leads various projects funded by industrial and public authorities, dealing with the interaction and communication of humans with technology.

Carsten Röcker is a senior researcher at the Human Technology Centre (HumTec) at RWTH Aachen University, working in the research program „eHealth – Enhancing Mobility with Aging". As part of an interdisciplinary team of researchers he is designing healthcare applications for supporting elderly people in ubiquitous computing environments. Previously, Carsten was a visiting PostDoc at the Media Computing Group, focusing on the evaluation of user requirements for smart work environments. Before joining RWTH Aachen University in 2008, he was a PostDoc at the Distributed Cognition and HCI Laboratory at the University of California in San Diego. From 2000 to 2006 he worked as a research associate at the Fraunhofer Integrated Publication and Information Systems Institute (IPSI) in Darmstadt. During this time he was involved in several projects designing novel information and communication technologies for intelligent home and office environments. He has an interdisciplinary background with academic degrees in the areas computer science (PhD), psychology (PhD), electrical engineering (Master) and management (Master).

***

Clemens Becker received his medical training at the University of Frankfurt and Gießen. He received his Medical Doctoral degree from the University of Heidelberg. His habilitation topic at the University of Ulm was on prevention of falls in long-term care (2005). He is a trained internist and geriatrician and is the medical director of the geriatric rehabilitation clinic of the Robert-Bosch-Krankenhaus in Stuttgart since 2003. Current research activities include gerontechnology and the use of body-fixed sensors and actuators for diagnostic and therapeutic purposes. More specifically the team aims to develop novel approaches for the prediction, prevention and recognition of falls in older people. The second main aim is to improve the understanding of physical activity (PA) patterns in order to develop methods to increase PA levels.

Stefan Beckers is M.D. and specialized in anaesthesiology and pre-hospital emergency medical care. He works in the Department of Anaesthesiology at the University Hospital of the RWTH Aachen University, Aachen, Germany. Besides he participated at several programms of the Harvard Macy Institute, Boston, MA, USA and is heading the local interdisciplinary skillslab facility of the Medical School. Since the beginning he is part of the group engaged in research and education in emergency medical care, with the special focus on applications of telemedicine in prehospital emergency settings.

Shirley Beul studied communication studies, politics and economics at RWTH Aachen University and obtained her final degree of a Magister Artium (M.A.) in 2009. She is a research assistant at the interdisciplinary Human Technology Centre (ehealth research group) and the department of Textlinguistics and Technical Communication. Shirley's research addresses the investigation of electronically mediated and media-based doctor-patient-communication. Her goal is to develop a tailor-made telemedical consultation service for chronically ill patients, which considers their needs, personal preferences, and communicative capabilities. She explores how human-centred interactions between physician and patient have to be realized, which factors this interaction influence and how susceptible it is. Her methodological competence regards the experimental and empirical evaluation of human computer interaction as well as surveys to detect user profiles.

Ilse Bierhoff, Msc. studied at the technical university of Eindhoven at the faculty Technical Innovation Science, department Human Computer Interaction. Her expertise is applying knowledge from social sciences on problems related to the introduction of new technologies. Research activities can be divided into three main areas. The first area is the implementation of the user centred design approach with a focus on the gathering of user requirements with innovative methods that allow an equal and creative interaction between user and experts. The second area is on a more practical level and focuses on giving guidance to the process of actually installing smart home technology and the evaluation of those projects with all the stakeholders. The third area focuses on the development of educational material on ambient assisted living for multidisciplinary teams of students.

Nicholas M. Boers is a Ph.D. candidate at the University of Alberta and has been involved in several projects related to wireless networking, including ad hoc sensor networks, and most notably the Smart Condo project. His work deals with software development for tiny devices, software specification, real-time systems, simulation, and performance evaluation. He received his B.Sc. in Computing Science from Vancouver Island University in 2004 and his M.Sc. in Computing Science from the University of Alberta in 2006. The Natural Sciences and Engineering Research Council (NSERC), the Informatics Circle of Research Excellence (iCORE), Alberta Advanced Education and Technology, and the Killam Trusts have provided funding for his research.

Tadeusz Brodziak received his Dipl.-Ing. degree in electrical engineering and information technology from the RWTH Aachen University in 2003. In 2003 he joined P3 solutions GmbH and he is currently the technical leader of the Med-on-@ix project group at P3 communications GmbH. In the past his work involved development of software systems, analysis of service quality in mobile networks and performing and team-leading field tests of mobile devices in EMEA. Since 2006 he is working at the project Med-on-@ix. His major work is the conceptual design and implementation of a secure and reliable communication link between "Telenotarzt-Zentrale" and emergency scene.

David Chodos is a PhD student in the Department of Computing Science at the University of Alberta. His research interests include virtual worlds, online education and training, service-oriented design, requirements engineering, and web-based software design. Two projects he is involved in are an interactive, virtual world-based training system for EMT students, and a "Smart Condo" that monitors a resident's actions unobtrusively, in order to provide at-home care for the elderly. He holds an NSERC scholarship, and has Bachelor's and Master's degrees in Computer Science from the University of Waterloo.

Cynthia L. Corritore is Professor of Information Systems and Technology in the College of Business at Creighton University. Her current research interests focus on two areas: how humans interact in a technology-enhanced world, and how technology and learning intersect. Specifically, she has focused on the topics of online trust in ecommerce and eHealth (including virtual worlds), mobile computing in business, and eLearning. She is also active in the business world, and does consulting in the areas of user experience, human-centered design and processes, and online learning pedagogy. She holds a US patent pending (2nd round) for a mobile technology.

Sarah Delaney is a senior research consultant at WRC with extensive experience in health and social services research. She graduated from Queen's University, Belfast with a BA in Social Anthropology in 1996. In 1999 she completed a Masters of Science Degree in Applied Social Research at University of Dublin, Trinity College. She is currently completing a PhD in Integrating Health and Social Care at the Royal College of Surgeons in Ireland. Key areas of experience include technology-supported health and social care services for older people, public participation in health and social care, service delivery models in health and social care, and informal care. Her work in this area has included a broad range of quantitative, qualitative and participatory research.

Katinka Dijkstra is an associate professor in cognitive psychology at the Erasmus University in Rotterdam. She obtained her Ph.D. degree from the University of Utrecht in 1992. Since then, she has worked as a post-doc and assistant professor at Florida State University in the United States at the Psychology Department, Department of Communication Disorders and at the Pepper Institute on Aging and Public Policy. In 2007, she joined the Brain and Cognition group in the Psychology Department at the Erasmus University in Rotterdam. Katinka Dijkstra's research focuses on autobiographical memory, aging and technology, and the effects of stress on cognitive functioning. She has published extensively in international peer-reviewed journals. With researchers from Florida State University, Georgia Technical University and the University of Miami, she has been part of CREATE II, a grant funded by the National Institute on Aging, to examine the role of technology in home, work, and health environments for the elderly population.

Harold Fischermann is Anesthetist at the Department for Anaesthesiology at the University Hospital Aachen Germany. Currently he is working on the surgical Intensive Care Unit of the University Hospital Aachen, and is a member of the telemedical research project med-on-@ix. This project focusses on the possibilities of a telemedical assistance system in the physician staffed emergency medical service of Aachen in order to improve the quality of prehospital patient care. Furthermore he did research in the analysis of the quality of documentation in emergency missions in emergency scenarios on a full scale human patient simulator.

James Fozard conducts research on aging and earlier directed the extended care patient treatment programs for the U.S. Department of Veterans Affairs. His research includes two longitudinal studies of aging - the VA Normative Aging Study and the National Institute on Aging Baltimore Longitudinal Study of Aging which he directed for 13 years. He is participating in the development of the scientific foundations of gerontechnology, a multidisciplinary field concerned with technology that benefits aging and aged persons. Currently on the faculty of the University of South Florida's School of Aging Studies, Fozard served on the faculty of the Johns Hopkins University, and Harvard Medical School. He earned his doctorate at Lehigh University and his post-doctoral training at the Massachusetts Institute of Technology. He is the author or coauthor of over 180 scientific articles and book chapters.

Nadja Frenzel has a bachelor's degree in "Health Sciences" from the Maastricht University, where she is currently earning a master's degree in "Health Policy, Economics and Management". She has been employed as a research assistant in the Department for Anesthesiology of the University Hospital Aachen since February 2009.

Pawel Gburzynski is a Computer Scientist (PhD in Informatics from the University of Warsaw, Poland) with interests in telecommunications, operating systems, performance evaluation, and simulation. Between 1985 and 2010 he was with the faculty of the Department of Computing Science, University of Alberta. In 2002, he co-founded Olsonet Communications (http://www.olsonet.com), where he currently acts as chief scientist. Dr. Gburzynski's contributions include SMURPH (a high-fidelity modeling/emulation package for communication systems), PicOS (an operating system for embedded applications) and TARP (a resilient ad-hoc routing scheme for low-cost sensor networks). He has devised a number of communication protocols, including ad-hoc wireless routing schemes and custom protocols for high-performance systems, and implemented many practical wireless networking solutions.

Lisa M. Guirguis, 1997 B.Sc. (Pharm) with Distinction, University of Alberta; 2001 M.Sc. (Pharmaceutical Sciences), University of Alberta, 2006 Ph.D. (Social and Administration Sciences in Pharmacy), University of Wisconsin, Major Specialization: Pharmacy Practice Research. Dr. Guirguis' expertise in the behavioural sciences and experience in community pharmacy underpins her work in three main areas: survey measurement, interprofessional practice, patient-pharmacist communication, and medication taking behaviours. Specific research and teaching interests address the role of pharmacists in providing care to patients with chronic diseases, practice change in community pharmacy, patient-pharmacist communications, the concordance framework in medication taking behaviours, and adapting techniques from the social sciences for research in pharmacy practice.

Brett Harnett joined the faculty at the University of Cincinnati as a Research Assistant Professor in 2004 and serves as the Division Director for Information Technology for the Department of Surgery. Prior to joining UC, Brett was the Director of Experimental Information Technology for a NASA-sponsored research program at Virginia Commonwealth University. Before moving to Virginia, he was a Systems Analyst for the Yale University School of Medicine in Connecticut. Activities include scientific review committees for the National Institutes of Health and a member of the Editorial Board for the Telemedicine and e-Health Journal. He received his undergraduate degree from Eastern Connecticut State University in Business Administration and his Master's degree in Information Systems from the University of Cincinnati. Over the past ten years he has published over a dozen peer-reviewed manuscripts, four book chapters and has been an invited speaker at various conferences and international meetings.

Jianzhao Huang graduated from University of Alberta in 2009 as a Master in Computing Science. His major research interests are software engineering and sensor network. Since 2008, he has been working on information systems that integrate sensing devices and provide visualization.

Luan Ibraimi received his Master Degree in Information and Communication Systems Security from the KTH Royal Institute of Technology, Sweden in 2007. He is currently a PhD Candidate at the EEMCS faculty of University of Twente. As part of his PHD he spent one year as a researcher at the Information and System Security group in Philips Research in Eindhoven (the Netherlands). His research interests are public key encryption and network security, especially on applying cryptographic techniques to securely manage electronic health records.

Joachim Jean-Jules is currently teaching business process modeling, research methodology and project management courses at the Université de Sherbrooke. He has taught a variety of courses at both the undergraduate and graduate levels at the University Quisqueya for several years. Before the current academic endeavour, he has spent many years in industry in a number of capacities. His current research interests focus on issues related to the areas of Technological innovation project management and the assimilation of large-scale IS requiring complex organizational arrangements. His works have been published in journal and proceedings of several international conferences including IJESMA, IRMA, Conf-IRM, AIM and AIMS.

Kai Kasugai is an architect working as a researcher in the eHealth Group at the Human Technology Centre at RWTH Aachen University, Germany. He studied architecture at the RWTH and at the Edinburgh College of Art, Scotland. After graduating, he worked as an architect and later as a researcher at the RWTH for a project funded by the Federal Office for Building and Regional Planning on the use of new technologies in an urban environment that is suitable for families and the elderly. He then received a postgraduate scholarship and lived in Tokyo for 18 months, where he first studied Japanese for 10 months to then work in two Tokyo-based architecture firms. After returning to Germany he joined the eHealth Team. Kai investigates how architecture, design, and HCI are redefining themselves in a world of ubiquitous computing. His current focus lies on interfaces between humans and technologically enhanced space.

William Kearns received his Ph.D. in psychology from the University of South Florida in 1989. He joined the faculty at the Louis de la Parte Florida Mental Health Institute in 1990 and was director of Information Technology from 1992 to 2003. He joined the Department of Aging and Mental Health Disparities in 2003 and is an Assistant Professor. He is an Associate Editor for the international journal Gerontechnology and is USF's Executive Liaison to the Internet2 Project, a consortium of over 200 Carnegie Research I institutions nationwide charged with developing enhanced network services supporting research and education. His interests include using automation to facilitate improved care for elders with dementia and using technology to improve access to mental health services and education. Dr. Kearns has been the PI on several grants including his recent grant from the DHHS Agency for Healthcare Research and Quality entitled "Evaluation and Integration of an Automated Fall Prediction System" #R21 HS18205-01

Lars Klack studied mechanical engineering at RWTH Aachen University (Germany) and the Technical University of Lisbon (Portugal) and specialized in biomedical engineering. As a PhD student he is now part of the eHealth research group (Human Technology Centre) at RWTH Aachen University. This group follows a multidisciplinary approach to develop innovative care strategies within the context of intelligent living environments. Currently Lars' research activities focus on the user-centered design of a medical assistance system for patients with chronic heart diseases and its integration in future home environments. This system should enable the heart patient to live independently at home and provide medical assistance in emergency situations without being visible at all times. The challenge of developing socially accepted systems that consist of highly reliable medical technologies enriched with the hedonic component of increasing the users satisfaction is prevalent in Lars' studies.

Vassiliki Koufi was born in Athens, Greece. She received a B.Sc. in Informatics from the University of Piraeus (2001), an M.Sc. in Data Communication Systems from Brunel University, UK (2003) and since 2003 she is a Ph.D candidate in the Department of Digital Systems at the University of Piraeus. Since 2002 she works as a network engineer in the Network Management Center at the University of Piraeus. Since February 2009 she is teaching fellow (under the provision of 407/80 Presidential decree) at the Department of Digital Systems, University of Piraeus. Ms. Koufi has been actively involved in several projects concerning the development of healthcare information systems and other web-based applications as well as the development and management of telecommunication services and applications. In addition, she has published several research papers in internationally refereed journals, international conferences and books. Her research interests include ubiquitous and pervasive healthcare, context-aware healthcare information systems, process-oriented web-based and cloud-based healthcare information systems, healthcare information systems security, personal health records systems and security issues arising in these systems.

Beverly Kracher is Professor of Business Ethics and Society at Creighton University's College of Business. She holds a Ph.D. in philosophy from the University of Nebraska-Lincoln. Her research and publications extend from online trust and ecommerce ethics to trust and ethics of leaders, business organizations, and governments. She writes an ethics column for the B2B magazine and workbooks for implementing organizational ethics programs. She has consulted on ethics and trust creation for national and international businesses and professional associations. Beverly is the executive director and president of the Business Ethics Alliance, a practitioner based organization that leads in building climates of ethical excellence in business communities.

Rosemarie Santora Lamm, Ph.D. ARNP, Licensed Mental Health Counselor is currently faculty at the University of South Florida Polytechnic, Arts and Science and U.S.F. School of Aging Studies. Dr. Lamm received her R.N. degree from the University of Buffalo and Buffalo General Hospital School of Nursing, B.A. from St. Leo University, Master of Arts in Gerontology, Master of Science in Nursing, and Ph.D. in Medical Anthropology from the University of South Florida. She is elected a fellow of the Society for Applied Anthropology and served as President of The Council of Nursing and Applied Anthropology. Dr. Lamm has been involved in research and assessment, "The Quality of Life Health Data" collection and analysis, utilized to promote awareness of educational and health needs. She has been the P.I. for grants from Retirement Research Foundation of Chicago, West Central Florida Area Agency on Aging, and Johnson and Johnson Society for Health Care and Healing. She has presented research related to health and aging both nationally and internationally in China, Germany and Brazil. She has her research results published in proceedings of The Society for Applied Anthropology.

Robert Lederer, Associate Professor of Design, is a graduate of Sydney College of the Arts. Australia. B.A.(i.d)1982, and the University of Alberta M.Des.1998. Robert Lederer has practiced as an Industrial Designer both as a staff designer and a freelance consultant in Australia and in Canada. He joined the University of Alberta as a sessional lecturer of Industrial Design in 1986 and as a FTC Assistant Professor and program Coordinator in 1999. His research at IRSM (Misericordia Hospital) has been examining "seamless technological interface" in patient treatment systems utilizing rapid –prototyping 3D imagery and other digital formats, as well developing test devices with researchers at the University Hospital MRI facility. A long term collaboration project with the Faculty of Rehabilitation Medicine in the development of student projects in the utilization of Universal design methodology and principles for the design of products for an aging population has received a commendation by the American Society on Aging for Exemplary Program in Industrial Design (2002). Professor Lederer teaches classes in design principles, advanced industrial design practice and human factors.

Lili Liu is Professor and Chair of the Department of Occupational Therapy, Faculty of Rehabilitation Medicine at the University of Alberta in Edmonton, Alberta, Canada. She earned a B.Sc. (Occupational Therapy) in 1984, M.Sc. (Rehabilitation Science) in 1988, and Ph.D. (Rehabilitation Science) in 1993, all from McGill University, Montreal, Quebec, Canada. Her research focuses on three related themes: technologies and aging (including telerehabilitation and virtual reality), Universal Design and aging, and rehabilitation outcome measures and interventions for older adults with cognitive impairment. Currently, she is a Research Affiliate with the Glenrose Rehabilitation Hospital (Alberta Health Services) and a Research Associate with CapitalCare.

Flora Malamateniou was born in Athens, Greece. She received the B.Sc degree in Statistics from the University of Piraeus in 1993 and the M.Sc and the Ph.D degree in Health Informatics from the University of Athens in 1995 and 1999, respectively. She has worked as a senior researcher at Research Academic Computer Technology Institute, Greece during 2000-2004 and at Informatics and Telematics Institute Centre for Research and Technology, Greece during 2004-2008. She has been actively involved in many national and EU-funded R&TD projects and in the European IST programmes, E2R I/II, TENCompetence, iCLASS, C-CARE and LIMBER. Currently, she is an Assistant Professor at the Department of Digital Systems of the University of Piraeus. Her current research interests include process-oriented, web-based healthcare information systems, pervasive healthcare, virtual healthcare records, information security and workflow systems.

Robert P. Marble is an Associate Professor of Decision Sciences in the College of Business at Creighton University. His Ph.D. is from the University of Illinois at Urbana-Champaign. His research interests and publications are in the areas of international information systems issues, information systems implementation, and applications of mathematical modeling and artificial intelligence techniques to information systems problems. A two-time Fulbright Scholar, he has spent several years as visiting researcher and guest professor at universities in the Federal Republic of Germany. He is a long-standing member of the Society for Information Management, the Decision Sciences Institute, the Association for Computing Machinery, the American Mathematical Society, and the Association for Symbolic Logic.

Arnd May, PhD, Ethicist, studied Philosophy in Goettingen and Bochum. He received his Ph.D. in 2000 and his dissertation was about Advance Directives. At the Institute for Advanced Study in the Humanities (KWI) he worked 2001-2003 in a project about ethics consultation in hospitals. In 2003/2004 he was appointed member of the consultation group of patients autonomy at the end of life of the Federal Ministry of Justice. In 2009 he was invited to write an expert opinion to the committee of legal affairs of the German Parliament. From 2007-2008 he was managing director of the clinical ethics committee (KEK) of the University Hospital Aachen. Since 2008 he is working about ethical aspects of the Research project Med-on-@ix. He is head of the consultation group about advance directives within the Department for Anesthesiology of the University Hospital

Ingo Meyer is a Sociologist with a Master (Magister Artium) degree from Bonn university. His studies focused on statistical methods (esp. non-linear methods), life-style research and social structure analysis. He lives in Bonn / Germany. He currently works as a research consultant and policy advisor for empirica (http://www.empirica.com) in issues relating to the Information Society, with a focus on its impacts on society and especially on older people, people with disabilities and other people at risk of exclusion. Other areas of professional activities include e-health, indicator development, statistics and benchmarking and the analysis of national and EU-level policies. In this capacity he was and is involved in several projects, including "MeAC - Measuring Progress of eAccessibility in Europe" (http://www.eaccessibility-progress.eu), "SOPRANO - Service-oriented Programmable Smart Environments for Older Europeans" (http://www.soprano-ip.org), "CommonWell - Common Platform Services for Ageing Well in Europe" (http://www.commonwell.eu), the Pilot on eHealth Indicators study (http://www.ehealth-indicators.eu) and the "eHealth Benchmarking" study (http://www.ehealth-benchmarking.eu).

Christian Möllering is a research assistant at the Human Technology Centre of the RWTH Aachen University within the eHealth group. Currently his research activities focus on building operation systems as well as the assessment and realization of new building related technologies applied in the area of medical services and energy efficiency. Besides a service platform with context awareness, the integrating of diverse technologies, taking into account the common user's requirements on tomorrow's technologies is a interesting challenge in a multi-disciplinary team. Christian studied physics at the Universities of Erlangen-Nürnberg and Oldenburg and is an expert in the field of innovative building automation, with work experience of more than 10 years. He worked on the German Reichstag as well as on projects towards energy efficiency (Balanced Office Building) and system integration.

Sonja Müller is research consultant at empirica (http://www.empirica.com). She holds a degree in geography, urban development, and economic sociology from Bonn University. Main fields of her research activity are ICT applications and their usage patterns amongst older people and people with special needs and the way ICTs impact on societal participation and inclusion of disadvantaged population groups. Since joining empirica in 2005 she has been involved in a number of projects focusing on the development and evaluation of technical systems in the area of Independent Living/Ambient Assisted Living and policy analysis in the area of eInclusion. Sonja Müller has authored and co-authored national and international publications.

In-Sik Na is anesthetist in the Department of Anesthesiology at the University Hospital in Aachen, Germany. In addition, he has further qualification as diving medicine physician and emergency physician, therefore he is working in a compression chamber since 2006 and also as emergency physician in the city of Aachen. As instructor of the "European Resuscitation Council (ERC)" and the "Pre Hospital Trauma Life Support (PHTLS)" he also takes part in the education of paramedics and emergency physicians. Actually he is working on the Surgical Intensive Care. Since 2007 he is involved in the Med-on-@ix Research project as researcher and emergency physician.

Ioanis Nikolaidis is a Professor with the Computing Science Department at the University of Alberta. He received his B.Sc. from the University of Patras, Greece, in 1989 and his M.Sc. and Ph.D. in Computer Science from Georgia Tech in 1991 and 1994, respectively. Between 1994 and 1996 he worked for the European Computer-Industry Research Center in Munich, Germany, in the area of distributed computing. He joined the University of Alberta in January 1997. He has published more than seventy articles in books, journals, and conference proceedings in the area of computer networking. His research interest range from network modeling and simulation, to large scale data delivery systems, to mobile and secure networking. He served for ten years (1999-2009) in the editorial board of the Computer Networks journal (Elsevier). Since 1999 he has been a member of the editorial board (and served as Editor in Chief between 2007 and 2009) of the IEEE Network magazine. He has served in the technical program committees of numerous conferences, including ICC, Globecom, INFOCOM, LCN, IPCCC, PerCom, IFIP Networking, and CNSR. He is in the steering committee of WLN (co-located annually with IEEE LCN) and in the steering committee of the ADHOCNOW conference.

Milan Petković is a part-time professor at the Eindhoven University of Technology and a senior scientist in Philips Research where he coordinates research in the domain of information security. He received his Dipl-Ing. and M.Sc. degrees in Computer Science from University of Niš, and his Ph.D. degree in Computer Science from University of Twente. Among his research interests are information security, trust management, databases and data management. He is a member of the emerging and future risk stakeholder group of ENISA - the European Network and Information Security Agency. He published more than 50 journal and conference papers as well as several books including a recent book on Security, Privacy and Trust in Modern Data Management. He is an active member of several standardization organizations including HL-7 and Continua Health Alliance.

Klaus Pfeiffer received the MSc degree in psychology at the University of Tuebingen, Germany, in 1997. He is currently research coordinator at the Clinic of Geriatric Rehabilitation which is a department of the Robert-Bosch-Hospital, Stuttgart. His research focuses on various aspects of applied gerontology. He has addressed aspects like coping with chronic diseases in the elderly, the development of family caregiver interventions, fear of falling, classification of fall prevention programs and user satisfaction with assistive and telehealthcare technologies.

Victor Pomponiu is a Ph.D. candidate and member of the Security and Network group at the Computer Science Department, Università degli Studi di Torino, Italy, since January 2009. He received his B.Sc. and M.Sc. in Computer Science from the Polytechnic University of Bucharest in 2006 and 2008 specializing in communication systems. His areas of research include image/signal processing, multimedia copyright protection and wireless sensor networks security, in particular cryptography, secure routing and intrusion detection.

Michael Protogerakis is a Research Assistant at the Centre for Learning and Knowledge Management and Department for Information Management in Mechanical Engineering at the RWTH Aachen University. He received his Diploma in Mechanical Engineering, in 2006. Since 2006 he is the project manager for the Med-on-@ix Research project on Telemedicine in Emergency Medical Services.

Rolf Rossaint is Professor and Head of the Department of Anaesthesiology at the University Hospital (since 1997) and Vice-Rector for Research at the Rheinisch-Westfälische Technische Hochschule in Aachen (since 2002), Germany. Dr. Rossaint studied medicine at the University of Düsseldorf and is board certified in Anaesthesiology. Prior to his present appointment, he was Associate Professor in the Clinics for Anaesthesiology and Surgical Intensive Care at the Humboldt University of Berlin. Dr. Rossaint was the recipient of the E.-K. Frey Prize (1993), the Pulmedica Prize (1996), the Annual Scientific Award (1996) from the European Academy of Anaesthesiology and the Poster Award of 25th International Symposium on Intensive Care and Emergency Medicine 2005. He has (co) authored over 300 articles in peer-reviewed journals. His clinical and research interests include pulmonary pathophysiology, ALI/ARDS/sepsis treatment, liver replacement therapy, xenon anaesthesia, coagulation management in trauma, and telemedicine in emergency medicine.

Cheryl Sadowski started her career in pharmacy in Manitoba, where she graduated from the U of M with her BSc (Pharm). After working briefly in community pharmacy, she started a Drug Information Specialty Industrial Pharmacy Residency at The Upjohn Company of Canada. After completing her residency she took a position as a staff pharmacist at North York Branson Hospital (North York, Ontario) where her clinical responsibilities included the psychiatry and geriatrics units. She completed her Doctor of Pharmacy degree at Wayne State University (Detroit, Michigan). Following her graduation, she began a one-year post-doctoral residency in geriatrics through Campbell University (North Carolina). Dr Sadowski was also a clinical instructor at Campbell University School of Pharmacy while completing her geriatrics training at The Sticht Center for Aging, Duke University Medical Centre, and

Dorothea Dix State Psychiatric Hospital in North Carolina. Dr Sadowski joined the Faculty of Pharmacy and Pharmaceutical Sciences, University of Alberta, in August 1999. She also has a clinical practice at the Misericordia Hospital, where she works in the Seniors Clinic and with the Geriatric Assessment Unit. Dr Sadowski's research interests include falls awareness and management of delirium, pain, and osteoporosis in acute hip fracture patients.

Lynn Schelisch, born 1981 in Wiesbaden, Germany, works as a scientific research assistant at the Research Area for Urban Sociology at the Technical University of Kaiserslautern. She holds a Diploma in spatial planning, focusing on urban sociology. Her main area of research is the user perspective in the field of Ambient Assisted Living. In a pilot project in Kaiserslautern she analyzed elderly people's experiences and acceptance of AAL technology, which was installed in their homes, using methods of empirical social research. She took part in the working group of the BMBF/VDE Innovationspartnerschaft AAL on education and further training in the field of AAL.

Marie-Thérèse Schneiders studied Communication Science at RWTH Aachen University. She is a full-time Ph.D. student and scientific assistant at the Centre for Learning and Knowledge Management and the Department of Computer Science in Mechanical Engineering (ZLW/IMA) at RWTH Aachen University. She is supporting software development projects with sociological research approaches especially in terms of user acceptance research. Within the national research project Med-on-@ix she is developing a change management approach to introduce the telematic support system into the emergency medical services of Aachen.

Andrew Sixsmith has been Professor and Director of the Gerontology Research Centre at Simon Fraser University since September 2007. Dr. Sixsmith is an executive board member of the International Society of Gerontechnology and is Chair of the 7th World Conference of the Society in Vancouver in 2010. He has been particularly involved in the strategic development of research in the area of technology for independent living. Since 2000, he has attracted funding for several prestigious research projects from the European Commission and the Engineering and Physical Sciences Research Council, Department of Health and Department of Industry in the UK and CIHR in Canada. Dr. Sixsmith has substantial teaching experience within gerontology and has been responsible for innovatory educational initiatives in the UK and internationally. He has published many papers in Journals such as the Gerontologist and Ageing and Society.

Max Skorning was born in 1975 in Aachen, Germany. He completed a professional education as a paramedic and afterwards started studying medicine in 1998. Since 2004 he is a resident physician in anaesthesiology and prehospital emergency medicine at the university hospital in Aachen, Germany. He achieved a doctor's degree in medicine in 2006. He published about cardiopulmonal resuscitation and emergency telemedicine in several national and international journals. Since 2004 he is in a leading position in the working group for prehospital telecare, resulting in the project Med-on-@ix that was sponsored by the German ministry of economics and technology. In addition Max Skorning is the representative of the scientific staff in the supervisory board of the university hospital since 2006 and the national representative of the physicians in training for specialisation in anaesthesiology in the German Society of Anaesthesiology and Intensice Care Medicine (DGAI). Max Skorning is a course director of the European Resuscitation Council (ERC) and a member of the executive committee of the German Resuscitation Council.

Annette Spellerberg was born in Bad Dribung, Germany and received her training in sociology, psychology and education science at the Free University of Berlin (Diploma 1987; PhD 1995). Annette Spellerberg worked as a researcher at the FU Berlin (1987-1989), at the Wissenschaftszentrum Berlin (WZB; Social Science Research Center)(1990-1997) and a research assistant at Bamberg University (2000-2002). In the academic year 1997-1998 she was a fellow at the Center for Advanced Study in the Behavioral Sciences in Stanford. From 2002 to 2008 she was an assistant professor and since then full professor of urban sociology at the Technical University of Kaiserslautern. Her areas of work are urban and regional sociology, social inequality, quality of life, lifestyles, and housing. Along with Prof. Dr. Lothar Litz from the Institute of Automatic Control at the Technical University of Kaiserslautern Spellerberg coordinated the pilot project "Assisted Living" in Kaiserslautern in which AAL technology was tested in real-world. Her task was the analysis of the user's experiences and acceptance of the implemented technology.

Sandra Sproll is a research associate in the field of human-computer interaction at the Fraunhofer Institute for Industrial Engineering in Stuttgart Germany. She holds a degree in Psychology and Economics. Her research interests are within the realm of Usability Engineering and User Experience focusing the overarching experience a person has as a result of interactions with a technical product or service. In several research and industrial projects she works on human-centered design, user-driven innovation and technology acceptance. In the area of ambient assisted living her research activities focus on methods for the development and evaluation of technical systems according to the special needs of elderly people.

Eleni Stroulia is a Professor and NSERC/iCORE Industrial Research Chair on Service Systems Management (w. support from IBM) with the Department of Computing Science at the University of Alberta. She holds M.Sc. and Ph.D. degrees from Georgia Institute of Technology. Her research addresses industrially relevant software-engineering problems with automated methods, based on artificial-intelligence techniques. Her team has produced automated methods for migrating legacy interfaces to web-based front ends, and for analyzing and supporting the design evolution of object-oriented software. More recently, she has been working on the development, composition, run-time monitoring and adaptation of service-oriented applications, and on examining the role of web 2.0 tools and virtual worlds in offering innovative health-care services. She has served as program-committee member for several Canadian and international conferences and workshops; she was the program co-chair for the Canadian AI in 2001, WCRE in 2003 and 2004, CASCON 2006 and ICPC 2007. She serves on the editorial board of the Computational Intelligence Journal and on the NSERC Discovery Grant adjudication committee 330 (2006-2008). She is a member of ACM, and IEEE.

George Vassilacopoulos was born in Athens, Greece, received his Ph.D. degree from the University of London, U.K. and he is currently a Professor at the Department of Digital Systems of the University of Piraeus. He has been an advisor of health informatics to the Greek Minister of Health, a member of the board of two major Athens hospitals and an advisor of informatics to the National Ambulance Service of Greece. He has actively participated in several research and development projects at both National and European levels. His research interests include healthcare information systems, workflow systems, healthcare systems security, web-based healthcare information systems and electronic patient records. He has authored numerous publications in these areas in international journals and refereed conferences. He is a member of BCS and IEEE.

Alain O. Villeneuve holds a DBA degree in Information Systems from Boston University. As a practitioner from 1975 to 1990, Dr Villeneuve has been involved in all stages of systems development and has actively participated in hundreds of systems implementation. Many IS projects into which he participated were in the area of healthcare management and networking. He has joined Université de Sherbrooke as a faculty in 1996. Dr Villeneuve's current research interests are in the area of knowledge management, knowledge creation and transfer, knowledge management supporting technologies, research methods, human expertise and decision-making. His works have been published in Decision Support Systems and Information and Management among others in addition to being presented at several international conferences. Dr Villeneuve was also an active member of KTE (Knowledge Transfer and Exchange) committee of the CIHR (Canadian Institutes for Health Research) for several years.

Susan Wiedenbeck is Professor of Information Science and Technology at the iSchool at Drexel University. Her current research encompasses trust on websites, particularly with respect to healthcare websites. In addition, she studies end-user development, with a strong emphasis on the interplay of people and technology, including an interest in trust and gender differences. She is a member of the Internet Public Library (IPL) research team at the iSchool, where she works on usability and user experience issues. She is Co-Editor-in-Chief of the International Journal of Human-Computer Studies, Senior Editor of the AIS Transactions on Human-Computer Interaction, and Associate Editor of the ACM Transactions on Computing Education.

Wiktoria Wilkowska is degree-qualified psychologist at RWTH Aachen University (Germany) and research assistant in the eHealth research group ("Enhancing mobility with aging") at the Human Technology Centre, Aachen, Germany. The eHealth research program explores interdisciplinary the field of Human-Computer Interaction with the particular interest in medical technologies in home environment. Wiktoria's current research addresses investigation of user diversity with regard to acceptance and usability of modern technologies applied in medical services. Following an user-centered approach her main objective is to learn about human motivation and greatest barriers in the usage of domestic medical assistance, which is meant to support older and chronically diseased people in their activities and everyday life. She is convinced that implementing the gained knowledge in medical systems would enhance the quality of living environment, and enable frail and ill persons to interact with an easy to use and as useful perceived technology.

Wiebren Zijlstra received the MSc degree in human movement sciences and a PhD degree at the University of Groningen, The Netherlands, in 1991 and 1997, respectively. He is currently senior researcher and assistant professor at the Center for Human Movement Sciences of the University Medical Center Groningen. His research focuses on different aspects of mobility, specifically on changes in mobility related activities with ageing and age-related pathology. In his research, he has addressed biomechanical, neuro-physiological, and cognitive aspects, as well as pathological and age-related aspects of the performance of mobility related tasks. The development and evaluation of interventions which aim to support or improve mobility in specific groups of older people, and the use of body-fixed-sensors for studying human motor functioning in a natural environment are main topics in his recent work.

Index

A

accelerometers 246, 247, 248, 261, 263, 265
access control 30, 31, 32, 44, 46, 48
accountability 24, 29, 42
activity monitoring 248
actor-network theory (ANT) 121
ad hoc networks 116
Advanced Audio Distribution Profile (A2DP) 276, 277
aging concept 93
aging in place 292, 309
aging societies 77, 78
AIXTRA 269, 274
ambient assisted living (AAL) 76, 81, 83, 84, 88, 89, 91, 92, 93, 195, 196, 198, 201, 212, 213, 214, 215, 217, 218, 225, 227, 228, 236, 238, 240, 242, 243
ambient assisted living environment (AAL Environment) 289, 290, 294
ambient intelligence (AmI) 90, 91, 92, 93, 297, 310, 311, 313, 314
ambient technology 196
American Academy of Pediatrics (AAP) 3
American College of Sports Medicine (ACSM) 252
AMIGO project 79
analog-to-digital converter (ADC) 97, 101
anonymity 24, 39, 40, 42, 45, 46
application programming interfaces (API) 289, 291, 298, 299, 301, 302, 303, 306, 308
Arthrosis 253
artificial intelligence (AI) 91, 92
assisted living 195, 196, 197, 212, 213, 214, 215, 289, 290, 292, 309, 310, 311, 312

assisted living facility (ALF) 144, 153, 155, 159
assistive medical devices 80
asynchronous communications 22
asynchronous monitoring 7
atrial fibrillation 7
audit trail 48
authentication 33, 34, 38, 39, 46, 48, 99, 101, 103, 104, 107, 108, 109, 110, 116, 117
authorization 116
availability 94, 99, 109
Aware Home 294, 310

B

barometric pressure sensor 246
Berg Balance Scale (BBS) 251
Bodily Wellbeing 218
body area networks (BAN) 95, 101
body sensor networks (BSN) 99, 115
Bottom-Up Processes 170, 194
BSN nodes 99
bureaucratic formalization 177
business process 137

C

Callon, Michel 121
care chains 25
care pathways 25
care provider organisation (CPO) 225
chronic disease management 124
Chronic Obstructive Pulmonary Disease (COPD) 253, 254, 264
Class 1 technologies 166
Class 2 technologies 166
Class 3 technologies 166

M

magnetic resonance imaging (MRI) 147
magnetometers 246, 247
Maslow, Abraham 81, 89
Maslow's hierarchy of needs 81
MavHome 295, 296, 297, 312
medical databases 26
medical engineering 77
Medication Event Monitoring Systems (MEMS) 293
Med-on-@ix 268, 269, 270, 271, 272, 273, 274, 275, 279, 280, 283, 284, 287
mental wellbeing 218
metadata 22
Microsoft 23, 27, 33, 35, 42
middleware 78, 93
miniature gyroscopes 246
mini-mental state examination (MMSE) 141, 145
MobiHealth system 99
mobile ad hoc networks (MANET) 96, 97, 98, 99, 108, 116
mobile nodes 96, 108, 116
mobile sensors 95

N

namespaces 22
national committee for quality assurance (NCQA) 9, 20
national electronic health record infrastructures 25
natural human movement 139
NHS Spine project 23, 25, 46
NICTIZ project 23, 25, 45
non-exercise activities with thermogenesis (NEATs) 251
non-zero sum games 53
Notarzt 268, 269

O

occupational therapy (OT) 298, 305
online health management 124
OpenAAL platform 79
Open Services Gateway Initiative (OSGi) 296
open source 22

OpenWings framework 79
operations support system (OSS) 298, 300, 301, 303
organizational assimilation 174, 176, 193
organizational climate 181, 191
organizational culture 126, 133
organizing vision (OV) 183, 184

P

Parkinson's Disease (PD) 140, 148, 155, 156, 254
passive infrared devices (PIR) 142, 143
patient-centered care 2, 16, 21
patient centered medical homes (PCMH) 1, 2, 4, 5, 6, 7, 11, 12, 13, 14, 15, 16, 17, 18, 20
patient centered medicine 2, 15, 18
patient centeredness concept 1, 2, 3, 4, 5, 7, 9, 10, 12, 14, 18, 19, 20, 21
patient registries 22
PC systems 99
Personal Assistive Unit for Living (PAUL) 195, 198, 199, 200, 201, 202, 203, 204, 205, 206, 207, 208, 209, 210, 211, 212, 214
personal digital assistants (PDA) 96, 98, 99, 100
personal healthcare domain 23
personal health records (PHR) 8, 9, 11, 15, 18, 23, 24, 26, 27, 28, 29, 33, 35, 41, 42, 48, 119, 120, 121, 122, 123, 124, 125, 127, 128, 129, 130, 131, 132, 136, 137
picture archiving and communications systems (PACS) 165
portable computers 96
pressure sensors 246
preventative medicine 2, 5
primary care physicians (PCP) 3, 14, 16, 17
Prisoner's Dilemma 53
privacy 23, 24, 29, 30, 32, 35, 40, 41, 42, 43, 44, 46
process-based healthcare system 137
process designs 125, 126
process reengineering 125, 126, 135
professional mobile Radio services (PMR) 277
proprietary technology 22

Breinigsville, PA USA
31 March 2011
258903BV00008B/6/P